Jensen and Swift's Diseases of Sheep

Jensen and Swift's Diseases of Sheep

CLEON V. KIMBERLING, DVM, MPH

College of Veterinary Medicine &
Biomedical Science
Colorado State University
Ft. Collins, Colorado

THIRD EDITION

LEA & FEBIGER

1988 • Philadelphia

Lea & Febiger
600 Washington Square
Philadelphia, PA 19106
U.S.A.
(215) 922-1330

First Edition, 1974
Second Edition, 1982

Library of Congress Cataloging in Publication Data

Jensen, Rue.
    Jensen and Swift's diseases of sheep.

    Rev. ed. of: Diseases of sheep. 2nd ed. 1982.
    Bibliography:
    Includes index.
    1. Sheep—Diseases.   1. Swift, Brinton L.
II. Kimberling, Cleon V.   III. Jensen, Rue.
Diseases of sheep.   IV. Title.   V. Title: Diseases
of sheep.
SF968.J45   1987   636.3'0896   87-3229
ISBN 0-8121-1099-4

PRINTED IN THE UNITED STATES OF AMERICA

Print No. 4 3 2 1

PREFACE

The earth sustains and the economy uses one billion sheep. Although widely distributed in all nations, these animals are numerically concentrated in the following countries: the Union of Soviet Socialist Republics (142 million), Australia (134 million), China (95 million), New Zealand (62 million), Turkey (44 million), India (41 million), and Argentina (35 million). During the last two decades, the numbers have declined in some countries. In the United States, the count decreased from 33 million in 1960 to 9.93 million in 1986, but during the same period, the total count for all nations remained nearly constant. The decline in the U.S. resulted from high costs of labor, mounting fees for grazing, and exorbitant rates of predation.

As grazers of plants that grow in subhumid and arid regions, sheep consume forage of low value and produce wool and meat of high value. Because of this direct conversion of natural feeds, peoples of many nations depend principally on sheep for both fiber and food. Despite the use of inexpensive feeds, economic profits to the industry have decreased because synthetic materials have acquired much of the fabric market, and red meats such as beef and pork have captured the food market. In addition to economic competition, sheep diseases of all causal categories, in addition to occasional devastation, continuously and insidiously drain numbers and quality and further reduce economic gains. Low prices for sheep products persistently threaten

not only viability, but also the survival of the industry. Producers cogently demand relief from these depressing conditions.

The purpose of this book is to provide veterinary assistance by increasing the availability of newly researched information for defining, describing, and controlling diseases. It is intended for both technical and general use. Advanced students with extensive training in biological sciences may use the volume for initial learning and later as practicing veterinarians for reviewing diseases of sheep. Producers and investors without technical education may use it for investigating and understanding specific maladies.

The primary structural units of the book are presented in three parts: Part I, Diseases of Breeding Sheep and Nursing Lambs; Part II, Diseases of Feedlot Lambs; and Part III, Diseases of Adult Sheep. Each primary part is subdivided into diseases of anatomic systems, such as the digestive system and the nervous system. For example, all diseases of feet, regardless of cause, are discussed in the same chapter, and the main diseases causing abortion are also given in a single chapter. The sequence of discussion for each disease is: definition, occurrence, etiology and pathogenesis, clinical signs and postmortem lesions, diagnosis, and prevention and treatment. References follow each disease section. Most technical details, required by veterinary students and practitioners, are contained in the sections on etiology, pathogenesis, and diagnosis. Under the remaining subheadings, non-technical details and general information can be studied independently without loss of subject continuity. For diseases such as ulcerative dermatosis, tetanus, and salmonellosis that occur in more than one primary part or may significantly affect several anatomic systems, the detailed discussion is located in the system category having the most serious involvement.

The third edition has maintained the same format as previous editions with expansion of the treatment, prevention, and management areas.

Ft. Collins, Colorado   Cleon V. Kimberling

ACKNOWLEDGMENTS

The third edition of Diseases of Sheep was written as a team effort. Dr. John M. Cheney revised the areas concerning parasites. Dr. Anthony Knight revised the areas concerning poisonous plants. The library search was conducted by Dr. Terresa Brennen, Dennis Sylvain and Lindsey Wess. Lisa Monzingo typed the manuscript and Marta Remmenga did the proofreading. The key supporting individual was Betty Kimberling, who took over our lambing and sheep operation plus became the weed control officer, allowing me time for uninterrupted concentration on review of the literature and incorporation into the text. This team performed admirably and from their efforts the third edition is a complete review and revision of current sheep research.

CONTENTS

PART II. Diseases of Feedlot Lambs

PART III. Diseases of Adult Sheep

PART **I** DISEASES OF BREEDING SHEEP
AND NURSING LAMBS

1

DISEASES OF RAMS

Cryptorchism

(Cryptorchidism; retained testis; undescended testis)

Cryptorchism, a developmental abnormality, is the failure of one or both testes to descend from the abdominal cavity into the scrotum. The affected organ may stop along a normal path of descent, or it may divert to an ectopic location; in either event, spermatogenesis fails, but androgen production proceeds. Even though unilateral cryptorchism may adversely affect semen quality, only bilateral cryptorchism results in sterility. Because of moderate prevalence and universal distribution, the condition causes considerable commercial damage to the sheep industry. Economic losses result from reduced fertility, sterility, maintenance of unproductive rams, and disqualification of rams from public shows and sales. The possibility of inheriting unilateral cryptorchism may extend losses to succeeding generations of rams. The losses can be reduced, however, by clinical examination of ram lambs and early elimination from the breeding flock of all affected animals.

OCCURRENCE. All breeds of rams appear to be susceptible to cryptorchism, but in some inbred families, the incidence may be significantly higher or lower than for the sheep population in general. A survey of the prevalence of cryptorchidism in 2,281 Merino rams of all ages was 0.18%. Even though rams of all ages may be affected, young animals have a higher incidence because some retained testes descend during early years of life and because some affected ram lambs are diagnosed and eliminated from the flock. In addition to sheep, cryptorchism affects all other species of domestic mammals, including man, and probably wild species.

Geographically, cryptorchism probably occurs in all countries where the sheep industry has developed into important animal agriculture.

ETIOLOGY AND PATHOGENESIS. Cryptorchism probably is genetically determined, either by an autosomal recessive gene or possibly by an autosomal dominant gene with incomplete penetrance. Postulated additional factors include mechanical obstructions such as fibrous adhesions and focal infections along the course of descent, especially near the inguinal ring where many cryptorchid testes locate, and hormonal unbalance. Whereas mechanical obstruction affecting one side only may frequently cause unilateral cryptorchism, improper amounts of gonadotropic hormone with systemic effects may cause bilateral cryptorchism.

The pathogenesis of ovine cryptorchism has not been determined and has been only slightly investigated. Research has been conducted in some mammals, especially laboratory rats and rabbits, and data from these studies have some application in understanding the development of ovine cryptorchism. In ovine fetuses, the right kidney develops in a position cranial to the left kidney, and the right testis, situated near the caudal pole of the right kidney, is more cranial than the left testis at the caudal pole of the left kidney. Because of the different anatomic position, the right testis, in descending to the scrotum, must migrate a longer distance than does the left testis; consequently, the right testis has greater opportunity and higher probability for encountering mechanical obstructions than does the left testis. Constriction or fibrosis near the right inguinal ring may interrupt right testicular movement and cause the organ to remain in the abdominal cavity near the ring.

Normal abdominal temperature exceeds normal scrotal temperature by approximately 5°C. Under the influence of abdominal temperature, the cryptorchid testis fails to develop functional seminiferous tubules, and spermatogonia, the primitive germinal epithelial cells, do not mature. The intertubular Leydig's cells, however, do synthesize and secrete androgens into the blood. Bilaterally cryptorchid rams, therefore, are sterile, but unilaterally cryptorchid rams may be fertile from spermatozoa produced in the scrotal testis. Following birth, some cryptorchid testes, under the influence of hormonal stimulation, ultimately descend into the scrotum.

CLINICAL SIGNS AND POSTMORTEM LESIONS. Neither bilateral nor unilateral cryptorchism produces clinical manifestations. Libido is normal, and physical features are masculine. Individual breeding records may show poor reproductive performance, and semen examination may indicate poor quality. Palpation of the scrotum, however, reveals the absence of one or both testes.

The incidence of cryptorchism among rams is approximately 0.5%. Among unilaterally cryptorchid rams, the right testis, in 90% or more of the animals, is retained in the abdomen.

At necropsy, the undescended testis may be found in the inguinal canal, near the inguinal ring, or between the kidney and the ring; rarely, it will be at an ectopic location, such as the femoral canal, perineum, or beside the prepuce.

Usually the cryptorchid organ is anatomically abnormal. The testis proper is small and soft. The average cryptorchid testis weighs approximately 19 g and the epididymis, 6 g; the average scrotal testis weighs 194 g and the epididymis, 35 g. The epididymis makes up approximately 30% of the testicular weight in the cryptorchid organ and only 18% in the scrotal organ. Most cryptorchid testes anatomically resemble scrotal testes (Fig. 1-1). Histopathologically, the seminiferous tubules are hypoplastic and may contain few or no spermatogonial cells. Sertoli's cells, however, do persist.

DIAGNOSIS. Both veterinarians and sheep producers diagnose cryptorchism by palpation of the scrotum. The clinical examination is made from behind the standing ram. Examination should include the proximal part of the scrotum as near as possible to the inguinal

Fig. 1-1. Cryptorchid testis. The testis is only slightly larger than the tail of the epididymis. × 1.0.

canal. One or both testes may be absent. The differential diagnosis should consider unilateral castration because of injury or disease. The history of the animal and the presence of an incision scar should facilitate the differentiation.

PREVENTION AND TREATMENT. Cryptorchid ram lambs can and should be identified and removed from breeding ram flocks. Such rams give subnormal breeding performance, but require the same maintenance investment as normal rams. In addition, the possibility of heritability of cryptorchism creates the risk of increasing cryptorchism among successive generations.

Some cryptorchid testes may be successfully treated by administering gonadotropic hormone or by surgical intervention. Treatment by either means is not feasible, however, and should not be practiced because of possible uneugenic effects on breeding lines.

Blackshaw, A.W. and Samisoni, J.I.: The testes of the cryptorchid ram. Res. Vet. Sci., 8:187-194, 1967.
Bratanov, K., Yassifov, K., and Tsekova, E.: Role of nucleic acids in animal reproduction. III. RNA and DNA in the epididymis and testicle of normal and cryptorchid lambs. Vet. Med. Nauki (Sofia), 5:7-11, 1968.
Claxton, J.H. and Yeates, N.T.M.: The inheritance of cryptorchism in a small flock of sheep. J. Hered., 63:141-144, 1972.
Dolling, C.H.S. and Brooker, M.G.: Cryptorchism in Australian Merino sheep. Nature, 203:49-50, 1964.
Watt, D.A.: Testicular pathology of Merino rams. Aust. Vet. J., 54:473-478, 1978.

Varicocele

Varicocele, a local disturbance in venous circulation, is characterized by saccular dilation and thromboses in the internal spermatic vein and probably is caused by excessive venous pressure. The condition may occur separately in either spermatic cord or simultaneously in both. Bilateral varicoceles of long duration may adversely affect semen quality and, when advanced in size, partially incapacitate affected rams for walking, grazing, drinking, and breeding. They eventually lead to intercurrent diseases and death. Because their incidence is low, varicoceles cause little material waste. Some economic losses, however, result from disqualification of affected rams for public

shows and sales, physical incapacitation for breeding, and high mortality.

Among domestic animals, varicoceles are unique and merit research for better understanding. Knowledge of their cause, pathogenesis, and heritability would significantly add to the scientific resources in veterinary science and may enable the development of a rational program for prevention and control.

OCCURRENCE. Varicoceles apparently occur in all breeds of rams. Animals 5 to 7 years of age, however, have a higher incidence than do rams 1 to 4 years of age. A survey of the prevalence of varicocele in 2,281 Merino rams of all ages was 0.09%. A prevalence of 1 to 2% has been reported in rams. Varicoceles in rams 1 year of age are rare because causative factors probably require more than 1 year to develop. To our knowledge, among domestic animals, varicoceles occur only in sheep. Humans, however, have a comparable condition.

Geographically, varicoceles probably occur in sheep of all countries. They have been reported in Australia, Britain, and in the United States in Colorado and Illinois.

ETIOLOGY AND PATHOGENESIS. The specific cause of varicoceles has not been determined. Conjectured causative factors include high blood pressure in the lumen and weakness in the wall of the internal spermatic vein at the anatomic area immediately proximal to the pampiniform plexus. The development of shunt channels connecting arterioles and venules and defective valves in the proximal part of the internal spermatic vein may materially enhance pressure, and congenital weakness in the wall of the vein may significantly predispose the animals to the condition.

Since the cause of varicoceles is not known, its pathogenesis cannot be fully understood; however, some of its aspects have been conjectured. As a result of testicular and epididymal lesions, such as abscesses, adhesions, orchitis, and epididymitis, arteriovenous shunts develop and convey blood from arterioles into venules. The direct connection, without intervening capillaries, transmits arteriolar pressure into the lumen of venules and sinuses of the pampiniform plexus. Much of the pressure continues into the internal spermatic vein. The absence of vein valves or the presence of defective valves may enhance pressure by placing the weight of the blood column on the susceptible part of the vein.

As a result of continuous pressure, the weak wall of the vein slowly but continuously dilates, and layers of fibrin form in the lumen of the vein. Although extensive thrombosis forms throughout the varicocele, some flow channels remain open. Even though varicoceles grow slowly, some acquire dimensions of up to 7×15 cm. The large masses exert pressure on surrounding tissues, including nerves, and cause considerable pain. Active physical movements, such as walking and breeding, exaggerate the discomfort and cause incapacitation.

After a long course, bilateral varicoceles may create hypoxia at the seminiferous tubules and thereby reduce sperm cell numbers and induce sperm cell deformities.

Most large varicoceles predispose affected rams to starvation and inanition. Eventually, other diseases, such as pneumonia, develop and cause death, or the owner, in despair, orders euthanasia.

CLINICAL SIGNS AND POSTMORTEM LESIONS. In affected rams, incipient and small varicoceles evince no clinical signs and apparently produce no inconvenience, but moderate and large-sized, especially bilateral, varicoceles often cause softened testes and severe and incapacitating pain. Affected rams are inclined to move more slowly or to become immobilized. An affected ram stands with the caudal limbs abducted and placed forward, with its back arched and its abdomen thin. Because of considerable immobility, the animal becomes isolated from the flock, consumes little food and water, and usually does not attempt copulation. Semen analysis may reveal a decline in the sperm cell count from 5×10^9 to 5×10^8 ml, reduced cell mobility, proximal cytoplasmic droplets, separated heads, and up to 50% abnormal acrosomes. Body temperature is normal unless an infectious disease intervenes. Palpation of the scrotum evokes pain and reveals the firm nodular mass in the spermatic cord.

The clinical course is prolonged and may extend through 1 to 3 years or more. Although the morbidity averages approximately 1%, most rams affected with large varicoceles usually die from disease complications.

At necropsy, varicoceles are found along the spermatic cords immediately dorsal to the pampiniform plexuses. They may be unilateral, with equal incidence on the right and left side, or bilateral. The size varies from small nodules to masses measuring 7×15 cm. Each moderate- to large-sized lesion consists of a firm, dark, lobulated, adhered, and circumscribed mass of convolutions in the internal spermatic vein (Fig. 1-2). The cut surface reveals the laminated thrombus, fibrous adhesions between convolutions, and cyanotic blood. Both the testicle and epididymis may be congested and mildly edematous.

Fig. 1-2. Varicocele in a spermatic cord. $\times$ 0.7.

Histopathologically, the affected vein is dilated and the vein wall attenuated. Fibrinous laminations with interspersed leukocytes, platelets, and erythrocytes form the thrombus, which occludes most of the lumen. Frequently, sinuses of the pampiniform plexus also are thrombosed.

DIAGNOSIS. Veterinarians diagnose varicoceles on the basis of clinical examination. Routine and systematic palpation of the scrotum reveals the firm, lobulated mass of variable size in the spermatic cord, and finding the typical lesion at necropsy confirms the clinical diagnosis.

The differential diagnosis requires consideration of abscesses and neoplasms, both rare lesions, in the spermatic cord. Abscess, a soft, diffuse, nonlobulated mass, provokes a measurable leukocytosis. Neoplasms, probably metastatic, are diffuse and nonlobulated. The primary neoplasm may be identified by skillful clinical examination.

PREVENTION AND TREATMENT. Veterinarians have developed no rational program for preventing or treating varicoceles. Because they assume that a propensity for varicoceles may be heritable, all affected rams should be identified by routine physical examination and eliminated from the breeding flock.

Gunn, R.M.C.: Studies in fertility in sheep. Seminal changes affecting fertility in rams. Aust. Vet. J., 18:94-106, 1942.

Jensen, R., Brown, W.W., and Flint, J.C.: Unpublished clinical records. Colorado State University, 1957.

Jensen, R., Flint, J.C., and Brown, W.W.: Arteriosclerosis and phlebosclerosis in testes of sheep. AJVR, 23: 480-488, 1962.

Miller, S.J. and Moule, G.R.: Clinical observations on the reproductive organs of Merino rams in pastoral Queensland. Aust. Vet. J., 30:353-363, 1954.

Murray, R.M.: Scrotal abnormalities in rams in tropical Queensland with particular reference to ovine brucellosis and its control. Aust. Vet. J., 45:63-67, 1969.

Ott, R., Heath, E., and Bane, A.: Abnormal spermatozoa, testicular degeneration, and varicocele in a ram. AJVR 42(2):241-245, 1982.

Watson, P.F.: Varicocele in the ram affecting spermatogenesis and sperm maturation. Vet. Rec., 95:343-345, 1974

Watt, D.A.: Testicular pathology of Merino rams. Aust. Vet. J. 54:473-478, 1978.

Epididymitis

(BE; Brucellary epididymitis)

(Ram epididymitis)

Epididymitis is a clinical or subclinical venereal disease of rams. It is characterized subclinically by poor semen quality with numerous leukocytes and clinically by enlargement and induration of the epididymis and atrophy of the testes. It is caused by a major bacterial pathogen of sheep. The disease results in economic losses for producers because of reduced fertility, shortened breeding life, necessary inspections, expensive immunizations, and increased labor. The most significant economic impact is lowered conception, extended duration of the lambing period, failure of a high percent of ewes to conceive, occasional abortions, and weak lambs. Even though losses are high, systematic use of preventive programs can significantly reduce the incidence or even eliminate the disease from an enterprise.

OCCURRENCE. BE occurs in all breeds, but animals with Merino and Suffolk breeding often appear to have high incidence. Most rams at and beyond the stage of sexual maturity probably are susceptible, and the incidence consequently increases directly with age because of its long course, cumulative effects, and repeated exposures.

The disease has been diagnosed in countries with wide geographic separation; these include Australia, New Zealand, Hungary, Yugoslavia, USSR, South Africa, Uruguay, Brazil, Peru and the United States. It probably occurs in other countries where the sheep industry constitutes an important segment of animal agriculture.

ETIOLOGY AND PATHOGENESIS. *Brucella ovis,* a specific cause of epididymitis, is a nonmotile, noncapsulating, nonsporing, gram-negative, slightly acid-fast coccobacillus that measures 0.5 to 0.7 × 0.06 to 1.5 μm. It does not ferment carbohydrates, change litmus milk, reduce nitrate, or produce H_2S or indole. It is catalase-positive. Initial isolations require enriched media and CO_2, but when established, they grow on basic fuchsin and thionin media.

The causative organism leaves the infected ram in the semen and enters susceptible rams through mucous membranes. Transmission, in order of importance, occurs through homosexual coitus, and heterosexual coitus. During nonbreeding seasons, ram herds often run together in unisexual bands containing both old diseased rams and young susceptible rams. Under such circumstances, rams commonly mount each other and deposit semen in the rectum and possibly on perineal skin and wool of mounted rams. Other rams may mount the same animal in rapid succession. Also, during a single estral period, a ewe may breed in succession with several different rams and receive a deposit of semen from each.

Thus, *B. ovis* bacteria in semen from infected rams may contact and penetrate susceptible mucous membranes of (1) the rectum of homosexually mounted rams, (2) the vagina of bred ewes, (3) the penis and prepuce of homosexually mounting rams, (4) the penis and prepuce of heterosexually breeding rams, and (5) the mouth and nose of feeding and drinking rams.

Regardless of the specific method of transmission, the disease begins at the mucous membrane. The pathogen penetrates the host tissue and enters the regional lymph nodes through afferent lymphatics. After causing hyperplasia of reticuloendothelial cells, some organisms pass through the nodes, enter the blood, spread to all organs, and localize in the epididymides, seminal vesicles, bulbourethral glands, and ampulas. Within 21 to 45 days after original exposure, the epididymides may have gross lesions, and by 60 days, most infections of lymph nodes, spleen, and liver have terminated.

Localization in the epididymides initiates a series of changes around the site of infection. Fluid accumulates in the interstitial tissue, and plasmacytes and lymphocytes assemble around blood vessels. Leukocytes, especially neutrophils, along with bacteria migrate into the epididymal duct. Epithelial cells lining the duct undergo hyperplasia, form obstructing folds in the lumen, and develop mural cysts. Masses of spermatids accumulate proximal to the occlusion and extravasate into interstitial tissue. Segments of spermatid-filled ducts and extravasated masses of spermatids provoke inflammatory reactions that become granulomas. Following complete occlusion of the epididymal duct, seminiferous tubules degenerate and the testes atrophy. Unfortunately for diagnosing the disease from gross lesions, the vesicular glands, more than epididymides, seem to be the target organ of infection. In a survey of 408 infected rams only 14% had gross palpable lesions. Semen quality varies in number of spermatozoan, leukocytes, bacteria, motility, and deformities irrespective of gross lesions. Infection may persist for up to 4 years.

Following infection, a serologic response develops. Bacteremia subsides after about 2 months, and serum antibodies can be detected in 2 weeks and persist for months or years. Other pyogenic bacteria may enter the tissue and induce abscesses.

CLINICAL SIGNS AND POSTMORTEM LESIONS. After an incubation period of 2 to 8 weeks, early lesions become detectable. Acute cases vary from slight enlargement and induration of the epididymides without testicular involvement to extremely painful and grossly swollen scrotal contents. As the case advances, however, the epididymis may further enlarge, become fibrotic and the testis become soft and atrophied. Some acute cases will subside leaving no gross lesions. Although lesions are usually in epididymal tails, they may be in the heads or bodies. Abscesses, if present, may fluctuate under digital pressure. Affected rams usually have normal libido and semen quality is extremely variable. Semen has reduced spermatozoa, increased number of leukocytes, decreased motility, increased separated heads and variable numbers of *B. ovis*.

At necropsy, changes are limited to the scrotal contents. The tunica vaginalis may adhere at one or more points to the epididymis. In early stages, the infected part of the epididymis is slightly enlarged and indurated, and the testis is near normal size, but in advanced stages, the infected epididymis is considerably enlarged and more firm. The cut surface demonstrates sperm cell granulomas with creamy to rubbery contents, fibrosis, and in some cases, abscesses and foci of mineralization. The testis is atrophic and soft (Fig. 1-3). Seminal vesicles are enlarged and firm.

Histopathologically, affected interstitial tissue presents fibroplasia and frequently sperm cell granulomas. The epididymal duct may be dilated and partially filled with spermatids and leukocytes. The hyperplastic lining epithelium often forms mural cysts (Fig. 1-4). Seminiferous tubules are atrophic to variable degrees. Some consist of a basement membrane lined with Sertoli cells, and others of collapsed basement membranes only.

A variety of changes occur in the epithelium and wall of the ampulla of the vas deferens. In the normal epithelium there are focal areas of necrosis. Neutrophils are present among the

Fig. 1-4. Vacuoles in epithelial membrane of the infected epididymis. Van Gieson's stain. × 125.

Fig. 1-3. Chronic epididymitis with abscesses in the head (a), sperm cell granulomas (b), and testicular atrophy (c).

epithelial cells and distribute among the spermatozoa in the lumen of the ampulla. In the seminal vesicles neutrophils distribute among the cells of the lamina propria of the septa and in the epithelium. These cells are present in the lumen of the ampulla. In the seminal vesicles neutrophils distribute among the cells of the lamina propria of the septa and in the epithelium. These cells are present in the lumen of saccular dilatations formed by the epithelium. Changes in the epithelium range from hyperplasia to karyolysis and pyknosis.

DIAGNOSIS. The identification of clinical and subclinical BE in individual rams of a herd requires three tests:

1. Examine each ram for gross lesions by simultaneously palpating both epididymides and both testes from a position behind the standing animal. The swelling and tenderness in lesions of early epididymitis and the enlargement and induration in lesions of advanced epididymitis can be detected. Identify and remove all diseased animals.

2. Test blood from all remaining rams for serum antibodies with an enzyme-linked immunosorbent assay (ELISA) using antigen from *B. ovis*. Identify and remove all reactors.

3. Culture semen from all remaining rams for *B. ovis*. Identify and remove all animals with positive results.

The differential diagnosis requires consideration of epididymo-orchitis, abscesses, testicular mineralization, and varicocele. Some of these diseases are clinically indistinguishable. The ELISA test may differentiate cases of brucellary epididymitis and epididymo-orchitis, and semen culture tests may identify specific causative bacteria. Abscesses from *Corynebacterium ovis* and occasionally other bacteria may occur in any part of the testis, epididymis, and tunica vaginalis. Such lesions may be large, may fluctuate from palpation, and may discharge exudate to the scrotal surface through a fistula. Small abscesses in the tail of the epididymis may be clinically indistinguishable from brucellary epididymitis and epididymo-orchitis. Testicular mineralization is usually unilateral. In generalized and advanced stages, the testis is hard as stone but may be of normal size, while the epididymis may be normal. Varicocele, or thrombosed varicosity of the internal spermatic vein, is a firm nodular mass in the spermatic cord proximal to the pampiniform plexus.

For technical assistance from a diagnostic laboratory, practitioners should submit blood, semen, and affected testes.

PREVENTION AND TREATMENT. Veterinarians and producers prevent BE by applying the principles of sanitation, immunization, identification, and culling of infected rams. The following procedures are effective for reducing the incidence and establishing clean herds:

1. Separate virgin ram lambs from older breeding and potentially infected rams. Never mix clean rams with infected rams.

2. Test all rams following the breeding program during the period of low sexual activity using the ELISA test for *B. ovis*. Identify and eliminate all positive rams. Repeat this procedure at 45 to 60 day intervals, during the period of low sexual activity, until the flock is free of *B. ovis*. Palpation of the epididymides should be done simultaneously with blood testing and eliminate rams with gross lesions. Transfer the clean rams to a clean environment. In each subsequent year repeat the blood test and clinical examination during the season of low sexual activity to determine the herd status.

3. Vaccinate ram lambs at 4 to 5 months of age with *B. melitinsis* Rev I vaccine. (In the United States the use of *B. melitinsis* Rev I and *B. abortus* strain 19 on sheep is legally prohibited.) The efficacy of *B. ovis* bacterin is extremely low and may interfere with blood tests in an eradication program. Therefore its use is not recommended.

4. Add newly purchased rams to the clean herd only after their clean status has been established (2 negative ELISA tests 45 to 60 days apart).

High cost in labor and materials precludes treatment except for notably valuable rams in early stages of infection. The daily administration for 3 weeks of 800 mg of chlortetracycline (Aureomycin) and 1 g of dihydrostreptomycin sulfate in some rams may eliminate infection and improve semen quality.

Afzal, M., Tengerdy, R., Kimberling, C., and Ellis, R.: Protection of rams against epididymitis by a *B. ovis*-vitamin E adjuvant vaccine. Vet. Immunol. Immunopath., 7:293-304, 1984.

Bagley, C., Burrell, G., Esplin, J., and Walters, J.: Effect of epididymitis on semen quality of rams. JAVMA, 185:876-877, 1984.

Biberstein, E.L., McGowan, B., Olander, H., II, and Kennedy, P.C.: Epididymitis in rams. Studies on pathogenesis. Cornell Vet., 54:27-41, 1964.

Buddle, M.B.: Vaccination in the control of infection in sheep. N.Z. Vet. J., 6:41-46, 1958.

Buddle, M.B.: Vaccination against *Brucella ovis* infection in sheep. N.Z. Vet. J., 5:43-50, 1957.

Buddle, M.B.: Studies on *Brucella ovis* (n. sp.), a cause of genital disease in sheep in New Zealand and Australia. J. Hyg., 54:351-364, 1956.

Buddle, M.B.: Observations on the transmission of brucella infection in sheep. N.Z. Vet. J., 3:10-19, 1955.

Buddle, M.B.: Production of immunity against ovine brucellosis. N.Z. Vet. J., 2:99-109, 1954.

Buddle, M.B. and Boyes, B.W.: A brucella mutant causing genital disease of sheep in New Zealand. Aust. Vet. J., 29:145-153, 1953.

Cameron, C.: Comparative efficacy of six Brucella vaccines in guinea pigs. Onderstepoort J. Vet. Res., 46:229-230, 1979.

FensterBank, R., Pardon, P., and Marly J.: Efficacy of Brucella melitensis Rev 1 vaccine against Brucella ovis infection in rams. Ann. Rech. Vet., 13(2):185-190, 1982.

Gunn, R.M.C.: Studies in fertility of sheep. Seminal changes affecting fertility in rams. Aust. Vet. J., 18:94-106, 1942.

Hartley, W.J., Jebson, J.L., and McFarlane, D.: Some observations on natural transmission of ovine brucellosis. N.Z. Vet. J., 3:5-10, 1955.

Jansen, B.: The pathology of bacterial infection of the genitalia in rams. Onderstepoort J. Vet. Res., 47: 263-267, 1980.

Jebson, J.L., Hartley, W.J., McClure, T.J., and McFarlane, D.: Pathology of brucellosis in rams in New Zealand. N.Z. Vet. J., 3:100-104, 1955.

Jebson, J.L., Hartley, W.J., and McFarlane, D.: Artificial infection of rams. N.Z. Vet. J., 2:80-89, 1954.

Kennedy, P.C., Frazier, L.M., and McGowan, B.: Epididymitis in rams: Pathology and bacteriology. Cornell Vet., 46:303-319, 1956.

Keogh, J., Doolette, J.B., and Clapp, K.H.: The epidemiology of ovine brucellosis in South Australia. Aust. Vet. J., 34:412-417, 1958.

Kimberling, C.: The economics and techniques of breeding soundness evaluation of rams. Proceedings Soc. for Theriogenology, 1984, pp. 102-110.

Kimberling, C., Schweitzer, D., and Butler, J.: Unpublished clinical records. Colorado State University, 1985.

Lee, K., Cargill, C., and Atkinson, H.: Evaluation of an enzyme-linked immunosorbent assay for the diagnosis of Brucella ovis in rams. Aust. Vet. J., 63:91-93, 1985.

Libal, M. and Kirkbridge, C.: Brucella ovis-induced abortion in ewes. JAVMA, 183:553-558, 1983.

McFarlane, D., Salisbury, R.M., Osborne, H.G., and Jebson, J.L.: Investigations into sheep abortion in New Zealand during 1950 lambing season. Aust. Vet. J., 28:221, 1952.

McGowan, B.: Epididymitis in rams. Effect of vaccination and culling on incidence. Cornell Vet., 69:67-76, 1979.

McGowan, B. and Shultz, G.: Epididymitis in rams: Clinical description and field aspects. Cornell Vet., 46: 277-281, 1955.

Miller, S.J. and Moule, C.R.: Clinical observations on the reproductive organs of Merino rams in pastoral Queensland. Aust. Vet. J., 30:353-363, 1954.

Murray, R.M.: Scrotal abnormalities in rams in tropical Queensland with particular reference to ovine brucellosis and its control. Aust. Vet. J., 45:63-67, 1969.

Rahaley, R., Dennis, S., and Smeltzer, M.: Comparison of enzyme-linked immunosorbent assay and complement fixation test for detecting Brucella ovis antibodies in sheep. Vet. Record, 113:467-470, 1983.

Ramos, A.A., et al.: Epididymitis in rams. A clinical survey in the state of Rio Grands do Sul, Brazil. Pesquisa Agropec. Braz., 1:211-213, 1967 (Abst. Vet. Bull., 38:137 [1968]).

Ris, D., Hamel, K., and Long, D.: Comparison of an enzyme-linked immunosorbent assay (ELISA) with cold complement fixation text for the serodiagnosis of Brucella ovis infection. N.Z. Vet. J., 32:18-20, 1984.

Simmons, G.C. and Hall, W.T.K.: Epididymitis of rams. Aust. Vet. J., 29:33-40, 1953.

Swift, B.L. and Weyerts, P.R.: Ram epididymitis: Study on infertility. Cornell Vet., 60(2):204-214, 1970.

Szabo, I. and Nyiredy, L.: Occurrence of epididymitis and orchitis of rams in Hungary. Magy. Allatorv. Lap., 22:439-443, 1967.

Walker, R., LeaMaster, B., Stellflug, J., and Biberstein, E.: Use of enzyme-linked immunosorbent assay for detection of antibodies to Brucella ovis in sheep. Field trial. AJVR, 46(8):1642-1646, 1985.

Webb, R., Quinn, C.A., Cockran, F., and Husband, A.: Evaluation procedures for the diagnosis of Brucella ovis infection in rams. Aust. Vet. J., 56:172-175, 1980.

Worthington, R., Stevenson, B., and deLisle, G.: Serology and semen culture for the diagnosis of Brucella ovis infection in chronically infected rams. N.Z. Vet. J., 33:84-86, 1985.

Worthington, R., Weddell, W., and Penrose, M.: A comparison of three serological tests for the diagnosis of Br. ovis infections in rams. N.Z. Vet. J., 32:58-60, 1984.

Epididymo-Orchitis

(Lamb epidiymitis)

(E-O; Actinobacillary epididymitis)

Epididymo-orchitis, a clinical or subclinical acute or chronic venereal disease of rams (especially ram lambs), is characterized by epididymitis and/or orchitis and is caused by Actinobacillus seminis and Actinobacillus like organisms. In endemic areas, this disease causes economic losses to producers from periods of inservice-ability, expensive treatments, and deaths in acute stages, and from reduced fertility, necessary inspections, and reduced marketability in chronic stages. The incidence can be reduced, however, by conscientious and persistent use of control programs.

OCCURRENCE. E-O occurs in rams of all breeds and all ages but predominantly in the 6 to 15 month age group. It is a major problem in stud flocks raising young rams in Australia, New Zealand, South Africa, Canada and the United States and has been reported in other major sheep producing countries. Although it occurs during all seasons, the highest incidence occurs when ram lambs are between 6 to 9 months of age. The most vigorous and best performing young rams kept in an intensive system on a high plane of nutrition are a high risk group likely to develop E-O.

ETIOLOGY. A variety of organisms cause E-O including *Actinobacillus seminis*, *A. actinomycetem-comintans*, *Haemophilus somnus* (ovis) and *Histophilus ovis*. An exact taxonomic classification for these organisms is lacking and the number of field strains are undetermined. A single taxon may be developed for this group. *Actinobacillus seminis*, the main cause of E-O is a nonmotile, nonsporing, gram-negative, pleomorphic bacterium that varies from coccoid forms to rods up to 6 mm in length and reside in the genital tracts and semen of rams. It does not ferment sugars, produce indole, split urea, produce B-galactosidase, lysine decarboxylase or arginine dihydrolase. It is catalase, oxidase, nitratase, and ornithine decarboxylase positive. It does not require CO_2 and on blood agar it forms round, pinpoint gray, nonhemolytic colonies in 24 hours of incubation. *Histophilus ovis*, another common causal organism, is catalase and arginine dihydrolase negative and oxidase, indole, nitratase and decarboxylase positive. Lysine decarboxylase reactions are variable. *Corynebacterium pyogenes*, a frequent isolate, is probably not the primary pathogen as it is usually isolated in conjunction with another pathogen.

The natural mode of transmission of *A. seminis* and related causal organisms has not been established.

PATHOGENESIS. The pathogenesis is not clearly understood. Entry via the mucous membrane through the lymphatics to the regional lymph nodes, through the blood and localizing in the genital organs is one hypothesis. A direct non-hematogenous route has been postulated. The organisms enter the preputial cavity from the environment, multiply and become established. As the ram lamb reaches puberty the development of the genital tract is under hormonal influence. A suitable environment is provided for spermatogenesis and spermatozoa survival. This environment is also suitable for the multiplication of bacteria and their spread from the preputial cavity to the rest of the genital tract. Thus they reach the accessory glands, and afterwards the epididymides and testes. Therefore, organisms which have no specific predilection for the accessory glands, epididymides and testes can initiate a pathologic process in these sites.

Localization of organisms in interstitial tissue of the epididymis attracts leukocytes that migrate, along with bacteria, into the epididymal duct. Epithelial cells lining the duct undergo hyperplasia, form obstructing folds in the lumen, and develop mural cysts. Masses of spermatids accumulate proximal to the occlusion and often extravasate into interstitial tissue. Segments of spermatid-filled duct and masses of extravasated spermatids provoke inflammatory reactions that become granulomas.

Localization of the organisms in intertubular stroma of the testes results in acute orchitis, with degeneration and necrosis of spermatogenic cells in seminiferous tubules. After healing, the testis is often sterile. Seminiferous tubular degeneration from either occlusion of the ductus epididymis or from acute orchitis may result in focal or general mineralization of the testis.

SIGNS AND LESIONS. *Actinobacillus seminis* infections of the genitalia can be classified into: 1. Carriers. 2. Subclinical cases. 3. Acute clinical cases. 4. Chronic clinical cases.

In carrier cases the ram is clinically normal although the organisms are present in the semen and prepuce. In endemic flocks rams excrete the organism from the onset of puberty and by 6 months of age the majority may be shedding the organisms. The defense mechanism eliminates the organism from genital tract of most rams by 12 to 15 months of age. In subclinical cases the ram palpates normal but has numerous neutrophils and bacteria in the semen. These rams have a higher risk of developing clinical lesions than carrier animals. Acute clinical cases occur most frequently in rams 6 to 9 months of age.

Rams with acute orchitis or acute epididymo-orchitis have a body temperature of 40 to 42°C, depression, immobilization, arched back, anorexia, leukocytosis, and unilateral or bilateral swelling and tenderness of the scrotal contents. Some animals die. Following abatement of systemic signs, the epididymis remains enlarged and becomes firm, and may excrete pus through a fistula to the scrotal surface, while the testis may atrophy or undergo mineralization. The affected testis becomes sterile.

Chronic clinical cases usually occur in older animals following a subclinical case or from partially resolved acute clinical cases.

At necropsy of animals in acute stages of E-O, the tunica vaginalis contains excess fluid, the epididymis and/or testis are swollen, and the surfaces, especially in the sinus epididymis, have deposits of exudate. In chronic stages, the tunica vaginalis may adhere to the epididymis and tunica albuginea at one or more points. The epididymis is enlarged and indurated and may contain abscesses and sperm cell granulomas.

DIAGNOSIS, PREVENTION AND TREATMENT. Clinical cases can be diagnosed by observation or palpation but are indistinguishable from *B. ovis* infections. The presence of neutrophils, easily observed under phase contrast microscopy, are suggestive of E-O in virgin ram lambs or older rams free of *B. ovis*. Serologic tests are supportive, but lack specificity and sensitivity. Bacteriologic examination of semen is required to confirm the identity of the etiologic agents. E-O can be prevented in ram lambs, under intensive management, with low level (100 to 150 mg per head per day) chlortetracycline in the feed. Subclinical and early acute clinical cases are best treated with therapeutic levels (5 to 10 mg/kg daily) of oxytetracycline over a course of 7 days. A satisfactory immunizing agent is not available although research with monoclonal antibodies may provide diagnostic and immunologic support to the control of E-O.

Baynes, I.D. and Simmons, G.C.: Clinical and pathological studies of Border Leicester rams naturally infected with *Actinobacillus seminis*. Aust. Vet. J., *44*:339-343, 1968.

Baynes, I.D. and Simmons, G.C.: Ovine epididymitis by *Actinobacillus seminis* (n. sp.). Aust. Vet. J., *36*:454, 1960.

Bruere, A., et al.: Genital infection of ram hoggets associated with a gram negative pleomorphic organism. N.Z. Vet. J., *25*:191-193, 1977.

Bulgin, M. and Anderson, B.: Association of sexual experience with isolation of various bacteria in cases of ovine epididymitis. JAVMA, *182*(4):372-374, 1983.

DeWet, J. and Erasmus J.: Epididymitis of rams in the central and southern districts of the Orange Free State. J. So. Afr. Vet. Assn., *4*:173-179, 1984.

Erasmus, J.: The usefulness of the API 20 classification system in the identification of *Actinobacillus actinomycetem comitans, Actinobacillus seminis* and Pasteurella haemolytica. Onderstepoort J. Vet. Res., *50*:97-99, 1983.

Healey, M., Kleinschuster, S., Gharpure, H., and Johnston, A.: Production and preliminary characterization of monoclonal antibodies to Actinobacillus sp. isolated from epididymitis lesions in a ram. Am. J. Vet. Res., *46*(6):1297-1302, 1985.

Jansen, B.: The etiology of ram epididymitis. Onderstepoort J. Vet. Res., *47*:101-107 1980.

Livingston, C.W. and Hardy, W.T.: Isolating *Actinobacillus seminis* from ovine epididymitis. AJVR, *25*:660, 1964.

Low, J. and Graham, M.: Histophilus ovis epididymitis in a ram in the UK. Vet. Rec., *117*:64-65, 1985.

Swanepoel, M.: A study for the differentiation of *Actinobacillus seminis, A. actinomycetem-comitans, Histophilus ovis* and *Pasteurella haemolytica*. Onderstepoort J. Vet. Res., *51*:41-46, 1984.

Van Tonder, E.M.: Actinobacillus seminis infection in sheep in the Republic of South Africa. I. Identification of the problem. Onderstepoort J. Vet. Res., *46*:129-133, 1979.

Van Tonder, E.M.: Actinobacillus seminis infection in sheep in the Republic of South Africa. II. Incidence and geographic distribution. Onderstepoort J. Vet. Res., *46*:135-140, 1979.

Van Tonder, E.M.: Infection of rams with *Actinobacillus seminis*. J. S. Afr. Vet Assoc., *44*:235-240, 1973.

Van Tonder, E.M. and Bolton, T.F.W.: Epididymitis in rams caused by *Actinobacillus seminis*. J. S. Afr. Vet. Assoc., *39*:87-90, 1968.

Walker, R., LeaMaster, B., Stellflug, J., and Biberstein, E.: Association of age of ram with distribution of epididymal lesions and etiologic agent. JAVMA, *188*(4):393-396, 1986.

Worthington, R.W. and Bosman P.P.: Isolation of *Actinobacillus seminis* in South Africa. J. S. Afr. Vet. Med. Assoc., *39*:81-85, 1968.

Ulcerative Posthitis

(UP; sheath-rot; pizzle-rot)

Ulcerative posthitis, a chronic and moderately contagious disease, is characterized by ulcers of the skin and mucosa of the prepuce and is caused by an interaction of high-protein diet (16 to 18%) and *Corynebacterium renale*.

In some enterprises it causes losses to producers from temporary incapacitation of rams, possible transmission to breeding ewes, extra labor, costly materials for treatment, and exclusion of affected animals from public shows and sales. Reduced production of wool and mohair is of economic significance.

OCCURRENCE. Ulcerative posthitis is prevalent among both wethers and rams of all breeds, but Merinos appear to be more susceptible than the British breeds. Angora goats are similarly affected. Wethers 3 years of age and older are commonly affected, and confined rams may develop infection before puberty as well as at older ages. In addition to sheep, UP also occurs in steers and bulls.

Seasonally, UP occurs during months of late spring and early summer when forage is abundant and high in protein content. Breeding rams may develop the disease during autumnal months when, in preparation for sales and breeding, they are fed high-protein diets, but it occasionally develops when dietary protein is as low as 12%.

Geographically, UP occurs in Australia, especially among wethers, but also in rams, and in America, South America, and the UK. The status of the disease in other countries is not known.

ETIOLOGY AND PATHOGENESIS. Ulcerative posthitis is caused by interaction of a high-protein diet and *Corynebacterium renale*. *Corynebacterium equi* and *C. hofmanni* have been reported; both produce urease. A diet containing 18% or more protein results in alkaline urine having increased concentration of urea. Compounded rations, especially those devised for finishing rams for public sales and shows and for breeding, and legume forage may contain a large amount of protein.

The diphtheroid bacterium, the second factor in the cause of UP, is a pleomorphic, aerobic, gram-positive, nonmotile, noncapsulated, nonsporing rod measuring 0.5 to 0.7 × 1.5 to 3 μm. It readily grows on most solid media and forms opaque punctiform colonies. In liquid media, it tolerates a pH range of 5.2 to 9.2 and a temperature range of 23° to 37°C. Although it hydrolyzes urea to ammonia, the urease does not accumulate in the extracellular fluid. Hydrogen sulfide and indole are not produced, and results of methyl red and Voges-Proskauer tests are negative. The organism occurs in ulcerated and normal skin of prepuces of sheep and cattle, and of vulvas of sheep.

Natural transmission of the organism probably is by direct and indirect contact, including copulation. Mating of ewes to infected rams may result in as high as a 50% incidence of vulvovaginitis.

As a result of high-protein diets, the urine contains as much as 4% urea. The diphtheroid bacteria, commonly inhabiting the skin near the preputial orifice, hydrolyzes the urea to ammonia, which severely irritates both preputial skin and mucosa. Epithelial cells surrounding the orifice necrotize and detach, leaving the ulcer. Necrotic tissue, inflammatory exudate, and bacteria dehydrate and form a crust on the ulcer. Although the ulcer usually localizes on the skin around the orifice, it may spread into the preputial cavity and there may form internal or mucosal ulcers. At the orifice, connective tissue may constrict and, together with exudate, close the opening. In this event, the decomposing urine and exudate distend the cavity and form sinus tracts from the mucosa to the skin surface. Following healing, the scarred orifice may cause permanent phimosis in rams. Since immunity does not follow infection, the disease may recur.

CLINICAL SIGNS AND POSTMORTEM LESIONS. Conditions favoring the development of UP include a change from low-protein to high-protein diet and the presence on the prepuce of the diphtheroid bacteria. Under these circumstances, ulcers may develop at the preputial orifice within 1 to 2 weeks after the change in diet. The external ulcers begin as areas of necrosis at points surrounding the orifice. The lesions usually spread circumferentially and laterally and may eventually involve 6 cm² of skin surface (Fig. 1-5). The ulcerated area, covered by soft or firm scab, does not inhibit preputial functions, such as micturition, and affected animals manifest little or no discomfort. External ulcers may extend through the orifice onto the mucosa. Fly strike, however, may occur.

Fig. 1-5. Necrosis at the preputial orifice in a ram with ulcerative posthitis. × 1.0.

the range is much higher. The mortality for external ulcers is zero, and for internal ulcers it is low; the course for external ulcers varies through a range of a few weeks to 6 months, and for internal ulcers through 2 to several weeks.

At necropsy of fatal or sacrificed animals, the preputial cavity is filled with exudate and urine, and the mucosa contains ulcers. Usually the anterior part of the mucosa contains a circular ulcer that cranially connects with the orifice and caudally extends along mucosal ridges. The urethral process may be necrosed and destroyed, and the glans may be ulcerated.

DIAGNOSIS. Veterinarians diagnose UP by clinical observation of typical ulcerations of the epithelium surrounding the preputial orifice and covered with a brownish crusty scab formation which, upon removal, produces minimal hemorrhage. Internal ulcerative posthitis is an extension of these lesions to the mucous membrane lining. Partial or complete occlusion of the preputial orifice causes enlargement and elongation and a thickening of the preputial wall. There is an accumulation of a foul-smelling mixture of urine and necrotic exudate. In the laboratory, *C. renale* can be isolated from the ulcers.

The differential diagnosis requires consideration of ulcerative dermatosis and urinary calculosis. The lesions of ulcerative dermatosis, while morphologically similar to those of UP, may in some animals locate on the face and/or feet, and lesion filtrates are infective. In calculosis, the preputial orifice is normal and may contain crystals precipitated from the urine. The distended urethra, over the ischial arch, pulsates, and the distended urinary bladder may be palpable.

PREVENTION AND TREATMENT. Producers and veterinarians prevent or reduce UP by management and medication. Planting judicious mixtures of grasses with legumes in improved pastures and careful planning of rations for rams can control the amount of dietary protein consumed. Removal of the wool or mohair from the preputial area aids in prevention. Implantation of wethers every 3 months with 70 to 100 mg of testosterone proprionate will

With internal ulcers, the prepuce becomes enlarged, swollen, and painful. In early stages, urine and exudate leak from the constricted but patent orifice and may stain surrounding wool. The affected animal kicks the prepuce and abdomen, stands with arched back, walks stiffly, and frequently alternates the standing and reclining positions.

Close examination of the prepuce reveals ulceration around the orifice and the presence of a mixture of malodorous urine and semisolid exudate in the distended preputial cavity. In advanced stages of the disease, the orifice may be completely occluded, and sinus tracts may drain contents from the posterior part of the prepuce to the skin surface. Internal ulceration also attracts fly strike. Death from uremia may occur.

Among rams, the morbidity for internal ulceration is low, but among wethers, it varies up to 20% or more, and for external ulceration, reduce the incidence and severity. Implanting with 12 mg zeranol will reduce the incidence but is not as effective. External ulcers should be treated, even though this is inconvenient, to avoid extension of lesions into the preputial cavity. Among wethers, the implanting of testosterone propionate pellets in the tissue lowers the disease incidence.

Treatment consists of (1) removal of the wool from the preputial area, debridement of affected tissue, application of ointment containing penicillin, bacitracin, or 5% copper sulfate, and transfer of the animals to a clean environment, or (2) surgical excision of a V-shaped part of the posterior wall of the prepuce for drainage, application of the same type of medicated ointment, and alterations in the diet to reduce protein intake.

Beveridge, W.I.B. and Johnstone, I.L.: Sheath-rot, noncontagious posthitis or chronic ulceration of the prepuce of sheep. III. Curative effect of reduced food consumption or surgical measures. Aust. Vet. J., 30:1-6, 1954.

Beveridge, W.I.B. and Johnstone, I.L.: Sheath-rot, noncontagious posthitis or chronic ulceration of the prepuce of sheep. I. Introduction and clinical observations. Aust. Vet. J., 29:269-274, 1953a.

Beveridge, W.I.B. and Johnstone, I.L.: Sheath-rot, noncontagious posthitis or chronic ulceration of the prepuce of sheep. II. Experiments on reproduction of the disease. Aust. Vet. J., 29:329-336, 1953b.

Brook, A.H., Southcott, W.H., and Stacy, B.D.: Etiology of ovine posthitis: Relationship between urine and the causal organism. Aust. Vet. J., 42:9-12, 1966.

Dent, C.H.R.: Ulcerative vulvitis and posthitis in Australian sheep and cattle. Vet. Bull., 41:719-723, 1971.

Doherty, M.: Outbreak of posthitis in grazing wethers in Scotland. Vet. Record, 116:372-373, 1985.

Filmer, J.F.: Ovine posthitis and balanoposthitis (pizzlerot): some notes on field investigations. Aust. Vet. J., 14:47-52, 1938.

Kimberling, C. and Arnold, K.: Diseases of the urinary system of sheep and goats. Vet. Clin. NA: LA Pract., 5(3):637-655, 1983.

Rojas, J.A.B. and Biberstein, E.L.: Diphtheroid agent of ovine posthitis. J. Comp. Pathol., 84:301-307, 1974.

Schild, A., et al.: Efficiency of implants of testosterone and zeranol in the control of ovine posthitis and their influence on weight gain and wool production. Pesq. Vet. Brasi., 2(2):55-59, 1982.

Shelton, M. and Livingston, C.: Posthitis in angora wethers. JAVMA, 167:154-155, 1975.

Southcott, W.H.: Etiology of ovine posthitis: description of a causal organism. Aust. Vet. J., 41:193-200, 1965.

Southcott, W.H.: The etiology of ovine posthitis. Aust. Vet. J., 39:212, 1963.

Southcott, W.H.: The etiology of ovine posthitis: transmission of the disease. Aust. Vet. J., 38:441-446, 1962.

Ulcerative Dermatosis

(UD; lip and leg ulceration; balanoposthitis; ovine venereal disease)

Ulcerative dermatosis, a contagious disease of sheep, is characterized by crusted ulcers of the skin of the face, feet, prepuce, penis, and vulva, and is caused by the UD virus, an unclassified agent. Of minor importance to the total sheep industry, the disease may cause financial waste to individual enterprises. Economic loss results from prolonged lameness, interference with feeding and breeding, incapacitation of rams, blindness of ewes and rams, expensive and troublesome treatment, and disqualification of affected sheep from public shows and sales.

OCCURRENCE.   UD occurs in all breeds and sexes of sheep. Although all ages are attacked, both sexes at breeding age suffer a higher incidence of the lesions. Seasonally, UD occurs most commonly during fall and winter. Breeding, commonly practiced during autumn, contributes to the incidence of the genital form, and grazing on winter ranges, often containing crusted snow and abrasive plants such as cacti, adds to the pedal form. Geographically, UD occurs in sheep of Britain, South Africa, and America. In the United States, the western intermountain region, especially Colorado, Idaho, Montana, Nevada, Oregon, Utah, and Wyoming, is an endemic area.

ETIOLOGY AND PATHOGENESIS.   The UD virus is unclassified, but in some respects it resembles the contagious ecthyma virus. It resists the action of ether and passes through Berkefeld V and N filters. All strains are antigenically homogeneous. In the laboratory, the virus adapts, although with difficulty, to cell cultures from embryonic bovine and ovine kidneys. It locates in lesion tissue and probably is transmitted by direct and indirect contact.

Commonly, bacteria inhabiting the skin surface, such as staphylococci and *Fusobacterium necrophorum,* contaminate and exacerbate the primary lesions.

The limited information on the pathogenesis of UD has derived from both clinical observations and experimental studies. Abrasions and lacerations of the skin of the feet, face, prepuce, and vulva, and of the mucous membrane of the penis facilitate growth of the virus in epithelial cells of those organs.

Discontinuities of the skin and mucosa have diverse mechanical causes. Walking through crusted snow and through spiny and sharp plants abrades the pedal skin, and grazing on dry piercing forage, such as brush and cacti, abrades and punctures the facial skin. Copulating, especially among sheep having grass awns and spiny seeds adhering to the wool near the genitals, lacerates the vulvar and preputial skin and the penile mucosa. Virus, entering the lacerated epidermis by direct or indirect exposures, multiplies in epithelial cells and, in conjunction with bacterial invaders, causes necrosis, pustules and destruction of all epithelial layers.

Fig. 1-6. Ulcers on facial skin from ulcerative dermatosis. × 0.6.

If undisturbed, the infected tissue within a few days forms a superficial ulcer covered by a firmly adhering scab. The continuation of abrasion, as often occurs, however, erodes the scab and necrotic tissue, and continued viral and bacterial infection in the floor and sides enlarges and deepens the ulcer.

Complications of the primary lesions include destruction of the urethral process, glans penis, and occasionally an eye, and the development of coffin joint arthritis. The penile damage at least temporarily incapacitates breeding rams, and the arthritis causes lameness for 12 to 18 months. Healing eventually occurs but may result in facial scars, blindness, and ankylosis of infected joints; penile scars may replace the glans and urethral process. Even after recovery, immunity appears to be of short duration.

CLINICAL SIGNS AND POSTMORTEM LESIONS. Following experimental inoculation of healthy sheep with UD virus, the incubation period varies from 2 to 5 days; after natural transmission, it may lengthen. An early detectable change is the formation of a pustule which, through necrosis of surrounding tissue, develops into an ulcer covered with a scab. The lesions, single or multiple, locate on the face, feet, or genitalia. In typical outbreaks, the lesions predominantly or exclusively develop in one anatomic location, but combinations of locations may exist.

Facial lesions form on the lips, nostrils, eyelids or other skin areas (Fig. 1-6). Each ulcer, circular in outline, varies from 5 to 30 mm in diameter and from 3 to 5 mm in depth. Unless continuously eroded by abrasions, a rigid and firmly attached scab forms. When the scab is forcibly removed, a granular and sometimes bleeding surface is exposed. A healed lesion leaves a depilated scar. Extensive lesions may interfere with prehension of feed. Histopathologically, the ulcer walls show necrosis, but not hyperplasia, of epithelial cells, and the floor granulation tissue. Colonies of bacteria frequently are discernible.

Pedal lesions locate on the skin between the hoof and carpus or tarsus and on the cranial or lateral surfaces (Fig. 1-7). From one to four feet may be infected. Each ulcer, again circular in outline, varies from 5 to 30 mm in diameter and 3 to 5 mm in depth. Abrasions from snow crust and range brush continuously remove the scab and maintain a raw surface. Severe ulcers cause lameness, and affected sheep separate from the flock and require special husbandry. In some feet, the ulcer invades the coffin joint capsule and causes prolonged swelling, lameness, and fistulation; healing by ankylosis eventually occurs. Owners, discouraged with affected sheep, may order euthanasia.

Genital ulcers on the skin of the vulva and prepuce cause acute swelling. Usually benign,

Fig. 1-7. Ulcer on pedal skin from ulcerative dermatosis. × 1.0.

Fig. 1-8. Ulcers on penis from ulcerative dermatosis. × 1.0.

the lesions develop scabs and heal. In some rams, however, the infected preputial orifice may prevent free micturition. Penile lesions usually locate on the glans penis (Fig. 1-8). Instead of a dry scab, moist exudate accumulates on the infected and swollen surface. The urethral process may necrotize, and urinary fistulas may form. These changes may cause either phimosis or paraphimosis and temporarily prevent breeding. Following healing, the urethral process may be absent, and part or all of the glans may be replaced by scar tissue (Fig. 1-9).

The morbidity for the facial form averages 20%; the pedal form, 25%; and the genital form, 80% of breeding ewes and rams. The mortality is low, and the rare deaths result from extensive bacterial infection. The course usually varies from 2 to 6 weeks; coffin joint arthritis, however, may persist for 12 to 18 months.

DIAGNOSIS. Veterinarians diagnose UD from evidence of typical lesions. In endemic areas, a high incidence of ulcerous skin lesions on the face, feet, or genitalia or a combination of these locations usually justifies a clinical diagnosis. In the laboratory, the causative virus can be isolated and grown on cell cultures from bovine or ovine embryonic kidneys. Histopathologic examination of lesions shows no epithelial hyperplasia.

The differential diagnosis requires consideration of contagious ecthyma, foot-and-mouth disease, and noninfectious posthitis. Contagious ecthyma, characterized by eruptive nodules on the skin of the lips, nostrils, and feet and on the oral and buccal mucosa causes epithelial hyperplasia that can be histopathologically identified. Ovine foot-and-mouth disease usually causes vesicles on the skin of the feet and on the mucosa of the dental pad. In the laboratory, the virus can be isolated and

Fig. 1-9. Penis healed after ulcerative dermatosis.
× 1.0.

Bosworth, T.J. and Glover, R.E.: Some observations on the nature of certain diseases of sheep. 49th Ann. Cong. Nat. Vet. Med. Assoc. Great Britain and Ireland, 1931, pp. 22-28.

Knowles, M.E.: Infectious lip and leg ulceration of sheep. Ann. Rept. Board Sheep Commissioners of Montana, 1907-08, pp. 17-28.

M'Fadyean, J.A.: Contagious disease of generative organs in sheep. J. Comp. Pathol. Ther., 16:375-376, 1903.

Mohler, J.R.: Lip and leg ulceration (necrobacillosis): Its cause and treatment. USDA, Bureau of Animal Industry. Cir., 160:12-35, 1910.

Roberts, R.S. and Bolton, J.F.A.: Venereal disease of sheep. Vet. Rec., 57:686-687, 1945.

Steyn, D.G.: Pisgoed or pisgras. Dir. Vet. Ser. Anim. Ind. Union S. Afr., 1930, pp. 417-420.

Tunnicliff, E.A.: Ulcerative dermatosis of sheep. AJVR, 10:240-249, 1949.

Tunnicliff, E.A. and Matisheck, P.H.: A filtrable virus demonstrated to be infective agent in ovine balanoposthitis. Science, 94:283-284, 1941.

Trueblood, M.S. and Chow, T.L.: Characterization of the agents of ulcerative dermatosis and contagious ecthyma. AJVR, 24:47-51, 1963a.

Trueblood, M.S., Chow, T.L., and Griner, L.A.: An immunologic study of ulcerative dermatosis and contagious ecthyma. AJVR, 24:42-46, 1963b.

identified. Noninfectious posthitis occurs in both rams and wethers, and the ulcerous lesions located at the preputial orifice.

PREVENTION AND TREATMENT. Veterinarians and producers reduce UD by applying appropriate sanitation and management principles. Prior to breeding, showing, or selling, both ewes and rams should be examined for characteristic lesions. Affected sheep should be isolated until all lesions have healed. Stock sheep should be protected against wool contamination with spiny seeds and abrading awns. If these foreign materials have been acquired, the wool around the genitalia should be clipped before breeding. No vaccine has been developed.

Treatment consists of lesion protection and topical medication. Confinement of sheep with pedal lesions protects the animals against further abrasions of the lesions, and soft-textured feed avoids further injury to facial lesions. After cleaning the lesion, ointment containing a tetracycline or penicillin antibiotic should be topically applied to control bacterial infection and to soften scabs.

Butting

(Fighting)

Butting, the method of fighting among rams, is the forward striking of the head and horns of a belligerent male against another male. The process has two forms: (1) congestive butting, in which two vying males charge through a distance of about 10 m and collide head-on, and (2) punitive butting, in which an aggressive male butts the body of another male. This behavioral problem results in economic losses for producers from deaths and injuries.

OCCURRENCE. Butting occurs in all breeds and ages of rams maintained in herds, but injuries develop most often in animals of the horned breeds 0.5 to 2 years of age being fed for rapid growth, early breeding, and auction sales. The activity is concentrated during late summer and early autumn, before the usual breeding time in the northern hemisphere. It occurs in all countries where sheep production is an important part of advanced animal agriculture.

ETIOLOGY AND PATHOGENESIS. A complex set of physiologic factors causes butting. Among these are individual belligerence, desire to dominate, and beginning of the breeding season.

Autumn is the normal breeding season in the northern hemisphere. Ram lambs, born during the previous winter and given special diet and care, at 8 months of age may weigh 90 kg, have fragile bones, and be sexually mature. Such animals readily engage in contestive butting with both peers and older, heavier, and stronger rams. In the process, the cervical vertebrae, especially if misaligned, may fracture or luxate and fatally injure the spinal cord. Punitive butting, with severe blows to the body, may fracture limb bones and ribs in rams of any age.

CLINICAL SIGNS AND POSTMORTEM LESIONS. During prebreeding and breeding time, the rams of a herd accelerate contestive butting. Occasionally, a herdsman observes a young ram collapse and fall to recumbency immediately after a collision. Usually, however, he simply finds the paralyzed or dead animal, with or without cutaneous excoriations between or anterior to the horns. Lameness from fractured limb bones also may be found. The mortality among young rams may reach 2%.

At necropsy of young rams, the fracture or luxation, with hemorrhage and spinal cord injury, can be identified. The usual location is between the second and seventh cervical vertebrae. Contused and fractured limbs also may be found.

DIAGNOSIS. Veterinarians identify butting injuries from reported observations of fighting by herdsmen and from injuries observed clinically or at necropsy. The differential diagnosis requires consideration of other types of trauma and lesions of caseous lymphadenitis along the vertebral column.

PREVENTION AND TREATMENT. Producers can reduce prebreeding butting by maintaining the young rams in small isolated groups, and they can prevent it by maintaining them in individual isolation, but isolation usually is not feasible management. Nonfatal limb fractures should be treated by standard methods for bone immobilization and rest.

RAM MANAGEMENT

RAM SELECTION. The majority of the genetic improvement in a flock results from proper ram selection. Selection of the ram(s) starts with establishing a set of goals and outlining the performance criteria necessary to meet those goals. Purchases should be made from breeders or ram testing cooperaters that provide appropriate performance data. Records are essential, including immunization status, herd health management, and medical history.

Fertility evaluation (testicular size, and spermatozoa quality) should be part of the selection criteria. Spermatozoa output is directly related to testicular size and weight which in turn are correlated with body condition. In ram lambs testicular growth correlates with body growth and levels off at maturity. Growth promotants have a detrimental effect on testicular development. The minimum scrotal circumference for a yearling (12 to 18 months) ram should be 33 to 34 cm and 30 to 31 cm for a ram lamb (6 to 9 months). The number and quality of spermatozoa are directly related to fecundity in the ewe. The semen should have a minimum of 30% progressively motile spermatozoa, 75% morphologically normal spermatozoa and no white blood cells.

A complete breeding soundness evaluation includes a thorough physical and conformational examination plus a negative ELISA test for *B. ovis* within 30 days of purchase. Purchased animals regardless of the source, should be isolated for an observation period of 30 days prior to introduction into the flock.

HEALTH MAINTENANCE. A herd health maintenance calendar and program should be developed for the specific needs of each ram flock including dates for: 1. Immunization. 2. Foot care. 3. Parasite control (internal and external). 4. Preparation for the breeding season (nutritional program, breeding soundness evaluation, shearing if applicable, etc.). 5. Management during the breeding season. 6. Management practices during the non-breeding season (such as ELISA testing for *B. ovis*). All rams should be permanently identified with a numbered flexible ear tag and records kept for each ram.

PREBREEDING MANAGEMENT. Spermatogenesis in rams has a duration of 49 days with an additional 11 days of maturation and transport through the epididymis and vas deferens. It is important to provide in the 2 months prior to breeding optimal management including adequate feed, water, shelter/shade and prevent exposure to conditions which will adversely affect these processes. Systemic diseases with elevated temperature and/or localized inflammation of the scrotum, high environmental temperatures and stress (shows and transportation) may cause spermatogenic dysfunction resulting in temporary infertility. Obese or thin rams have a lowered fertility. Close monitoring and a thorough physical examination of the rams will allow treatments or culling as the condition dictates. Nutrition has a direct relationship on testicular function, spermatogenesis and semen quality. Body condition is an indicator of the nutritional plane.

A good pasture with salt and mineral supplementation will provide adequate nutrition. If supplemental feeding is necessary follow the nutrient guidelines as outlined in "Nutrient requirements of sheep," sixth revised edition, Nutritional Academy Press, Washington, D.C., 1985. Measurement of libido and serving capacity is of minor importance if all rams are highly fertile and the rams are used in multisire breeding programs.

BREEDING SEASON MANAGEMENT. Teaser rams introduced 20 days prior to the breeding season will provide a degree of estrus synchronization. Thus increasing the number of lambs delivered in the first 16 days of the lambing period. Providing breeding rams with colored marking harnesses (change of color every 16 days) provides a monitoring system to assess the successfulness of the breeding program and give early indication of potential reproductive problems. The ram : ewe ratio should be one that fully exploits the ram's reproductive potential. Full utilization of the rams reproductive capabilities will maximize the genetic impact and minimize capital investment and maintenance expenses. Under good conditions maximum fecundity in mature ewes can be achieved by using 1% highly fertile rams. Ram lambs should be stocked at a rate of 3% and not used with mature rams. It is advisable to use only experienced rams and double the ram : ewe ratio on ewe lambs or first bred ewes. Breed ewe lambs separate from older ewes.

IMMUNIZATION CONSIDERATIONS. Clostridial infections are universally distributed wherever sheep are produced. With reported cases of Cl. perfringenes, Cl. novyi, Cl. haemolyticum, Cl. chauvoei, Cl. septicum and Cl. tetani it is advisable to immunize with a product containing these antigens. For maximum resistance the initial immunization should be followed by a second dose in 6 weeks and an annual booster. The primary course of shots should start at 10 to 12 weeks of age. Satisfactory protection against B. ovis is provided by one dose of B. melitensis Rev I antigen at 4 to 6 months of age. Bacterins for B. ovis, currently produced in the US, have poor efficacy (approximately 50%) and are not recommended. An immunization program for contagious ovine foot rot consisting of two initial doses 6 weeks apart followed by an annual booster 4 to 6 weeks prior to the period of high risk provides excellent protection (90% or greater). Immunization programs for diseases endemic to certain geographical areas such as foot and mouth disease, rinderpest, rift valley fever, etc., should be considered in the particular program area.

PARASITE CONTROL. Internal parasites are best controlled by a system of rotational grazing combined with an effective wormer where treated animals are rotated to clean pastures following treatment. External parasites are best controlled by timely (following shearing and other times as may be indicated) application of a pyrethroid spray or pour-on.

Dawe, S., et al.: The effect of ram percentage on the fertility of maiden ewes. Proc. Aust. Soc. Anim. Prod., 10:274-278, 1974.
Fitch, G., Brinks, J., Denham, A., and Kimberling, C.: Analysis of scrotal circumference growth curves in rams. Western Section, ASAS Proceedings, 36, 1985.
Hulet, C., Foote, W., and Blackwell, R.: Relationship of semen quality and fertility in the ram to fecundity in the ewe. J. Reprod. Fertil., 9:311-315, 1965.
Lightfoot, R. and Smith J.: Studies on the number of ewes joined per ram for flock matings under paddock conditions. Aust. J. Agric. Res., 19:1029-1042, 1968.
Lino, B.: The output of spermatozoa in rams. Aust. J. Biol. Sci., 25:359-366, 1972.
Pryor, W.: Feeding sheep for high reproductive performance. Morrow, D. (ed.): Current Therapy in Theriogenology. Philadelphia, W.B. Saunders Co., 1980.
Riesen, J., Beeler, B., Abenes, F., and Woody, C.: Effects of zeranol on the reproductive system of lambs. J. An. Sci., 45(2):293-298, 1977.
Walkley, J. and Barber, A.: The relationship between libido score and fertility in Merino rams. Proc. Aust. Soc. Anim. Prod., 11:141-144, 1976.

2

DISEASES OF EWES

Pregnancy Toxemia

(OPT; ketosis; lambing sickness; twin lamb disease)

Pregnancy toxemia is a metabolic disease of ewes in advanced pregnancy. Negative energy balance, hypoglycemia, and increased fat catabolism produce the characteristic ketonemia, ketonuria and neurologic signs of depression, inappetence, incoordination, impaired vision, and prostration which progresses to unconsciousness and death. The inciting factors are the stress of multiple fetuses, dietary restriction, or a traumatic change in environment. Because of its wide geographic distribution, general prevalence, and financial waste among farm and pasture flocks, the disease causes great concern to the entire sheep industry, and as production emphasis changes from range bands to farm flocks, it will acquire even greater importance. Economic losses result from deaths of affected ewes and unborn lambs and from the cost in materials and labor for preventive programs. The occurrence of a similar condition in humans adds interest and scientific significance to the disease. Although there are no recognized spontaneous toxemia-like states in animals which are completely analogous to human preeclampsia.

OCCURRENCE. OPT occurs in all breeds of ewes in their second and subsequent pregnancies. Thin ewes and over-conditioned ewes bearing twins or triplets develop the disease during the last month of pregnancy. Most cases are associated with a declining plane or interruption of nutritional intake due to storms, moving ewes to a new environment, or other stress factors. Ewes from farm and pastured flocks, especially over-conditioned ewes, have a higher incidence than ewes in range bands.

The disease probably occurs in all sheep-producing countries, but the prevalence is high in New Zealand, Australia, United States, Britain, and South Africa.

ETIOLOGY AND PATHOGENESIS. Rapid growth of twin or triplet fetuses, declining or interruption of ewe nutrition, and psychologic stresses cause OPT. Eighty percent of the lamb birth weight forms during the last 6 weeks of pregnancy. The growing fetuses exert an obligatory demand for 70 to 85 g of glucose per day. The normal non-pregnant sheep produces and uses 85 to 100 g of glucose per day for its maintenance. An inadequate supply of glucose for maternal and fetal tissues may result in OPT or in a delicate glycemic balance. The imposition of stress, such as transport, fast, change of feed, and intercurrent disease, often lowers the glucose state and initiates the disease.

The animal, however, institutes a series of glucose-conserving changes that rescue most ewes from profound and damaging hypoglycemia: (1) The animal may consume more feed, especially grains, and thereby increase the exogenous supply of glucose; (2) the liver converts glycogen to glucose; (3) maternal tissues hydrolyze fat, convert the resulting glycerol to glucose, and oxidize the fatty acids for energy, and in the oxidative process form ketone bodies—acetone, acetoacetic acid, and β-hydroxybutyric acid—which may accumulate to concentrations of hyperketonemia; (4) the tissues convert amino acids to glucose; (5) maternal organs may reduce the rate of glucose utilization for their own maintenance; and (6) the adrenal glands enlarge producing increased levels of blood cortisol, plasma renin, and blood aldosterone.

The exact pathogenesis of pregnancy toxemia is unclear although a disruption of the glucose homeostatic control mechanism is probably caused by the high glucose demands of multiple fetuses on an undernourished and stressed ewe. The impairment of maternal hepatic gluconeogenesis may also be restrained in the presence of a live fetus. An initial hypoglycemia is followed by increased fat catabolism with a resultant increase in the accumulation of lipids (predominantly triacylglycerols), giving rise to a fatty liver and increased ketone bodies in blood and urine. There is a high correlation between the levels of liver fat and plasma ketones suggesting that these changes are a consequence of fat mobilization caused by under nutrition. The stress and low caloric intake of OPT have a profound effect on the kidney and adrenal gland with a significant reduction in renal blood flow and glomerular filtration rate which raises plasma renin activities and elevates plasma cortisol levels. These high cortisol levels may inhibit glucose utilization by the tissues and cause the clinical manifestations (especially neurologic signs) associated with OPT. There is a correlation between the degree of elevation of plasma renin concentration and clinical severity. Serum levels of iron, magnesium and potassium are decreased, whereas blood urea nitrogen, creatinine, and the ratio of these components (Bun/Creatinine) are elevated. Serum bilirubin levels (total and direct) are higher. In the terminal stages of the disease fetal death is associated with a hyperglycemia. This may be due to a termination of glucose demand by the fetuses, a relatively high glu-

cose turnover rate and hepatocyte glucose production rate and a complete loss of glucose homeostasis. Renal failure, dehydration, and severe metabolic acidosis are most often irreversible causing death of the ewe.

CLINICAL SIGNS AND POSTMORTEM LESIONS. The signs of OPT may begin in a single animal or simultaneously in many ewes. The affected animal is either thin or obese. The ewe isolates from the flock, declines feed, shows incoordinate movements, elevates the head, and shows weakness. Eventually, the animal reclines in sternal recumbency and rises only with assistance; mucus discharges from the nose, and breathing accelerates. The acidic urine contains ketone bodies and protein. Neurologic signs, such as blindness, muscular tremors, convulsions, and coma, finally lead to death.

The morbidity ranges up to 20% of a flock, and the mortality of affected ewes reaches 80%. Recovery often results, however, from parturition by either natural birth or surgical intervention. The course varies from 2 to 10 days.

At necropsy, the uterus contains twin or triplet fetuses that may have died and decomposed before maternal death. The enlarged and friable liver is pale yellow from fatty degeneration. Chemical analysis of the liver may disclose an increase from a normal value of 3% fat to a pathologic value of 30%. The fatty liver syndrome is associated with advanced pregnancy as ewes without signs of OPT can have higher liver fat content than clinically affected ewes. The adrenals may also show enlargement by as much as 65%.

DIAGNOSIS. Veterinarians diagnose OPT on evidence of typical signs, necropsy lesions and laboratory findings. Blindness, anorexia, weakness, and incoordination in ewes in the last 3 weeks of pregnancy are suggestive signs, and twin or triplet pregnancies and fatty livers are indicative lesions. The measurement of blood glucose levels below 25 mg/dl (normal, 40 to 60 mg/dl) and ketonuria in early disease stages confirm the diagnosis.

The differential diagnosis requires consideration of hypocalcemia. Sheep with this disease show normal urine, straddling of the hind limbs, tremors, coma, and response to intravenous administration of calcium gluconate.

PREVENTION AND TREATMENT. OPT can be prevented by a well-planned nutrition and management program throughout pregnancy. The stages of fetal development dictates the nutritional requirements. Fetal growth during the first 15 weeks of gestation accounts for about 20% of the total development. The remaining 80% occurs during the last 6 weeks. During the first 15 weeks a 60-kg ewe in good condition carrying a single fetus should be fed to gain about 0.03 kg (0.066 lb) per day or 3.15 kg (7 lbs) over the 105-day period. During the last 6 weeks the ewe should gain 0.18 kg (0.4 lb) per day or 7.6 kg (16.5 lbs) over the 42-day period. A high quality hay, good pasture, or good crop aftermath will provide adequate energy intake for the first 15-week period. Total feed requirements for the single bearing ewe during the last 6 weeks is 1.5 × maintenance and 2.0 × maintenance for a twin bearing ewe. The additional energy for this period is best supplied by concentrate feeds as the rumen capacity is limited by fetal expansion.

Energy requirements during the last 6 weeks of pregnancy for the twin bearing ewe are approximately 180% greater than that of a single bearing ewe and 240% greater if she is carrying triplets. Ewes should be condition scored early in pregnancy and where possible separated into groups of thin, normal, or overconditioned and fed accordingly. The overconditioned ewe can be fed a submaintenance ration for the first 3½ months of pregnancy without harm. With the advent of the real time ultrasound for pregnancy diagnosis it is possible to determine single and multiple fetuses thus aiding in the nutritional management during the last 6 weeks of pregnancy. Although shearing is a stress condition, removal of the wool along with adequate energy intake seems to aid in metabolism and reduce the incidence of OPT especially in the over-conditioned ewe. The National Research Councils nutrient requirements for sheep should be used as a guideline for formulating rations to meet the energy, protein and mineral needs of the ewe during the various stages of gestation and lactation. The guidelines set forth do not provide the variations in climatic conditions when calculating the energy for maintenance. Temperature, wind, moisture, and the staple length of the wool must be considered as these effect the animals critical temperature and influence the body heat loss, thus increasing the demands for increased energy intake. Management practices such as shearing, vaccinating, drenching, trailing, or moving to a different location should be done well in advance of parturition to avoid undue stress which may precipitate OPT.

Treatment of OPT is directed towards correcting the energy, electrolyte, acid-base imbalance, correcting dehydration and stimulating a depressed appetite. Oral propylene glycol or corn syrup is a source of quick energy and should be given at a rate of 200 ml 4 times daily along with 3 to 4 liters of an electrolyte solution as used for dehydration in calf diarrhea (Life-Guard, Norden). Intravenous vitamin B mixtures or administration of 50 to 125 ml of a 20% solution of calcium borogluconate solution improves rumen motility and depression. Thirty mg trenbolone acetate (Finaject; Hoechst) intramuscularly once daily will aid in stimulating the appetite. These treatments must be accompanied by an intake of concentrate feeds. Hand feeding may be necessary. In more advanced cases give 250 to 500 ml of 10 to 20% glucose intravenously, correct the electrolyte imbalance, the metabolic acidosis and dehydration with intravenous fluids. In refractory cases termination of pregnancy may be necessary.

Bergman, E.N.: Glucose turnover rates in sheep. Nature, *202*:1333, 1964.

Bergman, E.N.: Quantitative aspects of glucose metabolism in sheep. Am. J. Physiol., *204*:147-152, 1963.

Bergman, E.N., Roe, W.E., and Kon, K.: Quantitative aspects of propionate metabolism in sheep. Am. J. Physiol., *211*:793-799, 1966.

Bergman, E.N., Starr, D.J., and Reulein, S.S.: Glycerol metabolism in normal and ketotic sheep. Am. J. Physiol., *215*:874-880, 1968.

East, N.: Pregnancy toxemia, abortions, and preparturient diseases. Vet. J. Clin. N.A.: Large Animal Practice, 5(3):601-618, 1983.

Ferris, T.F., Herdson, P.B., Dunnell, M.S., and Lee, M.R.: Clinical physiologic and pathologic study of pregnancy toxemia. J. Clin. Invest., *48*:1643-1655, 1969.

Gill, J.C. and Thompson, W.: The production of pregnancy toxemia in ewes. J. Agric. Sci., 45:229, 1954.

Groenwald, J.W., et al.: Pregnancy disease in sheep. Onderstepoort J. Vet. Sci. Anim. Ind., 17:246-251, 1941.

Hallford, D. and Swanson, D.: Serum profiles determined during ovine pregnancy toxemia. Agri-Practice, 4(4): 27-33, 1983.

Henderson, G., Read, L., and Schoswell, A.: Studies of liver lipids in normal, alloxan-diabetic and pregnancy-toxemic sheep. Biochemica et Biophysica Acta., 710: 236-241, 1982.

Hill, P., Caghlan, J., and Scoggins, Bryan G.: Functional and morphological studies of the adrenal cortex and kidney in ovine toxemia of pregnancy. J. Path., 144:1-13, 1984.

Holmes, J.R.: Pregnancy toxemia in grassland flocks. Vet. Rec., 65:299-303, 1953.

Hunt, E.R.: Treatment of pregnancy toxemia in ewes by induction of parturition. Aust. Vet. J., 52:540, 1976.

Jackson, H.D., Burtis, M.S., and Goetsch, G.D.: Effects of phlorhizin and heparin on fasted sheep. AJVR, 27: 885-890, 1966.

Kronfeld, D.S.: Fetal drain of hexose in ovine pregnancy toxemia. Cornell Vet., 48:394-404, 1958.

Kronfeld, D.S. and Raggi, F.: Plasma glucose and fatty acid concentrations in pregnancy toxemia in sheep. Res. Vet. Sci., 7:493, 1966.

McClymont, G.L. and Setchell, B.P.: Correlation hypoglycemic depth and induction of signs. Aust. Vet. J., 32:22-25, 1956.

McClymont, G.L. and Setchell, B.P.: Hypoglycemic encephalopathy in ovine pregnancy toxemia. Aust. Vet. J., 31:53-68, 1955.

M'Fadyean, J.: Fatty infiltration of liver in pregnant ewes. J. Comp. Pathol., 37:287, 1924.

Michael, D.T.: Survey of pregnancy toxemia. Vet. Rec., 69:595-598, 1957.

National Research Council. Nutrient requirements of sheep. National Academy Press, Wash., D.C., 1985.

Reid, R.L.: Adrenal glands in pregnancy toxemia. Aust. J. Agric. Res., 11:364-382, 1960.

Reid, R.L. and Hinks, N.T.: Feed requirements for preventing hypoglycemia in sheep. Aust. J. Agric. Res., 13:1092-1111, 1962.

Roderick, L.M., Harshfield, G.S., and Hawn, M.C.: The pathogenesis of pregnancy disease of sheep. JAVMA, 90:41-49, 1937.

Shulz, L. and Riese, R. Pregnancy toxemia in the ewe. Iowa St. Vet., 45(1):11-15, 1983.

Thompson, G.G.: Treatments for ovine pregnancy toxemia. N.Z. Vet. J., 4:136-144, 1956.

Wallace, L.R.: Growth of lambs before and after birth. J. Agric. Sci., 38:243-302, 1948.

Wastney, M., Arcus, A., Bickerstaffe, R., and Wolff, J.: Glucose tolerance in ewes and susceptibility to pregnancy toxemia. Aust. J. Biol. Sci., 35:381-392, 1982.

White, I., Russel, J., and Fowler, D. Real-time ultrasonic scanning in the diagnosis of pregnancy and the determination of fetal numbers in sheep. Vet. Rec., 115: 140-143, 1983.

Wierda, A., et al.: Effects of trenbolone acetate and propylene glycolon pregnancy toxemia ewes. Vet. Rec., 116:284-287, 1985.

Hypocalcemia

(HC; lambing sickness; milk fever; transport tetany)

Hypocalcemia, an acute metabolic disease of sheep, is characterized by tetany, incoordination, paralysis, and coma and is caused by an inadequate supply of metabolizable calcium. Because the disease has wide geographic distribution and occurs in pregnant ewes, lactating ewes, rams, and feedlot lambs and causes considerable financial waste, it concerns the sheep industry. Economic losses result from deaths, maternal neglect and abandonment of nursing lambs, and loss of live weight among feedlot lambs. The common development of HC among dairy cows and other domestic animals adds economic significance to the condition.

OCCURRENCE. HC occurs in all breeds and sexes of sheep beyond weaning age. Although the disease primarily affects fat ewes during the last 6 weeks of pregnancy and during the first week of lactation, it also occurs in rams and feedlot lambs following fast and transport. Most cases develop in ewes during the spring, in rams during summer and early fall, and in feedlot lambs during late summer and early fall when weaned lambs commonly move from western ranges to feedlots.

Geographically, HC probably develops in all major sheep-producing countries, but Australia, New Zealand, the United States, Britain, and South Africa have high incidences.

Hypocalcemia is the result of an increase in the rate of movement of Ca out of the blood plasma, which is not balanced by increases in the rate of absorption of Ca from the gut or in the rate of resorption of Ca from bone. The concentration of plasma Ca is controlled within narrow limits by a sensitive hormonal mechanism involving the hydroxylated metabolites of vitamin D, parathyroid hormone, and thyrocalcitonin. Magnesium has a regulatory relationship with calcium which may affect serum calcium concentrations. Parathyroid hormone and active vitamin D_3 are necessary for resorption of calcium from bone, for absorption of calcium from the intestine, and for

DISEASES OF EWES

renal tubular resorption of calcium. A low plasma magnesium level may cause refractoriness of bone to the action of parathyroid hormone.

The appearance of hypocalcemia in sheep and dairy cattle corresponds to the period of greatest calcium demand. The critical demand for calcium in the dairy cow occurs the last day or two of gestation and the onset of lactation. In contrast, the sheep's greatest demand for calcium occurs in the last 3 to 4 weeks of gestation when mineralization of the fetal skeleton is at its maximum and decreases following parturition. The presence of twin fetuses imposes almost twice the demand for Ca and P for mineralization of the fetal skeleton as a single fetus. Thus ewes bearing multiple fetuses are at higher risk of developing hypocalcemia. Hydroxyproline is important in skeletal metabolism and bone resorption. Serum levels of hydroxyproline increase the last 4 to 6 weeks before lambing mobilizing calcium from the bone. The level of hydroxyproline activity decreases with age as does the ability to mobilize calcium. This may partially explain the higher incidence of HC in older ewes.

ETIOLOGY AND PATHOGENESIS. The descent of plasma concentrations of calcium from normal values of 8 to 12 mg/dl to pathological values of 3 to 6 mg/dl undoubtedly causes clinical manifestations of HC. Associated with hypocalcemia is an increase in serum glutamic-pyruvic transaminase (SGPT), creatinine kinase (CK), and lactate dehydrogenase (LDH). Although veterinary scientists do not know the precise cause of these subnormal calcium levels, they do recognize several depressing factors: (1) prolonged consumption of calcium-deficient diets, which may lower the plasma calcium by 15 to 35%; (2) sudden change of diet from dry to lush pasture; (3) fasting from 2 to 6 days, especially when combined with transport, which may lower the calcium by 17 to 25%; (4) exercise, such as driving, which may lower the calcium by 15%; (5) late pregnancy and early lactation, which may lower the calcium by 50 to 60%; (6) minor surgical procedures, restrictive handling, and administration of epinephrine; (7) consumption

of oxalate containing feeds; and (8) severe weather conditions. These calcium-depressing factors, operating singly or together, in addition to the inability of the animal to mobilize calcium rapidly from the skeleton, result in serious and fatal hypocalcemia.

Other than low dietary intake of Ca, most Ca depleting events are associated with stress conditions. Stress increases norepinephrine corticosteroid secretion which antagonizes vitamin D, decreasing renal tubular resorption of calcium, decreases intestinal calcium absorption, and inhibits parathyroid hormone effect on bone, thus increasing calcium losses, decreasing calcium absorption, and decreasing calcium mobilization from the bone. If the calcium regulating mechanism fails to adjust, the plasma concentrations fall. When the level reaches a dangerous level near 3 to 6 mg/dl, irritability develops, followed by depression and coma. The parenteral administration of calcium maintains a required level until the affected animal adjusts its potential supply to its actual need for calcium. Except for calcium treatment, most animals with HC die.

CLINICAL SIGNS AND POSTMORTEM LESIONS. In all classes of affected sheep abrupt clinical signs are preceded by a decrease in ruminal motility and uterine tone in the case of the pregnant ewe. Poor uterine tone, associated with hypocalcemia has been correlated with cervico-vaginal prolapse and incomplete or non-dilation of the cervix. In marginal HC these signs may go undetected. The lack of ruminal motility reduces Ca absorption further depressing plasma calcium levels and precipitating apparent clinical signs. Motility of the abomasum decreases simultaneously with the development of clinical signs. Affected ewes in early stages show stiff and incoordinated movements and spraddled stance, especially in the hind limbs. Later muscular tremors, muscular weakness, apprehension, and rapid breathing are prominent. Ewes in advanced stages fall to sternal recumbency, with the head extended forward and the posterior limbs extended backward; they develop paralysis and pass into coma. Body temperature is normal. Up to 30% of ewes in affected flocks may develop the disease, and of these, 90% die unless treated. Death usually occurs after a course ranging from 4 to 48 hours. Rams, ewes, and feedlot lambs, following fast and transport, usually develop HC within 1 to 2 days after arrival at destination; some cases develop within a few hours after unloading. Lambs that fail to eat and drink on arrival at the feedlots suddenly, like affected ewes, become stiff, incoordinated, tremulous, weak, prostrated, paralytic, and comatose. In the gaunt, dehydrated, and unconscious lamb, the movements of ruminal fluid are clearly audible in the manipulated animal. The morbidity among feedlot lambs usually is 2 to 3%; these animals die unless they are treated. No gross or microscopic lesions are discernible.

DIAGNOSIS. Veterinarians diagnose HC from evidence of flock history, signs, and chemical analysis of the blood. A history of comatose ewes in advanced pregnancy of early lactation and of rams, ewes, and feedlot lambs recently fasted and transported is highly suggestive of the disease. Favorable response to intravenous administration of calcium gluconate provides more substantial evidence, and serum calcium levels measuring 3 to 6 mg/dl confirm the diagnosis.

The differential diagnosis requires consideration of hypomagnesemia, pregnancy toxemia, and enterotoxemia.

PREVENTION AND TREATMENT. Prevention of hypocalcemia in the pregnant ewe is accomplished by proper management avoiding those events or diets during late pregnancy that precipitate the disease syndrome. All procedures such as shearing, trailing, or transporting to a new environment, changes of feed, etc. should be accomplished at least 4 to 6 weeks prior to lambing. Adequate nutrition to meet the additional energy and mineral requirements should be provided. If ewes are to be trailed or transported long distances, a pelleted ration containing 5 parts of alfalfa and 1 part corn or other concentrate should be provided as it is impossible for the ewe to consume adequate amounts of loose hay or forage to satisfy the nutritional demands. Care must also be taken to provide adequate amounts of water and rest. A mineral supplement containing high levels of calcium and phosphorus (2:1) magnesium and vitamins A and D should be provided the last 6 weeks of gestation and early lactation. Lambs, rams and non-pregnant ewes that are subjected to long and stressful transportation should be supplied with good quality alfalfa hay, mineral supplementation to supply Ca, P, Mg and K and adequate water prior to and following transportation. Some lamb feedlots which encounter severe problems with transport tetany have greatly reduced the problem by providing a palatable buffered electrolyte in the water which contains Na, K, Ca, P, Mg, bicarbonate, sugars and flavoring. On arrival animals should be observed closely for the first 12 to 24 hours. These animals that appear listless and do not eat or drink should be separated, treated with 50 to 100 ml of 20% calcium gluconate intravenously, and placed in a small pen with access to loose alfalfa or grass hay away from competition of the healthy aggressive sheep.

Most sheep affected with HC promptly respond to intravenous or subcutaneous administration of 50 to 100 ml of 20% calcium gluconate. Some animals may require one or more additional treatments.

Asbury A.C.: Hypocalcemia in ewes. JAVMA, *141*:703-705, 1962.

Blumer, C.C., Madden, F.J., and Walker, D.J.: Hypocalcemia, grass tetany or grass staggers in sheep. Aust. Vet. J., *15*:24-27, 1939.

East, N.: Pregnancy toxemia, abortions, and periparturient diseases. Vet. Clin. N.A.: Large Animal Pract., *5*(3):601-618, 1983.

Franklin, M.C. and MacGregor, C.H.: Investigation of the cause of ram deaths after long journeys by rail. Aust. Vet. J., *20*:328-331, 1944.

Franklin, M.C., Reid, R.L., and Johnstone, I.L.: Dietary and other factors affecting serum-Ca levels in sheep. Aust. CSIRO Bull., 1948, p. 240.

Grieg, R.J.: Nature of lambing sickness. Vet. Rec., *9*:509, 1929.

Huber, T., et al.: Effect of hypocalcemia on motility of the ruminant stomach. Am. J. Vet. Res., *42*(9):1488-1490, 1981.

Hughes, L.E. and Kershaw, G.F.: Metabolic disorders associated with movement of sheep. Vet. Rec., *70*: 77-78, 1958.

Leslie, A.: Milk fever in New Zealand ewes. N.Z. Soc. Anim. Prod., *9*:153-155, 1949.

Lucas, M., Huffman, E., and Johnson, L.: Clinical and clinico-pathologic features of transport tetany of feedlot lambs. JAVMA, *181*(4):381-383, 1982.

Luthman, J., Persson, J., and Nilsson, G.: Effect of a high calcium metabolism and plasma gastrin levels in pregnant ewes. Zentralbl. Vet., 6:486-495, 1977.

McClymont, G.L.: Hypocalcemia and pregnancy toxemia of ewes. New South Wales Dept. Agric. Leaflet, 1947, p. 52.

Mosely, G. and Akford, R.F.E.: The effect of stress on the redistribution of calcium in sheep. J. Agric. Sci., 81:403-409, 1973.

Osguthorp, D.A.: Personal communications, 1973.

Pierson, R.E. and Jensen, R.: Hypocalcemia in feedlot lambs. Records Vet. Hosp., Colorado State University, 1972.

Sanson, B., Bunach, K., and Dew, S.: Changes in plasma calcium, magnesium, phosphorus and hydroxyproline concentrations in ewes from twelve weeks before until three weeks after lambing. Br. Vet. J., 138:393-401, 1982.

Schneider, K., Parkinson, J., Houston, J., and Leaver, D.: 1,25-dihydroxyvitamin D_3 increases plasma magnesium and calcium in sheep fed liquid diets low in calcium and magnesium. Aust. Vet. J., 62(3):82-84, 1985.

Shils, M.: Magnesium, calcium and parathyroid hormone interactions. Ann. New York Acad. Sci., 355:1622-1669, 1980.

Silva, J., Noakes, D.: The effect of experimentally induced hypocalcemia on uterine activity at parturition in the ewe. Thereo., 21(4):607-622, 1984.

Watt, J.A.A.: Sudden death in sheep. Vet. Rec., 72:998-1001, 1960.

Hypomagnesemia

(HM: grass tetany; grass staggers; wheat pasture poisoning)

Hypomagnesemia, an acute metabolic disease of pasture sheep and cattle, is characterized by excitative bearing and spastic tetany and is caused by a depressed supply of metabolizable magnesium from prolonged consumption of lush immature grasses. Because the disease has wide geographic distribution and causes extensive financial waste to grazing ewes, it has major importance and high concern for the entire sheep industry. As production emphasis shifts from range bands to pasture flocks, HM will acquire even more importance. Economic losses result from deaths, determent of full utilization of pasture feed, and the cost of preventive programs. Occurrence of the disease in greater proportions among cattle adds economic significance and scientific interest to the malady.

OCCURRENCE. HM occurs in all breeds of lactating ewes grazing early spring pastures. Although most cases develop in ewes during the first 4 weeks of lactation, other classes of sheep occasionally develop the disease. In the United States, western range bands, transferred from mountainous areas for fall and winter grazing on wheat pastures, also develop a high incidence of the disease. Most cases of HM occur during spring and autumn following rains and rapid growth of grasses, including young wheat plants and other cereal crops. Cases usually develop within 1 to 3 weeks after beginning the grazing.

Geographically, the disease probably occurs in all sheep-producing countries where grass and wheat grazing is an important part of sheep economy. The incidence is high in Australia, Britain, the Netherlands, Scandinavia, Canada, and America. In the United States, the majority of cases occur in the wheat belt of the high plains.

ETIOLOGY AND PATHOGENESIS. In normal sheep the plasma levels of magnesium and calcium are 2 to 3 mg/dl and 8 to 12 mg/dl, respectively. Magnesium and calcium homeostasis is controlled by a complex mechanism under the influence of the parathyroid and involving the synthesis of active vitamin D $(1,25(OH)_2D_3)$ in the kidney. Various factors that may contribute to a decrease in serum magnesium concentrations are norepinephrine, corticotropic hormone, increased mineral corticoid concentrations, increased glucagon concentration, increased dietary potassium intake, decreased carbohydrate intake, and excessive water intake. Exposure to cold along with inadequate energy intake synergistically reduces plasma magnesium levels. Cold stress alone has little effect on magnesium levels. The plasma magnesium levels normally increase during the last 3 weeks of pregnancy, but decrease abruptly at lambing and continue to decline for 2 to 3 weeks. Ewes with twins have lower magnesium levels for 2 to 3 weeks after lambing than ewes with singles.

The pathogenesis of HM begins with lush grasses, including young wheat plants, that rapidly grow after spring and autumn rains. These plants, especially those growing on ammonium-fertilized soil, contain high concentrations of protein, potassium, and aconitate.

Absorption of ammonia by plants results in reduced uptake of magnesium and calcium, with little effect on potassium, and produces high amide concentrations in plants with carbohydrate depletion. These factors combine in the animal to create high concentrations of free ammonia in the rumen, an increase in rumen pH, and depletion of carbohydrate and further reduces the availability of magnesium and calcium. The adult ewe has a reserve of magnesium in bone that can be mobilized into the extracellular fluid. Mobilization commences when the serum magnesium level falls below 1.8 mg/dl. When this reservoir is exhausted, the plasma level of magnesium falls; when the concentration reaches about 1.0 mg/dl, the plasma calcium level also declines. When it reaches 0.7 mg/dl, irritability develops, and when it reaches 0.5 mg/dl, fatal tetany and convulsions ensue. Death probably results from respiratory failure. Recovered animals are susceptible to recurrence of the disease.

CLINICAL SIGNS AND POSTMORTEM LESIONS. Clinical signs are of central origin and relate to reduction in magnesium of the cerebrospinal fluid. At the beginning of HM outbreaks, several ewes may develop characteristic signs. Affected animals are overly excited by ordinary stimuli, such as rapid driving, dog barking, physical restraint, lamb nursing, and loud noise. Breathing accelerates, tremors begin, and walking and running movements, because of muscular incoordination, become difficult. As the condition progresses and as strong stimuli continue, some ewes fall to a recumbent position, convulse, pass into coma, and finally die. Before the violent muscular actions, the body temperature is normal, but during convulsions it may rise to 43°C.

For mammals in general, the following proportionality expression applies:

$$\text{irritability} \propto \frac{[Na^+] + [K^+]}{[Ca^{++}] + [Mg^{++}] + [H^+]}$$

This formula means that irritability in sheep is directly proportional to the sum of the concentrations of the sodium and potassium ions and inversely proportional to the sum of the calcium, magnesium, and hydrogen ions.

The morbidity commonly reaches 20%, and the mortality of affected sheep, 80%. The course usually ranges from 2 to 24 hours.

At necropsy, petechial and ecchymotic hemorrhages commonly exist over serosal surfaces of the heart and intestines, but specific lesions are absent.

DIAGNOSIS. Veterinarians diagnose HM from evidence of clinical signs and laboratory findings. The history of excitement and convulsions among lactating ewes grazing lush grasses strongly suggests the disease. Plasma magnesium levels of 0.50 to 0.25 mg/dl in blood collected from live but affected animals confirm the diagnosis.

The differential diagnosis requires consideration of hypocalcemia and enterotoxemia. HM and hypocalcemia of lactating ewes are clinically similar diseases. Hypocalcemia favorably responds to intravenously administered calcium gluconate, and blood analysis shows plasma calcium levels as low as 3 mg/dl and magnesium levels near normal values. Enterotoxemia causes sudden deaths, and affected animals contain identifiable toxin in the small intestine.

PREVENTION AND TREATMENT. Prevention of HM is based upon supplying supplemental magnesium during the period when lush green forages are deficient in the compound and the parturient and nursing ewe normally has low plasma magnesium levels. Supplemental magnesium may be provided through a mineral mix containing:

400 kg calcium carbonate
150 kg magnesium oxide
 50 kg dehydrated molasses
200 kg trace mineral salt
200 kg ground corn or other concentrate

A 65 kg lactating ewe requires from 48 to 96 mg magnesium daily. The daily requirement is provided by consuming 7 to 14 g (¼ to ½ oz) of the above mineral mixture. The intake can be adjusted by altering the amount of molasses or concentrate. To assure adequate intake the mineral supplementation should be started a couple of weeks prior to moving onto lush pastures. Providing a small amount of alfalfa hay or other dry forage will also aid in preventing HM.

Successful treatment of hypomagnesemia depends on early diagnosis of the condition and prompt intravenous administration of one of the injectable products for HM which contains calcium borogluconate, dextrose, and magnesium borogluconate. Vitamin D_3 aids in magnesium absorption and mobilization. Supportive therapy provided by oral drenching with one of the electrolyte solutions such as Life-Guard (Norden) is also beneficial. The animals should be separated from others to reduce the competition for food and water.

Australian physiologists have developed a capsule formed from two hollow boat-shaped half-cylinders of magnesium and magnesium alloy. Inside the capsule is a steel wool cathode electrically connected to a magnesium anode. Magnesium ions are released by electrolysis in the acid rumen contents and are available to the animal.

Barrentine, B.F.: Grass tetany in ewes grazing winter oats. J. Anim. Sci., 7:535, 1948.

Barrentine, B.F. and Morrison, E.G.: Grass tetany in sheep grazing winter forages. Proc. Assoc. South. Agric. Workers, 50th, 1953, p. 64.

Bohman, V.R., Lesperance, A.L., Harding, G.D., and Grunes, D.L.: Induction of experimental tetany in cattle. J. Anim. Sci., 29:99-102, 1969.

Burau, R. and Stout, P.R.: Trans-aconitic acid in range grasses in early spring. Science, 15:766, 1965.

Care, A.D. and Ross, D.B.: Gastrointestinal absorption of Mg in sheep. Proc. Nutr. Soc., 21: No. 1, X, 1962.

Commonwealth Scientific and Industrial Research, CSIRO. 26th Annual Report. East Melbourne, 3072 Australia, 1973-1974.

Fontenot, J.P., Miller, R.W., Whitehair, C.K., and Mac-Vicar, R.: Effect of high-protein high-potassium ration in lambs. J. Anim. Sci., 19:127-133, 1960.

Gardner, J.A.A.: Control of serum magnesium levels in sheep. Res. Vet. Sci., 15:149-157, 1973.

Hemingway, R.G. and Ritchie, N.S.: Importance of hypocalcemia in developing hypomagnesemia tetany. Proc. Nutr. Soc., 24:54-63, 1965.

Herd, R.P.: Supplementary magnesium for preventing grass tetany in sheep. Aust. Vet. J., 42:369-373, 1966.

Herd, R.P.: Hypomagnesemia and grass tetany in sheep. Aust. Vet. J., 38:455-456, 1962.

Hoflund, S.: Deficiency diseases of sheep. North Am. Vet., 23:27-31, 1942.

Inglis, J.S.S., Weipers, M., and Pearce, P.J.: Hypomagnesemia in sheep. Vet. Rec., 71:755-763 1959.

Kemp, A., Deijs, W.B., and Hemkes, O.J.: Intake and utilization of Mg from herbage by cows. Neth. J. Agric. Res., 9:134-158, 1961.

Kiesel, G.K., Alexander, H.D., and Brooks, G.: Serum enzyme and electrolyte values of lambs fed Mg-deficient ration. AJVR, 30:381-391, 1969.

L'Estrange, J.L. and Axford, R.F.E. Study of serum mineral in grazing lactating ewes. J. Agric. Sci., 62:341-351, 1964.

Lucas, M., Huffman, E., and Johnson, L.: Clinical and clinico-pathologic features of transport tetany of feedlot lambs. JAVMA, 181(4):381-383, 1982.

Meyer, H.: Pathogenesis of the clinical symptoms of hypomagnesemia in ruminants. Vet. Sci. Commun., 1:1, 1977.

Meyer, H. and Scholz, H.: Pathogenesis of hypomagnesemic tetany. I. Relationships between the magnesium contents of blood and cerebrospinal fluid. DTW, 78:55-61, 1972.

Rook, J.A.F.: Spontaneous and induced Mg deficiency in ruminants. Ann. N.Y. Acad. Sci., 162:727, Art. 2, 1969.

Rook, J.A.F. and Balch, C.C.: Mg metabolism during spring grazing. J. Agric. Sci., 51:199-207, 1958.

Sanson, B., Bunach, K., and Dew, S.: Changes in plasma calcium, magnesium, phosphorous and hydroxyproline concentrations in ewes from twelve weeks before until three weeks after lambing. Br. Vet. J., 138:393-401, 1982.

Schneider, K., Parkinson, G., Houston, J., and Leaver, D.: 1,25 dihydroxy vitamin D_3 increases plasma magnesium and calcium in sheep fed liquid diets low in calcium and magnesium. Aust. Vet. J., 62(3):82-84, 1985.

Schuster, N.H., Watts, H.J., Webster, M.E., and Campbell, R.W.: Grass tetany in ewes. Aust. Vet. J., 45:508-516, 1969.

Sjollema, B.: Nature and therapy of grass tetany. Vet. Rec., 10:425-450, 1930.

Suttle, N.F. and Field, A.C.: Effect of K and Mg intakes on development of hypomagnesemia in sheep. Br. J. Nutr., 23:81-90, 1969.

Terashima, Y., et al.: Plasma magnesium levels as influenced by cold exposure in fed or fasted sheep. J. Nutr., 112:1914-1920, 1982.

Contagious Agalactia

Contagious agalactia, an acute or chronic disease of sheep and goats is characterized by early septicemia followed by localized infection in the udder, eyes, and joints and is caused by *Mycoplasma agalactiae*. In endemic areas of Europe, the Balkans, Africa, and Asia this prevalent and recurring disease has major economic importance to the sheep industry. Even though not fully measured, the waste to individual enterprises as well as to the sheep industry is high. Economic losses result from deaths, reduced physical condition, lowered milk production, abortions, and expensive preventive programs and treatment procedures.

OCCURRENCE. All breeds and sexes of sheep are susceptible to contagious agalactia. Pregnant ewes, especially during the last trimester of gestation are more susceptible than other groups. Although lambs can contract the disease, they are more resistant than adult sheep. Goats of all breeds, sexes, and ages are more susceptible than corresponding groups in sheep. In an endemic area, both sheep and goats usually develop the disease.

The US Public Health Service and the US Department of Agriculture (USDA) Administrative Policy classify *Mycoplasma agalactiae* as an exotic class 5 agent: "Forcing animal pathogens that are excluded from the United States by law or whose entry is restricted by USDA administrative policy." *Mycoplasma agalactiae* has been reported in the US from goats on two occasions but it has not been reported in sheep.

Although contagious agalactia may occur in isolated cases throughout the year, the highest incidence is during November, December, and January, and again during May and June.

Geographically, the disease exists in Spain, Portugal, France, Italy, Switzerland, Rumania, Yugoslavia, Albania, southern USSR, Greece, Morocco, Algeria, Libya, Turkey, Syria, Lebanon, Israel, Iran, West Pakistan, India, and Mongolia.

ETIOLOGY AND PATHOGENESIS. *Mycoplasma agalactiae*, the specific cause of contagious agalactia, is pleomorphic and consists of globules, granules, rings, and filaments. The dimensions range from 125 to 150 μm $\times$ 0.2 to 0.8 μm. Lacking a cell wall, the organism is gram-negative in staining affinity and is advantageously differentiated with Giemsa stain and dark-field illumination.

The organism of contagious agalactia grows on many types of laboratory media enriched with 10 to 20% serum. It also grows in milk and produces acid from lactose, mannitol, and erythritol, but not from glucose, fructose, galactose, raffinose, arabinose, xylose, sucrose, and maltose. On blood agar, the organism hemolyzes erythrocytes and forms a characteristic brown discoloration. The flat, circular, and translucent colonies measure up to 1 mm in diameter, and the center grows into the medium.

The antigenic structure appears to be homogeneous, and cross-agglutination between this and other related species does not occur.

The pathogenesis of contagious agalactia has been scientifically studied only in some aspects and, consequently, many parts are still conjectural. The causative agent enters a new susceptible sheep through the alimentary tract as a contaminant of feed and water or through the conjunctivae from accidental instillation of contaminated droplets or dust particles of soil and manure.

At some point along the alimentary tract, possibly in the small intestine, the organism penetrates the mucous membrane, where it grows and multiplies. After approximately 24 hours from the time of inoculation, the organism invades the blood and maintains septicemia for 12 hours. The blood transports the organism to all organs, and by the fifth day, organisms locate in the liver, spleen, pancreas, and brain and establish foci of infection in the udder, eyes, joints, and gravid uterus. In the udder, the organisms cause interstitial mastitis, which results in gradual destruction of glandular epithelium, in replacement with fibrous connective tissue, and, finally, in chemical changes in the milk and loss of milk production.

Pathologic changes in one or both eyes begin with congestion and swelling of the conjunctiva and the cornea. Later, punctiform keratitis forms, with each opaque focus measuring up to 1 mm in diameter. Eventually, purulent keratitis and iridocyclitis develop, and these pathologic changes obstruct the canal of Schlemm at the filtration angle, increase the pressure of the aqueous humor, and cause rupture of the weakened cornea, with extrusion of aqueous humor and iris.

Changes in infected joints occur both in the cavity and in connective tissue around the joint capsule. In the joint cavity, the synovium may be increased and clouded and may contain flakes of fibrin. After a prolonged course, articular surfaces may erode and ankylose. Some joint capsules rupture and discharge infected exudate to the surface. The periarticular connective tissue becomes edematous and swollen, and these changes cause joint enlargement and lameness. Uteruses, especially those in the third trimester of gestation, often develop placentitis and abort the infected lambs. Recovered animals are immune to subsequent attacks.

Viable forms of *M. agalactiae* discharge from infected sheep and goats into the external environment as contaminants in milk, ocular secretions, nasal secretions, feces, urine, exudate from open joints, and vaginal discharges following abortion. The organisms spread to other animals by direct contact and move to new locations by contaminating mobile vehicles.

CLINICAL SIGNS AND POSTMORTEM LESIONS. Following an incubation period of 5 to 7 days from subcutaneous inoculation and up to 60 days from natural exposure, body temperature rises to a range from 41 to 42°C. The period of fever corresponds to the time of septicemia. During early stages, infected animals become depressed and anorectic, and some may die. As it progresses, the disease usually develops signs of keratitis and arthritis and, in female sheep, mastitis and abortion.

The acidity of the milk from infected udders changes from a normal pH 6.8 to pH 7.8, becomes yellow in color and, on standing, separates into a light green supernatant layer and a grumous sediment. Gradually, the udder atrophies and the milk yield diminishes. Joints, especially carpal and tarsal, become swollen, painful, and lame. In some animals, a joint may rupture and discharge exudate.

One or both eyes may become infected, leading to impaired vision and blindness. Depending on the stage of disease development, the infected eye may show congestion and swelling, punctiform keratitis with each opaque focus measuring up to 1 mm in diameter, keratitis with yellow opacity of the cornea, or rupture of the cornea (Fig. 2-1).

Ewes in the third trimester of gestation may abort either dead or living infected lambs and later develop vaginal discharges. Some outbreaks show a preponderance of either udder,

eye, or joint involvement. Israeli veterinarians assert that the disease in their country rarely causes abortion.

At necropsy, animals that have died during early acute stages often present generalized peritonitis. In sacrificed sheep, the pathologic changes vary with the stage of lesion development. The infected udder is grossly atrophic in either one or both halves of the organ. Microscopically, the chronic inflammatory reaction in the stroma shows increased fibrosis and a reduced number of glandular acini.

Infected joint capsules are edematous, and the synovium may contain clumps of fibrin. Articular surfaces may be eroded and occasionally ankylosed. In early stages of keratitis, the cornea is edematous and infiltrated with leukocytes. In advanced stages, abundant purulent exudate infiltrates both cornea and the ciliary body. If corneal rupture has occurred, anterior synechia may have formed.

DIAGNOSIS. Veterinarians diagnose contagious agalactia on the basis of characteristic signs and lesions and with assistance from laboratory findings. In endemic areas, fever with eye, joint, and udder lesions strongly suggests the disease. Laboratory confirmation can be obtained by isolating *M. agalactiae* from the blood, milk, or tears. *Mycoplasma agalactiae* can be identified by direct immunofluorescent

Fig. 2-1. Infected eye from ewe with contagious agalactia. × 1.2.

procedure using fluorescein conjugate prepared against *M. agalactiae*. Its status in the US as a class 5 agent prohibits all but federal agencies to study this mycoplasm or to prepare diagnostic reagents which makes diagnosis and identification difficult.

The differential diagnosis requires consideration of chlamydial polyarthritis and other abortifacient diseases, such as vibriosis, salmonellosis, and enzootic abortion.

PREVENTION AND TREATMENT. Veterinarians and sheep producers employ the most appropriate preventive method for the circumstance. Disease outbreaks in regions where contagious agalactia has not previously existed should be eradicated by identifying and slaughtering all infected and exposed sheep and goats, by cleaning, disinfecting, and resting infected premises, and by quarantining the infected area until no additional cases develop in test sheep or goats placed in the quarantined premises.

In endemic areas, attendants should maintain cleanliness. Infected sheep and goats should be isolated from healthy animals, owners should avoid adding new sheep of questionable health status, communal pastures should be avoided, and all contaminated manure, bedding, feed, dead animals, and placentas should be burned or buried. Susceptible sheep should be immunized against the disease either with killed vaccine or with live vaccine containing attenuated *M. agalactiae*. If possible, vaccine should be administered before breeding and repeated annually.

None of the currently available drugs gives fully satisfactory results in treating contagious agalactia. The tetracyclines, however, give some benefits and, until clinical improvement occurs, should be administered daily at the rate of 11 mg per kg of body weight. Tylosin and erythromycin have been effective in goats.

Animal Health Yearbook. FAO-WHO-OIE (Italy), 1970.

Arisoy, F., Erdag, O., Cottew, G.S., and Watson, W.A.: Investigations into agalactia of sheep and goats in Turkey. Turk. Vet. Hekim. Dern. Derg., 37:11-17, 1967.

Bory, G. and Entessar, F.: Etude sur l'agalaxie contagieuse des chèvres et des moutons en Iran. Bull. Off. Int. Epizoot., 57:399-420, 1962.

Bridre, J. and Donatien, A.: Le microbe de l'agalaxie contagieuse du mouton et de la chèvre. Ann. Inst. Pasteur, 39:925-951, 1925.

Cottew, G.S., et al.: Differentiation of *Mycoplasma agalactiae* from other Mycoplasmas of sheep and goats. J. Comp. Pathol., 78:275-282, 1968.

Curasson, G.: Maladieuse des animaux domestique. Tome I et II. Paris, Vigot Frères, 1946.

DaMassa, A.: Recovery of *Mycoplasma agalactiae* from mastitic goat milk. JAVMA, 183(5):548-549, 1983.

Foggie, A., Ethridge, J.R., Erdag, O., and Arisoy, F.: Contagious agalactia of sheep and goats. Studies on live and dead vaccines in lactating sheep. J. Comp. Pathol., 81:165-172, 1971a.

Foggie, A., Ethridge, J.R., Erdag, O., and Arisoy, F.: Contagious agalactia in sheep and goats. Immunity of lactating ewes vaccinated before mating with live or dead vaccines. J. Comp. Pathol., 81:393-400, 1971b.

Foggie, A., Ethridge, J.R., Erdag, O., and Arisoy, F.: Contagious agalactia of sheep and goats. The serial passage in goats of an attenuated strain of *Mycoplasma agalactiae* A1K40. Res. Vet. Sci., 11:477-479, 1970a.

Foggie, A., Ethridge, J.R., Erdag, O., and Arisoy, F.: Contagious agalactia of sheep and goats. Preliminary studies on vaccines. J. Comp. Pathol., 80:345-358, 1970b.

Kuliev, A.V.: Transmission of contagious agalactia in sheep and goats. Dokl. Vsesoyus Akad. Selskokhoz. Nauk., 15:42-46, 1953.

Perran, P.: Contagious agalactia syndrome in goats due to *Mycoplasma mycoides Subsp. Capri.* New observations. Bull. Acad. Vet. France, 47:179-188, 1974.

Popovici, I. and DeSimon, M.: Vaccination against contagious agalactia of sheep and goats in Romania. Arch. Vet., 1:21-28, 1966.

Watson, W.A., Cottew, G.S., Erdag, O., and Arisoy, F.: The pathogenicity of Mycoplasma organisms isolated from sheep and goats in Turkey. J. Comp. Pathol., 78:283-291, 1968.

Zavagli, V.: Contagious agalactia of sheep and goats. Bull. Off. Int. Epizoot., 36:336-362, 1951.

Zavagli, V.: Contagious agalactia in sheep and goats. Experimental research. Zooprofilassi, 1: No. 1, 3-6; Nos. 2-3, 12-26, 1946.

Mastitis

(*Bluebag; garget*)

Mastitis, an infectious, noncontagious disease of lactating ewes, effects the mammary gland with a wide range of insults and subsequent tissue damage, a resultant decrease or cessation of milk production, and in some cases death of the animal. A broad clinical classification of mastitis may be: (1) acute clinical mastitis, (2) subclinical mastitis, (3) chronic indurative mastitis. Mastitis is a universal problem wherever sheep are produced. The causal agent will vary due to the influence of climate, environment, and management. *Staphylococcus aureus* and *Pasteurella hemolytica* are most prevalent. The economic significance has not been well documented. Clinical cases pose obvious economic loss from the cost of labor and therapy, incapacitation of the mammary gland, starvation of lambs and death of ewes. Recovered clinical cases, subclinical cases, and chronic indurative cases are of far greater economic significance due to premature culling of ewes with udder abnormalities, lamb death from starvation, and reduced milk production with an ultimate decrease in live lamb production.

OCCURRENCE. Mastitis occurs in all breeds of farm and range ewes. The incidence increases with age of the ewe and the number of lactations. The disease develops during the period between parturition and weaning.

Geographically, mastitis probably occurs in all sheep-producing countries, but especially among ewes of New Zealand, Australia, United States, Britain, Norway, France, Germany, Italy, Yugoslavia, and Bulgaria.

ETIOLOGY AND PATHOGENESIS. A variety of organisms may be isolated from the infected udder with *Staphylococcus aureus* and *Pasteurella hemolyticum* being the predominant organisms in severe acute clinical mastitis. *Staphylococcus aureus* is most frequently associated with gangrenous mastitis, although in severe clinical cases it is impossible to differentiate clinically between *Staph. aureus* and *P. hemolyticum*. Bacteria of secondary importance include other coagulase negative staphylococcus spp., *Corynebacterium pyogenes, Streptococcus* spp., *Pasteurella multocida, Escherichia coli, Pseudomonas aeruginosa, Bacillus* spp., *Proteus* spp., micrococcus, recently *Histophilus ovis*, and *Actinobacillus seminis. Staph. aureus*, a nonmotile, noncapsulating, nonsporing, gram-positive, spherical, aerobic bacterium, measures 0.8 × 1.0 μm, and forms single, paired, chained, and clustered groupings. It grows on most standard laboratory media, and on solid media it forms round, smooth, glistening, yellow or gray colonies.

Although *Staphylococcus aureus* is the most frequently isolated causative organism, *P. hemolyticum* is reported to be the predominant organism in range ewes. Bacillus spp, usually considered a contaminate, has been reported as the causal agent in clinical and subclinical mastitis in ewes at weaning time under grazing conditions. Environment, management systems (intensive, extensive or a modification of both) and the period of production (periparturient, early lactation or weaning) play a profound role on the bacterial challenge and the severity of the condition. Table 2-1 illustrates the significance of the two major organisms *Staph. aureus* and *P. hemolytica*. It is interesting to note that Tunnicliffs work was with ewes under extensive manage-

TABLE 2-1. *Bacterial Causes of Mastitis*

No. of Cases	Pathogens Isolated			References
	Staph. Aureus	*P. Haemolytica*	Other Species	
36	24	4	8	Leyshon, 1929
17	16	1	—	Hauke, 1960
270	252	1	17	Saeter and Eieland, 1961
238	171	28	39	Tsonev and Mateev, 1961
369	231	—	138	Katitch et al., 1967
27	3	23	1	Miessner and Schoop, 1932
117	3	113	1	Tunnicliff, 1949
23	14	4	5	Madel, 1983
50	8	4	38	Baswell and Watson, 1983
126	33	—	93	Gibson and Hendy, 1976

ment systems. Recent reportings in the US and Europe describe a chronic indurative mastitis associated with the ovine progressive pneumonia virus (OPPV) or the maedi/visna virus.

As an environmental bacterium, *Staph. aureus* resides on animal skins and mucosal membranes. Besides gangrenous mastitis, it associates with many other diseases, such as abscesses, dermatitis, arthritis, and pyemia. The organism, resistant to inimical environments, is killed in 30 minutes by temperatures of 60 to 80°C, in 35 minutes by 1% phenol, in 60 minutes by 0.5% mercuric chloride, and in 10 minutes by 10% formalin. It is sensitive to the action of penicillin, tetracycline, and chloramphenicol.

P. haemolytica, an aerobic, nonmotile, nonsporing, encapsulated, gram-negative, bi-polar, pleomorphic rod, measures 0.2 to 0.4 × 0.6 to 2.6 μm. On serum agar it forms round, moist, smooth colonies and ferments dextrose, levulose, mannitol, sorbitol, sucrose, and xylose. This delicate bacterium is destroyed in 10 minutes at 60°C and in 15 minutes by 0.5% phenol, but endures for several weeks in moist soil and dead tissues. It commonly inhabits the upper respiratory tract of normal sheep and the lungs of pneumonic sheep.

The transmission of mastitis among ewes probably occurs by mechanical means. Indiscriminate nursing by some lambs enables the lips and mouths, especially those with contagious ecthyma lesions, to transfer pathogens from the teats of carrier ewes to the teats of susceptible ewes. In addition, insects, such as houseflies with sponging mouth parts, may successively feed first on infected and then on susceptible teats and, in the process, transmit pathogenic bacteria.

Acute clinical mastitis begins with entrance of either *Staph. aureus* or *P. haemolytica* into the teat canal. Skin lesions, such as vesicles and pustules from contagious ecthyma on the teats of the ewe or on the mouth of the lamb, enable the pathogens to grow on the teat surface and to penetrate the teat orifice. Either of the pathogens, following entrance into the lactiferous sinus, rapidly spreads throughout the gland. Acute inflammation develops, and milk secretion ceases.

In staphylococcal mastitis, bacterial toxins form and vessels thrombose; the resulting intoxication and ischemia cause gangrene of the affected gland. After 2 to 3 days the dead tissue sloughs. In most surviving cases of pasteurellal mastitis, the infection finally localizes and forms an abscess, which may rupture and discharge infective exudate onto the surface. In either form of mastitis, death results from toxemia and shock. In surviving ewes, the diseased gland is permanently incapacitated.

CLINICAL SIGNS AND POSTMORTEM LESIONS OF SEVERE ACUTE CLINICAL MASTITIS.   Following an incubation period of 1 or 2 days, body temperature rises to 41 to 42°C. The affected sheep separates from the flock, declines feed, becomes gaunt, and forbids nursing but, because of pain, remains standing and walks with reluctance and lameness.

Most infection is unilateral. In staphylococcal mastitis, the gland and preglandular abdomen becomes edematous. After 2 to 3 days of reaction, the skin, especially around the teat, becomes black, cold, and doughy. Fragments of the darkened and malodorous gland slough and temporarily hang from the animal by attached skin. In pasteurellal mastitis, the affected gland, acutely swollen, painful and firm, is red in early stages but may become cyanotic in late stages (Fig. 2-2). The milk rapidly diminishes in volume and becomes serous and flocculent. Surviving ewes often develop udder abscesses, which may rupture onto the surface and finally fibrose and heal. The loss of wool frequently follows acute mastitis.

The morbidity rate commonly reaches 5% but may go higher, and the mortality for staphylococcal and pasteurellal mastitis, except for treated ewes, is near 80 and 50%, respectively. The course in fatal cases ranges from 1 to 4 days.

At necropsy, gross lesions are limited to the affected udder. Fly strike and screwworm infestation may be superimposed on gangrenous mastitis.

Fig. 2-2. Left half of udder enlarged from pasteurellal mastitis. × 0.2.

SUBCLINICAL MASTITIS

Culling rate in flocks average about 20% per annum with udder abnormalities being the predominant cause of loss. The shortened productive life of the ewe along with a decrease in milk production leads to starvation or decreased lamb weights contributing to the economic wastage in the industry. The mode of entry, virulence of the causal agent (usually *Bacillus* spp., coagulase negative staphylococci and other secondary organisms), and pathogenesis is not clearly understood. The end result is damaged glandular tissue which becomes fibrosed or abscessed with a resultant decrease in milk production.

CHRONIC INDURATIVE MASTITIS

Chronic indurative mastitis is characterized by a high morbidity and low mortality in affected flocks often with subclinical character, a chronic course, and a decrease in milk production. Affected flocks may have an annual culling rate from 5 to 20%. Clinically the udder appears full, the halves are uniform palpably firm with subnormal to minimal milk flow. The

milk presented appears normal and free from bacteria or mycoplasmas. The causal agent is a retrovirus identical to ovine progressive pneumonia virus (OPPV) or the virus of maedi/visna. There is a marked lymphoid hyperplasia and periductal lymphoid proliferation with follicle formation. Lymphoid follicles are found in the alveolar parenchyma along with atrophy or disappearance of alveolar tissue. These lymphocytic accumulations possibly contribute to inhibiting milk flow through the duct system. Infiltration of the interstitium with mononuclear cells cause slight to moderate fibrosis of the parenchyma producing the uniform firmness of the gland. Ovine progressive pneumonia is characterized by similar lymphocytic proliferation.

DIAGNOSIS OF ACUTE CLINICAL MASTITIS. Veterinarians diagnose both staphylococcal and pasteurellal mastitis from evidence of signs, lesions, and laboratory findings. Fever, depression, and unilateral swelling of the udder are indicative signs. Udder changes such as black discoloration, environmental temperature, and sloughing characterize gangrenous mastitis. The isolation of *Staph. aureus* or *P. haemolytica* from the udder's secretion or from diseased udder tissues confirms the diagnosis.

Subclinical Mastitis

As there are no apparent systemic clinical signs the condition is diagnosed by somatic cell counts or diligent palpation of the mammary gland. Somatic cell counts in normal secretions average about 340,000 cells/ml and 4.0×10^6 cells/ml in mastitis. Increasing age and later stages of lactation will increase the somatic cell count of normal milk. Routine palpation of the udder following weaning, prior to breeding and prior to lambing is a useful screening procedure to detect subclinical mastitis.

Chronic Indurative Mastitis

Chronic indurative mastitis is diagnosed by a history of insufficient lamb growth while nursing a ewe with udders which appear full of milk. On examination little or no milk can be expressed. The milk expressed is usually normal in consistency. Palpation reveals a diffusely undurated udder with both halves equally affected. Positive serology or viral isolation confirm the diagnosis of chronic indurative mastitis caused by OPPV or maedi/visna.

PREVENTION AND TREATMENT OF ACUTE CLINICAL MASTITIS. Clean surroundings, good husbandry practices and prevention of sore mouth aid in preventing acute clinical mastitis. Some producers file the sharp edges from the central incisors to prevent injury to the teats thus reducing the risk from bacterial build up in sores.

Local immunization of the mammary gland with antigens produced from killed *Brucella abortus* or *Staphylococcus aureus* enhance the neutrophil response to staphylococcal infection. Local immunization of the mammary gland holds promise but needs further development. Early treatment of staphylococcal mastitis with penicillin at the rate of 5000 units/kg of body weight given at daily or more frequent intervals, and of pasteurellal mastitis with streptomycin at the rate of 2 g the first day, followed by half that dose on each of 2 subsequent days, gives satisfactory results. Sulfamethazine, orally administered at the daily rate of 5 to 10 g per animal, is also effective. Treatment may be with both antibiotic and sulfonamide compounds. In the case of a valuable ewe, administer oxytocin every 2 hours, milk out the secretion and infuse with penicillin or other intramammary infusions. Although gentomycin is efficacious in treating mastitis it is not approved for use in sheep and goats.

Subclinical mastitis is effectively and economically treated following weaning by the infusion of 1 tube of a dry cow treatment per ewe. These usually contain penicillin and streptomycin or cloxacillin. Sanitary procedures of cleaning and disinfecting the teat orifice must be practiced.

Maintaining an OPPV free flock is the only preventive measure for chronic indurative mastitis.

Al-Samarrae, S., Sharman, V., and Yousif, A.: Mastitis in sheep in Iraq. Vet. Rec., *116*:323, 1985.

Alsenosy, A. and Dennis, S.: Pathology of acute experimental Actinobacillus seminis mastitis in ewes. Aust. Vet. J., *62*:234-237, 1987.

Anderson, B., Bulgin, M., Adams, S., and Duelke, B.: Firm udder in periparturient ewes with lymphocytic accumulations, retrovirus infection, and milk unavailable at the teat. JAVMA, *186*:391-393, 1985.

Beauregard, M. and Higgins, R.: Ovine mastitis due to *Histophilus ovis*. Can. Vet. J., *24*:284-286, 1983.

Colditz I. and Watson, D.: Humoral and cellular factors affecting the neutrophil response of the locally immunized mammary gland to staphylococcus infection. Vet. Imm. Immunopath., *8*:107-118, 1985.

Gross, J.J., Pollak, E.J., Anderson, J.G., and Torrell, D.T.: Incidence and importance of subclinical mastitis in sheep. J. Anim. Sci., *46*:1-8, 1978.

Hauke, H.: Epidemiology and microbiology of infectious mastitis in sheep. Mh. Vet. Med., *15*:688-694, 1960.

Hendy, P. and Pugh, K.: Prevention of post weaning mastitis in ewes. Vet. Rec., *109*:56-57, 1981.

Jensen, R.: Gangrenous mastitis in range ewes. Unpublished records. Colorado State University, 1928-1937.

Korukov, G.: Carriage of staphylococci by ewes. Vet. Med. Nauki (Sofia), *4*:61-67, 1967.

LeGall, A. and Plommet, M.: Experimental staphylococcal mastitis in ewes. Ann. Biol. Anim. Biochim. Biophys., *5*:113-130, 1965.

Leysohn, W.J.: An examination of cases of ovine mastitis. Vet. J., *85*:286-300, 1929.

Madel, A.: *Mastitis: Diseases of Sheep*. Edited by W.B. Martin. London, Blackwell Scientific Publications, 1983, pp. 153-158.

Marsh, H.: Ovine mastitis from pasteurella. JAVMA, *81*:376-382, 1932.

Miessner, H. and Schoop, G.: Contagious ovine mastitis. DTW, *40*:69-75, 1932.

Nocard, E. Gangrenous mastitis in sheep. Ann. Inst. Pasteur, *1*:416, 1887.

Quinlevan, T.D.: Bacteriology of ovine mastitis in New Zealand. N.Z. Vet. J., *16*:153-160, 1968.

Saeter, E.A. and Eieland, E.: Ovine mastitis in Norway. Nord. Vet. Med., *13*:32-44, 1961.

Seddon, H.R.: Diseases of domestic animals in Australia. Part 5, Vol. II. Commonwealth of Aust., Dept. Health, 1965, pp. 14-15.

Shoop, D. and Myers L.: Serological analysis of isolates of *Pasteurella haemolytica* and *Staphylococcus aureus* from mastitic ewes. Am. J. Vet. Rec., *45*:1944-1946, 1984.

Tsonev, T. and Mateev, M.: Causes of ovine infectious mastitis. Izv. Vet. Inst. Zaraz. Parazit. Bolesti (Sofia), *2*:199-202; 203-219, 1961.

Tunnicliff, E.A.: Pasteurella mastitis in ewes. Vet. Med., *44*:498-506, 1949.

Vander Molen E., Vecht, U. and Houwers, D.: A chronic indurative mastitis in sheep, associated with maedi/visna virus infection. Vet. Quart., *7*:112-119, 1985.

Webb R.: Clinical findings and pathological changes in *Histophilus ovis* infection of sheep. Res. Vet. Sci., *35*:30-34, 1983.

3

DISEASES CAUSING ABORTIONS

Rift Valley Fever

(RVF; enzootic hepatitis)

Rift valley fever, an infectious zoonosis of sheep, with undetermined contagiousness, is characterized by short incubation period, fever, hepatitis, high morbidity and mortality in lambs under 1 week of age and high abortion rates and is caused by a virus. Even though it is limited to the African continent, this devastating disease, through recurring epizootics, causes enormous waste of livestock, seriously affects regional sheep industry and poses a threat to sheep populations throughout the world. Economic losses result from abortions, deaths of both lambs and ewes, protein deficiencies among sheep-dependent people, and cost of preventative programs.

Besides sheep, the disease attacks cattle, goats, and people. Although seldom fatal, human RVF causes temporary incapacitation, physical misery, and reduced income and thus adds to the total losses. Veterinary and public health officials of the Union of South Africa alleged that the outbreak in that country during 1951 infected 20,000 people and killed 100,000 sheep and cattle.

During the 1977 Egyptian epizootic there were 18,000 human cases with 598 deaths. A 1978 serosurvey, extrapolated to the official population figures, estimated over a million infections of man.

OCCURRENCE. European breeds of sheep and cattle are highly susceptible. Ruminants indigenous to Africa are also susceptible to some degree but little is known of their clinical response. Seroepidemiologic surveys indicate that sheep, cattle, goats, camels, donkeys, and man may be involved. Viral isolations and measurable antibody titers have not been associated with a clinical response in camels, although abortion has been linked to serologic response. The dry ecosystems, commonly inhabited by camels, do not normally support the insect populations and densities associated with epizootics of RVF. Only when unusual wet conditions exist are there reports in ruminants from these areas becoming infected with RVF. Under experimental conditions, puppies and dogs, kittens and cats, monkeys, mice and hamsters are also susceptible to the disease.

RVF had been a pathogen of domestic animals and humans in sub-Saharan Africa. During the Egyptian epizootic the virus demonstrated its ability to spread and cause extensive disease in a totally new ecologic context, thus opening the potential for spread to other parts of the world where ecologic conditions might prove receptive to a similar epizootic. RVF was first discovered in Kenya in 1931. Subsequent research suggests that the virus exists throughout most of the continent in a poorly understood natural cycle. Periodic epizootics occur when climatic conditions (usually high rainfall) favor an increased density of arthropod vectors and a corresponding susceptible population.

ETIOLOGY. The RVF virus is a member of the Phlebovirus genus of the family Bunyaviridae. These viruses are three-segmented, with a negative sense RNA genome and mature into approximately 100-nm lipid-enveloped virus particles in the region of the cellular Golgi apparatus, and replicate in the cytoplasm of hepatic cells. Some studies have indicated a smaller diameter and the absence of an envelope. Persisting for a considerable time on fomites, the virus is most stable in solutions at pH 7 to 8. When lyophilized and stored at low temperatures, viability persists for many months. Although strains vary in virulence, they are uniform in antigenic structure. In the laboratory, the virus grows in embryonating chicken eggs and in both adult and suckling mice and hamsters. During fever, it locates in the blood and later in liver and spleen of susceptible mammals, and in vectoring mosquitoes.

TRANSMISSION. Evidence suggests that arthropods (Culicoides, mosquitoes, and black flies [Simulium]) are the major transmitters of RVF, although their exact role and the mode of transmission is not fully understood. Continuation of the virus between epizootics in other species or inapparent carriers is speculative. Human cases usually occur after necropsy or slaughter of RVF infected animals where transmission is thought to be by direct contact or aerosols. Fulminating epizootics commonly occur at 4- to 5-year intervals; many infected cattle and sheep die, but most survivors are immune. During years between outbreaks the sheep, cattle, and other ruminants become susceptible.

PATHOGENESIS. An infective dose of virus is probably attained by the feeding of massive numbers of mosquitoes, sand flies, or black flies on infected and then susceptible hosts. The virus is then distributed via the blood to all organs. In the liver the hepatotropic virus penetrates the cytoplasm, where it replicates and causes death of the host cell. Eventually, most hepatic cells die. Death results from shock and hepatic insufficiency. In pregnant ewes, the virus enters the placenta, damages cells, and causes abortion. Following the formation of viremia, the body temperature rises and the fever persists for 2 to 3 days. At the beginning of fever, leukocytosis develops, but leukopenia follows promptly. In nonfatal cases, complement-fixing antibodies appear approximately 10 days after beginning fever, reach a titer peak at 30 days, and may persist 6 to 8 weeks and then decline. Neutralizing antibodies appear 30 days after fever, reach a titer peak in 30 days, and persist at a significant level for a year or longer.

CLINICAL SIGNS AND POSTMORTEM LESIONS. In young lambs the incubation period varies from 20 to 72 hours. Some lambs suddenly die without manifesting signs. Usually, however, the affected lambs develop fever, decline feed, physically weaken, recline, and die after a course of 24 hours. Mortality often reaches 95%. The most constant clinical finding in adult animals is abortion.

In adult sheep, RVF is less severe than in lambs. Some ewes develop asymptomatic RVF. After a short incubation period, however, most sheep show fever of 41 to 42°C, abortion, and vomiting. During fever, severe leukopenia, especially of neutrophils, forms. The course extends through a few days, and mortality approximates 20%. Frequently, cattle and people associating with the infected sheep contract the disease. Cattle show signs similar to sheep with abortions among pregnant cows and death of calves. Infected people develop dengue-like symptoms and recover after 3 to 4 days of misery and incapacitation. Complaints during the Egyptian epizootic included retinal vascular disease, encephalitis, and hemorrhagic fever.

At necropsy of infected lambs, the prominent lesions are limited to the liver. In early stages of the disease, the liver is swollen, friable, and mottled. The parenchyma contains multiple gray-yellow foci, each surrounded by a red zone of congestion. In advanced stages, the entire liver is gray-yellow on both capsular and cut surfaces. A few foci of hemorrhage may be discernible through the capsule. The subendocardium and subepicardium, as well as other serosal surfaces, may contain hemorrhages. Other findings include splenomegaly and lymphadenopathy. In adult ewes, hepatic changes are similar but less severe. Mottling predominates. The uterus may show evidence of recent abortion.

Histopathologic changes in lambs and adult ewes are similar. During early stages, the hepatic tissue changes are focal in distribution. Aggregates of neutrophils accumulate in sinusoids. Later, groups of necrotic liver cells form near the leukocyte accumulations. Still later, foci of necrosis coalesce, until nearly all hepatic cells within a lobule and even the organ are necrotic. Cells at the periphery of lobules retain viability longer than cells in other lobular zones. A wide range of degenerative and necrotic changes are seen in hepatocytes. The most conspicuous include prominent nuclear changes (clumping and margination of chromatin, pyknosis, karyorrhexis, karyolysis), cytoplasmic fragmentation of disintegration, focal cytoplasmic degradation and sequestration and the formation of acidophilic cytoplasmic bodies (inclusion-like). The enlarged nuclei may show margination of chromatin and the formation of acidophilic inclusion bodies. Similar extensive liver damage occurs in humans that die from the disease.

DIAGNOSIS. Veterinarians clinically diagnose RVF from evidence of characteristic signs and lesions. In enzootic areas fever, short course, high mortality in lambs, abortions and 20% mortality of adult ewes, mottling and/or generalized yellowing of liver in lambs and ewes, similar disease in associating calves and cows, and influenza-like disease among attending people all suggest RVF. Similar extensive liver damage occurs in humans that die from the disease. Finding histopathologic changes in the liver gives further diagnostic evidence. Isolation and identification of the RVF virus confirm the diagnosis. Virus isolation may be achieved by inoculating infected blood, liver, or spleen into embryonating chicken eggs and unweaned mice. Virus neutralization with known antibodies and the complement-fixation test help identify the virus. Indirect fluorescent antibody tests, immunodiffusion tests, hemagglutination test, and hemagglutination-inhibition tests are also used to detect circulating RVF-specific antibody.

PREVENTION. Susceptible animals can be protected by immunization, but a comprehensive control program is complicated by variations in ecosystems, a lack of understanding of the quantitative determinants of the epizootic disease (vector density, vector competence, vector biology, host factors), and often a delay in diagnosis due to insufficient specific tools for field diagnosis. WHO sets forth a detailed set of recommendations including diagnosis, surveillance, a vaccination scheme, and the control of animal movement for the areas beyond the sub-Saharan enzootic range and for sub-Saharan Africa. Two types of vaccine are currently involved, the modified live virus vaccines (MLVV) and attenuated vaccines. The modified live virus vaccines cost less to produce, maintain a longer time of immunity (up to 12 months) and require only one initial immunization and can be stored for extended periods of time (10 years) in the lyophilized state. The MLVV will cause abortions and has the potential for reversion to a virulent strain. Its use is therefore restricted to enzootic and epizootic areas. The inactivated vaccines are effective and safe, but are more expensive to produce, unable to be stored for extended periods (6 months), and require at least 2 doses for optimal immune response. These vaccines are recommended for use in areas beyond the enzootic or epizootic range. Using technologic advances, the cloning of genetic information for the immunogenic membrane protein into a bacterium will greatly reduce the cost, improve the antigenicity, eliminate abortions, and reversion to virulence. Attenuated vaccines are available for humans in high risk situations.

Alexander, R.A.: Rift Valley fever in the Union. J. S. Afr. Vet. Med. Assoc., 22:105-109, 1951.
Animal Health Yearbook. FAO-WHO-OIE (Italy), 1970.
Assaad, F., et al.: The use of veterinary vaccines for prevention and control of Rift Valley Fever: Memorandum from WHO/FAO meeting. Bulletin WHO, 61: 261-268, 1983.
Ayoub, N. and Allam, I.: The immunodiffusion test in Rift Valley fever. Bull. Off. Into. Epiz., 93:1395-1400, 1981.
Broom, J.C. and Findlay, G.M.: The filtration of Rift Valley fever virus through graded collodion membranes. Br. J. Exp. Pathol., 14:179-181, 1933.

Coetzer, J. and Ishak, K.: Sequential development of the liver in newborn lambs infected with Rift Valley River virus. I. Macroscopic and microscopic pathology. Onderstepoort J. Vet. Res., 49:103-108, 1982.

Coetzer, J., Ishak, K., and Calvert, R.: Sequential development of the liver lesions in newborn lambs infected with Rift Valley fever virus. II. Ultrastructural findings. Onderstepoort J. Vet. Res., 49:109-122, 1982.

Daubney, R., Hudson, J.R., and Garnham, P.C.: Epizootic hepatitis or Rift Valley fever. An undescribed virus disease of sheep, cattle and man from East Africa. J. Pathol. Bacteriol., 34:545-579, 1931.

Davies, F., Koros, J., and Mbugua, H.: Rift Valley fever in Kenya: The presence of antibodies to the virus in camels (Camelus dromedarius). J. Hyg., Camb., 94:241-244, 1984.

Easterday, B.C. and Murphy, L.C.: The growth of Rift Valley fever virus in cultures of established lines of cells. Cornell Vet., 53:3-11, 1963.

Easterday, B.C., Murphy, L.C., and Bennett, D.G.: Experimental Rift Valley fever in lambs and sheep. AJVR, 23:1231-1240, 1962.

Eisa, M.: Preliminary survey of domestic animals of the Sudan for precipitating antibodies to Rift Valley fever virus. J. Hyg., Camb., 93:629-637, 1984.

Findlay, G.M., Stefanopoulo, G.J., and MacCollum, F.O.: Presence d'anticorps contre la fievre de la Vallee du Rift dans le sang des Africains. Bull. Soc. Pathol. Exot., 29:986-996, 1936.

Gear, J., et al.: Rift Valley fever in South Africa. S. Afr. Med. J., 29:514-518, 1955.

Harrington, D.F., et al.: Evaluation of a formalin-inactivated Rift Valley fever vaccine in sheep. AJVR, 41:1559-1564, 1980.

Kitchen, S.F.: The development of neurotropism in Rift Valley fever virus. Ann. Trop. Med. Parasitol, 44:132-145, 1950.

Lecatsas, G. and Weiss, K.E.: Electron microscopic studies on BHK21 cells infected with Rift Valley fever virus. Arch. Gesamte. Virusforsch., 25:58-64, 1968.

Lupton, H., Peters, C., and Eddy, G.: Rift Valley fever: Global spread or global control? Proc. Eighty-Sixth Ann. Mtg. U.S. An. Health Assn., 1982, pp. 261-275.

McGavran, M.H. and Easterday, B.C.: Rift Valley fever virus hepatitis. Light and electron microscopic studies in the mouse. Am. J. Pathol., 42:587-607, 1963.

McIntosh, B.M.: Rift Valley fever. I. Vector studies in the field. J. S. Afr. Vet. Assoc., 43:391-395, 1972.

Pini, A., Lund, L.J., and Davies, F.G.: Fluorescent and neutralizing antibodies to infection by Rift Valley fever virus. J. S. Afr. Vet. Assoc., 44:161-165, 1973.

Plowright, W. and Ferris, R.D.: Rift Valley fever. Tissue culture. East Afr. Vet. Res. Org. Ann. Rept., 1957, p. 28.

Saddington, R.S.: In vitro and in vivo cultivation of the virus of Rift Valley fever. Proc. Soc. Exp. Biol. Med., 31:693-694, 1934.

Smithburn, K.C.: Rift Valley fever. The neurotropic adaptation of the virus and the experimental use of this modified virus as a vaccine. Br. J. Exp. Pathol., 30:1-30, 1949.

Smithburn, K.C., Haddow, A.J., and Gillett, J.D.: Rift Valley fever. Isolation of the virus from wild mosquitoes. Br. J. Exp. Pathol., 29:107-121, 1948.

Smithburn, K.C., Haddow, A.J., and Lumsden, W.H.R.: Rift Valley fever; transmission of the virus by mosquitoes. Br. J. Exp. Pathol., 30:35-47, 1949.

Walker, J.S., et al.: Clinical aspects of Rift Valley fever virus in household pets. I. Susceptibility of dog. J. Infect. Dis., 121:9-18, 1970a.

Walker, J.S., et al.: Clinical aspects of Rift Valley fever virus in household pets. II. Susceptibility of cat. J. Infect. Dis., 121:19-24, 1970b.

Weiss, K.E.: Rift Valley fever—a review. Bull. Epizoot. Dis. Afr., 5:431-458, 1957.

Yedloutschnig, R., Dardiri, A., Mebus, C., and Walker, J.: Abortion in vaccinated sheep and cattle after challenge with Rift Valley fever virus. Vet. Rec., 109:383-384, 1981.

Wesselsbron Disease

(WD)

Wesselsbron disease, an infectious but noncontagious zoonosis, is characterized by fever, abortion, and hepatitis and is caused by Wesselsbron virus, a member of the family Togaviridae, transmitted by mosquitoes, Aedes caballus and A. circumluteolus. The disease closely resembles Rift Valley fever in all clinical and pathologic aspects, although Wesselsbron disease and Rift Valley fever are caused by antigenically different viruses.

Occurring in the Union of South Africa, Malawi, and Zimbabwe, and as evidenced by viral antibodies, in Cameroun and Chad, the disease attacks lambs 1 to 8 days of age, ewes in advanced pregnancy, possibly other ruminants, horses, swine, and people. In the laboratory both unweaned and adult mice are susceptible to infection.

The spherical virion contains a core of single-stranded RNA, measures 30 to 45 nm, and multiplies in the cytoplasm of liver cells. Under natural conditions as well as in the laboratory, the mosquitoes (Aedes caballus and A. circumluteolus) probably transmit the virus to susceptible mammals.

Both young lambs and ewes in advanced pregnancy contract clinical WD. After an incubation period of 24 to 72 hours, young lambs develop fever and die within 1 to 2 days. Lambs have severe icterus, hepatomegaly, petechia in the abomasum, and generalized lymphadenopathy. Mortality approximates 100%. Pregnant ewes also develop fever and, after 6 to 14 days, may abort or produce still-born lambs. The mortality among infected ewes varies from 5 to 20%. At necropsy, both lambs and ewes show enlarged, friable, and yellow or mottled livers, and histologically widespread necrosis of hepatocytes. Intranuclear inclusions and cytoplasmic Councilman-like bodies are found.

Veterinarians suspect WD when, in endemic areas, the following conditions prevail: (1) ewes abort or bear dead lambs, (2) lambs 1 to 8 days of age and some ewes sicken and die, (3) dead ewe and lamb livers show degenerative changes, and (4) people associated with the diseased sheep develop influenza-like conditions. A positive diagnosis, however, requires isolation and identification of the WD virus; it can be isolated from the blood, brain, and liver of infected lambs and ewes and from vectoring mosquitoes.

Veterinarians and producers prevent WD by reducing vectoring mosquito populations and by vaccinating adult sheep. In endemic areas, avianized live-virus vaccine should be administered annually before breeding. Vaccination of pregnant ewes may induce abortion.

Belonje, C.W.A.: Field observations on Wesselsbron disease. J. S. Afr. Vet. Med. Assoc., 29:1-12, 1958.
Coetzer, J.A.W., Theldoridis, A., and Van Heerden, A.: Wesselsbron disease, pathological, hematological, and clinical studies in natural cases and experimentally infected new-born lambs. Onderstepoort J. Vet. Res., 45:93-106, 1978.
Lecatsas, G. and Weiss, K.E.: Formation of Wesselsbron disease virus in BHK21 cells. Arch. Gesamte. Virusforsch., 27:332-338, 1969.
LeRoux, J.M.W.: The histopathology of Wesselsbron disease in sheep. Onderstepoort J. Vet. Res., 28:237-243, 1959.
Maurice, Y.: Wesselsbron disease and Rift Valley fever among sheep and wild ruminants of Chad and Cameroun. Rev. Elev. Med. Vet. Pays Trop., 20:395, 1967.
Muspratt, J., Smithburn, K.C., Paterson, H.E., and Kokernot, R.H.: Studies on arthropod-borne viruses of Tongaland. X. The laboratory transmission of Wesselsbron virus by the bite of Aedes circumluteolus. Afr. J. Med. Sci., 22:121, 1957.
Neitz, W.O.: Viral diseases of sheep. Rept. FAO/OIE Int. Conf. on Sheep Diseases (Rome), 1966, pp. 43-54.
Smithburn, K.C., Kokernot, R.H., Weinbren, M.P., and de Meillon, B.: Studies on arthropod-borne viruses of Tongaland. IX. Isolation of Wesselsbron virus from a naturally infected human being and from Aedes circumluteolus. S. Afr. J. Med. Sci., 22:113, 1957.
Parker, J.R. and Stannard, L.M.: Intracytoplasmic inclusions in fetal lamb kidney cells infected with Wesselsbron virus. Arch. Gesamte. Virusforsch., 20:469-472, 1967.
Weiss, K.E., Haig, D.A., and Alexander, R.A.: Wesselsbron virus—a virus not previously described, associated with abortion in domestic animals. Onderstepoort J. Vet. Res., 27:183-195, 1956.

Tick-Borne Fever

(TBF)

Tick-borne fever, an acute infectious but noncontagious disease, is characterized clinically by fever and abortions and pathologically by the presence of colonies of organisms in the cytoplasm of leukocytes. It is caused by a rickettsia transmitted by ticks. Even though the disease has little importance to the entire sheep industry, to enterprises in endemic areas it causes economic losses from abortions and stillbirths, deaths of aborting ewes, market depreciation of affected land, and the cost of tick control.

OCCURRENCE. TBF occurs in all breeds, sexes, and ages of sheep and goats. Animals raised in TBF-free areas are especially susceptible and, when placed in tick-infested pastures, contract severe and often fatal infection. In addition to sheep, both cattle and goats are naturally susceptible. Most cases develop during spring and autumn and correlate with times of extensive and vigorous tick activity. Besides the highlands of Scotland, TBF occurs in the tick-infested forest pastures of Ireland, Norway, Finland, and India.

ETIOLOGY AND PATHOGENESIS. *Ehrlichia (cytoecetes) phagocytophilia,* the specific cause of TBF, locates within cytoplasmic vacuoles of granulocytes and monocytes. The pleomorphic organisms, single or aggregated, are round, oval, or rod-shaped and vary in size from 1 to 3 μm in diameter, and color gray, black, and blue with Romanowsky, polychrome methylene blue, and Macchiavello stains. Larger particles each contain a cell wall, plasma membrane, ribosome-like granules, and a nucleoid. The organism, when stored in blood or splenic tissue at 20, 4, and $-79°$C, remains viable for 10, 13, and 550 days, respectively. Ovine strains reside in sheep blood from time of incipient fever through 2 to 3 weeks after fever declines, and they differ antigenically from bovine strains.

Natural transmission occurs through the bite of the vectoring tick, *Ixodes ricinus,* in Britain and Europe, but by *Rhipicephalus haemophysaloides* in India. The organism passes trans-stadially, but not transovarially, within the ticks, and, consequently, both nymphae and adults, but not larvae, can transmit infection to new mammalian hosts. Experimentally, scientists can transmit TBF by injecting infective blood from reacting sheep into susceptible animals.

During blood-feeding, the rickettsiae, along with saliva, pass from the infected tick into the blood of the susceptible host. After entering the cytoplasm of granulocytes and monocytes, the organisms form vacuoles, replicate, and discharge substances that provoke a febrile reaction and suppress leukocytopoiesis. Ingestion by hematophagous arthropods returns the organisms to the environment. Ewes in the third trimester of pregnancy may abort, presumably from placental damage. Death results from acute uterine infections following abortion. Clinically recovered sheep temporarily resist reinfection with the same antigenic strain of rickettsiae.

CLINICAL SIGNS AND POSTMORTEM LESIONS. Following an incubation period of 2 to 6 or more days, the body temperature rises to 41 to 42°C, maintains the high level for 1 to 2 days, and then gradually declines over 2 to 3 weeks. Concurrent with the temperature rise is a tachycardia, moderate depression, slight anorexia, and ruminal stasis with a loss of condition. Adult ewes show muscular stiffness and lameness. Organisms persist in the blood for several weeks. During the stage of high fever, as many as 95% of the granulocytes and monocytes contain rickettsiae, and leukopenia may form and persist for a few days. A lymphocytopenia results from a transient depletion in numbers of circulating B-lymphocytes and only a small reduction in T-lymphocytes and is associated with a depletion of lymphoid tissues in the spleen and lymph nodes. The re-

sultant reduction in B-lymphocytes causes suppression of the humoral immune response acting as an immunosuppressant. A significant feature of TBF is the effect upon immune response to vaccinations and the complication or concurrence with other diseases especially pneumonias. Approximately 30% of ewes in the third trimester of pregnancy abort, and 23% of these die. Although the morbidity may reach 25 to 50% of a flock, the overall mortality is low. The clinical course extends over several weeks.

At necropsy, the gross changes are reduced body weight and, in some ewes, abortion or stillbirths. The histopathologic changes evince the presence of single organisms or colonies of particles in the cytoplasm of leukocytes.

DIAGNOSIS. In endemic areas, veterinarians diagnose TBF on evidence of tick parasitism, fever, depression, and abortions. Finding typical rickettsiae in the cytoplasm of granulocytes or monocytes confirms a clinical diagnosis. Specific complement-fixing antibody has been demonstrated and high titers suggest the animal may be in the carrier state of infection.

The differential diagnosis requires consideration of other abortifacient diseases, especially louping-ill, because that viral disease and TBF are transmitted by the same species of tick and, consequently, may occur together in a flock or individual. Louping-ill produces locomotor disturbance and specific neuropathologic changes, but not rickettsiae in the leukocytes. The louping-ill virus can be isolated from blood and brain tissue and grown in embryonating chicken eggs and cell cultures. Cotyledonary smears, stained with modified Ziehl-Neelsen preparation, should be examined for enzootic abortion of ewes, and for brucella and vibrio bacteria.

PREVENTION AND TREATMENT. Veterinarians and producers prevent or reduce TBF by avoiding heavy exposure of susceptible sheep to parasitism of vectoring ticks. Susceptible ewes in advanced pregnancy should not enter tick-infested pastures. Residing in an infected area during periods of low tick activity gradually acclimatizes sheep to this ecologic disease and enables animals to acquire natural immunity before the time of heavy tick exposure. Individual sheep may be effectively treated by administering oxytetracycline for several days at the daily rate of 11 mg/kg of body weight. Ethoxyethylglyoxal dithiosemicarbazone administered at the onset of parasitemia reduces fever, depresses parasitemia, and eliminates relapses. Therapeutic doses (1 mg/kg) of corticosteroid (betamethasone) provides significant but transitory (6 to 12 hours) reduction in temperature, an increase in total leukocytes (primarily granulocytes) and a transient reduction in lymphocytes.

Batungbacal, M., Scott, G., and Barrels, C.: The lymphocytopenia in tick-borne fever. J. Comp. Path., 92: 403-407, 1982.
Batungbacal, M. and Scott, G.: Suppression of the immune response to clostridial vaccine by tick-borne fever. J. Comp. Path., 92:409-413, 1982.
Batungbacal, M. and Scott, G.: Tick-borne fever and concurrent parainfluenza-3 virus infection in sheep. J. Comp. Path., 92:415-428, 1982.
Collins, J.D., Hannan, J., Ferguson, A.R., and Wilson, J.O.: Tick-borne fever in Ireland. Irish Vet. J., 24: 162-166, 1970.
Evans, A.T.: Preliminary observations on the chemotherapy of tick-borne fever of sheep and cattle. Trans. R. Soc. Trop. Med. Hyg., 66:547, 1972.
Foggie, A.: Studies on the infectious agent of tick-borne fever in sheep. J. Pathol. Bacteriol., 63:1-15, 1951.
Foggie, A. and Allison, C.J.: A note on occurrence of tick-borne fever in cattle in Scotland with comparative studies of bovine and ovine strains of the organism. Vet. Rec., 72:767, 1960.
Foggie, A., Lumsden, W.H.R., and McNeillage, G.J.C.: Preservation of the infectious agent of tick-borne fever in the frozen state. J. Comp. Pathol., 76:413-416, 1966.
Gilmour, N., et al.: Tick-borne fever and pasteurellosis in sheep. Vet. Rec., 11:512, 1982.
Gordon, W.S., Brownlee, A., Wilson, D.R., and MacLeod, J.: Third Int. Cong. Microbiol. New York, 1939.
Gordon, W.S., Brownlee, A., Wilson, D.R., and MacLeod, J.: Tick-borne fever (a hitherto undescribed disease of sheep). J. Comp. Pathol. Ther., 45:301-307, 1932.
Jamieson, S.: Tick-borne fever as a cause of abortion in Sheep. II. Vet. Rec., 62:468, 1950.
Littlejohn, A.I.: Tick-borne fever as a cause of abortion in sheep. Vet. Rec., 62:577-579, 1950.
MacLeod, J. and Gordon, W.S.: Studies in tick-borne fever in sheep. I. Transmission by the tick Ixodes ricinus, with a description of the disease produced. Parasitology, 25:273-283, 1933.
Raghavachari, K. and Reddy, A.M.K.: Cytoecetes ovis var. decanni (n. sp.) as the cause of tick-borne fever in sheep in India. Indian J. Vet. Sci. Anim. Husb., 29:69-86, 1959.
Snodgrass, D.R. and Ramacosandran, S.: A complement fixation test for tick-borne fever of sheep. Br. Vet. J., 9:127, 1971.
Stamp, J.T. and Watt, J.A.: Tick-borne fever as a cause of abortion in sheep. I. Vet. Rec., 62:465, 1950.
Tuomi, J. and Von Bonsdorff, C.H.: Electron microscopy of tick-borne fever agent in bovine and ovine phagocytizing leukocytes. J. Bacteriol., 92:1478-1492, 1966.
VanMiert, A., VanDuin, C., Schotman, A., and Franssen, F.: Clinical haematological and blood biochemical changes in goats after experimental infection with tick-borne fever. Vet. Parast., 16:225-233, 1984.
Watson, W.A.: Infertility in the ram associated with tick-borne fever infection. Vet. Rec., 76:1131-1136, 1964.
Woldheiwet, Z. and Scott, G.: Immunological studies on tick-borne fever in sheep. J. Comp. Path., 92:457-467, 1982.
Woldheiwet, Z. and Scott, G.: Corticosteroid therapy of tick-borne fever. Vet. Rec., 110:151-152, 1982.

Enzootic Abortion of Ewes

(EAE; chlamydial abortion)

Enzootic abortion of ewes, a subacute contagious disease, is characterized by fever, abortions, stillbirths, and weak lambs and is caused by a chlamydia. Because of universal geographic distribution and high flock incidence, the disease has major importance to the industry and often causes severe economic losses. In addition to abortion, the chlamydia may cause conjunctivitis, polyarthritis, epididymitis, pneumonia, and diarrhea.

OCCURRENCE. Although EAE occurs in all breeds of mature ewes, animals 2 years of age have higher incidence than other age groups. Following contact of susceptible ewes with aborting sheep, abortion among the newly exposed ewes is especially high during the next two lambing crops. In addition to sheep, the natural disease occurs occasionally in pregnant goats and cows and rarely in people. High incidence correlates with the months of parturition, which in the United States are March, April, and May. Sheep confined to crowded lambing facilities, such as buildings or pens, develop higher transmission rates and consequently have a greater incidence than sheep lambing on open grazing range or large pasture. The disease may be accompanied by vibriosis.

Even though EAE occurs in nearly all major sheep-producing countries, the disease is common in Scotland, France, Germany, Bulgaria, Yugoslavia, Rumania, and America. In the United States, EAE is widespread, but more prevalent among sheep of western states of the intermountain area.

ETIOLOGY AND PATHOGENESIS. *Chlamydia psittaci* causes EAE. This gram-negative, non-motile, obligate parasite inhabits cytoplasmic vacuoles of host cells, where it may remain for a period of prolonged and even lifetime latency. The infectious particle, consisting of a cell membrane and nucleoid, measures 0.3 nm in diameter and contains both DNA and RNA. The cell contains lipid and mucopeptide and, like some bacteria, its growth is inhibited by penicillin and cycloserine. The mature particles color purple with Giemsa's stain and red with Macchiavello's stain. The organism inactivates in 10 minutes at 60°C, and in 30 minutes, 24 hours, and 24 hours when exposed to ether, 0.1% formalin, or 0.5% phenol, respectively, but it maintains infectivity for many months or years when lyophilized and stored at −50 to −70°C. The organism is cultivated in the yolk sac of embryonating chicken eggs and in cell cultures of the fetal lamb.

Like many other chlamydiae, the agent of EAE possesses two antigens—group and specific—associated with the cell wall. The group antigen, common to all chlamydiae, resists heat, nucleases, and proteases but inactivates from the action of lecithinase. The specific antigen is shared by a limited group of related chlamydiae, is detectable with immunofluorescence and gel-diffusion reactions, and is neutralized by specific antibodies. Strains from different clinical sources classify into two antigenic groups: (1) Immunotype 1 from cases of EAE, from normal ovine intestines, and from cases of epizootic bovine abortion; and (2) Immunotype 2 from cases of ovine polyarthritis, from intestines of polyarthritic sheep, from cases of ovine conjunctivitis, and from cases of bovine polyarthritis. Strains within each group are antigenically related, but strains of group 1 antigenically differ from strains of group 2.

The transmission of EAE from infected to susceptible sheep occurs at the time of parturition and abortion. Infected ewes discharge—

along with placentas, fetuses, and uterine exudate—vast numbers of viable chlamydiae to the external environment. The organisms contaminating feed and water enter susceptible ewes or lambs through the alimentary tract, and those contaminating dust and fluid droplets disperse into the air and enter susceptible animals through the respiratory system.

Crowding in lambing facilities, such as buildings and small pens, facilitates spread. Transmission to ewes between 30 and 120 days of gestation may result in placentitis, fetal injury and abortion, or birth of weak lambs, but transmission to ewes in the last month of pregnancy usually does not induce abortion. Transmission to nonpregnant ewes, ewes in the last month of gestation, and lambs may result in latent infection of somatic tissues and abortion during the next pregnancy.

Although the pathogenesis of EAE has received some attention from investigators, many aspects of the disease development remain obscure and conjectural. The chlamydiae possess a strong predilection for the placenta. Following entrance of the organism into the alimentary or respiratory systems, or activation of latent infection of pregnant sheep, the agent, transported by blood to the placenta, traverses the maternal capillary walls in the septal extremities, and enters the extravasated blood in the lacunae.

The septal tips normally hyalinize during the second month of pregnancy, and this change, predisposing hemorrhage into the lacunae, facilitates passage of microorganisms through capillary walls. From the lacunae, the chlamydiae penetrate chorionic epithelial cells, multiply, and form colonies of elementary bodies in cytoplasmic vacuoles. As a result, the parasitized cells lyse and detach, and masses of organisms discharge into surrounding mesenchymal tissue and intraepithelial capillaries of chorionic villi and into the intervillus-septum space. Organisms entering the chorionic capillaries are distributed to fetal viscera, and organisms released into the intervillus-septum space enter and parasitize new epithelial cells.

By this multiplying process, the infection gradually and radially spreads along chorionic villi and maternal septa toward the placentomal base and periplacentomal tissue. The infection provokes inflammation in both cotyledon and caruncle. Neutrophils infiltrate the tissue, and necrosis, partly from thrombosis, develops. These changes separate the chorionic villi from maternal septa and interfere with transplacental exchange of maternal and fetal substances. Abortion results from a combination of placental damage and fetal injury.

Complement-fixing antibodies form within 7 to 10 days after beginning active infection and may persist for 30 months. Low titers of neutralizing antibodies form later and persist longer than the complement-fixing antibodies. Recovered ewes are immune to subsequent attacks. The chlamydiae discharge to the external environment through infected placentas, aborted fetuses, and uterine discharges.

CLINICAL SIGNS AND POSTMORTEM LESIONS. Following natural transmission, the incubation period usually varies from 50 to 90 days. The clinical signs are abortion, stillbirths, and weak lambs. The abortions occur during the last month of pregnancy. After parturition, affected ewes may discharge uterine exudate for a few days. Some ewes die as a result of secondary bacterial metritis. The first disease outbreak in a flock causes abortion, ranging from 20 to 30%, but thereafter 5% annually abort. An individual ewe aborts only once.

At necropsy, the chorion, rarely available, is edematous and blood-stained. The interplacentomal chorion contains plaques of granular, opaque, and blood-tinged exudate, and cotyledons show a change in color from purple-red to gray. Brown hemoglobin, derived from hemolysis of blood in the hematoma, may be diffused throughout the periplacentomal transudate.

Histopathologic alterations occur in the caruncle, cotyledon, and fetus. In early stages, changes are concentrated in the hilar zone of placentomes: the extremities of some septa are necrotic and infiltrated with leukocytes; some chorionic epithelial cells bulge with cytoplasmic masses of elementary bodies; the edematous chorionic mesenchyma is infiltrated with leukocytes. From this anatomic site, infection gradually and radially spreads throughout the placentome. In advanced stages, areas of necrosis, involving both villi and septa, may extend from the hilar zone towards the cotyledonary base; most chorionic epithelial cells are infected; and detached epithelial cells and inflammatory exudate separate villi from septa. Fetal lesions consist of a diffuse or focal reticuloendothelial hyperplasia and an accumulation of giant cells (megakaryocytes and Langhans' giant cells) in the mesenteric lymph nodes. Adrenal glands show a proliferation of lymphoid cells, plasmablasts, and neutrophils. Liver changes are of diagnostic value and consist of perivascular lymphohistiocytic proliferations as well as lymphohistiocytic proliferation in the walls of the interlobular veins. Similar proliferations are found in kidneys, hearts, and lungs.

DIAGNOSIS. A history of abortions, stillbirths, and weak lambs during the last month of pregnancy along with characteristic necropsy findings suggest EAE. The aborted fetuses are clean and well preserved with varying degrees of subcutaneous petechial hemorrhages, congested livers (sometimes with focal areas of necrosis appearing as white spots) and enlarged lymph nodes. Hemorrhage occurs in the thymus, lymph nodes, muscles, and subcutis with subcutaneous edema and ascites. These findings are variable depending on the age of the fetus at the time of the infectious insult. The cotyledons show a characteristic gray-brown necrosis with a leathery gray-brown or clay colored roughened surface at the peri- and intercotyledonary chorion. A gray brown to reddish brown uterine discharge may persist for a few days. A laboratory confirmation is necessary to support the clinical diagnosis. Isolation via chick embryo or cell culture confirms a diagnosis but is time consuming, expensive, and difficult to isolate as these pathogens are readily inactivated in the process that ultimately leads to abortion. The successful isolation of chlamydia depends on the correct specimen being inoculated into tissue cultures as quickly as possible. A few grams of cotyledons is the tissue of choice. A transport media consisting of sucrose (74.69/l), K2HPO4 (1.237 g/l), L-glutamic acid (0.721 g/l), fetal calf serum (10% v/v), vancomycin and streptomycin (100 μg/ml) and nystatin and gentamicin (50 μg/ml) will maintain the organism viable for up to 30 days without refrigeration. Exfoliative cytology provides an excellent, inexpensive and rapid means of diagnosis. Impression smears are made from affected cotyledons, pieces of chorion from the margin of placental lesions, or cut surfaces of lungs, spleen, kidneys, or lymph nodes, stained by the Giemsa method and observed for elementary bodies in heavily infected trophoblasts.

Microscopic demonstration of elementary bodies in impression smears of placentas is conclusive evidence of chlamydial infection. The same tissues as mentioned above can be used for the direct and indirect fluorescent antibody test which is specific and sensitive with good antibody preparations. Serologic tests i.e. (complement fixation and enzyme-linked immunosorbent assay) are good indicators to evaluate the antibody response. Paired serum samples, taken at the time of abortion and 14 to 21 days later, should have a significant rise in titer as maximum antibody titers are reached at 14 to 21 days after parturition in infected ewes. A delayed hypersensitivity skin test for EAE indicates a cell mediated immune response which may be indicative of infection before clinical signs become apparent.

The differential diagnosis requires consideration of vibriosis, brucellosis, and salmonellosis. Stained smears differentiate the causes, and causative bacteria can be isolated and identified.

PREVENTION AND TREATMENT. The epidemiologic factors in an outbreak of EAE involve a primary case or cases that abort, contaminating feed and water with infected placenta and uterine discharge. The infective organisms enter establishing infection. If these events occur early in pregnancy, abortion is likely. Delivery of a normal lamb usually occurs if the exposure occurs during the last trimester, but the subsequent pregnancy is in jeopardy. Early detection and isolation of aborting ewes with proper

disposal of fetuses, placenta, and discharges plus disinfection of the premises or area with standard germicides such as 2% lye, 2% cresol, or quaternary ammonia will prevent entry of the organism into a new host. As it is difficult to eliminate the organism once it has contaminated the environment, alteration of the susceptibility of the host is a logical alternative.

Immunization should be done prior to conception. The economics related to sheep biologics in the U.S has not permitted extensive research into improving immunogens for EAE. Effective experimental vaccines have been prepared with cell culture techniques and temperature-sensitive mutants. A commercially produced vaccine combining chlamydia psittaci and campylobacter is available. The manufacturer's recommendation is one dose 6 weeks prior to breeding followed by a second shot in 2 to 4 weeks with an annual booster. Antibiotic treatment with tetracycline is usually ineffective and disappointing as irreversible placental and fetal damage has taken place by the time clinical signs and abortions occur. However, on a flock basis, an early diagnosis, followed by an initial treatment of 20 mg/kg of terramycin/LA200 and maintained on 400 to 450 mg/head/day of tetracycline in the feed will reduce the abortions and number of weak lambs. In flocks where EAE is endemic 100 to 150 mg of tetracycline per head per day in the feed for 2 to 3 weeks prior to breeding is recommended. The ultimate control of EAE depends on the development of an effective vaccine. Treatment, if attempted, should include the parenteral administration of oxytetracycline for 2 to 4 days at the daily rate of 12 mg/kg of body weight.

Animal Health Yearbook. FAO-WHO-OIE (Italy), 1970.

Beer, J.: Untersuchungen an und mit komplementbinden antigenen des virus-aborts der schafe. Zentralbl. Veterinaermed., 5:305-308, 1958.

Blewett, D., et al.: Ovine enzootic abortion: the acquisition of infection and subsequent abortion within a single lambing season. Vet. Rec., 11:499-501, 1982.

Dane, D.S. and Clapp, K.H.: Complement-fixing antibodies to the psittacosis-lymphogranuloma group of virus in south Australian sheep. Aust. Vet. J., 32:91-93, 1956.

Djorov, A.: Histological changes in the foetus in ovine enzootic abortion. Zentralbl. Veterinaermed., 19B: 578-587, 1972.

Faye, P., et al.: Study of a strain of ovine abortion virus isolated directly in chick embryos. Bull. Acad. Vet. Fr., *37*:263-267, 1964.

Faye, P., et al.: Chlamydial enzootic abortion in goats. Bull. Acad. Vet. Fr., *44*:61-64, 1971.

Frank, F.W., et al.: Artificially induced immunity to enzootic abortion in ewes. AJVR, *29*:1441-1447, 1968.

Fraser, G. and Horne, H.H.: Growth and development of the agent of enzootic abortion of ewes in tissue culture. Vet. Rec., *77*:884-885, 1965.

Hall, R., Waldhalm, D., and Delong, W.: The prevention of chlamydial abortion in sheep and goats. Proc. 3rd Intn'l Conf. on Goat Prod. and Dis., *540*, 1982.

Johnson, F., Clarkson, M., and Spencer, W.: Direct isolation of the agent of enzootic abortion of ewes (*Chlamydia psittaci*) in cell cultures. Vet. Rec., *113*:413-414, 1983.

Kawakami, Y., et al.: Miyagawanella: psittacosis-lymphogranuloma group of viruses, isolation of a virus from feces of naturally infected sheep. Bull. Natl. Inst. Anim. Health, *36*, 1958.

Lvey, N., Munoz, A., and McCormick, W.: Enzyme-linked immunosorbent assay for the detection of antibody to *Chlamydia trachomatis* and *Chlamydia psittaci*. J. Lab. Clin. Med., *102*:918-925, 1983.

McKercher, D.G., et al.: Isolation of the virus of enzootic abortion of ewes from California and Oregon sheep. JAVMA, *145*:564-569, 1964.

Mendlowski, B. and Segre, D.: Polyarthritis in sheep. I. Description of the disease and experimental transmission. AJVR, *21*:68-73, 1963.

Mitscherlich, E.: Control of virus abortion in ewes. Berl. Muench. Tieraerztl. Wochenschr., *78*:81-88, 1965.

Novilla, M.N.: Dissertation: Placental pathology of experimentally induced enzootic abortion in ewes. Colorado State University, 1967.

Novilla, M.N. and Jensen, R.: Placental pathology of experimentally induced enzootic abortion in ewes. AJVR, *31*:1983-2000, 1970.

Parker, H., Hawkins, W.W., and Brenner, E.: Epizootiologic studies of ovine virus abortion. AJVR, *27*:869-877, 1966.

Popovici, V.: Ovine virus abortion. I. Incidence and diagnosis. II. Epidemiology. Lucr. Ist. Cerc. Vet. Bioprep. Pasteur, *1*:339-347, 1962.

Roberts, W., Grist, N.R., and Giroud, P.: Human abortion associated with infection by ovine abortion agent. Br. Med. J., *4*:37, 1967.

Rodolakis, A. and Bernard, F.: Vaccination with temperature-sensitive mutant of *Chlamydia psittaci* against enzootic abortion of ewes. Vet. Rec., *114*:193-194, 1984.

Rodolakis, A. and Souriau, A.: Response of ewes to temperature-sensitive mutants of *Chlamydia psittaci* (var ovis) obtained by NTG mutagenesis. Ann. Rech. Vet., *14*:155-161, 1983.

Rodolakis, A., et al.: Efficacy of a long-acting oxytetracycline against chlamydial ovine abortion. Ann. Rech. Vet., *11*:437-444, 1980.

Romvary, J.: Virus abortion in Hungarian sheep. Magy. Allatorv. Lap., *13*:81-83, 1958.

Semerdzhiev, B., Ognyanov, D., and Makaveeva-Simova, E.: Virus abortion in a flock of goats. Vet. Med. Nauki (Sofia), *3*:115-121, 1966.

Spencer, W. and Johnson, F.: Simple transport medium for the isolation of *Chlamydia psittaci* from clinical material. Vet. Rec., *113*:535-536, 1983.

Storz, J.: *Chlamydia and Chlamydia-induced Diseases.* Springfield, Ill., Charles C Thomas, 1971.

Storz, J.: Chlamydial abortions. Lab Diag. of abortion in food animals (edited by C. Kirkbride). Am. Assn. Vet. Lab. Diagnosticians, 34-43, 1984.

Storz, J.: Psittacosis agents as cause of polyarthritis in cattle and sheep. Vet. Med. Rev., *2/3*:125-139, 1967.

Storz, J.: Psittacosis-lymphogranuloma infection of sheep. Antigenic structures. J. Comp. Pathol., *76*:351-362, 1966.

Storz, J.: Superinfection of pregnant ewes latently infected with a psittacosis-lymphogranuloma agent. Cornell Vet., *53*:469-480, 1963.

Storz, J. and McKercher, D.G.: Etiological studies of epizootic bovine abortion. Zentralbl. Veterinaermed., *9*:411-427, 1962.

Storz, J., Pierson, R.E., Marriott, M.E., and Chow, T.L.: Isolation of psittacosis agents from follicular conjunctivitis of sheep. Proc. Soc. Exp. Biol. Med., *125*:857-860, 1967.

Studdert, M.J.: Bedsoniae associated with abortion in sheep and cattle. Diss. Abst., *26*:6276, 1966.

Studdert, M.J. and Kennedy, P.C.: Enzootic abortion in ewes. Nature, *203*:1088-1089, 1964.

Studdert, M.J. and McKercher, D.G.: Bedsonia abortion of sheep. I. Etiological studies. Res. Vet. Sci., *9*:48-56, 1968a.

Studdert, M.J. and McKercher, D.G.: Bedsonia abortion of sheep. II. Pathology and pathogenesis with observations on the normal ovine placenta. Res. Vet. Sci., *9*:57-64, 1968b.

Waldhalm, D., Delong, W., and Hall, R.: Efficacy of a bacterin prepared from *Chlamydia psittaci* grown in cell culture for experimental immunization of ewes. Vet. Microb., *7*:493-498, 1982.

Wilsmore, A., Abduljalil, S., Parsons, U., and Dawson, M.: Observations on a skin sensitivity test for ovine enzootic abortion. Br. Vet. J., *140*:468-476, 1984.

Young, S., Parker, H., and Firehammer, B.D.: Abortion in sheep due to a virus of the psittacosis-lymphogranuloma group. JAVMA, *133*:374-379, 1958.

Younger, R.L. and Parker, H.D.: Distribution of ovine virus abortion in the United States. JAVMA, *139*:108-110, 1961.

Brucellosis

(*Mediterranean fever*)

Brucellosis, an acute or chronic contagious disease, is characterized by septicemia followed by localization of infection in the lymph nodes and genital organs and is usually caused by bacterial pathogens that attack most mammals, including man. In the United States the disease, because of low incidence, has minor economic importance to the industry, but for some countries, especially those located in southern Europe, northern Africa, and the Middle East, brucellosis has major significance for both the sheep industry and public health. Economic losses result from abortions, stillborn lambs, early death of lambs, unthriftiness and death of adult sheep, condemnation of carcasses, and from the cost of preventive and eradicative programs. Athough *B. abortus,* one of the causes of brucellosis in sheep, has a host preference for cattle, sheep may be naturally infected for more than 40 months. Additional losses come from prolonged misery, incapacitation, and treatment of infected people.

OCCURRENCE. Although all breeds and sexes of sheep are susceptible to brucellosis, animals from endemic areas appear to possess more resistance to the disease than sheep from brucellosis-free areas.

The incidence of ovine brucellosis is higher during April, May, and June because lambing is scheduled for that time, and aborting ewes excrete contaminated milk and vaginal discharge into the environment of susceptible animals. The contamination of feed and water commonly results in spread of the infection.

Geographically, brucellosis occurs in the sheep-producing areas of Algeria, Morocco, Tunisia, Ethiopia, Congo, Kenya, Burundi, Mozambique, South Africa, Guatemala, Mexico, The Netherlands, France, Spain, Italy, Germany, Portugal, Yugoslavia, Israel, West Pakistan, and Mongolia. In some countries, the incidence of ovine brucellosis is low and sporadic. *B. melitensis* has been eradicated from the United States.

ETIOLOGY AND PATHOGENESIS. The genus *Brucella* contains four species of major importance to veterinary medicine: *B. melitensis* with infection reservoirs in goats and sheep, *B. abortus* with infection reservoirs in cattle, *B. ovis* with infection reservoirs in sheep, and *B. suis* with infection reservoirs in swine. Although strains within species vary, the species generally have some differentiating characteristics (Table 3-1).

B. melitensis and *B. abortus,* the causes of brucellosis in sheep, are nonmotile, nonsporing, gram-negative, aerobic coccobacilli that measure 0.5 to 2.0 $\times$ 0.5 μm. After a period of adaptation, the organisms grow well on artificial media at pH 6.6 to 7.2, but initial isolations, especially for *B. abortus,* require an increase in the partial pressure of CO_2. When grown on suitable media for 1 to 2 days, the translucent colonies measure 1 to 2 mm in diameter and may dissociate into smooth, rough, smooth intermediate, mucoid, and smooth mucoid strains.

Each species of brucella is further subdivided into biotypes. *B. melitensis* has at least 3 biotypes. Biotype 3 is most commonly associated with abortions. Further study is needed on the pathogenesis and epidemiology of the various biotypes.

The smooth strains possess a constant antigenic structure. The species share some major antigens, but also possess some minor differences in agglutinins. A delayed-type hypersensitivity develops as a result of infection and is used in diagnosing previous contacts of an individual animal with brucella organisms.

TABLE 3-1. *Differentiating Characteristics for Species of Brucella*

Species	Colony Type	H$_2$S Production (days)	Need for CO$_2$	Urease Activity	Growth on Serum Agar Plus					
					Thionine			Basic Fuchsin		
					1:25 $\times$ 10^3	1:50 $\times$ 10^3	1:1 $\times$ 10^5	1:25 $\times$ 10^3	1:50 $\times$ 10^3	1:1 $\times$ 10^5
B. melitensis	S	−	−	+ +	+	+	+	+	+	+
B. abortus	S	+	2	−	−	−	−	+	+	+
B. ovis	R	+	−	−	±	+	+	−	±	±
B. suis	S	−	4	+ + +	+	+	+	−	−	−

The bacteria commonly are found in blood, milk, vaginal discharges, spleen, lymph nodes, placentas, and fetuses of infected sheep. The duration of infection in these tissues and secretions varies usually from 20 to 90 days.

Although scientists have studied the pathogenesis of ovine brucellosis only slightly, they have investigated the development of the same disease in cattle and goats, and the knowledge from all studies helps to clarify brucellosis in sheep. The animal may contract the disease in four ways: (1) through the alimentary tract in contaminated feed or water, (2) through the respiratory system in contaminated dust or droplets, (3) through the genital system in contaminated semen, and (4) through the skin and conjunctivae from contaminated dust or droplets.

When the bacteria penetrate tissues in small numbers, they enter and localize in the regional lymph nodes, but when the organisms are numerous, they pervade the lymph nodes and pass into the blood, where they maintain septicemia for 30 to 50 days. Through the blood, the bacteria enter all organs and may establish infection in lymph nodes, spleen, liver, brain, vertebrae, joints, synovial sheaths, gravid uterus, udder, and male genitalia. In most infected sheep, the infection is self-limiting, and spontaneous recovery occurs in approximately 90 days.

Commonly, the bacteria localize in genital organs and cause extensive tissue damage. When they enter the placenta, especially during the third trimester of pregnancy, the organisms pass from maternal blood through septal vessel walls and enter the cytoplasm of chorionic epithelium. The latter cells may necrotize, and the bacteria may enter capillaries of chorionic villi and distribute to all fetal organs. Necrosis in the placenta interferes with the passage of nutrient elements and compounds from maternal blood to fetal blood and with the passage of waste compounds from fetal blood to maternal blood.

The combined effect of placental damage and fetal infection may result in abortions, stillbirths, or infected lambs. Following parturition, the sheep excretes B. melitensis cells through vaginal discharge, milk, and occasionally urine. Infection with brucella cells stimulates immunity from both humoral antibodies and cell-mediated responses.

CLINICAL SIGNS AND POSTMORTEM LESIONS. Following a variable incubation period, some infected ewes develop fluctuating body temperatures with peaks of 42°C. During febrile periods, the animals are depressed and slightly anorectic. In many outbreaks of brucellosis, the first clinical sign is abortion by ewes in the third trimester of pregnancy; stillbirths and weak lambs may also occur. Some ewes become lame and show swelling of some joints and synovial sheaths. Central nervous system disturbances and paralysis, especially of the posterior limbs, occasionally develop.

The abortion rate within a flock varies from a low number up to 60 to 70%. Approximately 20% of infected ewes abort twice, and another 20% bear weak or dead lambs. Ewe mortality is low, but deaths may occur from spondylitis or pneumonia. Infected rams may develop orchitis and pneumonia. Following parturition, discharges and secretions are heavily contaminated during the first few days, but then the numbers of bacteria gradually decrease. Infected ewes excrete B. melitensis cells in milk and vaginal discharge for 3 months and in urine for 2 months.

At necropsy, most gross lesions are located in the genital and skeletal systems. The infected uterus is swollen and edematous and may have recently aborted or lambed. Parts of the placenta may be retained. Intact placentas show severe edema of the chorioallantoic membranes (Fig. 3-1). Opaque exudate surrounds some placentomes and hemoglobin from hemolyzed blood of hematomas imparts a brown color to edematous fluid in and around the placentomes. Some sheep, especially those showing clinical paralysis, have spondylitis and meningitis of adjacent spinal cord. Some joints and tendon sheaths are swollen and contain an increased amount of synovium and flakes of exudate.

Aborted fetuses and stillborn lambs evince variable degrees of changes. In many, generalized edema is extensive throughout all

Fig. 3-1. Edema and necrosis in placentome infected with *B. melitensis*. × 1.0.

on sera of affected sheep. Using the tube-agglutination test, a titer of 1:160 or higher is positive for brucellosis. The agglutination test may also be performed on milk or whey.

In areas inaccessible to laboratory facilities, the intrapalpebral allergic test is a simple and reliable screening test in infected flocks.

The differential diagnosis requires consideration of all other abortifacient diseases including infections, such as vibriosis, salmonellosis, leptospirosis, enzootic abortion of ewes, Rift Valley fever, and tick-borne fever, and intoxications, such as *Astragalus* poisoning. Differentiation of the infectious diseases requires laboratory identifications of the causative organisms. *Astragalus* poisoning results from pregnant ewes feeding on excessive amounts of *Astragalus* plants.

PREVENTION. Veterinarians and sheep producers control brucellosis by applying the most appropriate preventive methods for the prevailing circumstance. Ovine brucellosis out-

tissues, especially the subcutis and intermuscular fasciae. The peritoneal and pleural cavities contain serofibrinous exudate. The infected liver and spleen are swollen, and hemorrhages are abundant on serosal surfaces.

The histopathologic changes are most advanced in the hilar zone of placentomes. In this area, colonies of *B. melitensis* accumulate in lacunae between maternal septa and fetal villi. Masses of bacteria penetrate and grow in the cytoplasm of chorionic epithelial cells (Fig. 3-2). Villi are edematous, and fetal capillaries may contain colonies of bacteria. Necrosis and detachment of chorionic epithelial cells may be extensive.

DIAGNOSIS. Veterinarians diagnose brucellosis on the basis of abortions, bacterial isolations, serologic tests, and allergic reactions. In the laboratory, scientists culture and identify *B. melitensis* from septicemic blood, vaginal discharges, urine, milk, spleens, lymph nodes, placentas, and aborted fetuses, especially from abomasa.

Enzyme immunoassay, complement-fixation, and agglutination tests may be performed

Fig. 3-2. Chorionic epithelial cells filled with *B. melitensis*. Giemsa's stain. × 1550.

breaks in areas where the disease has not previously existed should be eradicated by identifying and slaughtering all infected and exposed sheep and goats, by cleaning, disinfecting, and resting infected premises, and by quarantining the infected area until no additional cases develop in test sheep and goats placed in the quarantined premises.

To prevent disease spread in endemic areas, attendants should maintain cleanliness, infected sheep and goats should be isolated from healthy animals, owners should avoid adding to the flock new sheep of questionable health status, communal pastures and ranges should be avoided, and all contaminated manure, bedding, feed, dead animals, and placentas should be buried or burned. Susceptible sheep should be immunized with live vaccine containing *B. melitensis* strain Rev 1, if available, or *B. abortus* strain 19. If possible, the vaccine should be applied before breeding and repeated annually. (In the United States, the use of *B. abortus* strain 19 and *B. melitensis* strain Rev 1 on sheep and goats is prohibited.)

Alessandrini, A.: Incidence of brucella infection in Italy with special reference to Arezzo Province. Ann. Hygiene, *48*:205-223, 1938.

Allsup, T.N.: Abortion in sheep associated with *Brucella abortus* infection. Vet. Rec., *84*:104-108, 1969.

Ariel, M.: On the morbid anatomy of abortion of sheep caused by *Brucella melitensis*. In *Brucellosis in Sheep*. Moscow. VIEM Publ. Dept., 1937a, pp. 129-149; 1937b, p. 176.

Biggi, P.: *Brucella melitensis* in the blood, milk and serum of experimentally infected sheep. Ann. Fac. Med. Vet. (Pisa), *9*:264-270, 1956a; 271-277, 1956b; 287-311, 1956c.

Bruce, E.A.: Brucellosis in sheep. JAVMA, *76*:841-842, 1930.

Dubois, C.: Rev. Vet., Toulouse, *35*:540, 1910.

Ebabi, A. and Zowghi, E.: The use of allergic test in the diagnosis of *Brucella melitensis* infection in sheep. Br. Vet. J., *139*:456-461, 1983.

El-Ghani, M., El-Hamid, S., Nada, S., and Osman, K.: Identification of species and biotypes of the Brucella genus in apparently healthy and aborted ewes and goats in Egypt. Int. J. Zoon., *11*:139-144, 1984.

Entessar, F., Ardalan, A., Ebadi, E., and Jones, L.M.: Effect of living Rev. 1 vaccine in producing long-term immunity against *Brucella melitensis* in sheep. J. Comp. Pathol., *77*:367-376, 1967.

Erdem, R., Williams, C.F., and Stableforth, A.W.: *Brucella melitensis* Rev. 1 vaccine experiments on the duration of immunity. Pendik Vet. Kontrol Ara. Enst. Derg., *2*:20-32; 33-38, 1969 (Abst. Vet. Bull., *40*:691, 1970).

Farina, R. and Biggi, P.: *Brucella melitensis* in the vaginal secretions of experimentally infected sheep. Ann. Fac. Med. Vet. (Pisa), *9*:278-283, 1956.

Huddleson, I.F.: *Brucellosis in Man and Animals*. New York, The Commonwealth Fund, 1943.

Itabashi, K., et al.: II. Epizootiological observations on the ovine brucellosis amongst sheep in Manchoukuo. J. Jpn. Soc. Vet. Sci., *16*:456-467, 1937 (Abst. Vet. Bull., *8*:136, 1938).

Ivanov, M.M.: Specific prophylaxis of sheep brucellosis. 17th World Vet. Cong. Proc., *1*:577-579, 1963.

Molello, J.A., Flint, J.C., Collier, J.R., and Jensen, R.: Placental lesions of sheep experimentally infected with *Brucella melitensis*. AJVR, *24*:905-911, 1963a.

Molello, J.A., Jensen, R., Collier, J.R., and Flint, J.C.: Placental lesions of sheep experimentally infected with *Brucella abortus*. AJVR, *24*:915-922, 1963b.

Mustafa, A., Roberts, R., and Corbel, M.: Isolation of *Brucella melitensis* from sheep in Syria. Vet. Rec., *117*:277, 1985.

Paltrinieri, S., Farina, R., and Andreani, E.: Vaccination trials against ovine brucellosis due to *Br. melitensis*, using strain Rev. 1. Zooprofilassi, *23*:241-262, 1968.

Renoux, G.: Vaccination des brebis contre l'infection à *Br. melitensis*. Arch. Inst. Pasteur (Tunis), *35*:251-274, 1958.

Renoux, G.: Brucellosis in goats and sheep. Adv. Vet. Med., *3*:250, 1957.

Shaw, W.B.: *Brucella abortus* infection in sheep. I. Field case. Br. Vet. J., *32*:18-27, 1976.

Stoenner, H.G.: Isolation of *Brucella abortus* from sheep. JAVMA, *118*:101-102, 1951.

Striter, V., Voskresenskii, B., and Kotljarova, H.: On the bacteriology of sheep brucellosis under natural and experimental conditions of infection. In *Brucellosis in Sheep*. Moscow. VIEM Publ. Dept., 1937, pp. 23-35.

Tarasov, I. and Versilova, P.: A bacteriological examination of the aborted fetus for the presence of *Brucella melitensis*. In *Brucellosis in Sheep*. Moscow. VIEM Publ. Dept., 1937, pp. 37-44; 69-93.

Taylor, R.M., Lisbonne, M., Vidal, L.F., and Hazemann, R.H.: Quelques notes epidemiologiques sur l'infection des chèvres et des brebis par *Br. melitensis*. Rev. Med. Vet., *90*:188-205, 1938.

Thoen, C.O.: Use of an enzyme immunoassay test for characterizing the A and M antigens of brucella. J. Clin. Microbiol., *9*:485-487, 1979.

Unel, S., Erdem, R., Williams, C.F., and Stableforth, A.W.: *Brucella melitensis* Rev. 1 vaccine. Res. Vet. Sci., *10*:254-259, 1969.

Van Drimmelin, G.C.: *Brucella melitensis* isolated from karacul sheep of southwest Africa. S. Afr. J. Sci., *49*:299-302, 1953.

Young, S.: Preliminary report on a brucella infection in a ewe. Vet. Rec., *65*:247-248, 1953.

Zammit, T.: *Report of Commission Investigation of Mediterranean Fever*. III. London, Harrison and Sons, 1905, p. 83.

Zdrodovskii, P.F.: Investigations of the VIEM expedition. In *Brucellosis in Sheep*. Moscow. Viem Publ. Dept., 1937.

Abortion from *Brucella ovis*

In most sheep-producing countries, *Brucella ovis* causes epididymitis and also abortion in New Zealand and the United States. Field outbreaks of the disease cause lamb losses from abortions and stillbirths varying from 2 to 20% and averaging approximately 9%. The ages of aborting ewes vary from 1 to 4 years.

Although the exact method of natural disease transmission has not been determined, recent research indicates some pertinent probabilities. A major source of the infecting bacteria probably is semen from rams affected with epididymitis. The intraconjunctival sac inoculation of ewes within 1 to 21 days after breeding interferes with conception, but inoculation of ewes either into the conjunctival sac or intravenously within 21 to 90 days after breeding results in placentitis, abortion, and stillbirth.

Either natural or induced infection from *B. ovis* has some characteristic features. Abortions occur during the third trimester of gestation, and the membrane surfaces between placentomes contain gross plaques of yellow-white exudate. Infected cotyledons easily detach from caruncles, and the chorioallantois is thickened with edema of interstitial tissue. When pregnant ewes are intravenously inoculated with viable *B. ovis,* the organisms are cleared from maternal lymph nodes, spleen, liver, lungs, kidneys, and mammary gland within 50 days, but the bacteria persist within the infected placenta and fetal stomachs.

Veterinarians diagnose the disease on the basis of placental lesions and laboratory findings. Large amounts of placental edema and plaques of exudate between placentomes in membranes from late gestation abortions have diagnostic significance. Smears of placental exudate, vaginal discharge, and fetal stomachs usually reveal the small, mildly acid-fast bacteria. In the laboratory, *B. ovis* can be isolated from infected cotyledons, interplacentomal plaques, uterine discharges, aborted fetuses, and stillbirths.

The high incidence of *B. ovis* ram epididymitis in large range flocks with concurrent abortions and weak lambs are indications of a *B. ovis* abortion problem. Sera of both rams and ewes should be tested with the enzyme-linked immunosorbent assay (ELISA) test for *B. ovis* antibodies. Abomasal contents and lung of the aborted fetus are the tissues of choice for attempted *B. ovis* isolation.

Since infected semen from rams affected with epididymitis is a likely source of *B. ovis* transmitted to ewes, the elimination from flock rams of all animals having clinical epididymitis and/or a positive titer for complement-fixing antibodies specific to *B. ovis* should protect ewes against exposure. Clean flocks should be protected against reinfection by avoiding the purchase and addition of diseased rams or diseased pregnant ewes.

Collier, J.R. and Molello, J.A.: Comparative distribution of *Brucella abortus, Brucella melitensis* and *Brucella ovis* in experimentally infected pregnant ewes. AJVR, *25:*930-934, 1964.

Hartley, W.J., Jebson, J.L., and McFarlane, D.: The artificial infection of sheep with brucella-like organism. N. Z. Vet. J., *2:*80-89, 1954.

Libal, M. and Kirkbride, C.: *Brucella ovis*-induced abortion in ewes. JAVMA, *183:*553-554, 1983.

McFarlane, D., Salisbury, R.M., Osborne, H.G., and Jebson, J.L.: Investigations into sheep abortions in New Zealand during 1950. Aust. Vet. J., *28:*221-226, 1952.

Meinershagen, W.A., Frank, F.W., and Waldhalm, D.G.: *Brucella ovis* as a cause of abortion in ewes. AJVR, *35:*723-724, 1974.

Molello, J.A., Jensen, R., Flint, J.C., and Collier, J.R.: Placental pathology. I. Placental lesions of sheep experimentally infected with *Brucella ovis*. AJVR, *24:* 897-904, 1963.

Osburn, B.I.: Pathologic and immunologic responses of the ovine fetus to *Brucella ovis*. Diss. Abst., *26:*2146, 1965.

Plant, J.W.: *Brucella ovis* infection and flock fertility. New South Wales Vet. Proc., *13:*36-38, 1977.

Salmonellal Abortion

(*SA; paratyphoid abortion; salmonellosis*)

Salmonellal abortion, an acute contagious disease characterized by metritis and abortion, is caused by salmonella serotypes of bacteria that commonly reside in the alimentary tracts of carrier animals and in contaminated feed and water. Although not common in any one geographic area, the disease probably exists in all sheep-producing countries and causes significant economic losses to the entire sheep industry. Financial waste results from abortions, stillbirths, deaths among newborn lambs and affected ewes, and damage to the wool of recovered sheep. The occurrence of salmonellosis among people as food poisoning and among feedlot lambs as acute dysentery adds both public health significance and economic importance to the disease.

OCCURRENCE. SA occurs in all breeds of ewes. Although most adult ages may be attacked, old ewes, because of encountering salmonellas and acquiring immunity, usually experience lower disease incidence than do young ewes. Animals in the third trimester, and especially the last month, are more susceptible than ewes in other stages of pregnancy. Most mammals and birds are susceptible, and some of these animals become symptomless carriers and excrete salmonella-infected feces.

SA usually occurs during those months when sheep reach the third trimester of pregnancy. In the United States, the disease develops during late winter and early spring because lambing is usually scheduled for those seasons.

Although veterinarians have diagnosed SA in Germany, Hungary, France, Britain, Cyprus, Italy, Yugoslavia, Australia, and the United States, the disease probably occurs in all countries where the sheep industry is prominent.

ETIOLOGY AND PATHOGENESIS. *Salmonella typhimurium, S. abortus ovis, S. montevidio,* and *S. dublin,* the usual causative serotypes, are not host-specific. They are widely distributed and commonly found in the alimentary tracts of sheep, cattle, and other animals and occasionally in contaminated feed and water. Gram-negative in staining affinity, these motile, aerobic, nonsporing bacilli measure 0.5 to 0.8 × 1 to 3 μm. They grow readily on many laboratory media and ferment glucose, maltose, mannitol, dulcitol, and sorbitol, but not lactose, saccharose, or salicin.

Factors that may increase ewe susceptibility to SA include several debilitating situations. Shipment over long distances and fasting for long periods may initiate the disease. Inclement weather may add to the ill effects of travel and hunger. Crowding and inadequate feeding during times of shearing, dipping, or other manipulative operations may expose ewes to large numbers of salmonellae in contaminated feed or water and result in a disease outbreak.

Since the pathogenesis of SA has received little scientific study, the details on the mechanism of disease development are largely conjectural. The causative organisms inhabit the alimentary tract and gallbladder of some normal but carrier sheep. Slowly growing and multiplying, the bacteria mix with feces and discharge to the exterior; other host animals, such as cattle, horses, rodents, poultry, and carnivorous birds, also may become carriers and excrete salmonella to the exterior.

The organisms spread by the migration of excreting carrier animals and by transport of contaminated feed and water. In the external environment, the bacteria are susceptible to the lethal effects of dehydration and sunlight, but they survive for many weeks in water and in moist soil, manure, and feed; along with these media, the organisms then enter the alimentary tracts of pregnant ewes.

In the small intestine, virulent salmonellal cells penetrate the mucous membrane. On invasion of the lymphatics, the bacteria enter Peyer's patches, mesenteric lymph nodes, and finally the systemic blood, which transports them to all organs. Colonization may occur in lymph nodes, spleen, liver, and placentas. In the hilar zone of the placentome, the organisms leave the maternal blood and enter the extravasated blood in the lacunae. The growing and multiplying bacteria penetrate chorionic epithelial cells, perhaps by active phagocytosis, and eventually enter the blood capillaries of the fetal circulation. Fetal septicemia results in necrosis, hemorrhage, and inflammation throughout most of the visceral organs. The infected fetus and/or ewe may die.

Fetuses may die in the uterus and become either abortions or stillbirths, or they may survive parturition as sick lambs that often die during the first week of life. Prenatal death probably results from necrosis of chorionic epithelial cells, interference to exchange of maternal nutrients and fetal excretions, shock, and fetal damage. Postnatal death of infected lambs results from pneumonia, toxemia, peritonitis, abomasitis, and starvation.

Most infected ewes recover. Following elimination of metritis, the ewe may carry and excrete salmonella-infected feces. After a few weeks to 4 months, most carrier ewes eliminate the inapparent infection and become immune. Fatalities among infected ewes result from septicemia, toxemia, metritis, and shock.

CLINICAL SIGNS AND POSTMORTEM LESIONS. Susceptible ewes in the third trimester of pregnancy may abort or bear stillborn lambs within 6 to 36 days after ingesting virulent *S. montevidio, S. typhimurium, S. abortus ovis,* or *S. dublin* in contaminated feed or water. Prior to abortion or stillbirth, affected ewes develop fever of 41 to 42°C, anorexia, and depression. Some, but not all, show diarrhea. A vaginal discharge may form a few days before and continue for a few days after abortion. In an outbreak of the disease the daily number of abortions and/or stillbirths is low during early stages, high during intermediate stages, and low again during terminal stages. Living lambs born with infection are weak, depressed, and recumbent and may be diarrheic. They do not nurse and usually die within 1 to 7 days of age. Affected ewes may also die either after abortion or without abortion. The herd outbreak usually extends through 10 to 15 days. The abortion and stillbirth rate ranges up to 60%, and an additional lamb mortality may also reach 10%. Usually 5 to 7% of aborting ewes die.

At necropsy, aborted or stillborn lambs and lambs that die during the first week of life evince signs of septicemia. The placental, fetal, and lamb tissues show edema and hemorrhage, and the swollen liver and spleen may contain pale foci of infection. Dead ewes evince acute metritis. If abortion or stillbirth has occurred, the swollen uterus usually contains retained placenta, necrotic tissue, and serous exudate.

Young ewes experimentally inoculated before breeding with *S. abortus ovis* resist reinfection during the second half of the ensuing pregnancy. Hence, yearling ewes exposed to reinfection when mass abortions had previously occurred are likely to be immune during the subsequent pregnancy.

DIAGNOSIS. Veterinarians diagnose SA on evidence of typical signs, characteristic lesions, and laboratory findings. The development of diarrhea in some aborting ewes and diarrhea in sick surviving lambs indicate the disease. Lesions of septicemia in both aborted lambs and fatally infected ewes provide further significant evidence. Smears from cotyledons and from peritoneal fluids of lambs may contain gram-negative bacilli. The isolation of salmonellae from maternal blood, feces, or vaginal discharge, and from placenta or fetal organs confirms the diagnosis. Serum from convalescent and recovered ewes agglutinates the isolated salmonella in dilutions varying from 1:50 to 1:2000.

The differential diagnosis requires consideration of other abortifacient diseases, including vibriosis, listeriosis, brucellosis, enzootic abortion, leptospirosis, and, in some areas, Rift Valley fever. Although some of these infectious diseases present suggestive signs and lesions, their positive diagnoses require isolation and identification of the specific cause or the demonstration of a rising titer of antibodies against specific organisms.

PREVENTION AND TREATMENT. Programs for preventing SA are based on sanitary principles that protect pregnant ewes from ingesting virulent salmonellae in contaminated feed and water. Feces from carrier animals, aborted lambs, and placentas as well as vaginal discharges are the main sources of infection. By applying the following procedures, losses from disease outbreaks may be averted or reduced:

1. Prevent contamination of feed and water with feces by avoiding feeding on the ground or watering from stagnant contaminated pools.

2. Prevent contamination of feed and water with rodent feces by controlling the numbers of rats and mice.

3. Avoid exposing susceptible ewes to public stockyards where salmonellae may be present.

4. Avoid crowding, shipping, and fasting of susceptible ewes.

5. Isolate aborting and discharging ewes from the main flock.

6. Dispose of infected dead fetuses, lambs, and ewes, and infected placentas and litter by incineration or deep burial in quicklime.

7. Vaccinate with salmonella bacterin before anticipated and unavoidable exposure of susceptible ewes to the disease.

Because extra labor is required and animal response is often disappointing, treatment of ewes for salmonellosis is usually unsatisfactory to both owners and veterinarians. Furacin and electrolytes added to the water may give some benefit. Until improvement has occurred, individual ewes should daily receive 10 mg of tetracycline per kg of body weight.

Baker, J.R., Faull, W.B., and Rankin, J.E.F.: An outbreak of salmonellosis in sheep. Vet. Rec., 88:270-277, 1971.

Bosworth, T.J. and Glover, R.E.: Contagious abortion in ewes. Vet. J., 81:319-334, 1925.

Bozinovic-Saljinski, T. and Gramatikovski, G.: Incidence of Salmonella abortus ovis infection in Macedonia (in Croat). Vet. Glasn., 14:251-253, 1960.

Dennis, S.M. and Armstrong, J.M.: Ovine abortion due to Salmonella typhimurium in western Australia. Aust. Vet. J., 41:178-181, 1965.

Gramatikovski, G., Dzekov, R., and Evtimov, I.: Salmonellosis in sheep and lambs in Macedonia. Vet. Glasn., 24:963-968, 1970.

Hunter, H.G., Carrigall, W., Matheson, A.D., and Scott, J.A.: An outbreak of Salmonella typhimurium in sheep and its consequences. Vet. Rec., 98:126-130, 1976.

Iliev, T., et al.: Significance of preliminary mass infection of flocks in the epidemiology of salmonella abortion in sheep. Nauchni and Trudove Vissh Veterinaromeditsinski Institut Sofia, 22:37-44, 1972.

Lesbouyries, Dadot, and Berthelon: Avortment paratyphique de la brebis. Bull. Acad. Vet. Fr., 86:318-321, 1933.

Linklater, K.: Abortion in sheep associated with Salmonella montevidio infection. Vet. Rec., 112:372-374, 1983.

Malyavin, A.G., Polnikova, A.N., and Fisenko, O.F.: Rearing young stock. Specific prophylaxis and therapy of salmonellosis in lambs and sheep. Trudy nauchnokontrol. Inst. Vet. Prepator, 12:272-280, 1964.

Manley, F.H.: Contagious abortion of sheep and goats in Cyprus. J. Comp. Pathol. Ther., 45:293-300, 1932.

Meinershagan, W.A., Waldhalm, D.G., and Frank, F.W.: Salmonella dublin as a cause of diarrhea and abortion in ewes. AJVR, 31:1769-1771, 1970.

Mlinac, F.: Infectious abortion among ewes in southern Serbia, caused by a microorganism closely related to Salmonella typhi. Vet. Arch., 8:362-372, 1938.

Pegreffi, G.: Avortement des brebis du aux B. paratyphique. Bull. Sez. Ital. Soc. Intern. Microbiol., 6:280-283, 1934.

Schermer and Erlich: Berl. Tieraerztl. Wochenschr., 37:171, 1921.

Shearer, G.C.: An outbreak of abortion in ewes due to Salmonella dublin. Vet. Rec., 69:693-695, 1957.

Smith, H.W. and Buxton, A.: Isolation of salmonellae from feces of domestic animals. Br. Med. J., 1:1478, 1951a.

Smith, H.W. and Buxton, A.: An outbreak of Salmonella schwartzengrund infection in poultry. J. Pathol. Bacteriol., 63:459, 1951b.

Suhaci, I. and Isopescu, I.: Paratyphoid abortion of ewes in Rumania. Arch. Vet., 29:17-27, 1937.

Suveges, T. and Toth, I.: Incidence of Salmonella abortus ovis in ewes in Hungary, Magy. Allatorn. Lap., 17:401-405, 1962.

Vickers, C.L., et al.: Paratyphoid dysentery and paratyphoid abortion in a flock of bred yearling ewes. JAVMA, 132:22-23, 1958.

Watson, W.A.: Salmonella dublin infection in a lambing flock. Vet. Rec., 72:62-65, 1960.

Campylobacteriosis

(Vibriosis)

Ovine campylobacteriosis, an acute contagious disease, is characterized by late abortions, stillbirths, and weak lambs and is caused by Campylobacter fetus subsp. fetus. As a result of its wide geographic distribution and high rates of abortion, the disease has major importance to the sheep industry and often causes severe financial waste to individual enterprises. Economic losses come from abortions during the last trimester of pregnancy, stillbirths, weak lambs, deaths among some aborting ewes, and from the cost of immunization. The occurrence of vibriosis in cattle and people adds both economic importance and public health significance to the malady.

OCCURRENCE. Campylobacteriosis occurs in all breeds of pregnant ewes held in partial or complete confinement. Animals in the third trimester of gestation, especially in the last month, are highly susceptible. Aborting ewes and animals extensively exposed to the organism during an outbreak do not abort the following year. Most outbreaks of vibriosis occur during spring months because for many flocks that is the time of scheduled parturition.

Geographically, vibriosis sporadically occurs in Iceland, Britain, Scandinavia, The Netherlands, USSR, Hungary, Greece, Iran, New Zealand, Ecuador, and America. In the United States, most outbreaks develop among flocks of the western states.

ETIOLOGY AND PATHOGENESIS. *Campylobacter fetus* subsp. *fetus,* a pleomorphic, curved or coccoid, motile, noncapsulating, nonsporing, granular, gram-negative bacterium, measures 0.2 to 0.5 × 1.5 to 5 μm in young cultures. On serum or blood agar in an atmosphere of 10% CO_2, it forms bluish raised colonies 1 to 3 mm in diameter. Cysteine and numerous other amino acids enhance growth. Organisms of serotype C form catalase but do not produce H_2S.

Eight genetically different variants of *C. fetus fetus* have been identified in New Zealand by restrictive endonuclease analysis, a new technique for typing bacteria. Serologic examination by the tube agglutination, protein A staphylococcus agglutination and gel diffusion tests show evidence for the existence of two major serogroups (A/B and C/D).

Pathogenic organisms in the environment are sensitive to drying, sunlight, and standard disinfectants. They are killed in 5 minutes at 58°C and are sensitive to streptomycin but resistant to bacitracin and polymyxin.

The serotypes pathogenic for sheep locate in the placenta, fetus, uterine exudate, and, following abortion in some ewes, in the alimentary tracts. They reside, between lambing seasons, in the gallbladders and intestines of carrier sheep and shed into the environment. Transmission of organisms between flocks occurs through movement of carrier sheep, contaminated equipment and caretakers, and carnivorous birds from infected to susceptible flocks. Transmission between members of a flock occurs following the first abortions. Aborting ewes discharge vast numbers of *C. fetus fetus* in the aborted tissues. The bacteria enter susceptible ewes by way of the alimentary tracts through contaminated feed and water, and through the practice of curious

Fig. 3-3.   Edema and necrosis in a cotyledon infected with *Campylobacter fetus*. × 0.7.

ewes nosing and licking aborted fetuses and placentas.

The pathogenesis of vibriosis begins when the causative organisms enter the alimentary tract of a susceptible ewe. The bacteria penetrate the mucosa at unknown points and establish a bacteremia, which persists 1 to 2 weeks. The blood transports the organisms to the gravid uterus, where they induce placentomal infection. At the hyalinized tips of the uterine septa, the bacteria pass through the walls of maternal capillaries, invade the extravasated blood in the lacunae, enter the cytoplasm of chorionic epithelial cells, and finally move into the fetal blood.

Most severely infected uteruses abort the damaged, dead, or weakened fetuses; the precise mechanism that initiates and executes abortion is not known. Some ewes die from retained dead fetuses and peritonitis. During and following abortion, some organisms localize in the gallbladder and produce carrier sheep. Recovered animals form specific agglutinins and are immune to new attacks for at least 2 years.

CLINICAL SIGNS AND POSTMORTEM LESIONS. The epidemiologic sequence starts in the last trimester of pregnancy with an index case or cases which abort contaminating the environment and exposing susceptible pregnant ewes. Following a 1- to 3-week incubation period numerous secondary cases develop and abort. Although most aborting ewes show no premonitory signs, some animals develop a genital discharge before and after abortion. Most aborting ewes rapidly recover, but some die from retention of dead fetuses, metritis, and peritonitis.

The morbidity among fully susceptible flocks ranges up to 70% and averages 20 to 25%. Approximately 5% of affected ewes die. Within a flock, abortions may occur over several weeks.

At necropsy, dead ewes show acute metritis, often with decomposing fetuses. Uterine fluids may discharge, through necrotic perforations in the wall, into the peritoneal cavity. Aborted and stillborn lambs frequently are swollen along the abdominal wall from the accumulation of sanguineous fluids beneath the skin and between muscles. Infected lambs that live a few days often contain discrete or confluent pale foci, 2 to 3 cm in diameter, in the liver. Fetal placentas, also thickened from blood-stained fluids, contain soft gray cotyledons (Fig. 3-3).

Histopathologic changes are concentrated in the hilar zones of placentomes. Septa show arteriolitis, necrosis, and leukocytic infiltration. Bacteria are abundant in extravasated blood of the lacunae. In advanced stages of the disease, colonies of C. fetus locate in the cytoplasm of chorionic epithelial and endothelial cells (Figs. 3-4 and 3-5).

DIAGNOSIS. Veterinarians diagnose vibriosis on evidence of typical signs, lesions, and laboratory findings. Multiple abortions among ewes in the last 6 weeks of pregnancy and subcutaneous edema of aborted fetuses sug-

Fig. 3-4. Photomicrograph of cotyledon infected with *C. fetus* subsp. *fetus* showing normal hyalinized tip of endometrial septum (a), inflammation and necrosis in septum (b), normal villus (c), and normal hemorrhage between septum and villus (d). HE stain. × 115.

Fig. 3-5. Chorionic villus containing colonies of *C. fetus* in epithelial and endothelial capillaries. Giemsa's stain. × 544.

gest vibriosis. A positive diagnosis, however, requires the identification of *C. fetus* in the infected tissues. Smears from uterine exudate, cotyledons, and fetal stomachs, differentiated in Ziehl-Neelsen stain or Giemsa's stain, should be examined for the curved organisms (Fig. 3-6). Culture of *C. fetus* from the fetal stomach or other tissues is necessary for a definitive diagnosis.

The differential diagnosis requires consideration of other abortifacient infections, such as brucellosis, listeriosis, enzootic abortion of ewes and salmonellosis; the diagnosis of these diseases requires laboratory identification of the causative organisms.

COMPOUNDS OR OTHER EFFECTIVE DISINFECTANT. Modifying the susceptibility of the host is the other alternative. A commercial vaccine is available in the U.S. and is recommended for use at breeding time. In situations of high exposure a second vaccination is recommended at the last trimester. Vaccination in face of an outbreak

with simultaneous antibiotic therapy will usually provide favorable control. The antibiotic regimen is daily injections of a penicillin-streptomycin preparation for 2 to 5 days or 400 mg/head/day of tetracycline in the feed for 5 days followed by 100 mg/head/day for the rest of the lambing period. The current state of the art in identifying antigenic variants of *C. fetus fetus* will aid in developing immunogens specific for the needs of a particular sheep population. Protective immunity established against a given strain may not be effective against different serotypes possibly explaining some vaccine failures.

Berg, R.L., Jutila, J.W., and Firehammer, B.D.: A revised classification of *V. fetus*. AJVR, *32*:11-22, 1971.

Bird, M., Stephens, D., Wall, E., and deLisle, G.: Serology of *Campylobacter fetus fetus* strains from four outbreaks of ovine abortion. N.Z. Vet. J., *32*:14-17, 1984.

Bryans, J.T. and Shepard, B.P.: Isolation of *Vibrio fetus* from feces of lambs and pen contact transmission of infection. Cornell Vet., *51*:376-383, 1961.

Bryner, J.H., Estes, P.C., Foley, J.W., and O'Berry, P.A.: Infectivity of three *Vibrio fetus* biotypes for gallbladder and intestines of cattle and sheep. AJVR, *32*:465-470, 1971.

Collins, D. and deLisle, G.: Typing of *Campylobacter fetus fetus* isolates from sheep abortions in New Zealand. N.Z. Vet. J., *33*:52-53, 1985.

Collins, D. and Ross, D.: Restriction endo-nuclease analysis of campylobacter strains with particular reference to *Campylobacter fetus fetus* subsp. *fetus*. J. Med. Microbiol., *18*:117-124, 1984.

Firehammer, B.D., Lovelace, S.A., and Hawkins, W.W.: The isolation of *V. fetus* from the ovine gallbladder. Cornell Vet., *52*:21-35, 1962.

Firehammer, B.D., Marsh, H., and Tunnicliff, E.A.: The role of the ram in vibriosis of sheep. AJVR, *17*:573-581, 1956.

Hoff, H.: Inoculation experiments with ovine *Vibrio fetus* strains on pregnant guinea pigs and pregnant heifers. Nord. Vet. Med., *5*:859, 1953.

Jensen, R., Miller, V.A., Hammerlund, M.A., and Graham, W.R.: Vibrionic abortion in sheep. I. Transmission and immunity. AJVR, *18*:326-329, 1957.

Jensen, R., Miller, V.A., and Molello, J.A.: Placental pathology of sheep with vibriosis. AJVR, *22*:169-185, 1961.

Lee, A.M. and Scrivner, L.H.: Experimental work upon recent outbreaks of abortion in ewes. AJVR, *2*:50, 1941.

Lee, A.M. and Scrivner, L.H.: An investigation of severe losses from abortion in ewes. JAVMA, *92*:68, 1938.

M'Fadyean, F. and Stockman, S.: Report of Departmental Committee on epizootic abortion. Board of Agriculture and Fisheries, 1913.

McFarland, D., Salisbury, R.M., Osborne, H.G., and Jebson, J.L.: Investigations into sheep abortion in New Zealand. Aust. Vet. J., *28*:221, 1952.

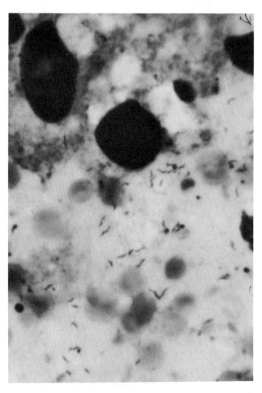

Fig. 3-6. Smear of uterine discharge showing *C. fetus*. Giemsa's stain. × 1200.

Marcis, A.: Contagious abortion of sheep. Allatorv. Lapok, 57:313, 1934.

Markovic B., Ilic, M., Trbic, B., and Olujic, M.: *Vibrio fetus* infection in sheep in Serbia. Vet. Glasn., *18*:519-521, 1964.

Marsh, H. and Firehammer, B.D.: Serological relationships of twenty-three ovine and three bovine strains of *V. fetus.* AJVR, *14*:396, 1953.

Meinershagen, W.A., Waldhalm, D.G., Frank, F.W., and Scrivner, L.H.: Magpies as a reservoir of infection for ovine vibriosis. JAVMA, *147*:343-345, 1965.

Miller, V.A. and Jensen, R.: Experimental *Vibrio fetus,* adjuvant vaccine. AJVR, *24*:65-68, 1963.

Miller, V.A. and Jensen, R.: Experimental immunization against ovine vibriosis. AJVR, *22*:43-46, 1961.

Miller, V.A., Jensen, R., and Gilroy, J.J.: Bacteremia in pregnant sheep following oral administration of *V. fetus,* AJVR, *20*:677-679, 1959.

Spiegl, A.: DTW, *33*:118, 1925.

Storz, J., et al.: Prevention of vibriosis, by vaccination. AJVR, *27*:115-120, 1966.

Veron, M. and Chatelain, R.: Taxonomic study of the genus *Campylobacter fetus* (Smith and Taylor) Sebald and Veron. Int. J. System. Bacteriol., *23*:122-134, 1973.

Wallace, G., McNerney, D., and Orbell, W.: Typing of *Campylobacter fetus fetus* isolated from sheep abortions in New Zealand. N.Z. Vet. J., *33*:107, 1985.

Welch, H. and Marsh, H.: Vibrionic abortion in sheep. JAVMA, *65*:203, 1924.

Leptospirosis

(*Icterohemoglobinuria*)

Leptospirosis is thought to be the most widespread zoonosis in the world with increasing public health significance for people in high risk occupations or recreational exposure to leptospiral contaminated surface water. In sheep leptospirosis is characterized by clinical responses ranging from the benign transient case to acutely severe cases with fever, hemolytic icterus, hemoglobinemia, hemoglobinuria, abortion, and death. Economic losses may occur in endemic areas from abortions, loss of production, deaths, and cost of preventive programs. The occurrence of leptospirosis in other domestic animals, especially cattle and swine, lend significant economic importance to the disease.

OCCURRENCE. Leptospirosis occurs worldwide in all breeds and sexes of sheep. The prevalence of leptospirosis is higher in younger animals. Epidemiologic studies indicate that cattle, swine, raccoon, opossum, hedgehog, and other wildlife species are the maintenance host or reservoir of leptospirosis with sheep being the accidental host. Serologic surveys show a higher prevalence of leptospiral antibodies in sheep in areas of high cattle populations. The ecologic and environmental relationships with the reservoir hosts directly influence the transmission and prevalence of leptospirosis in sheep.

ETIOLOGY AND PATHOGENESIS. Taxonomists classify all pathogenic leptospires in one species, *Leptospira interrogans,* with 160 leptospiral serotypes (serovars), which are subdivided into 21 serogroups. Isolations of 7 serovars from 5 serogroups have been made from livestock in the United States. The major serovars in the U.S. include pomona, hardjo, canicola, grippotyphosa, and icterohaemorrhagiae. The prevalence of a particular serovar differs from country to country and within countries due to climatic and ecological variations. Important serovars for sheep will be the ones of highest prevalence in cattle and the reservoir hosts.

Serovars are morphologically and culturally similar. Measuring $7.4 \times 0.1 \,\mu$m, these organisms each contain numerous coils and a hook at either or both ends, consist of a central axial filament surrounded by a protoplasmic cylinder and membrane, and differentiate with Giemsa's and Levaditi's stains. They grow in Korthof's and Stuart's fluid media enriched with 5 to 10% rabbit serum. In infected sheep, the organisms locate in blood and liver during leptospiremic stages and in the kidneys and urine during leptospiruric stages. Outside the animal body, they survive drying for 0.5 hour, freezing for 2 hours, soil-drying for 0.5 hour, and soil-water mixtures for 183 days.

Carriers of *L. hardjo, L. pomona* and *L. icterohaemorrhagiae,* the main causative serotypes of ovine leptospirosis, include cattle and swine and probably other species of domestic and wild animals. During leptospiruric stages, both bovine and porcine urines contain high concentrations of leptospires. Susceptible sheep cohabiting with infected cattle and/or swine, therefore, have ample opportunity for receiving the urinary leptospires directly through the skins and membranes or indirectly through contaminated feed or water.

Following exposure of sheep to pathogenic leptospires the organisms enter blood vessels and, for 3 to 5 days, produce leptospiremia, fever, and hemolysis. Plasma antibodies become detectable within 6 days of infection, reach peak titers in 10 days, and gradually diminish after 40 to 50 days. Because of early antibody production, the leptospires leave the blood within 5 to 10 days and localize in some convoluted tubules of the renal cortex. From these locations, the organisms shed into urine and void to the exterior. Leptospiruria may persist for 60 days, and in the absence of antibody titers.

CLINICAL SIGNS AND POSTMORTEM LESIONS. Following an incubation period of 5 to 7 days, body temperature rises to 42 to 43°C. Some sheep become depressed and decline feed. Because of hemolysis, the hemoglobin levels descend from normal values of 12 to 14 g/dl to pathologic values as low as 6 to 7 g/dl, hemoglobinuria develops, and icterus forms in varying degrees. Ewes in the last 8 weeks of pregnancy may abort. The morbidity may reach 25% among ewes and 50% among lambs, and the mortality among affected animals may be 60%.

At necropsy, pregnant ewes may show recent abortion or fetal death. Following subsidence of acute stages, the kidneys contain pale foci in the cortices. During leptospiremic stages, small numbers of organisms may be found in the liver and kidneys, and during leptospiruric stages large numbers may be in some convoluted and collecting tubules of the nephrons.

DIAGNOSIS. Veterinarians diagnose leptospirosis on evidence from signs, lesions, and laboratory findings. Fever, anemia, hemoglobinuria, icterus, and abortions strongly suggest the disease. Diagnostic confirmation includes: (1) isolation of leptospires from fetal or placental tissues or urine of the aborting ewe within about 14 days after abortion, (2) demonstration of the leptospires by darkfield microscopy, fluorescent antibody or histologic technique from the same tissues, (3) demonstrating maternal or fetal antibody titers by use of the microscopic agglutination microtitration test or the enzyme-linked immunosorbent assay test.

The differential diagnosis requires consideration of chronic copper poisoning, protozoan blood diseases, and abortifacient infections. Sheep with chronic copper poisoning show abnormally high levels of copper in the plasma and liver. Erythrocytic parasites can be identified in stained blood films. Abortifacient organisms, such as species of *Brucella*, *Campylobacter*, *Listeria*, and *Chlamydia*, can be isolated and identified in the laboratory.

PREVENTION AND TREATMENT. A prevention program is based upon a knowledge of the host-environment relationship and the prevalence of the disease in the area. Introduction of potential carriers should be prohibited. Separation of classes of livestock should be practiced. Any clinical cases should be isolated and treated with disinfection of contaminated areas. Sanitary feeding and watering practices will reduce the potential transmission. Many management systems do not lend themselves to such rigorous sanitary procedures, therefore increasing the resistance of the susceptible host by a vaccination regimen is necessary. To be effective the bacterin should be adequately potent and contain only serovars endemic in the area of use. These products are commercially available and can be used in a preventive program or in combination with antibiotics in a therapeutic program. Vaccination of an infected animal will reduce shedding but probably not eliminate shedding of the organism. Vaccination regimens will differ (frequency and time of vaccination) depending on the management and degree of contamination of the environment (usually at 6- or 12-month intervals). Treatment regimens are dictated by the value of the animals involved. Parental dihydrostreptomycin (25 mg/kg) given twice daily for 3 to 5 days or tetracycline in the feed (on a continuous basis for 2 to 3 weeks) to provide 200 to 400 mg/head/day to a 60 kg ewe are effective treatments. Electrolytes administered in the water or as a drench are helpful supportive treatments.

Alder, B., Faine, S., and Gordon, L.: The Enzyme-Linked Immunosorbent Assay (ELISA) as a serological test for detecting antibodies against *Leptospira interrogans* serovar *Hardjo* in sheep. Aust. Vet. J., *57*: 414-417, 1981.

Aliev, A.G.: Pathogenesis of leptospirosis in sheep. Veterinariia (Moscow), No. 4, 1959, pp. 41-42.

Andreani, E., Santarelli, E., and Diligenti, R.: Leptospirosis in sheep. Natural infection by the hardjo serotype. Ann. Fac. Med. Vet. (Pisa), *27*:33-40, 1975.

Beamer, P.D., Hardenbrook, H., Jr., and Morrell, C.C.: Studies on leptospirosis in domestic sheep. Vet. Med., *48*:365-366, 1953.

Biancifiori, F. and Cardaras, P.: Enzyme-linked immuno assay in the diagnosis of leptospirosis in domestic animals using peroxidase-conjugated protein A. Comp. Immun. Microbial. Infect. Dis., *6*:57-65, 1983.

Bokori, J., Kemenes, F., and Szemeredi, G.: *Leptospira pomona* infection in Hungary. Magy. Allatorv. Lap., *13*:352-354, 1958.

Chappell, V.E, Hanson, L.E., and Garrigus, U.S.: Leptospiral antibodies in sera from Illinois sheep. Cornell Vet., *51*:369-375, 1961.

Chulovskii, I.K.: Leptospirosis in western Siberia. Veterinariia (Moscow), No. 2, 1971, pp. 66-68.

Ellinghausen, H., Thiermann, A., and Sulzer, C.: *Leptospirosis in Diagnostic Procedures for Bacterial, Mycotic and Parasitic Infections.* 6th Edition. Edited by A. Balows and W. Hausler. Washington, D.C., Am. Public Health Assn., 1981.

Ellis, W., et al.: Possible involvement of leptospirosis in abortion, stillbirths and neonatal deaths in sheep. Vet. Rec., *112*:291-293, 1983.

Fraga de Azevedo, J. and Palmeiro, J.M.: First case of leptospirosis in Portugal. Bolm. Pecur, *32*:113-125, 1964.

Hansen, L. and Tripathy, D.: Research for resolution of leptospiral field problems. Proc. U.S. An. Heal. Assn., 192-202, 1981.

Hartley, W.J.: Ovine leptospirosis. Aust. Vet. J., *28*:169-170, 1952.

Hathaway, S., Wilesmith, J., and Little, T.: Some population parameters of *Leptospira interrogans* serovar hardjo infection in sheep. Vet. Rec., *114*:428-429, 1984.

Kingscote, B.: Leptospirosis in sheep in Western Canada. Can. Vet. J., *26*:164-168, 1985.

Kirkbridge, C.: Leptospiral abortions. Am. Assn. Vet. Lab. Diag., 54-76, 1984.

Marshall, R.B., Broughton, E.S., and Hathaway, S.C.: Protection of sheep by vaccination against artificial challenge with leptospira interrogans serovar hardjo. N.Z. Vet. J., *27*:195-196, 1979.

Morse, E.V., Morter, R.L., Langham, R.F., et al.: Experimental ovine leptospirosis. J. Infect. Dis., *101*:129-136, 1957.

Okazaki, W. and Ringen, L.M.: Effects of environment on survival of *L. Pomona*. AJVR, *18*:219-223, 1957.

Report of Leptospira Subcommittee. Stockholm. Int. Bull. Bact. Nomen. Taxon., *13*:159-160, 1963.

Sessi, P.: Incidence of leptospirosis of sheep and goats in Tuscany, Italy. Ann. Fac. Med. Vet. (Pisa), *10*:117-132, 1958.

Thiermann, A.: Leptospirosis immunization. JAVMA, *183*: 838-839, 1983.

Waitkins, S.: Update on leptospirosis. Br. Med. J., *290*: 1502-1503, 1985.

Toxoplasmosis

Toxoplasmosis has emerged as one of the most important zoonotic diseases involving sheep, humans, domestic cats, and other felidae.

Toxoplasmosis in the non-pregnant ewe is mild or asymptomatic and thus undiagnosed. The clinical effects in pregnant ewes are characterized by early embryonic death and resorption, fetal death and mummification, abortion, stillbirth, and neonatal death. Toxoplasmosis is the leading cause of abortion in many sheep producing countries, thus a disease of major economic significance to the sheep industry. In humans toxoplasmosis may be subclinical, can cause significant disease, or transplacental infections with congenital abnormalities when a woman is infected for the first time during pregnancy. The vast geographic distribution and the variety of susceptible hosts adds to the significance of this zoonotic disease.

OCCURRENCE. The domestic cat and other felidae are the only definitive hosts for the causative agent *Toxoplasma gondii*. Domestic and wild animals, rodents, and man serve as the intermediate and in most cases the dead end host. Most domestic animals and especially sheep are highly susceptible. Prevalence rates are higher where sheep cohabit in ecologic systems that have been contaminated with the environmentally resistant oocysts. Serologic surveys show that the prevalence of infection is influenced by management and rainfall, with a higher prevalence of infection in flocks kept under intensive or semi-intensive systems of management. Serologic surveys on cats and other animals in arid areas of Australia have been negative indicating that drying is not conducive to survival and transmission of the oocyst. The extreme difference between the rates of clinical cases and serologic cases in all host species indicates that disease, for the most part, goes undiagnosed. Clinical ovine toxoplasmosis is relatively common and is diagnosed more frequently as awareness increases and diagnostic techniques improve. The prevalence of toxoplasma antibodies is generally higher in sheep than other domestic animals which poses questions of species susceptibility and transmission. Toxoplasma and chlamydia are often found in the same placenta, which poses the possibility of a mechanism by which one organism potentiates the pathology of the other.

ETIOLOGY AND PATHOGENESIS. The life cycle of *Toxoplasma* has three basic forms (1) the proliferative form where the tachyzoites are found in a multitude of cells and corresponds to the parasitemic phase, (2) the encysted form where the bradyzoite is found in muscle, nerve, and other tissue in the form of a cyst with a well-defined parasitic membrane, and (3) the oocyst (the end product of gametogony), a zygote within a two-layered wall found in the feces of the definitive host and fecal-contaminated environments. Cats become infected by ingesting oocysts (from the contaminated environment), bradyzoites (tissue cysts from raw meat of infected animals or from tachyzoites (from ingestion of small mammals that are in the parasitemic or acute phase). The prepatent period (the time for development within the host to the release of the oocyst) varies according to the particular stage ingested, from 3 to 24 days. Nearly all cats shed oocysts after ingesting tissue cysts (bradyzoites) but 50% or less of the cats infected with the oocyst or tachyzoite stage will shed oocysts. Cats may eliminate a few thousand up to 260 million oocysts per day. Oocyst shedding occurs for 10 to 15 days in a young susceptible cat, immunity develops, and shedding ceases, although in some debilitating conditions and following corticosteroid administration shedding may recur. The unsporulated oocyst must sporulate, forming two sporocysts each containing four sporozoites to become infective. This usually takes 2 to 3 days. Sporulation requires an optimal temperature (20 to 38°C) and humidity; drying kills the cyst. Under an optimal environment of shade and moisture the sporulated, infective oocyst can survive for more than 1 year and if ingested by a susceptible cat the cycle starts again. The oocyst is also infective for the intermediate host. Reproduction in the definitive host is by gametogony (sexual reproduction within the epithelial cells on the tips of the villa of the small intestine called an enteroepithelial cycle) or in the definitive and intermediate host an extraintestinal cycle by endogeny (asexual reproduction by internal budding in the lamina propria, invasion of the lymphatics, dissemination to most organs and tissues via macrophages in the blood and formation of the tissue cyst containing the bradyzoites). These cysts produce little if any tissue reaction but they do elicit an antibody response which may last indefinitely.

Sheep, being herbivores, become infected by ingesting oocyst from feed or water sources contaminated by infected cat feces. The asexual extraintestinal reproductive cycle develops. The bradyzoites are distributed via the blood to tissues throughout the body but the pathologic damage to the gravid uterus and fetus is most significant. The effects depend upon the age of the fetus at the time of infection. In the first 2 months of pregnancy infection commonly causes embryonic death with resorption. Infections in mid-pregnancy (20 to 100 days) may cause death of the fetus with either mummification or abortion. If the fetus survives this period, it may be stillborn at term or weak and die within hours of birth. Ewes infected in late pregnancy (110 days to term) produce congenitally infected lambs.

CLINICAL SIGNS AND POSTMORTEM LESIONS. Up to 50% of adult sheep and 20% of feedlot lambs of the western U.S. have positive titers (1:64 or higher dilutions) by the indirect hemagglutination test. The clinical signs of toxoplasmosis correlate with affected organs. Ewes with encephalitis show circle walking, incoordinated movements, muscular rigidity, and prostration. With oculitis, they evince impaired vision and altered pupillary reflexes, and with metritis and placentitis they abort during the last month of pregnancy or bear stillborn and weak lambs. Congenitally infected lambs are mentally dull, physically weak, muscularly incoordinated, and unable to nurse. Death results from starvation.

On necropsy, gross changes are seen in placentas and fetuses. Some swollen cotyledons contain gray foci 1 to 2 mm in diameter

(Fig. 3-7), and some fetal brains show chalky areas of necrosis in the white matter of the cerebrums. Histopathologic changes consist of (1) cotyledonary necrosis, leukocytosis and toxoplasma tissue-cysts, and leukoencephalomalacia with tissue-cysts in the corpus callosum, septum pellucidum, internal capsule, and anterior cerebellar peduncles in fetuses, and (2) necrotizing granulomas with pseudocysts in retina, ciliary body, myocardium, diaphragm, liver, and kidney in adults.

DIAGNOSIS. Veterinarians diagnose toxoplasmosis on evidence of signs, lesions, and laboratory findings. Abortions during the last month of pregnancy and the presence of gray foci in the cotyledons strongly suggest toxoplasmosis. Positive diagnoses, however, require proof of the presence of toxoplasmas in infected placentas or fetal brains by inoculation of the tissues into mice, embryonating eggs or cell cultures, or by visualization of the parasite in sections of infected tissues with regular or fluorescent antibody stains. Positive complement-fixation, Sabin-Feldman cytoplasm-modifying antibody tests, indirect hemagglutination (IHA), or enzyme-linked immunosorbent assay (ELISA) assist in flock diagnosis of the malady.

The differential diagnosis requires consideration of all other abortifacient infections, such as listeriosis, brucellosis, vibriosis, enzootic abortion, leptospirosis, and salmonellosis; each of these diseases is diagnosed by identifying the specific causative organism or by demonstrating rising titers of antibodies specific to the particular causes.

PREVENTION AND TREATMENT. Veterinarians and producers reduce the amount of toxoplasmosis by avoiding contamination of sheep feed and water with cat feces and by preventing cats from eating raw meat.

Vaccines for sheep and cats are being investigated and may be useful tools in future preventive programs. Chemoprophylaxis in cats with 200 mg/kg monensin suppresses oocyst shedding and establishes an immunity to reinfection. Similar chemoprophylactic trials to prevent development of the disease in sheep have not been reported. Active or chronic infection of toxoplasmosis has been shown to have an immunosuppressant effect decreasing the effectiveness of other immunogens given during the time of infection.

Behymer, E., et al.: Epidemiologic study of toxoplasmosis on a sheep ranch. Am. J. Vet. Res., 46:1141-1144, 1985.

Beverley, J.K.A. and Mackey, R.R.: Ovine abortion and toxoplasmosis in East Midlands. Vet. Rec., 74:499-501, 1962.

Beverley, J.K.A. and Watson, W.A.: Ovine abortion and toxoplasmosis in Yorkshire. Vet. Rec., 73:6-11, 1961.

Beverley, J.K.A., Watson W.A., and Payne, J.M.: The pathology of the placenta in ovine abortion due to toxoplasmosis. Vet. Rec., 88:124-128, 1971a.

Beverley, J.K.A., Watson, W.A., and Spence, J.B.: The pathology of the fetus in ovine abortion due to toxoplasmosis. Vet. Rec., 88:177-178, 1971b.

Blewett, D.: The epidemiology of ovine toxoplasmosis. Vet. Ann., 25:120-124, 1985.

Blewett, D.: The epidemiology of ovine toxoplasmosis. I. The interpretation of data for prevalence of antibody in sheep and other host species. Br. Vet. J., 139:537-545, 1983.

Boniolo, A., Dovis, M., Malvano, R., and Zannino, M.: ELISA for specific anti-toxoplasma IgM antibodies: aspects related to serum interference. J. Immuno. Meth., 59:113-119, 1983.

Buxton, D., Gilmour, J., and Angus, K.: Perinatal changes in lambs infected with *Toxoplasma gondii*. Res. In. Vet. Sci., 32:170-176, 1982.

Fig. 3-7. Gray foci of necrosis and inflammation in cotyledon of ewe with toxoplasmosis. (Courtesy of Dr. J.W. Hartley)

Buxton, D., et al.: Immunosuppression in toxoplasmosis: studies in sheep with vaccines for chlamydia abortion and louping-ill virus. Vet. Rec., *109*:559-561, 1981.

Cole, C.R., Sanger, V.L., Farrell, R.I., and Kornder, J.D.: The present status of toxoplasmosis in veterinary medicine. North Am. Vet., *35*:265, 1954.

Dreesen, D.: The life cycle of *Toxoplasma gondii*: an illustrative view. Cont. Ed., *5*:456-560, 1983.

Dubey, J.P. and Frenkel, J.K.: Cyst-induced toxoplasmosis in cats. J. Protozool., *19*:155-177, 1972.

Frenkel, J.K., Dubey, J.P., and Miller, N.I.: *Toxoplasma gondii* in cats: fecal stage identified as coccidian oocysts. Science, *167*:893-896, 1970.

Frenkel, J.K., Dubey, J.P., and Miller, N.I.: *Toxoplasma gondii*: fecal forms separated from nematode *Toxocara cati*. Science, *164*:432-433, 1969.

Frenkel, J. and Smith, D.: Immunization of cats against shedding of toxoplasma oocysts. J. Parasitol., *68*: 744-748, 1982.

Frenkel, J. and Smith, D.: Inhibitory effects of monensin on shedding of toxoplasma oocysts by cats. J. Parasit., *68*:851-855, 1982.

Hartley, W.J. and Kater, J.C.: The pathology of *Toxoplasma* infection in the pregnant ewe. Res. Vet. Sci., *4*:326-332, 1963.

Hartley, W.J. and Marshall, S.C.: Toxoplasmosis as a cause of perinatal mortality. N.Z. Vet. J., *5*:119-124, 1957.

Hutchinson, W.M., Dunachie, J.F., Siim, J.C., and Work, K.: Coccidian-like nature of *Toxoplasma gondii*. Br. Med. J., Jan. 17, 1970, pp. 142-144.

Jakob-Hoff, R. and Dunsmore, J.: Epidemiological aspects of toxoplasmosis in southern western Australia. Aust. Vet. J., *60*:218-219, 1983.

Janitsche, K.: Experimental toxoplasmosis in the intestinal tract of cats. Zentralbl. Bakteriol. (Orig.), *218A*:517-524, 1971.

Koestner, A. and Cole, C.R.: Neuropathology of ovine and bovine toxoplasmosis. AJVR, *22*:53-66, 1961.

Konishi, E. and Takahashi, J.: Reproducible enzyme-linked immunosorbent assay with a magnetic processing system for diagnosis of toxoplasmosis. J. Clin. Microb., *17*:225-231, 1983.

Munday, B.L.: The epidemiology of toxoplasmosis in Tasmania. Aust. Dept. Agric., 1970, p. 95.

Nicolle, G. and Manceaux, L.: Infection à corps de Leishman du gondii. C. R. Acad. Sci., *147*:763-766, 1908.

Olafson, P. and Monlux, W.S.: Toxoplasma infection in animals. Cornell Vet., *32*:176-190, 1942.

Osborne, H.G.: Abortion in sheep associated with toxoplasma. Aust. Vet. J., *35*:424-425, 1959.

Ovedulve, J.P.: The probable identity of *Toxoplasma* and *Isopora*. T. Diergeneesk, *95*:149-155, 1970.

Piper, R.C., Cole, C.R., and Shadduck, J.A.: Ocular toxoplasmosis in animals. Am. J. Ophthalmol., *69*:662-676, 1970.

Plant, J., Freeman, P., and Saunders, E.: Serological survey of the prevalence of *Toxoplasma gondii* antibodies in rams in sheep flocks in New South Wales. Aust. Vet. J., *59*:87-89, 1982.

Rakhimov, T.Kh., et al.: Toxoplasmosis in animals. Nauchno-Issledovatelskii Vet. Inst. Samarkand SSR, 1971, pp. 15-16.

Sheffield, H.G. and Melton, M.L.: *Toxoplasma gondii* transmitted through feces without *Toxocara cati* eggs. Science, *164*:431-432, 1969.

Sikes, R.: Toxoplasmosis. JAVMA, *180*:857-859, 1982.

Weiland, G. and Dalchow, W.: Toxoplasmosis in animals in Turkey based on serology. Berl. Muench. Tieraerztl. Wochenschr., *83*:65-68, 1970.

Wilkins, M. and O'Connell, E.: Effect of lambing percentage of vaccinating ewes with *Toxoplasma gondii*. N.Z. Vet. J., *31*:181-182, 1983.

Work, K.: Toxoplasma transmission and life history. Acta. Path. Microbiol. Scand. (B), 1971, p. 51.

Locoweed Poisoning

(*Locoism*)

Locoweed poisoning is a chronic degenerative toxicosis of sheep, is characterized by behavioral deviations, sensory abnormalities, muscular incoordination, reduced weight, abortions, and fetal malformations. It is caused by chronic habitual consumption of certain species of locoweeds, common plants of western North America. Because locoweeds grow in vast range areas used for sheep, locoism can cause extensive financial waste in some years. Economic losses result from unthriftiness, deaths, abortions and fetal malformations. Further losses result from the inefficient use of range land heavily infested with locoweeds. Horses and cattle may also be poisoned by locoweeds. Overall, the locoweeds cause more widespread economic loss to the livestock industry in the western United States than any other group of poisonous plants.

OCCURRENCE. Locoism occurs in ewes of all breeds and ages of sheep, including fetuses, and may recur in the same animals. Outbreaks of the disease develop during late autumn, winter, and early spring in occasional years when climatic conditions support winter growth of locoweeds on winter ranges. Geographically, locoweeds grow in the plains and western states of the United States, and even though sporadic locoism occurs throughout the plant ranges, epizootic outbreaks usually develop among grazing sheep in mild-winter areas, such as may prevail at the valleys and low hills of the Colorado Plateau and Basin-Range geologic provinces. Many normal years may intervene between epizootics of a given area.

ETIOLOGY AND PATHOGENESIS. Two closely related genera of the family Leguminosae—*Astragalus* and *Oxytropis*—are responsible for locoism in livestock. Approximately 263 species of the 372 North American species of Astragalus and Oxytropis are known to be toxic. The nontoxic species provide useful livestock forage in semiarid areas. The precise means by which locoweeds cause disease is not fully understood, but the signs of poisoning in all probability relate to the effects of either the indolizidine alkaloids, nitro-containing glycosides, or selenium content of the plants. Rarely does a single species contain more than one of these toxic compounds. Table 3-2 classifies a few of the more common locoweeds as to their toxic components.

The nitro-containing astragalus species contain glycosides which are either metabolized in rumen to 3-nitropropanol (3-NPOH) or 3-nitropropionic acid (3-NRA) (Table 3-2). Species containing 3-NPOH (Miserotoxin) are generally more toxic than those containing 3-NPA, although the latter is present in greater quantity. Toxicity of these compounds is due in part to their ability to oxidize hemoglobin to methemoglobin. However, not all clinical signs of toxicity are due to the degree of methemoglobinemia suggesting other metabolites of 3-NPOH have toxic effects on the animal.

Cattle are severely poisoned with as little as 4.8 g/kg body weight of *Astragalus miser,* whereas sheep require 3 to 4 times this dose to develop toxicity. Rapid consumption of a toxic dose of the plant may cause sudden dyspnea and death, but if a toxic dose is consumed over a period of time, more recognizable signs of weakness, ataxia, and respiratory difficulty become apparent. Pregnant ewes may abort at any stage of gestation, or produce malformed lambs.

A second distinct neurologic syndrome occurs in sheep grazing Astragalus and Oxytropis species containing indolizidine alkaloids that resemble classical locoism encountered in horses and cattle habitually grazing locoweed. Swainsonine, the indolizidine alkaloid present in locoweeds and the cause of locoism, was first identified in the Australian Darling pea (*Swainsona canescens*). It is an inhibitor of alpha-mannosidase, a lysomal enzyme involved in oligosaccharide metabolism. When this enzyme is inhibited by Swainsonine, mannose-rich saccharides accumulate in lysosomes impairing cellular metabolism. Locoism is therefore essentially a lysosomal storage disease characterized histologically by the presence of cytoplasmic vacuoles in cells of the nervous system, liver, kidney, and lymphocytes.

TABLE 3-2. *Classification of Common* Astragalus *spp. According to Type of Toxin*

Selenium Accumulators	Indolizidine Alkaloids (Locoweeds)	Nitro-containing Glycosides[a]
A. bisulcatus	A. argillophilus	A. atropubescens (3-NPOH)
A. racemosus	A. bisulcatus	A. canadensis (3-NPA)
A. pectinatus	A. earlei	A. cibaria (3-NPA)
A. pattersonii	A. lentiginosus	A. convallarius (3-NPOH)
	A. mollissimus	A. diversifolius (3-NPOH)
	A. nothoxys	A. falcatus (3-NPA)
	A. pubentissimus	A. miser (3-NPOH)
	A. thurberi	A. pterocarpus (3-NPOH)
	A. wootonii	
	Oxytropis lambertii	
	Oxytropis sericea	
	(= O. lambertii var. sericea)	

[a] The glycosides are metabolized in ruminants to 3-NPOH or 3-NPA as indicated for each species in parentheses.

Animals must consume locoweed containing the indolizidine alkaloid swainsonine for several months before signs of toxicity develop. Sheep generally avoid eating locoweeds unless forced to do so under adverse situations. However, once sheep are accustomed to eating the plants, they will habitually and selectively seek out locoweeds, even in subsequent growing seasons. Signs of locoism develop when sheep consume 90% of their body weight in locoweed. Progressive neurologic degeneration characterized by depression, excitement when disturbed, loss of herding instinct, and abnormal behavior may be seen in affected sheep. Pregnant ewes may either abort or produce lambs with deformed limbs (carpal flexion). The most striking teratogenic effects of locoweeds occur when they are eaten by the ewe between 90 to 120 days of pregnancy, causing enlargement of the heart, spleen, and thyroid glands of affected lambs.

The third aspect of Astragalus toxicity relates to the accumulation of selenium in some species (Table 3-2). Chronic selenium toxicity as it occurs in other livestock is not commonly encountered in sheep. Acute selenium poisoning occurs sporadically in sheep that eat large quantities of selenium accumulator plants over a short period. In such cases sheep die acutely from respiratory failure. It is probable that the syndrome of selenium toxicity (blind staggers) historically attributed to eating selenium accumulating locoweeds is in fact due to the effects of either the indolizidine alkaloid or nitro-containing glycoside content of the plants, and not due to the selenium content.

Astragalus and Oxytropis species are perennial herbs with woody roots, pinnately compound leaves and racemose, pealike flowers ranging in color from white to purple (Fig. 3-8). Oxytropis species are differentiated by the distinctly pointed flower keel from which the common name "point locoweed" is observed. Variable numbers of kidney shaped seeds are produced in leguminous pods. The glycosides and alkaloids are present in greatest quantity in the leaves and remain stable in the dried plant.

Fig. 3.8. *Oxytropis sericea,* white locoweed.

Frequently sheep consuming locoweeds containing indolizidine alkaloid (Table 3-2) are observed to develop a higher incidence of pneumonia, keratoconjunctivitis, and foot rot. This may result from some impaired lymphocyte function and immunosuppression induced by lymphocytic vacuolization, present in locoweed toxicity.

CLINICAL SIGNS AND POSTMORTEM LESIONS. After several weeks of the animals' daily feeding on small amounts of locoweed, the clinical signs begin. In early stages affected sheep elevate their heads and move with a trotting gait. They concentrate their appetites on locoweeds and disregard other forages. As the disease progresses, animals weaken, lose weight, stumble, and fall. Vision and hearing are impaired, and disorientation finally supervenes. During terminal periods of recumbency, the limbs perform ambulating movements. Throughout the disease course, abortions of any gestational stage may occur. Serum aspartate aminotransferase activity increases. Up to 80% of pregnant ewes abort, and as many as 70% of fetuses, stillbirths, and lambs show anatomic malformations, such as variable amounts of contracted limb tendons, overextension of fetlock joints, rotation of the forelimbs, and small body size (Fig. 3-9). The morbidity ranges up to 50% and the mortality of affected sheep may reach 90%. The clinical course varies from one to several weeks.

At necropsy, affected ewes show emaciation but no specific gross lesions. Affected fetuses and lambs manifest various teratologic defects. Both ewes and lambs may reveal cytoplasmic vacuoles in neurons of the central nervous system, epithelial cells of renal convoluted tubules, epithelial cells of the thyroid gland, and chorionic epithelial cells of the placenta and lymphocytes.

DIAGNOSIS. Locoweed poisoning is diagnosed on evidence of grazing access to locoweeds, the manifestations of clinical signs, abortions, and congenital limb deformity in lambs. Vacuolization in peripheral blood lymphocytes and in tissues of the nervous system, heart, kidneys, thyroids etc. is characteristic of locoweed poisoning. The differential diagnosis requires consideration of other chronic intoxications.

PREVENTION AND TREATMENT. Producers prevent locoism by monitoring the winter growth of locoweed and avoiding the grazing of sheep in areas of weed stands. Providing supplementary feed, such as alfalfa pellets, may reduce hunger and the desire of sheep for green feed. Treatment consists of early exclusion of locoweed from the diets by relocating the animals where locoweed does not exist and substituting nutritious feed for the damaging weed.

Balls, L.D. and James, L.F.: Effects of locoweeds on reproduction of ewes. JAVMA, *162*:291-292, 1973.

Hartley, W.J. and James L.F.: Microscopic lesions in fetuses of ewes ingesting locoweed (*A. lentiginosis*): AJVR, *34*:209-211, 1973.

Huxtable, C.R. and Dorling, P.R.: Poisoning of livestock by Swainsona spp.: current status. Austr. Vet. J., *59*:50-53, 1982.

James, L.F.: Effect of locoweed (*A. lentiginosus*) feeding on fetal lamb development. Can. J. Comp. Med., *40*:350-354, 1976.

James, L.F.: Syndromes of Astragalus poisoning in livestock. J. Am. Vet. Med. Assoc., *158*:614-618, 1981.

James, L.F. and Hartley, W.J.: Effects of milk from animals fed locoweed on kittens, calves, and lambs. AJVR, *37*:1263-1265, 1977.

James, L.F., Hartley, W.J., Williams, M.C., and Van Kampen, K.R.: Field and experimental studies in cattle and sheep poisoned by nitro-bearing *Astragalus* or their toxins. Am. J. Vet. Res., *41*:377-392, 1980.

James, L.F., Shupe, J.L., Binns, W., and Keeler, R.F.: Abortive and teratogenic effects of locoweed on sheep and cattle. AJVR, *28*:1379-1388, 1967.

James, L.F. and Van Kampen, K.R.: Effect of locoweed toxin on rats. AJVR, *37*:845-846, 1976.

James, L.F., Van Kampen, K.V., and Hartley, W.J.: *Astragalus bisulcatus*—a cause of selenium or locoweed poisoning. Vet. Hum. Tox., *25*:86-89, 1983.

Kingsbury, J.M.: *Poisonous Plants of the U.S. and Canada.* Englewood Cliffs, N.J., Prentice-Hall, 1964.

Marsh, C.D., Clawson, A.B., and Eggleston, W.W.: Locoweed disease. USDA Farmer's Bull., 1936, p. 1054.

Mathews, F.P.: Locoism in domestic animals. Tex. Agric. Exp. Stat. Bull., *456*:1-27, 1932.

Molyneux, R.J. and James, L.F.: Loco intoxication: Indolizidine alkaloids of spotted locoweed (*Astragalus lentiginosus*). Science, *216*:190-191, 1982.

Sharma, R.P., James, L.F., and Molyneux, R.J.: Effect of repeated locoweed feeding on peripheral lymphocytic function and plasma proteins in sheep. Am. J. Vet. Rec., *45*:2090-2093, 1984.

Stermitz, F.R., Norris, F.A., and Williams, M.C.: Miserotoxin, a new naturally occurring nitro compound. J. Am. Chem. Soc., *91*:4599-4600, 1969.

Van Kampen, K.R. and James, L.F.: Sequential development of lesions in locoweed poisoning. Clin. Toxicol., *5*:575-580, 1972.

Van Kampen, K.R. and James, L.F.: Ophthalmic lesions in locoweed poisoning of cattle, sheep, and horses. AJVR, *32*:1293-1295, 1971a.

Van Kampen, K.R. and James, L.F.: Ovarian and placental lesions in sheep from ingesting locoweed. Pathol. Vet., *8*:193-199, 1971b.

Van Kampen, K.R. and James, L.F.: Pathology of locoweed poisoning in sheep. Pathol. Vet., *6*:413-423, 1969.

Fig. 3-9. Lamb with congenital deformity of anterior limbs from maternal intoxication by *A. pubentissimus*.

Williams, M.C. and James, L.F.: Poisoning in sheep from Emery milkvetch and nitro compounds. J. Range Manag., *29*:165-167, 1976.

Williams, M.C., James, L.F., and Bond, B.O.: Emory milkvetch (*Astragalus emoryanus var emoryanus*) poisoning in chicks, sheep and cattle. Am. J. Vet. Res., *40*:403-406, 1979.

Goiter

(*Iodine deficiency*)

Goiter, a subacute or chronic deficiency disease, is characterized by an enlarged thyroid gland and is caused by a deficiency of biologically available iodine, a trace mineral. The frequency of the disease is generally low because of the common practice of including KI in prepared salts and feeds, but it may still be high and wasteful in some individual enterprises. Economic losses accrue from unthriftiness, low reproductive efficiency, fetal and lamb deaths, and poor quality of wool. Occurrence of the disease in other domestic mammals and people adds economic importance and public health significance to the general malady.

OCCURRENCE.   Goiter develops in all breeds, sexes, and ages, but more often in adult ewes than adult rams, and more frequently in fetuses and lambs than in yearlings and older sheep. Geographically, it coexists with iodine-deficient soils, which generally are found in highland regions of the continents. In the Americas, deficient areas include the western provinces of Canada, the northeastern and northwestern states of the U.S., and the western states of Latin America, Venezuela, and Columbia.

ETIOLOGY AND PATHOGENESIS.   Goiter is usually caused by (1) inadequate intake of iodine in feed and water and (2) excessive consumption of goitrogenic compounds in plants.

Ionized iodine is absorbed through gastric and jejunal mucosae into the plasma, where it forms iodides. These compounds are distributed to all tissues and are actively concentrated and stored in the thyroid gland. Within gland follicles, the iodine oxidizes and combines with tyrosine to form monoiodotyrosine and diiodotyrosine. These two compounds couple together to produce the hormones triiodothyronine and thyroxine, which conjugate with proteins to form thyroproteins, mostly thyroglobulins, that accumulate in the colloid. As needed, the thyroproteins hydrolyze, and the released hormones pass into the blood, bind to globulins or albumins, and transport to cells for action. Eventually, about 80% of the iodine is removed from the hormones in the liver, with conservation and reuse of the iodine, but the remaining 20% is excreted in the bile. Iodides are excreted in the urine.

Deficient consumption of iodine results from a series of related events. Heavy rainfall gradually removes iodine from highlands, especially from areas with sandy soils. Heavy fertilization accentuates the deficiency. Soil deficiencies lead to plant deficiencies and then to animal deficiencies. Insufficient iodine in the feed and then in the plasma interrupts the accumulation or trapping of iodides in the thyroid and thus disables the synthesis of thyroid hormones.

Some forage plants contain antithyroidal compounds. Essentially, all species of *Cruciferae* (mustard family), as well as soybeans and peanuts, contain thiocyanates and other chemical radicals that prevent or reduce the trapping of iodides in the thyroid. In addition, plant goitrin, along with related compounds of thiourea and thiouracil, interferes with iodination of tyrosine and related chemical processes.

When goitrogenic factors—deficiencies or compounds—operate, the synthesis of thyroid hormones is suppressed. The resulting low blood level allows the anterior pituitary to release its thyroid stimulating hormone, which stimulates the thyroid to produce more of its hormones, and the strong effort results in follicular hyperplasia and glandular enlargement.

CLINICAL SIGNS AND POSTMORTEM LESIONS. Iodine deficiency induces a subnormal basal metabolic rate, generally with profound systemic effects. Growth rates and routine activities are depressed. The dry skin has poor-quality wool and hair, and the neck is variably enlarged in the laryngeal area. Adult rams show reduced libido and low semen quality. Ewes have irregular estrus and abnormal conception rates, and may resorb embryos, abort, or produce goitrous stillborn and weak lambs. Affected lambs have thick, scaly skin with sparse wool. The neck is thickened, in some cases bulging, and breathing may be difficult and noisy.

At necropsy, adult sheep show bilateral enlargement of the thyroid gland and, in advanced stages, edema in and around the gland. Glands may be enlarged by a factor of up to three. Neonatal lambs also have enlarged thyroids (Fig. 3-10) that are commonly edematous. These glands may be increased by a factor of up to ten or more. Body cavities may contain fluids, and anatomic deformities may be present. Histologically, thyroid follicles are lined with tall hyperplastic epithelial cells that invaginate into lumina. Colloid may be absent from some.

DIAGNOSIS. Veterinarians suspect goiter from evidence of typical signs and lesions, especially in animals residing in endemic regions, and they confirm the diagnosis histologically. The differential diagnosis requires

consideration of other, particularly infectious abortifacient diseases, avitaminosis-A, and neoplasms. For technical assistance from a diagnostic laboratory, practitioners should submit aborted, stillborn, and weak lambs.

PREVENTION AND TREATMENT. Producers prevent and treat deficiencies by providing adequate amounts of dietary iodine. Commonly, salt mixtures containing trace minerals are fed at the level of 0.5% of the diet and have approximately the following composition: NaCl, 97.00%; cobalt, 0.015%; copper, 0.023%, iodine, 0.070%; iron, 0.117%; manganese, 0.225%; sulfur, 0.040%; and zinc, 0.008%. The formula ingredient can be calcium iodate. Ewes feeding continuously on cruciferous goitrogens such as kale may require higher levels of iodine. Seriously goitrous neonatal lambs seldom respond to treatment.

Andrews, F.N., et al.: Iodine deficiency in new-born sheep and swine. J. Anim. Sci., 7:298, 1948.
Church, D.C. and Pond, W.G.: Basic animal nutrition. Corvallis, Ore., C.D. Church, 1974.
Furgeson, K.A., Schinckel, P.G., Carter, H.B., and Clarke, W.H.: Influence of thyroid on wool follicle development in lambs. Aust. J. Biol. Sci., 9:575, 1956.
Gross, J.: Iodine and bromine. In *Mineral Metabolism*. Part B, Vol. II. New York, Academic Press, 1962.
Kingsbury, J.M.: *Poisonous Plants of the U.S. and Canada*. Englewood Cliffs, N.J., Prentice-Hall, 1964.
Rudert, C.P. and O'Donovan, W.M.: Iodine supplementation of ewes grazing *Cynodon aethiopicus*. Rhod. J. Agric. Res., 12:141-148, 1974.
Wilson, J.G.: Hypothyroidism in ruminants with special reference to fetal goiter. Vet. Rec., 97:161-164, 1975.

AKABANE DISEASE

Akabane disease (AD) is an insect transmitted viral disease of sheep, goats, and primarily cattle characterized by a nonapparent disease in nonpregnant animals and abortions, hydroencephaly, arthrogryposis, microencephaly, and proencephaly of the fetus in the pregnant animal. AD has been reported since the 1940s in endemic areas of Australia and Japan with other reported incidences in Israel, Korea, Turkey, Kenya, and South Africa. The causal agent is a member of the simbu serogroup of Bunyaviridae and is transmitted by the insect vector *Culicoides breuitaris* and possibly other

Fig. 3-10. Dorsal view of lateral lobes (a) of the thyroid gland from a newborn lamb with fatal goiter.

culicoides and mosquitoes. Following transmission and the establishment of a viremia, the sheep host produces serum neutralizing antibodies and becomes immune in about 14 days with no apparent clinical signs.

In the pregnant ewe the virus becomes established in the placentoma tissue and is capable of infecting the fetus at the time of placental attachment (about 31 days of gestation). Viral invasion of the fetus can take place over an extended development period invading the rapidly dividing cells of the nervous system causing a wide range of developmental deformities. As the fetus gains immune competence (as early as 64 days) serum neutralizing antibodies are produced eliminating the virus. The virus is of low cytopathogenicity allowing the infected fetus to survive while producing developmental defects. The clinical syndrome may result in increased abortions with or without CNS developmental abnormalities or a decrease in the number of pregnant ewes at the expected lambing period. At parturition the lambs may exhibit arthrogryposis (fixed flexion or extension of one or more limbs), hydroencephaly (large portions of the brain replaced by fluid causing blindness and dummy lambs), and microencephaly causing a variety of neurologic disorders. The lesions may be mild to severe depending on the timing and severity of the viral attack and can produce a combination of developmental disorders.

Virus isolation is impossible at the time of full term parturition, therefore, diagnosis is based on the detection of precholesterol serum neutralizing antibodies from the lamb, serum from the dam, and pathologic evidence. Histologic examination of the brain and spinal cord reveals a diffuse loss of myelinated fibers from the lateral and ventral horn neurons and loss of nerve fibers from ventral spinal nerves aids in making a diagnosis. The condition must be differentiated from genetic, chemical, and plant teratogens.

Prevention is based on exposure of susceptible animals early in life or during a nonbreeding period. A killed vaccine is available in Japan and may be useful in endemic areas. New and susceptible introductions into an endemic area should be done prior to the breeding season to allow the immunity to be established during the nonbreeding period.

Della-Porta, A.: Akabane disease in sheep and goats. *Current Veterinary Therapy*. 2. Edited by J. Howard. Philadelphia, W.B. Saunders Co., 1986, pp. 526-527.

Akabane Disease: In *Merck Veterinary Manual*. 6th Edition. Rahway, Merck & Co. Inc., 1986, pp. 351-352.

Parsonson, I., et al.: Akabane virus infection in the pregnant ewe. 1. Growth of virus in the foetus and the development of the foetal immune response. Vet. Microb., *6*:197-207, 1981.

Parsonson, I., Della-Porta, A., and Snowdon, W.: Akabane virus infection in the pregnant ewe. 2. Pathology of the foetus. Vet. Microb., *6*:209-224, 1981.

4

DISEASES OF NURSING LAMBS

DISEASES OF THE DIGESTIVE SYSTEM

Hemorrhagic Enterotoxemia

An acute contagious toxemia of newborn lambs, hemorrhagic enterotoxemia is characterized by sudden deaths and hemorrhagic enterocolitis and is caused by beta toxin of *Clostridium perfringens* type C, a bacterium commonly residing in soil and manure. Since hemorrhagic enterotoxemia has a low incidence and a limited geographic distribution, the disease, even in endemic regions, has minor economic importance to the sheep industry. Some individual sheep enterprises, however, may experience considerable economic waste from the disease. Financial loss results from deaths of most affected lambs, mastitis in ewes of deceased lambs, and the cost of preventive programs and of disposal of dead lambs. Struck, a disease of adult sheep also caused by *C. perfringens* type C, is considered in Chapter 12.

OCCURRENCE. Hemorrhagic enterotoxemia occurs in all breeds and sexes of lambs. Animals 12 to 72 hours of age are highly susceptible; beyond that age, the morbidity rapidly diminishes and few lambs die. Most outbreaks develop in late winter and early spring during periods of cold, wet, and windy weather. Lambing sheds and barns, especially those facilities that have been used for lambing on previous and successive years, favor the disease. Lambs of ewes maintained on range or

large open pastures during parturition do not develop hemorrhagic enterotoxemia.

The known geographic distribution of the disease is limited to the western part of the United States, especially Colorado, Wyoming, and Montana. Since the causative organism is widely distributed in many sheep-raising countries, the disease probably could occur wherever newborn lambs, the organism, and environmental factors favor disease transmission and development. In addition to sheep, veterinarians have diagnosed hemorrhagic enterotoxemia among young calves and swine; in these animals, the disease has high incidence and considerable economic importance because most affected animals die.

ETIOLOGY AND PATHOGENESIS. *Clostridium perfringens* type C, the cause of hemorrhagic enterotoxemia, lives in soil, manure, and the alimentary tracts of some sheep and cattle. This anaerobic bacterium is a gram-positive, nonmotile, encapsulated, spore-bearing bacillus that measures 4 to 8 × 0.8 to 1.5 μm. The bacterium ferments most sugars except mannitol and produces both acid and gas. On the basis of toxin-antitoxin neutralization tests, the species is divided into 6 types: A, B, C, D, E, and F. The species produces 12 exotoxins, which are named with letters of the Greek alphabet. Each type produces one major toxin and one or more minor toxins. The major toxin of type C is beta toxin, which is necrotizing in effect. (For types, toxins, and diseases, see Table 6-1.)

73

Only fragmentary information is available on the pathogenesis of hemorrhagic enterotoxemia. The specific information on this disease, together with knowledge of related infections, however, enables the development of a plausible hypothesis on pathogenesis. Soil, manure, and equipment surfaces of lambing sheds and barns become heavily seeded with viable spores of C. perfringens type C. With strong resistance to drying and heat, these organisms endure in the environment through periods when pens are unused. When pregnant or parturient ewes enter the infected pens, the bacterial spores contaminate teats, lips, and other skin surfaces of the ewes.

They also contaminate the hands and instruments of laborers who care for the animals. In some enterprises, caretakers routinely open the lambs' mouths with either fingers or instruments and assist the animals with the first nursing. From ewes, caretakers, and pens, virulent bacteria soon move to the lips and mouths of the lambs. The mixture of ingested bacteria and large feedings of milk enters the stomach and eventually passes into the small and large intestines. Within these organs and acting on the milk substrate, the bacteria rapidly multiply and form beta toxin.

Because of its necrotizing effect, the toxin injures epithelial cells of the mucous membrane. Many cells undergo necrosis and slough into the gut lumen. Some blood capillaries rupture and produce hemorrhage. Leukocytes accumulate in the tissue. Under circumstances of intestinal injury, the beta toxin is absorbed into the blood and produces acute toxemia. Many vital neurons may be injured. In some lambs, the intestinal changes cause diarrhea; in this event, the loss of water, Na^+, Cl^-, K^+ and HCO_3^- through the fluid feces results in dehydration and acidosis. Shock, neuronal injury, dehydration, and acidosis cause early death.

Bacteria return to the exterior through infected feces and decomposing tissues, sporulate, and re-enter the soil. Immunized ewes accumulate specific antibodies in the colostrum, and during early feeding, the lambs ingest and absorb the antibodies in sufficient amounts for protection against the formation and action of the beta toxin.

CLINICAL SIGNS AND POSTMORTEM LESIONS. Following an incubation period of 12 to 24 hours, infected lambs decline feed, become depressed, develop tremors, and manifest abdominal pain. Some animals display diarrhea and physical weakness. Fluid feces usually contain small amounts of blood, which gives a brownish discoloration to the excretion. In advanced stages of the disease, the lambs convulse, pass into coma, and die.

The disease course varies from a few to 12 hours, and the morbidity ranges from 10 to 30%. Most affected lambs die. Lambs infected with sublethal amounts of bacteria and toxin may escape detection of signs, recover, and develop specific antibodies.

At necropsy, severe lesions are limited to the digestive system. The abomasum commonly contains considerable milk that may or may not be coagulated. Reddened from congestion and hemorrhages, the mucous membrane is covered with adherent mucus. From the exterior, the small intestine, especially the jejunum and ileum, the colon, and cecum appear red or dark brown from congestion and hemorrhage into the lumen (Fig. 4-1). Some discrete subserosal hemorrhages may be discernible.

On opening the gut, the fluid contents are stained brown or pink from hemorrhages. The swollen, necrotic, and hemorrhagic mucosa is rough and irregular. The mesenteric lymph nodes are swollen and reddened. Petechial hemorrhages may discolor the serosal surfaces of many organs, especially the subepicardium, subendocardium, and thymus. The pericardial sac usually contains an excessive amount of fluid and a few strands of fibrin. Beta toxin can be demonstrated in intestinal contents by injecting filtrate with and without neutralizing antitoxin into mice.

Histopathologically, the intestinal mucous membrane shows swelling, congestion, hemorrhage and necrosis. Numerous C. perfringens cells are in the contents as well as on the mucosal surface. In some lambs, extensive necrosis has destroyed many villi of the small intestine.

Fig. 4-1. Intestines from a lamb with hemorrhagic enterotoxemia. × 0.2.

DIAGNOSIS. Veterinarians diagnose hemorrhagic enterotoxemia on the basis of typical signs and lesions. Depression and short disease course in shed-confined lambs 12 to 72 hours of age strongly suggest the disease. At necropsy, the darkened and hemorrhagic intestines and the milk-filled stomach are significant findings. In the laboratory, the gram-positive *C. perfringens* bacteria are demonstrable in stained smears, and beta toxin in intestinal contents can be identified for confirming or establishing a diagnosis of the disease.

The differential diagnosis requires consideration of lamb dysentery, colibacillary diarrhea, and mechanical injury. For technical assistance from a diagnostic laboratory, practitioners should submit ileal and jejunal content cooled in a clean container, as well as affected intestine opened and fixed in 10% formalin.

PREVENTION. Veterinarians and owners prevent or reduce hemorrhagic enterotoxemia by immunization and sanitation. An effective commercial vaccine containing beta toxin antigen is readily available. The pregnant ewe should receive 2 inoculations, with the last administered 2 to 4 weeks prior to lambing. An annual booster is recommended. As an alternative to vaccination of ewes, lambs in an exposing environment should receive beta antitoxin at the time of birth. Moving pregnant and parturient ewes from infected facilities to a grazing range or open pasture avoids exposing the young lambs to large numbers of *C. perfringens* type C and thus may prevent the disease. After an outbreak of the disease in a lambing facility, the premise should be vacated, cleaned, disinfected, and rested at least several months before reuse. Infected manure and dead lambs should be incinerated or buried in quicklime.

Bailey, D.: Sheep flock health management. *Current Veterinary Therapy 2. Food Animal Practice*. Philadelphia, W.B. Saunders Co., 1986.

Griner, L.A. and Baldwin, E.M.: Further work on hemorrhagic enterotoxemia of infant calves and lambs. Proc. Meeting Am. Vet. Med. Assoc. 1954, pp. 45-50.

Griner, L.A. and Bracken, F.K.: *Clostridium perfringens* type C in acute hemorrhagic enteritis of calves. JAVMA, *122*:99-102, 1953.

Griner, L.A. and Johnson, H.W.: *Clostridium perfringens* type C in hemorrhagic enterotoxemia of lambs. JAVMA, *125*:125-127, 1954.

Colibacillosis

(*Escherichia coli infection*)

An acute and mildly contagious infection in young lambs, colibacillosis is characterized by gastroenteritis and/or septicemia and is caused by specific pathogenic strains of *Escherichia coli*, a species of bacteria commonly residing in the alimentary tracts of animals. Because of its wide geographic distribution and apparent increasing prevalence, the disease possesses considerable economic importance to the entire sheep industry and, in the future, may gain additional significance. Financial losses result from deaths among newborn lambs and mastitis among ewes of dead lambs, and from the cost of preventive programs such as sanitary lambing facilities, extra labor, and disposal of dead animals. Understanding the disease requires knowledge of its two clinical forms: enteric infection and septicemic infection.

OCCURRENCE. Colibacillosis of lambs occurs among flocks that lamb in facilities where crowding and unsanitation prevail. Habitually used lambing sheds that are not cleaned and disinfected between successive occupants are commonly associated with the disease. Sheep flocks that lamb in open uncrowded pastures and ranges do not develop colibacillosis.

All breeds and sexes of lambs are susceptible to the disease, but lambs 2 to 3 days of age more commonly develop the enteric form, and lambs 2 to 6 weeks of age commonly contract the septicemic form.

Although the disease may develop during any season, the prevalence is high among lambs born during late winter and early spring. Outbreaks are highly correlated with moist inclement weather. For this reason, lambs born during this seasonal period require protection against inclement weather.

The geographic distribution of colibacillosis is wide and may be increasing. In the United States, the disease occurs among flocks in the western states and possibly other states. In other countries, outbreaks have been reported in Britain, Australia, Argentina, Italy, New Zealand, and Russia.

ETIOLOGY AND PATHOGENESIS. *Escherichia coli* is ubiquitous in nature. It is a normal and beneficial inhabitant of the intestinal tract of man and domestic animals. Exposure of the susceptible animal to a pathogenic *E. coli* under ideal circumstances allowing the organism to attach and colonize on the lining of the intestinal tract produces clinical disease. Characterization of the organism is by a complex scheme of serotyping. There are 3 classes or types of antigen (O, K, and H). There are approximately 170 O antigens, 56 H antigens and 103 K antigens depending on the classifying techniques applied. The O antigens occur on the bacterial cell walls and the H antigens occur on the flagella. The K antigens are surface antigens of 2 types, acidic polysaccharides or proteins. The polysaccharide K antigens occur as capsular antigens with poor immunogenic properties. The proteinaceous K antigens exist as hair-like processes extending from the cell walls (pilus antigens). These

pilus antigens facilitate attachment to the intestinal mucosal surface and colonization which are necessary for pathogenicity. Some polysaccharide K antigens also enhance colonization. The pilus antigens (of which K99 and F41 are significant in sheep) are highly immunogenic and are important in inducing protective immunogenic responses during natural infections or after immunization. The *E. coli* organism is further characterized into: (1) enteropathogenic *E. coli* (EPEC), (2) enterotoxigenic *E. coli* (ETEC) and (3) enteroinvasive *E. coli*, each requiring serotyping or other techniques for identification. The enterotoxigenic strains of *E. coli* elaborate two enterotoxins, heat-stable (ST) and heat-labile (LT) toxins which either singly or together cause diarrhea. The ST fraction provides the pathogenicity in lambs. The enteric form of colibacillosis occurs in the first 24 to 48 hours of life when the newborn lamb receives an oral inoculation of enterotoxigenic *E. coli* (ETEC) organisms by nursing contaminated teats, nibbling contaminated pen litter, and from both the contaminated instruments and hands of caretakers who assist with the first nursing. The ETEC attach to the mucosal lining of the intestine, colonize, produce enterotoxins (the heat stable [ST] fraction is the pathogenic form for lambs) which penetrate the mucosal cells and cause fluid secretion into the intestine resulting in diarrhea. Colostrum deprived and stressed lambs which have not absorbed sufficient colostral antibodies are highly susceptible.

If the bacteria remain localized to the alimentary tract, the enteric form of colibacillosis develops, but if the bacteria invade the lymphatic system via the tonsils and enter the systemic blood, the septicemic form develops. In enteric colibacillosis, death results from severe dehydration, acidosis, shock, and possibly some toxemia. In septicemic colibacillosis, the organisms localize and produce lesions in joints and the central nervous system, especially meninges and brain, and these lesions cause death.

CLINICAL SIGNS AND POSTMORTEM LESIONS. Clinical signs in lambs affected with colibacillosis vary with the two disease forms. Lambs with enteric infection usually are born in a lambing building and manifest the beginning illness at about 24 to 36 hours of age. Initially, the feces become semifluid and yellow to gray in color; later, they become more fluid and are occasionally stained with blood. In an attitude of abdominal pain, the back is arched and the tail extended. Finally, the depressed and weakened lamb prefers recumbency and dies after a disease course of 24 to 36 hours. Morbidity may be high, and the mortality varies from 15 to 75% of affected animals.

Lambs affected with the septicemic form of colibacillosis vary in age from 2 to 6 weeks and usually come from a flock in which some lambs manifest diarrhea as a result of enteric form. Affected animals have a body temperature ranging from 41 to 42°C and show strong evidence of central nervous system involvement. During early stages of the disease course, the limbs of affected lambs may have stiff and uncoordinated movements. Often the head is deflected to one side, and vision is impaired.

After the early stages, depression supervenes, and the animal reclines continuously. The head extends in opisthotonos, and one or more limbs perform paddling movements. Some joints, especially of the limbs, may be swollen and painful. During terminal stages, the lamb becomes comatose and, because of beginning pneumonia, may breathe rapidly. During the time of clinical signs, the cerebrospinal fluid is opaque, and *E. coli* usually can be isolated from the fluid and blood.

At necropsy, the lesions also vary with the two forms of colibacillosis. In lambs affected with the enteric form, the tail and wool are stained and soiled with feces. Most tissues are severely dehydrated, and the lamb has lost weight. Internally, the primary lesions are in the alimentary tract. The abomasum, small intestine, especially the ileum, and large intestine contain considerable yellow to gray semifluid feces, and the tissues are congested and slightly swollen. The mesenteric lymph nodes are swollen and reddened. In some lambs, the lungs may show the beginning stages of pneumonia.

Lambs that have died from septicemic colibacillosis show evidence of generalized infection. The peritoneal, thoracic, and pericardial cavities may contain fibrin and excessive amounts of fluid. Some joints, commonly the elbow and carpal, are enlarged, and the synovial fluid is opaque and may contain flakes of fibrinopurulent exudate (Fig. 4-2). In the central nervous system, meninges of the brain are congested and may contain numerous small hemorrhages. Sulci over the cerebrum often contain conspicuous amounts of purulent exudate. Histopathologically, the affected peritoneal surfaces, joints, and meninges show hyperemia, hemorrhages, fibrinous or purulent exudate, and gram-negative bacteria. The inflammatory reaction may extend into the brain.

DIAGNOSIS. Veterinarians diagnose colibacillosis on the basis of typical signs and lesions and through laboratory findings. In lambs with enteric colibacillosis, the history of shed-lambing and the development of fatal diarrhea in animals 1 to 4 days of age represent

Fig. 4-2. Infected hock joint from a lamb earlier affected with acute colibacillosis. × 0.8.

significant evidence. At necropsy, the yellow-gray fluid of the small and large intestines also indicates the disease.

In the laboratory, virulent strains of *E. coli* can be isolated from the intestines and sero-typed. In lambs affected with septicemic coli-bacillosis, the fever, lameness, and central nervous system disturbances in lambs 2 to 6 weeks of age constitute strong evidence of the disease. At necropsy, finding peritonitis, arthritis, and/or meningo-encephalitis gives further evidence. The existence of diarrhea among young lambs in the affected flock also adds to the collective indication of colibacillosis. Laboratory confirmation is obtained by isolating and identifying virulent strains of *E. coli*.

The differential diagnosis requires consideration of lamb dysentery, hemorrhagic enterotoxemia, and enterotoxemia of suckling lambs.

PREVENTION AND TREATMENT. Veterinarians and producers prevent colibacillosis among lambs by applying standard principles of sanitation. Whenever weather conditions permit, parturition should take place in open uncrowded pastures, fields, and ranges. This practice tends to avoid exposure of newborn lambs to most pathogens, including *E. coli*.

Under some circumstances of weather, however, the lambs must receive protection during the first few days of life. Lambing facilities should possess built-in portability or should be easily cleaned and disinfected. The building should be properly ventilated to avoid excessive amounts of condensing moisture from accumulating in the interior; floors should be kept dry. At the end of a lambing season, the facility should be cleaned and disinfected and, if possible, moved to a new location and exposed to direct sunlight. During a lambing season, the individual pens within the facility should be cleaned and disinfected between uses by successive occupants.

Caretakers should wear rubberized gloves and boots and should clean and disinfect them before moving between individual pens and lambs. All sick lambs and ewes should be isolated from the main flock and lambing facility, and all dead lambs and ewes as well as con-

taminated manure and bedding should be incinerated or deeply buried in quicklime.

In large shed operations where sanitary conditions may be compromised due to time, labor, and weather conditions protection of the lamb can be attained via colostral antibodies. The ewe should be immunized twice 2 to 4 weeks apart with the last immunization at least 2 weeks prior to parturition with a vaccine containing K99 and F41 antigens. These vaccines have been shown to be effective. To obtain maximum protection from colostral antibodies the lamb must receive colostrum within the first 1 to 2 hours of birth. If the lamb has had a difficult and delayed delivery, is weak or exposed to hypothermia, it will delay the time from delivery to nursing or reduce the absorption of colostrum from the gut. In these cases the ewe should be milked and the colostrum administered via a stomach tube. A 14-gauge French catheter and bulb syringe works well for this procedure. Strict sanitary procedure must be followed. The catheter should first be measured and marked to assure that when inserted the tip is in the rumen. Inserting the catheter is done by gently passing the catheter in the space between the incisors and the premolars, over the base of the tongue and down the esophagus. The catheter can be palpated with the fingers as it passes down the esophagus. Once in place one should aspirate on the free end of the catheter. If properly placed the esophagus or rumen will cover the holes in the catheter making it impossible to aspirate air. Aspiration of air through the catheter indicates that it is in the trachea. The newborn lamb should receive from 60 to 120 ml of colostrum within the first 2 hours of birth. Bovine colostrum from a cow that has been immunized with K99, F41 and clostridial antigens will provide a good source of passive protection if the ewe's colostrum is inadequate or not available. The donor cow should be immunized, with the desired antigens, twice 2 to 4 weeks apart with the last immunization about 4 weeks prior to parturition. Collect only the first milking and freeze into 30-ml aliquots (ice cube size) and store in a plastic container in the freezer to be used at lambing time. Thaw gradually in warm water (do not microwave). Many producers treat colibacillosis with 1 ml of spectinomycin or other antibiotic orally with good results. The key to success of this treatment is early diagnosis and prompt treatment before the actual scours appear. The first sign producers notice may be a slight depression.

Botes, H.J.W.: Fatal enterobacterial septicemia in lambs. J. S. Afr. Vet. Med. Assoc., 37:17-25, 1966.

Clarkson, M., Faall, W., and Kerry, J.: Vaccination of cows with clostridial antigens and passive transfer of clostridial antibodies from bovine colostrum to lambs. Vet. Rec., 16:467-469, 1985.

Ducket-Suchaux, M., Bertin, A., DeRycke, J., and Lechopier, P.: Experimental Escherichia coli diarrhea in colostrum deprived lambs. Ann. Rec. Vet., 13:259-266, 1982.

Giovanelli, D.N., et al.: Colibacillosis in lambs. Gac. Vet., 21:147-152, 1959.

Gregory, D., Cardella, M., and Myers, L.: Lamb model in the study of immunity to enteropathogenic Escherichia coli infections. Am. J. Vet. Res., 44:2073-2076, 1983.

Hughes, L.E., Heath, G.B.S., and Barr, M.: Disease associated with E. coli in lambs. Vet. Rec., 74:350-351, 1962.

Kater, J.C., Davis, E.A., Haughey, K.G., and Hartley, W.J.: Escherichia coli infection in lambs. N.Z. Vet. J., 11:32-38, 1963.

Klipstein, A.: Escherichia coli enterotoxins and cross-linked toxoid vaccines. Proc. Path. Sc. GB and Ireland. I, 1985.

Marsh, H. and Tunnicliff, E.A.: Dynasty of newborn lambs. Montana Agric. Exp. Stat. Bull., July, 1938, p. 361.

Mondini, S.: Outbreak of Escherichia coli infection in lambs. Atti Soc. Ital. Sci. Vet., 17:683-684, 1963.

Phillips, R.W. and Knox, K.L.: Water kinetics in entire disease of neonatal calves. J. Dairy Sci., 52:1664-1668, 1969.

Phillips, R.W., Lewis, L.D., and Knox, K.L.: Alterations in body water turnover and distribution in neonatal calves with acute diarrhea. Ann. N.Y. Acad. Sci., 176:231-243, 1971.

Rees, T.A.: Studies on Escherichia coli of animal origin. II. Escherichia coli from young lambs. J. Comp. Pathol. Ther., 68:399-401, 1958.

Roberts, D.S.: Further observations on E. Coli disease in lambs. Aust. Vet. J., 34:152-156, 1958.

Roberts, D.S.: Escherichia coli infection in lambs. Aust. Vet. J., 33:43-45, 1957.

Rowe, B.: Serotyping and approaches to enterotoxin detection. Proc. Path. Soc. B and Ireland. I, 1985.

Shaw, W.B.: Escherichia coli in newborn lambs. Br. Vet. J., 127:214-219, 1971.

Sojka, W.J.: Enteric diseases in newborn piglets, calves and lambs due to Escherichia coli infection. Vet. Bull. 41:509-522, 1971.

Sutton, E.G. and Gee, B.D.: Escherichia coli infection in lambs. Vet. Rec. 75:390, 1963.

Terlecki, S. and Shaw, W.B.: Escherichia coli infection in lambs. Vet. Rec., 71:181-182, 1959.

Terlecki, S. and Sojka, W.J.: The pathogenicity for lambs of E. coli of certain serotypes. Br. Vet. J., 121:462-470, 1965.

Volkova, A.A.: Bacterium coli infection in lambs, Tr. Uzbek, Nauch, 9:48-58, 1938 (Vet. Bull., 10:578, 1940).

Lamb Dysentery

(Bloedpens)

Lamb dysentery, an acute contagious toxemia of newborn sheep, is characterized by short course, diarrhea, and ulcers in the small intestine and is caused by toxins from anaerobic bacteria commonly residing in soil. Because of its limited geographic distribution, the disease has minor importance to the sheep industry, but because of local severity, it may cause heavy financial losses in endemic regions. Some sheep enterprises may lose as many as 20 to 30% of lambs in a flock. The routine vaccination of ewes in endemic areas, however, has reduced the incidence to insignificance.

OCCURRENCE. Lamb dysentery occurs in lambs of all breeds and sexes. During initial outbreaks on a property, the disease attacks lambs 1 to 3 days of age; with successive years of existence on the same property, it occurs in animals up to 2 weeks of age. Although the disease may develop during any season, high incidence occurs during late winter and spring, especially when accompanied by considerable precipitation. Geographically, the malady occurs in Britain, South Africa, and possibly Kenya. Even though the disease has been suspected in the United States, convincing clinical and laboratory evidence has not been reported.

In addition to lambs, the malady rarely occurs in calves and foals.

ETIOLOGY AND PATHOGENESIS. Clostridium perfringens type B, the cause of lamb dysentery, lives in soil, manure, and the alimentary tracts of some animals. This anaerobic bacterium is a gram-positive, nonmotile, encapsulated, sporing bacillus that measures 4 to 8 × 0.8 to 1.5 μm. Except for mannitol, the bacterium ferments most sugars and produces both acid and gas. On the basis of toxin-antitoxin neutralization tests, the species is subdivided into 6 types: A, B, C, D, E, and F. The species produces 12 exotoxins named with Greek letters. Each type produces one major toxin and possibly one or more minor toxins. The major toxin of type B is beta toxin, a necrotizing substance.

Accumulated information makes possible an hypothesis for pathogenesis. The causative bacteria reside for long periods in the soil of infected properties and numerically concentrate around corrals and lambing facilities. From the soil, organisms contaminate feed and water and enter the alimentary tracts of ewes; some of these animals become carriers and excrete the organisms to the exterior.

During the first few days following birth, the bacteria enter the alimentary tracts of susceptible lambs by contaminating teats of the ewes, hands of caretakers, and faces of the newborn sheep. In the small intestine, especially the ileum, the organisms multiply and colonize in microscopic breaks or crevices of the mucosa. In these areas, the bacteria produce beta toxin, which causes expanding necrosis around each infected focus. Detachment of some necrotic tissue produces ulcers measuring 1 to 2 mm in diameter. Injury by toxin to surrounding capillaries results in hemorrhage at the periphery of each ulcer.

Bacterial and toxinal irritation to the intestines increases peristaltic movements and results in diarrhea. In calf diarrhea, a similar disease, the fluid feces contain bacteria, water, Na^+, Cl^-, K^+, HCO_3^-. After a disease course of a few days, the infected calves lose an average of 12% of their total body water, and 50% of the lost water comes from the plasma. The loss of water results in severe dehydration, and the loss of HCO_3^- results in acidosis. Death comes from shock, toxemia, dehydration, and acidosis.

The bacteria return to the soil through feces and decomposed tissues. In the few surviving lambs, the intestinal ulcers heal, and the beta toxins and other toxins provoke the formation of specific antitoxins, which protect hosts against subsequent attacks. Lambs born to immunized ewes ingest sufficient antibodies contained in the colostrum for passive and temporary immunization.

CLINICAL SIGNS AND POSTMORTEM LESIONS. According to degrees of severity, lamb dysentery is classified into four forms: acute, subacute, chronic, and mild. The acute form prevails during the first few lambing seasons after a property becomes infected. Onset of the disease is sudden, and flock masters find dead lambs without having observed their illnesses. Sick lambs separate from other sheep, decline feed, and prefer recumbency. Manipulation is painful. The fluid feces are yellow, but become brown from the presence of blood. After a short course, coma supervenes, and the lambs die. Morbidity varies up to 30%, and mortality is nearly 100% of affected lambs.

The subacute form of lamb dysentery develops in most lambs after a property has experienced the disease on each of several successive lambing seasons. Some lambs, however, continue to contract the acute form of the disease. Affected lambs separate from the flock, tend to immobilize and recline, and decline feed. When forced to walk, affected lambs arch their backs and display pain. The dehydration of skin and eyes becomes prominent. The fluid feces, yellow in early stages, become brown and may contain discernible blood. The severely depressed lamb passes into terminal coma before dying. The morbidity is high, and nearly 100% of affected lambs die. Chronic lamb dysentery occurs on farms after many successive years of the disease on the property.

At necropsy, the entire carcass, as well as individual organs, is dehydrated, and feces soil the tail and wool. The small intestine, especially the ileum, is congested and usually contains multiple ulcers, each 1 to 2 mm in diameter. A zone of hemorrhage surrounds each ulcer, but only rarely does an ulcer perforate the gut wall.

DIAGNOSIS. Veterinarians diagnose lamb dysentery on the basis of typical clinical signs, postmortem lesions, and laboratory findings. Persisting and fatal diarrhea, short clinical course, and small ulcers with peripheral hemorrhage have diagnostic significance. In the laboratory, scientists confirm or establish a diagnosis by isolating *C. perfringens* type B and identifying beta toxin in ileal contents.

PREVENTION. An effective vaccine is commercially available and should be administered to pregnant ewes in endemic areas. Two doses with an interval of 4 to 6 weeks may be necessary for the first immunization. The maternal antibodies accumulate in the colostrum and, during early feedings, transfer to the lambs. Sanitary management practices help to avoid or reduce the disease. The environment of the lambs should be kept clean and dry; caretakers with contaminated hands or instruments should avoid opening lambs' mouths. Relocating pregnant ewes, just prior to parturition, to clean facilities reduces exposure of the young lambs to *C. perfringens* type B. All dead lambs should be incinerated or buried in quicklime.

Dalling, T.: Anaerobic infections of sheep. Vet. Rec., *48*:1477-1480, 1936.

Dalling, T., Mason, J.H., and Gordon, W.S.: Lamb dysentery prophylaxis. Vet. J., *84*:640-648, 1928a.

Dalling, T., Mason, J.H., and Gordon W.S.: Lamb dysentery prophylaxis. Vet. Rec., *40*:532, 1928b.

Gaiger, S.H. and Dalling, T.: Bacillary dysentery in lambs. J. Comp. Pathol. Ther., *36*:120-125, 1923.

Gaiger, S.H. and Dalling, T.: Bacillary dysentery in lambs. J. Comp. Pathol. Ther., *34*:79-105, 1921.

Henning, M.W.: *Animal Diseases in South Africa.* South Africa, Central News Agency, 1956, pp. 465-474.

Hepple, J.R.: Necrotic enterotoxemia in a calf due to *Clostridium perfringens* type B. Vet. Rec., *64*:633-634, 1952.

Montgomerie, R.F. and Rowlands, W.T.: "Lamb dysentery" in a foal. Vet. Rec., *49*:398-399, 1937.

Phillips, R.W. and Knox K. L.: Water kinetics in enteric disease of neonatal calves. J. Diary Sci., *52*:1664-1668, 1969.

Phillips, R.W., Lewis, L.D., and Knox, K.L.: Alterations in body water turnover and distribution in neonatal calves with acute diarrhea. Ann. N.Y. Acad. Sci., *176*:231-243, 1971.

Walker, J.: Annual Report, Dep. of Agriculture, Kenya, 1922-1923.

Wilsdon, A.J.: Relationship of *"Bacillus ovitoxicus"* (Bennetts) to the *Clostridium welchii* group. Third Ann. Rep. Univ. of Cambridge Instit. Anim. Pathol., 1933.

Enterotoxemia of Suckling Lambs

(*Pulpy kidney disease; milk colic; dirt-eating disease*)

An acute infectious but noncontagious disease of suckling lambs, enterotoxemia is characterized by sudden deaths, convulsions, and hyperglycemia and is caused by anaerobic bacteria commonly found in soil and manure. Because the disease has wide geographic distribution and attacks the fattest lambs of the flock, enterotoxemia has considerable importance to the sheep industry. Economic losses result from deaths of rapidly growing and fattening lambs and from mastitis that may form in lactating ewes following the loss of young lambs.

OCCURRENCE. Enterotoxemia of suckling lambs occurs in all breeds and sexes, but more commonly among ewe than wether lambs, and almost exclusively in single rather than in twin lambs. Young sheep consuming mothers' milk, supplementary concentrate feed, and succulent young forage are highly vulnerable to attack. Usually, only rapidly growing and excellently conditioned animals are affected. Although all ages of suckling lambs are susceptible, uncastrated and undocked animals 3 to 8 weeks of age have the highest incidence. Other susceptible species include kids and probably calves.

The seasonal incidence is higher during spring and early summer, especially when rainfall or irrigation has provided sufficient moisture for fast growth of nutritious plants.

Geographically, enterotoxemia occurs in New Zealand, Australia, England, Wales, Tasmania, and probably South Africa. In the United States, it occurs among lambs on pasture and range in Colorado, Wyoming, Oregon, California, Texas, and probably other states.

ETIOLOGY AND PATHOGENESIS. *Clostridium perfringens* type D, the cause of enterotoxemia of suckling lambs, lives in soil, manure, and the alimentary tracts of animals. This anaerobic bacterium is a gram-positive, nonmotile, encapsulated, spore-bearing bacillus that measures 4 to 8 × 0.8 to 1.5 μm. Except for mannitol, the bacterium ferments most sugars and produces both acid and gas. On the basis of toxin-antitoxin neutralization tests, the species is subdivided into 6 types: A, B, C, D, E, and F. The species produces 12 exotoxins, which are named with Greek letters. Each type produces one major toxin and possibly one or more minor toxins. The major toxin of type D is epsilon prototoxin, which is converted to lethal epsilon toxin by trypsin. For the types, toxins, and diseases, see Table 6-1.

Although some aspects of enterotoxemia are unknown, sufficient information exists to support an hypothesis on pathogenesis. Spores of *C. perfringens* type D reside in soil and manure for prolonged periods, and soils around corrals, feedlots, bedgrounds, and watering and feeding facilities become heavily seeded with the organisms. Along with contaminated feed and water, as well as soil eaten by lambs, the spores enter the alimentary tracts. Some viable organisms pass through the stomachs into the small intestines. Under normal circumstances, the bacteria slowly multiply and form small amounts of epsilon toxin.

Ordinarily, peristaltic movements propel the contents to the exterior and thus prevent high concentrations of bacteria and toxin from accumulating in the gut. Rapidly growing and fattening lambs, however, consume large quantities of milk, succulent grass, and supplementary feed concentrate such as grain. Under these circumstances of overeating, some particles of undigested food pass through the abomasum into the small intestine.

In the ileum, the vegetative cells of *C. perfringens* type D, acting on the starch substrate, rapidly multiply and swiftly form epsilon prototoxin. Trypsin converts prototoxin into epsilon toxin, which may attain concentrations of 10,000 mouse-minimum-lethal-doses per gram. These high concentrations slow intestinal mobility and enhance intestinal permeability, and such changes facilitate the passage of toxin into blood capillaries of the portal system. Glucosuria results from passage of sugar from the plasma into the urine.

In many affected lambs, injury to vital neurons and shock cause death. Sublethal doses of toxin stimulate the production of specific antibodies in the surviving animal. Along with feces and decomposing tissues, the bacteria pass to the exterior, form spores, and re-enter the soil. Surgical operations such as docking, castrating, and marking cause discomfort, and this circumstance prevents or retards overeating, a necessary factor in the development of enterotoxemia. For this reason, castration stops outbreaks of disease in male lambs. Some producers maintain that losses seldom occur after docking and castrating.

CLINICAL SIGNS AND POSTMORTEM LESIONS. The course of illness in suckling lambs affected with enterotoxemia is short and may develop during the night; consequently, husbandmen commonly find the dead lambs during morning inspections. Occasionally, however, producers and veterinarians observe sick lambs through the entire disease course. Affected animals separate from the flock and, during warm weather, seek the shade. Respirations are rapid and may include oral breathing. Saliva drips from the mouth, and the body temperature elevates. The animal alternates between standing and recumbency and may manifest abdominal pain. Short, repetitive convulsions with intervening periods of depression are common. Finally, coma supervenes, reflexes cease, the limbs paddle, and the lamb dies.

The disease course commonly lasts 1 to 2 hours, but may occasionally extend to 12 hours. Morbidity averages 5 to 10%, but in some flocks may be as high as 30%. Most affected lambs die.

At necropsy, the abomasum contains a large amount of undigested feed and may include ingested dirt. The gastric mucous membrane may be congested and spotted with small hemorrhages. The subserosa of the intestines, thymus, lung, or diaphragm and the subepicardium and subendocardium often contain numerous small hemorrhages. The pericardial sac is distended by clear fluid containing strands of fibrin. The lungs contain fluid and congested blood. The fluid contents of the ileum contain demonstrable toxin, and smears reveal numerous vegetative cells of *C. perfringens*.

DIAGNOSIS. Veterinarians diagnose enterotoxemia of suckling lambs on the basis of typical signs and lesions. Sudden unexpected deaths in excellently conditioned lambs, convulsions, and a short course are important suggestive signs. At necropsy, a large amount of undigested feed in the abomasum, distention of the pericardial sac with clear fluid, and hemorrhages on the heart and thymus are characteristic findings.

The urine contains glucose. In the laboratory, scientists confirm the diagnosis by identifying epsilon toxin in contents of the ileum or in the blood. As soon as possible after death of the lamb, samples for laboratory study should be removed from the ileum, placed in a clean glass container, and refrigerated.

The epsilon toxin of *C. perfringens* type D is identified by the mouse intravenous neutralization test or by counter immunoelectrophoresis. *C. sordellii* is being isolated with increased frequency in lambs with enterotoxemia.

The differential diagnosis requires consideration of blackleg, anthrax, and cyanogenic plant poisonings.

PREVENTION. Flocks that encounter losses from enterotoxemia should start an immunization program in the ewes prior to lambing. Initially it is necessary to immunize the ewes with a good *C. perfringens* type D toxoid twice 2 to 4 weeks apart, the last immunization to be given about 4 weeks prior to lambing. After this initial sensitizing procedure an annual booster given about 4 weeks prior to lambing will assure maximum antibody production and concentration of these protective antibodies in the colostrum. With the increasing frequency of *C. sordellii* in cases of enterotoxemia and problems with other clostridia in some flocks, it may be advisable to incorporate these into an immunization program. Excellent results have been obtained from using commercial products which contain as many as 8 clostridial antigens. To receive maximum protection the newborn lamb must receive and absorb the colostral antibodies in the first couple of hours of life. Care should be taken to see that the ewe has adequate milk at lambing time and the lamb is able to stand and nurse within the first hour or two. A detailed description on the passive transfer of antibodies from cows colostrum and the procedure for providing colostrum to the weak or hypothermic lamb is given under the colibacillosis section.

Bennetts, H.W.: Infectious entero-toxemia of sheep in Western Australia. Council for Scientific and Industrial Research Bulletin, 57, 1932.

Bosworth, T.J. and Glover, R.E.: The effect of *Clostridium welchii* on the substance present in the normal intestine. Fourth Rep. Dir. Instit. Anim. Pathol. Cambridge, 4:79, 1934-1935.

Boughton, I.B. and Hardy, W.T.: Infectious enterotoxemia (milk colic) of lamb and kids. Tex. Agric. Exp. Stat. Bull. No. 598, 1941.

Boughton, I.B. and Hardy, W.T.: Infectious enterotoxemia of young lambs. Tex. Agric. Exp. Stat. Forty-Ninth Ann. Rep., 1936, pp. 278-279.

Bullen, J.J.: Enterotoxemia of sheep. J. Pathol. Bacteriol., 64:201-206, 1952.

Bullen, J.J. and Batty, I.: Experimental enterotoxemia of sheep. J. Pathol. Bacteriol., 73:511-518, 1957.

Bullen, J.J. and Scarisbrick, R.: Experimental reproduction of enterotoxemia in sheep. J. Pathol. Bacteriol., 73:495-509, 1957.

Clarkson, W., Faull, W., and Kerry, J.: Vaccination of cows with clostridial antigens and passive transfer of clostridial antibodies from bovine colostrum to lambs. Vet. Rec., 116:467-469, 1985.

Dayfus, C.V.: Vaccination of ewes against "pulpy kidney" (infectious enterotoxemia) in lambs. N.Z. J. Agric., 54:65-70, 1937.

Dayfus, C.V.: Vaccination of ewes against "pulpy kidney" (infectious enterotoxemia) in lambs. N.Z. J. Agric., 52:289-292, 1936.

Gill, D.A.: Infectious enterotoxemia and *Clostridium welchii* in lambs. N.Z. J. Sci. Tech., 18:106-119, 1936.

Gill, D.A.: Report on pulpy kidney disease of lambs. N.Z. Dep. Agric. Ann. Rep., 1933, pp. 30-49.

Gill, D.A.: Pulpy kidney disease of lambs. N.Z. J. Agric., 42:300, 1931.

Gilruth, J.A.: Acute renal congestion (pulpy kidney) in plethoric lambs. N.Z. Dep. Agric. Fifteenth Rep., 1907, pp. 387-389.

Gordon, W.S., Stewart, J., Holman, H.H., and Taylor, A.W.: Blood changes and post mortem findings following injection of sheep with culture filtrates of *Cl. welchii* types A, C and D. J. Pathol. Bacteriol., 50:251-269, 1940.

Harshfield, G.S., Cross, F., and Hoerlein, A.B.: Further studies on overeating (enterotoxemia) of feedlot lambs. AJVR, 3:86, 1942.

Henderson, T.: The detection of *Clostridium perfringens* type D enterotoxin in the intestinal contents of animals by counter immunoelectrophoresis. N.Z. J. Sci., 27:423-426, 1984.

Hepple, J.R. and Chodnik, K.S.: Immunization of lambs against *Cl. welchii* type D enterotoxemia with purified toxoid. Vet. Rec., 71:201-207, 1959.

McGowan, B.: Effect of constant intake of chlortetracycline on pneumonia, enterotoxemia and production in nursing lambs. JAVMA, 130:350-352, 1957.

Montgomerie, R.F. and Rowlands, W.T.: Pulpy kidney disease of young lambs in North Wales. Vet. J. 87:401-410, 1931.

Muth, O.H.: Control of pulpy kidney disease of lambs. JAVMA, 104:144-147, 1944.

Oxer, D.T.: "Pulpy kidney" in lambs. Commonwealth of Aust. Coun. Sci. Ind. Res. Pamphlet No. 35, 1932.

Popoff, M.: Bacterial examination in enterotoxemia of sheep and lamb. Vet. Rec., 114:324, 1984.

Richards, S. and Hunt, B.: Clostridium sordellii in lambs. Vet. Rec., 111:22, 1982.

Roberts, R.S.: Braxy-like diseases of sheep. Vet. Rec., 50:591-604, 1938.

Stewart, J.: High protein diet and renal disturbance in young lambs. Vet. J., 85:209, 1929.

Wilsdon, A.J.: The relationship of "Bacillus ovitoxicus" (Bennetts) to the Clostridium welchii group. Third Ann. Rep. Univ. of Cambridge Instit. Anim. Pathol., 1933.

Wilsdon, A.J.: Observations on the classification of Bacillus welchii. Univ. of Cambridge Instit. Anim. Pathol. Second Rep., 1931.

Nematode Gastroenteritis

(Helminthosis; gastrointestinal parasitism)

Gastrointestinal parasitism is primarily a disease of grazing sheep of all ages. At least 10 genera of nematodes develop in the gastrointestinal tract of sheep. Table 4-1 compares the morphologic difference of these 10 genera from the abomasum, small intestine, and large intestine of sheep.

A number of factors will determine if the disease is subacute, acute, or chronic. In general, younger sheep are more susceptible to acute infections, whereas chronic infections are more common in older sheep. Sheep grazing pastures in warm wet regions are more susceptible to heavier infections than sheep grazing pastures in hot and/or arid regions. Sheep on a good plane of nutrition can also withstand the harmful effects of parasitism far better than sheep in a poor plane of nutrition. Immunity to gastrointestinal parasitism in sheep is slow to develop, and may not be fully expressed until 1 year of age, making young animals more susceptible to acquiring heavy infections than older animals.

Economic losses in sheep production are manifested in a number of ways. Gastrointestinal parasitism causes a reduction in food intake, liveweight gains and wool growth in all ages of animals. In lactating ewes there is a decrease in milk production. In heavily parasitized animals there may be a high mortality, especially in young animals. The cost incurred in treating and controlling parasitic infections also adds to the cost of production.

OCCURRENCE. To understand the occurrence of gastrointestinal infections in sheep, it is necessary to be knowledgeable regarding the epidemiology of infections. All gastrointestinal nematodes produce eggs which are passed in the feces of infected sheep. These eggs, except for nematodirus, hatch into first stage larvae L_1 which molt into second stage larvae (L_2) and into infective third stage larvae (L_3). Under optimal conditions this entire free living cycle takes place in 7 to 10 days. At temperatures above 10°C (50°F) larval development is prolonged and at temperatures below 5°C (41°F) development ceases. The egg and L_3 will, however, withstand moderate freezing and can overwinter in most temperate climates. At temperatures above 25.8°C (78.4°F) most of the infective larvae on the pastures are destroyed.

Infective larvae remain trapped in the fecal material until there is adequate moisture for their migration onto the pastures. Infective larvae only migrate a short distance from the fecal material, 10 to 20 cm. Movement of infective larvae further from the fecal material occurs when the fecal material is broken up and spread by farm equipment, animal hooves, or flood irrigation. Moist infective larvae are present on the herbage in the early part of the day when the dew is on the grasses. At this time the larvae can migrate up the herbage for a short distance and sheep are capable of grazing them off.

Once the infective larvae (L_3) are ingested, development to the fourth (L_4) and fifth (L_5) larvae (young adults) takes place in 15 to 22 days for most gastrointestinal parasites (prepatent period). At this time mating occurs and eggs are again passed in the feces.

The development from the L_4 to L_5 can, however, be delayed for weeks to months (arrested development or hypobiosis). Hypobiosis occurs when conditions in the environment

TABLE 4-1. *Important Species of Gastrointestinal Helminths*

Anatomic Location	Names		Dimensions		
	Scientific	Common	Adults (mm)	Spicules (mm)	Eggs (μm)
abomasum	Haemonchus contortus	large stomach worm	F 18–30 M 10–20	0.46–0.50	70–85 × 41–48
	Ostertagia circumcincta	medium stomach worm	F 10–12 M 7–8	0.28–0.32	80–100 × 40–50
	Trichostrongylus axei	stomach hairworm	F 4–6 M 3–5	r 0.08–0.09 l 0.11–0.15	79–92 × 31–41
small intestine	Trichostrongylus colubriformis	intestinal hairworm	F 5–7 M 4–5	0.13–0.15	79–101 × 39–47
	Nematodirus spathiger	thread-necked worm	F 15–23 M 10–15	0.7–1.21	175–260 × 106–110
	Cooperia curticei	small intestinal worm	F 5–6 M 4–5	0.13–0.14	63–70 × 30–32
	Strongyloides papillosus	threadworm	F 3–6 M 3–6	—	40–60 × 20–25
	Bunostomum trigonocephalum	hookworm	F 19–26 M 12–17	0.6–0.7	79–97 × 47–50
large intestine	Oesophagostomum columbianum	nodular worm	F 15–21 M 12–17	0.8–0.9	73–89 × 34–45
	Chabertia ovina	large-mouthed bowel worm	F 17–20 M 13–14	1.3–1.7	90–105 × 50–55
	Trichuris ovis	whipworm	F 35–70 M 50–80	5.0–6.0	70–80 × 30–42

are not favorable for the survival of the free living stages. In the northern temperate regions of the United States, in Britain and in western Europe hypobiosis occurs in the late fall and winter due to the cool weather. In the southern United States and northern Africa hypobiosis occurs during the hot dry weather of the summer months. Hypobiosis is an extremely important epidemiologic phenomenon because it allows the parasite to survive adverse weather conditions which would destroy most of the free living stages. It also allows for the development of new infections and is responsible for the biggest source of pasture contamination during the next grazing season. Hypobiosis occurs to a marked degree with *Haemonchus, Ostertagia,* and *Nematodirus,* but to a lesser degree with *Trichostrongylus.*

ETIOLOGY. Although 10 genera of gastrointestinal nematodes infect sheep, only 3 genera,

Haemonchus, Ostertagia, and *Trichostrongy-lus,* are major pathogens. In some areas in England *Nematodirus battus* can be a major pathogen in young lambs. This parasite has recently been reported in sheep from western Oregon.

Although sheep commonly are simultaneously infected by several genera, each type is herein separately considered.

1. *Haemonchus contortus.* This widely distributed worm, a major metazoan pathogen of sheep 2 to 24 months of age, inhabits the abomasum, and feeds by sucking blood from the mucosa. Clinical hemonchosis develops during wet summers and early autumns. Free-living stages of the life cycle begin with expulsion of eggs in feces to the exterior. Under favorable humidity and temperature, eggs hatch within 24 hours and, after two successive molts and 4 or 5 days, form infective larvae, which ascend forage and await ingestion by a sheep.

Parasitic stages start with ingestion of infective larvae. After passing into the abomasum, the larvae attach to the mucosa, feed on blood, grow to maturity through a prepatent period of 14 to 29 days, and continue patency for 1 to 2 months. A prolific female produces 5000 to 10,000 eggs daily, and 2000 to 10,000 worms constitute a heavy burden. On pasture, few larvae survive winters in temperate zones or more than 3 months of dry summer. During summer and autumn, the proportion of inhibited fourth-stage larvae rapidly rises from 50% in July to nearly 100% in November.

The clinical signs in infected sheep relate to the loss of blood. Heavily infected animals become anemic and may die when the hemoglobin level descends to 4 g/dl. Ewes lose weight, reduce milk production, and often develop intermandibular edema; lambs grow slowly, lose weight, develop cervical and intermandibular edema, and may die. Diarrhea seldom develops. At necropsy, both emaciation and worms are discernible (Fig. 4-3). Besides sheep, goats and cattle are attacked.

2. *Ostertagia circumcincta.* Following ingestion the infective larvae exsheath in the rumen and pass to the abomasum. In the ab-

Fig. 4-3. *Haemonchus contortus* in ovine abomasum. Ingesta was separated from the worms. × 1.5.

omasum the larvae enter the gastric glands. In the gastric glands the third and fourth molt occurs and the young adult emerges 17 to 20 days following infection unless hypobiosis of the L_4 larvae occurs.

Larvae in the gastric glands causes a severe hyperplastic gastritis with raised nodules in the mucosa. Just prior to emerging from the gastric gland the L_4 molts to the L_5. The growth of the larvae at this time causes a destruction of the pepsinogen and parietal cells which are replaced with nonfunctional cells. As this occurs the pH in the abomasum rises from 2 to 7 resulting in the severe diarrhea seen in ovine ostertagiasis. At this time plasma protein leaks into the abomasum and gastric pepsinogens enter the plasma. The rise in pH also allows additional bacteria growth in the abomasum and digestion diminishes.

The clinical signs of ovine ostertagiasis in ewes include diarrhea, unthriftiness, decreased milk production, weight loss, and slight anemia. In lambs there is a diarrhea, decrease in feed intake, loss of weight, and moderate anemia. At necropsy the wall of the abomasum is thick and edematous. The mucosa contains numerous small umbilicated plaques giving it a morocco leather or cobblestone appearance (Fig. 4-4). Both sheep and goats are affected.

3. *Trichostrongylus axei* and *T. colubriformis*. These prevalent nematodes commonly attack sheep, goats, cattle, and antelope and are pathogenic to lambs and young sheep of all breeds and sexes. Trichostrongylosis usually develops during cool seasons, especially

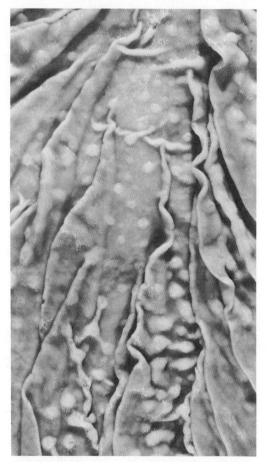

Fig. 4-4. Abomasum of a lamb with multiple umbilicated nodules or plaques caused by larval *O. circumcincta*. × 1.3.

autumns. The free-living stages of the life cycle begin with expulsion of segmented eggs to the exterior. Under favorable conditions, they hatch within 1 day and after two successive molts and 3 to 4 days, develop into infective larvae, which ascend plants and await ingestion by a suitable host.

Parasitic stages start with ingestion of infective larvae. *T. axei* inhabits the abomasum and *T. colubriformis* the duodenum. The larvae enter the mucosa, molt, and mature during a prepatent period of 3 weeks. On pasture, the larvae develop and endure best during cool autumnal temperatures, and moderate numbers survive winters in temperate zones and dry summers.

In trichostrongylosis, severity of the signs varies directly with the number of infecting worms. Heavily parasitized sheep show depression, unthriftiness, anorexia, and diarrhea. The production of meat, milk, and wool diminishes, and many sheep die from malnutrition, dehydration, and intercurrent diseases. At necropsy, gastroenteritis and emaciation are prominent changes. In nursing lambs, weaned lambs, and adult ewes, 2000, 15,000, and 30,000 worms, respectively, are significant burdens.

4. *Nematodirus spathiger* and *Nematodirus battus* are common nematodes in sheep but are rarely pathogenic by themselves. Clinical infections are confined to young lambs especially with *N. battus* infections. The L_3 develops within the egg shell and is resistant to freezing weather and can survive for up to 2 years. Pathogenic infections of *N. battus* infections occur because almost all of the eggs hatch at the same time following a period of cold and/or freezing weather. As a result large numbers of L_3 are present on the foliage at the same time. Clinical disease in young lambs with *N. battus* usually occur in the late spring and early summer.

Following ingestion the L_3 enter the mucosa of the anterior small intestine. In the mucosa two parasitic molts occur and the young adults emerge in about 15 days. Clinical signs of nematodirasis are related to the development of the larvae in the mucosa.

The clinical signs in lambs begin with a partial anorexia about 1 week following infection. The lambs soon stop nursing and grazing but continue to drink. A diarrhea begins about 2 weeks following infection and there is a rapid loss of weight and dehydration.

The pathologic change of clinical infections is one of acute enteritis. The small intestine is inflamed and has superficial erosions. The carcass shows signs of emaciation.

DIAGNOSIS.   Treatment and control of nematode gastroenteritis in sheep must be based on an accurate diagnosis, which includes many factors. Most producers and veterinarians base their diagnosis on previous history of the herd or flock, clinical signs, and fecal egg examinations. While all of these factors are important, they can be misleading at times.

The clinical signs seen with nematode gastroenteritis, anemia, unthriftiness, retarded growth, and diarrhea, must be considered but are not always diagnostic by themselves. The same clinical signs can be seen with malnutrition and other disease.

The history of the herd or flock should always be considered when making a diagnosis and recommending treatment and control. Sheep grazing lush pastures when the stocking rate is high and there is adequate moisture are more susceptible to clinical disease than sheep grazing mountains in parts of the United States. Young sheep are more susceptible to clinical infections than older animals. Most nematode infections in a given area occur on a seasonal basis each year and outbreaks of parasitism can be predicted.

In the live animal, examination of the fecal material for nematode eggs is the only way to determine if the animals are infected. Fecal examinations alone may, however, be misleading for several reasons. The number of eggs produced by a single adult worm vary greatly between various genera. The larval stages of some nematodes are more pathogenic than are the adults. The consistency of the feces also influences the egg counts. Fecal examinations should always be done on individual animals and several animals in the herd or flock should be examined.

Necropsy examination of dead or sacrificed animals provides the best diagnostic information regarding the degree of infection and which parasites are involved. In the examination, the abomasum, small intestine, and large intestine should be tied off and opened separately, saving the contents, since many of the worms are small and difficult to see. Several small aliquots of the diluted contents must be examined. This can be done by placing the controls in a glass dish and adding water until the material is diluted sufficiently to see the small worms.

5. *Cooperia curticei.*   This slightly pathogenic nematode attacks the small intestine of lambs from 2 to 12 months of age and, when present in large numbers, causes clinical disease. Under favorable conditions, the expelled eggs hatch within 1 day and develop into infective larvae within 5 to 6 days. Following ingestion, the larvae enter the small intestine, penetrate the mucosa, molt and, through a prepatent period of 3 weeks, develop to maturity. They feed on blood and other nutrients and cause both hemorrhage and malnutrition. On pasture, the larvae show moderate resistance to desiccation during dry summers.

Lambs severely affected with cooperiosis show anemia, reduced live weight, depression, and diarrhea. At necropsy, variable amounts of enteritis and the parasites are present. Goats also are affected.

6. *Strongyloides papillosus.*   This widespread nematode commonly infects the small intestine of lambs and young sheep. Even though clinical strongyloidosis occasionally occurs, the causative worm has low pathogenicity. Expelled eggs contain larvae that form either a generation of free-living females and males or a generation of parasitic females only. The latter enter the host either through the alimentary tract or through the skin. Larvae, after penetrating the derma, invade the veins, transport to the lungs, ascend the trachea, and finally enter the alimentary tract.

In the small intestine, the larvae penetrate the mucosa and develop into adult females, which reproduce by parthenogenesis. Worm burdens of 9000 to 26,000 may damage the mucosa and thereby induce unthriftiness, diarrhea, live weight loss, slow growth, and death. In addition to sheep, the parasites attack goats, cattle, and some wild ruminants.

7. *Bunostomum trigonocephalum.* Hookworms prevail in moist warm climates but seldom attack range sheep of the semiarid western and southwestern states of America. They are pathogenic, however, and in heavy infections cause disease outbreaks during autumns. Expelled eggs, under favorable conditions, hatch in 24 to 36 hours and, after two molts over 7 days, form infective larvae.

Transmission to sheep may occur directly through the alimentary tract or indirectly through the skin, blood, lungs, trachea, and then into the alimentary tract. After passing into the small intestine, the larvae suck blood, molt again, and grow to maturity through a prepatent period of 2 months. On pasture, they are sensitive to low temperature and humidity, and, consequently, seldom survive cold winters or dry summers. Most outbreaks occur during cool autumns.

Heavy hookworm infection causes unthriftiness, anemia, diarrhea, fecal blood flecks, loss of live weight, edema, and retarded growth. At necropsy, enteritis and the worms are discernible. Hookworms also attack most other species of domestic mammals.

8. *Oesophagostomum columbianum.* This pathogenic nematode commonly infects the large intestine and, to a lesser extent, the small intestine of sheep 3 to 24 months of age. Attacks often begin in the autumn and continue for 6 months or more. Losses result from impaired growth, unthriftiness, and deaths.

The free-living stages of the life cycle begin with expulsion of eggs in feces. Under conditions of favorable moisture and temperature, the eggs hatch within 24 hours and, after two molts and 6 or 7 days, the larvae become infective. Following ingestion by susceptible sheep, the larvae penetrate the mucosa of the small or large intestines, where they again molt and remain for 1 week to many months. After emerging, the larvae molt the fourth time, attach to the mucosa, and mature through a prepatent period of 6 weeks.

During the free-living stages, larvae, like those of *H. contortus,* are highly sensitive to low temperatures and desiccation, and consequently, few if any survive 5 months of winter or 3 months of dry summer; they develop and endure best in cool climates of temperate zones.

The pathogenesis begins with invasion of the intestinal wall by larvae. Some worms limit penetration to the mucosa; others push into the submucosa, muscularis, and subserosa. In some young sheep experiencing their first exposure to the worm, the reaction is mild; in others, possibly because of sensitization from previous contacts, the reaction is strong. If the strong reaction occurs, neutrophils, eosinophils, lymphocytes, and giant cells accumulate around the larvae, causing nodulation, caseation, and finally mineralization; during nodulation, the larvae may emerge and complete their cycles.

Lesions may endure for a year or more, and during this time they ulcerate the mucosal surface and occasionally the serosal surface. The intestinal lesions cause accelerated peristalsis with diarrhea in early stages and decelerated peristalsis with constipation in advanced stages. Usually 80 to 90 worms in 3- to 6-month old lambs and 200 to 300 worms in adult sheep constitute significant burdens.

Clinical signs of oesophagostomumosis begin with soft or fluid feces and inappetence and may be followed by alternating episodes of diarrhea and constipation. Affected sheep are weak, stiff, and unthrifty and may lose as much as 50% of live weight. At necropsy, the carcass is emaciated, and the thickened large intestine contains large amounts of mucus and up to several hundred caseated and mineralized nodules that measure 1 to 5 mm in diameter. In addition to sheep, goats and antelope are attacked.

9. *Chabertia ovina.* This minor parasite occupies the colon, where it attaches and feeds by prehending mucosal tissue in its voluminous mouth. Damage to hosts is slight and of little economic importance.

Following expulsion, the eggs hatch in 24 hours and after two molts form infective larvae within 5 to 6 days. Ingested third-stage larvae have a histiotropic phase in the wall of the small intestine prior to the third ecdysis. The fourth-stage larvae and fourth ecdysis occur in the cecum, and fifth-stage larvae reach maturity in the colon. Prepatency extends through about 49 days. The worm feeds by sucking fluids from orally prehended tissue. On pasture, the larvae appear sensitive to cold winters and desiccating summers. Most natural outbreaks of chabertiosis develop during cool autumnal climates.

Heavily infected sheep may show diarrhea with mucus and blood in the feces, weakness, some loss of live weight, and some anemia. At necropsy, the carcass may show some emaciation, colitis, and worms. Besides sheep, goats and cattle are affected.

10. *Trichuris ovis*. This slightly pathogenic nematode, anatomically attenuated throughout the anterior three-fourths of its length, occupies the cecum and attaches to the mucosa. Although cecitis results from infection, host damage from natural infection appears to be clinically insignificant.

The life cycle begins with expulsion of unsegmented eggs which, under favorable conditions, embryonate in 3 weeks and develop into infective larvae within the shells. Following ingestion, hatching occurs; the larvae enter the cecum, attach to the mucosa, feed on blood, and mature through a prepatent period of 1 to 3 months. During the free-living stages, the shell-protected larvae strongly resist desiccation and freezing and may retain viability for several years. Under natural conditions, clinical infection seldom occurs. At necropsy, a mild cecitis and attached adult worms are discernible. Individual sheep harbor as many as 300 worms.

DIAGNOSIS. Veterinarians diagnose nematode gastroenteritis on the basis of evidence of clinical signs, postmortem lesions (Fig. 4-5), and laboratory findings. Unthriftiness, retarded growth, anemia, and diarrhea among lambs and young adults are indicative signs. Fecal examinations for numbers and genera of parasite eggs give further evidence. Results of fecal studies alone, however, often provide

Fig. 4-5. Foci of nematode penetration in abomasum. × 1.3.

unreliable information because of variance in: (1) egg production within a species of parasite, (2) egg production between strongyle species, (3) mixing and excreting eggs and feces, and (4) methods for collecting and identifying eggs. At necropsy, the abomasum, small intestine, and large intestine can be separately washed and the worms collected, counted, and identified; these data, along with other necropsy findings, establish, confirm, or modify clinical diagnoses.

The differential diagnosis requires consideration of coccidiosis, pneumonia, salmonellosis, oral poisoning, and acidosis. For technical assistance from a diagnostic laboratory, practitioners should submit separate fecal samples from each of several animals of a suspect flock.

PREVENTION AND TREATMENT. The goal of nematode control in sheep is to prevent pasture contamination with eggs which later develop into infective larvae. All too often treatment and control programs are directed at removal of the worm burden from the infected animal with little or no regard for reducing exposure of animal to the infection. All effective control programs must, therefore, take into consideration the epidemiology of nematode infection in the area. Consideration must be given to the seasonal development of infective larvae, the inhibited or hypobiotic larvae, the worm turnover, the periparturient rise in fecal egg counts, the survival of infective larvae on the pastures, and the immune status of the animal.

The initial infection acquired by sheep when first placed on a pasture is from the larvae which survived the previous grazing season. In many cases these pastures have undergone severe weather changes, either cold and freezing or hot and dry conditions. Many of the infective larvae will have died off because of these changes but some will survive to provide this initial infection. These infections are picked up early in the grazing season and usually do not cause clinical disease but are one source of later pasture contamination. The next and much larger infection is acquired by the animal as the result of pasture contamination from the development of hypobiotic larvae and the periparturient rise in the ewe. This usually occurs later in the grazing season when weather conditions permit the development of larvae numbers of the infective larvae. Clinical disease, if it develops, is usually the result of this infection. Since young animals are on the pastures at this time, they are particularly susceptible to clinical disease because of their lack of immunity at this time.

It is not possible to design one parasite control program that is universally applicable in all situations and at the same time cost effective. Ideally, if sheep are treated at the time they are removed from the pastures with an anthelmintic which will remove adult and immature worms, the animals will be free of parasites. The animals will then remain free of nematode infection if they are turned out on pastures free of infection or kept in dry lots. In many mountain pastures in the western part of the United States, this may be the only treatment required. In the midwestern part of the United

States, it is recommended that in addition to this treatment sheep be treated at 3 weeks after they are turned out on pastures to remove the infection they pick up from overwintering larvae. Usually 3 or 4 treatments are required to remove the infections picked up from overwintering stages.

Veterinarians and producers worldwide have a large number of anthelmintic available to treat sheep. Unfortunately only three of these are approved for use in sheep in the United States (phenothiazine, thiabendazole, and levamisole).

Phenothiazine is one of the oldest anthelmintics available for treating nematode infections in sheep. Because of prolonged usage many sheep nematodes have developed resistance to phenothiazine. Phenothiazine has good anthelmintic efficacy for *Haemonchus* and *Oesophagostomum* but rather poor efficacy for other abomasal and small intestinal nematodes in sheep. The drug is not effective against larval stages. The dose of phenothiazine for lambs under 50 pounds is 12.5 g and 25 g for adult sheep.

Thiabendazole was the first broad spectrum benzimidazole anthelmintic developed for use in sheep. Thiabendazole is 95 to 100% effective against adult *Haemonchus, Trichostrongylus, Bunostomum, Strongyloides, Chabertia,* and *Oesophagostomum*. It is somewhat less efficacious for adult *Ostertagia, Cooperia,* and *Nematodirus*. It has little or no activity against the larval stages of nematodes in sheep. Again because of its prolonged usage since 1960 and probably because of misusage, several sheep nematodes have developed a resistance to thiabendazole. Nematodes resistant to thiabendazole also show some resistance to other benzimidazole anthelmintic (parabendazole, cambendazole, mebendazole, fenbendazole, oxibendazole, oxfenbendazole, albendazole) and the pro-benzimidazoles (febantel and thiophanate). The dose of thiabendazole in sheep is 44 mg/kg body weight.

Fenbendazole is another benzimidazole anthelmintic with 95 to 100% efficacy for all gastrointestinal nematodes of sheep including trichuris and lungworms. It is also highly efficacious against the sheep tapeworm *Moniezia*. It is also one of the few anthelmintics which has efficacy against the immature and inhibited stages of gastrointestinal nematodes. The dose of fenbendazole for gastrointestinal nematodes and tapeworms is 5 to 10 mg/kg body weight.

Albendazole is another benzimidazole anthelmintic used in sheep with 95 to 100% efficacy for adult gastrointestinal nematodes and lungworms in sheep except *Trichuris*. It is somewhat less efficacious against immature and inhibited stages of these nematodes. It is the only broad spectrum anthelmintic which is efficacious against adult liver flukes. Albendazole also has some activity against *Moniezia*. The dose of albendazole for roundworms, lungworms, and tapeworms is 5–10 mg/kg and for adult liver flukes 10–20 mg/kg body weight.

Other benzimidazole anthelmintics used in sheep are cambendazole, mebendazole, and oxfendazole. These anthelmintics have activity similar to albendazole for gastrointestinal nematodes, lungworms, and tapeworms. They do not have activity against liver flukes, however. The dose of cambendazole is 10–15 mg/kg, mebendazole 10 mg/kg, and oxfendazole 5 mg/kg body weight.

Febantel and thiophanate are two probenzimidazole anthelmintics used in sheep. Both of these anthelmintics are converted to benzimidazole in the host. Nematodes resistant to the benzimidazole anthelmintics are usually resistant to the probenzimidazoles. The activity of these two anthelmintics is reported to be greater than 90% for gastrointestinal nematodes except *Trichuris* and *Strongyloides*. Febantel also has activity against lungworms and tapeworms but thiophanate does not have this activity. The dose of febantel in sheep is 5 mg/kg and the dose of thiophanate is 100 mg/kg body weight.

Levamisole is an imidazothiazole anthelmintic which has been widely used in sheep since the early 1960s. It has greater than 95% activity against all gastrointestinal nematodes of sheep except *Trichuris* and *Strongyloides*. Reports vary on its efficacy for immature and inhibited gastrointestinal stages in sheep. Levamisole is also effective against adult and immature lungworms but has no activity against tapeworms. Since levamisole is not related to the benzimidasole anthelmintic, it is usually effective against nematodes which show resistance to this group of anthelmintics. In some countries the injectable form of levamisole is available in combination with clostridial vaccines. The dose of levamisole in sheep is 7.5 mg/kg body weight.

Haloxon is the only organophosphate approved for use as an anthelmintic in sheep. It has greater than 90% efficacy for abomasal and small intestinal parasites in sheep but poor efficacy for large intestinal nematodes. It is not effective against lungworm or tapeworms in sheep. The dose of haloxon in sheep is 50 mg/kg body weight.

Morantel tartrate is a broad spectrum anthelmintic which has greater than 95% efficacy for all gastrointestinal parasites except *Ostertagia* and *Trichuris*. The efficacy for *Ostertagia* is about 90%. It has high efficacy against third stage larvae but not inhibited stages. It has no activity for lungworms and tapeworms. A sustained release rumen bolus has been developed for cattle which protects pastured cattle for up to 90 days. The dose of morantel in sheep is 10 mg/kg body weight.

Ivermectin is the newest of the broad spectrum anthelmintics used in sheep. The efficacy for all gastrointestinal parasites and lungworms approaches 100% except for *Nematodirus* and *Trichuris*. It is the most effective anthelmintic marketed for immature and inhibited larval stages. It has no activity against tapeworms and flukes. In addition to its anthelmintic activity, Ivermectin has activity against several arthropod parasites of sheep including all larval stages of *Oestrus*, and mange mites. The dose of Ivermectin in sheep is 0.2 mg/kg body weight.

Andrews, J.S.: Pathology from *Haemonchus contortus* in lambs. J. Agric. Res., *65*:1-18, 1942.

Armor, J. and Bogan, J.: Anthelmintics for ruminants. Br. Vet. J., *138*:371-382, 1982.

Armor, J., and Bairden, K.: Anthelmintic efficiency of Ivermectin against naturally occurring gastrointestinal nematodes in sheep. Vet. Rec., *111*:80-81, 1982.

Baldock, F. G. and Green, P.E.: Worms in sheep—Anthelmintics choose and use wisely. Queensland Ag. J., 111:89-91, 1985.

Barton, N.J. and Brimblecombe, C.J.: The effects of anthelmintic treatment and season on the quantity and quality of wool grown by merino sheep. Aust. J. Agric. Res., 34:557-568, 1983.

Boag, B. and Thomas, R.J.: Epidemiology of nematode parasites in sheep. Res. Vet. Sci., 12:132-139, 1971.

Brunsdon, R.V.: Spring rise phenomenon. N.Z. Vet. J., 18:47-54, 1970.

Brunsdon, R.V.: Parasites and sheep production. Ruakura Farmers Conf., 1965, pp. 43-57.

Brunsdon, R.V. and Vlassoff, A.: Postparturient rise. N.Z. Vet. J., 19:32-37, 1971.

Coop, R.L., Angus, K.W., Hutchison, G., and Wright, S.: Effect of anthelmintic treatment on the productivity of lambs infected with the intestinal nematode, Trichostrongylus colubriformis. Res. Vet. Sci., 36:71-75, 1984.

Cornwell, R.L. and Jones, R.M.: Field trials in sheep with the anthelmintic morantel tartrate. Vet. Rec., 86: 465-469, 1970.

Gordon, H.M.: Gastroenteritis of sheep. Aust. Vet. J., 26:14-28; 46-52, 1950.

Heath, G.B.S.: Epidemiology of parasitic gastroenteritis. Vet. Rec., 85:305-308, 1969.

Helle, O.: Survival of sheep nematodes on pasture. Acta Vet. Scand., 12:504-512, 1971.

Herd, R.P.: Parasite life cycle of Chabertia ovina in sheep. Int. J. Parasitol., 1:189-199, 1971.

Herd, R.P.: Epidemiology and control of nematodes and cestodes in small ruminants. In Vet. Clin. N. Am.—Food Animal Practice, Parasites: Epidemiology and Control. Edited by H.C. Gibbs, R.P. Herd, and K.D. Murrell. Philadelphia, W.B. Saunders Co., 1986.

Herd, R.P., Streitel, R.H., McClure, K.E., and Parker, C.F.: Control of hypobiotic and benzimidazole-resistant nematodes of sheep. JAVMA, 184(4):726-730, 1984.

Herd, R.P.: Nematode infections—cattle, sheep, goats, swine. In Current Veterinary Therapy—Food Animal Practice. Edited by J.L. Howard. Philadelphia, W.B. Saunders Co., 1986.

Kates, K.C.: Survival of sheep nematodes on pasture. Proc. Helminthol. Soc. Wash., 17:39-58, 1950.

Kates, K.C.: Overwinter survival of sheep nematodes on pasture. Proc. Helminthol. Soc. Wash., 10:23-25, 1943.

Kates, K.C. and Turner, J.H.: Pathogenicity of Nematodirus spathiger in sheep. AJVR, 14:72-81, 1953.

Leyva, V., Henderson, A.E., and Sykes, A.R.: Effect of daily infections with Ostertagia circumcinta larvae on food intake, milk production and wool growth in sheep. J. Agric. Sci., 99:249-259, 1982.

Losses in Agriculture. Agric. Handbook No. 291 ARS, 1965, p. 79.

Marquardt, W.C., Fritts, D.H., Senger, C.M., and Seghetti, L.: Effect of weather on development and survival of N. spathiger. J. Parasitol., 45:431, 1959.

Marsh, H.: Weekly parasite egg counts in lambs and yearlings. J. Parasitol., 22:379-385, 1936.

O'Sullivan, B.M. and Donald, A.D.: Nematode parasites in lactating ewes. Parasitology, 61:301-315, 1970.

Pandey, V.S., Cabaret, J., and Fikri, A.: The effect of strategic anthelmintic treatment on the breeding performance and survival of ewes naturally infected with gastrointestinal strongylus and protostrongylus. Ann. Rech. Vet., 15(4):491-496, 1984.

Preston, J.M.: Ivermectin and control of nematodiasis in sheep. Prev. Vet. Med., 2:309-315, 1984.

Reveron, A.E., Topps, J.H., and Pratt, G.: Effect of nematodes on metabolism in lambs. Proc. Nutr. Soc., 30:19A-20A, 1971.

Roberson, E.L.: Antinematodal drugs. In Veterinary Pharmacology and Therapeutics. 4th Edition. Edited by J.M. Jones, N.H. Booth, and L.E. McDonald. Iowa State University Press, 1977.

Salisbury, J.R. and Arundel, J.H.: Relation of lactation and postparturient rise in ewes. Aust. Vet. J., 46: 267-271, 1970.

Seghetti, L.: Environmental survival of Tr. colubriformis. AJVR, 9:52-60, 1948.

Seghetti, L. and Senger, C.M.: N. spathiger in lambs. AJVR, 19:642-644, 1958.

Swan, G.E., et al.: Efficacy of Ivermectin against internal parasites of sheep. J. So. Afr. Vet. Med. Asso., 55:165-169, 1984.

Thomas, R.J. and Boag, B.: Epidemiological studies on gastrointestinal nematode parasites of sheep. Infection patterns. Res. Vet. Sci., 13:61-69, 1972.

Thomas, H.: The efficacy of febantel on gastrointestinal nematodes in sheep. Res. Vet. Sci., 25:290-293, 1978.

Threlkeld, W.L.: Cycle and pathogenicity of Chabertia ovina. Virginia Agric. Stat. Bull. 111, 1948.

Turner, J.H. and Wilson, G.I.: Strongyloidosis in lambs. Vet. Med., 22:132-133, 1955.

Waller, P.J. and Thomas, R.J.: Inhibition of Haemonchus contortus in sheep. Parasitology, 71:285-291, 1975.

Woodhouse, C.A.: Pathogenicity of Strongyloides. JAVMA, 113:242-243, 1958.

Yazwinski, T.A., et al.: Anthelmintic efficacy of fenbendazole in sheep. Vet. Med./Small Ani. Cli., 78:243-244, 1983.

Zimmerman, G. and Hoberg, E.: Sheep parasite found for time in United States. JAVMA, 188(5):478, 1986.

Liver Fluke Disease

(LFD; fascioliasis; distomatosis; liver rot)

Liver fluke disease, a sequence of acute parenchymal hepatitis and chronic cholangitis, is characterized by unthriftiness, loss of weight, anemia, edema, and eosinophilia and is caused by four species of trematodes, all of the liver. Because the disease has worldwide distribution and high incidence in endemic areas, attacking all classes of grazing sheep and causing extensive financial waste, it is of major concern to the sheep industry. Economic losses result from inefficient conversion of feed, retarded growth, deaths, condemnation of infected livers, costs of preventive and treatment programs, reduced wool production, predisposition to other diseases, restricted use of infested lands, and protein deficiencies among sheep-dependent people. Occurrence of the disease among goats, cattle, camels, and wild ruminants adds importance to the malady.

The disease has two clinical forms: (1) acute LFD, a traumatic invasion of liver parenchyma by immature flukes, and (2) chronic LFD, a biliary fibrosis resulting from prolonged residence of adult flukes.

OCCURRENCE. Although all breeds, sexes, and ages of sheep are susceptible to LFD, animals 4 to 12 months old probably are more vulnerable than animals of other age groups. Most new outbreaks develop during the summer and autumn, but once established, the infection may persist at low levels through all seasons of several successive years. LFD occurs in all areas where sheep, snails, moisture, and temperature favor the parasite. Table 4-2 gives the geographic distribution. Feedlot lambs, because of their selection for obvious

gainability, seldom are clinically diseased, but often they are subclinically affected with low to moderate numbers of the parasite acquired from grazing infested pastures and ranges.

ETIOLOGY AND PATHOGENESIS. Four species of trematodes—*Fasciola hepatica, Fasciola gigantica, Fascioloides magna,* and *Dicrocoelium dendriticum*—cause LFD. Table 4-2 gives their adult dimensions and hosts. Each species contains sexual stages represented by adults and asexual stages represented by miracidia, rediae, cercariae, and metacercariae. Each species invades sheep livers and inflicts variable amounts of damage.

1. *Fasciola hepatica.* The common liver fluke, the most pathogenic and prevalent of the flukes, has great economic importance. The hermaphroditic adults—leaf-shaped, double-suckered, spiny, and gray—occupy the lumina of bile ducts. The life cycle begins with the passage of eggs, mixed with bile and feces, to the exterior. In a moist habitat at 18°C or higher, eggs hatch in 2 to 3 weeks but do not develop at temperatures below 10°C. The resulting miracidia, ciliated and free-swimming,

TABLE 4-2. *Statistics on Four Species of Liver Flukes*

| Species | Dimensions | | Hosts | | Geographic Distribution |
	Adults mm	Eggs μm	Intermediate	Definitive	
Fasciola hepatica (common liver fluke)	20–30 × 8–15	130–150 × 63–90	*Lymnaea truncatula* *L. bulimoides* *L. tomentosa*	sheep, goats cattle, elk, rabbit, deer	Cosmopolitan; U.S.: West Coast, Rocky Mts., Gulf Coast, Great Lakes
F. gigantica (giant liver fluke)	25–75 × 5–12	156–197 × 90–104	*L. auricularia*	sheep, goats, cattle, deer	Africa, India, Hawaii
Fascioloides magna (large American fluke)	23–100 × 11–26	109–168 × 75–96	*Lymnaea* *Fossaria* *Pseudosuccinea* *Stagnicola*	sheep, cattle, deer, elk	Canada; U.S.: Great Lakes, West Coast, Gulf Coast, Rocky Mts.; Europe
Dicrocoelium dendriticum (lancet fluke)	6–10 × 1.5–2.5	36–45 × 20–30	1. *Cionella lubrica* 2. *Formica fusca*	sheep, goats, cattle, horses, deer, elk, rabbit, woodchuck	Cosmopolitan; Canada; U.S.: Northeast, Great Lakes

actively seek suitable freshwater snails, which they penetrate, as intermediate hosts, and successively form sporocysts, rediae, and cercariae.

The cercariae, after about 50 days, emerge, swim in water, and within a short time locate on grass, discard their tails, secrete protective coverings, and become metacercariae. These inactive forms await ingestion and may live 6 months or longer. Following their ingestion by sheep and excystation in the small intestine, the young flukes traverse the intestinal wall and move through the abdominal cavity to the liver, especially the ventral lobe. By burrowing movements and enzymatic actions, they migrate through the parenchyma and, after 5 to 6 weeks, locate in lumina of bile ducts, where they mature and live for 3 to 4 years. Some migrating flukes accidentally enter hepatic veins and are carried by the blood into the lungs, where they may continue to migrate, but in this anomalous location, they usually fail to complete their life cycle.

Injury to the host occurs at each anatomic area occupied by the parasite, and the amount of damage varies directly with the number of parasites present. In the liver, about 300 parasites cause clinical states, and smaller numbers produce subclinical states. The passage of large numbers of young flukes into and through the peritoneal cavity may, along with introduced bacteria, cause peritonitis.

In acute LFD, migrations traumatize the liver parenchyma and cause necrosis, hemorrhage, inflammation, and later, fibrosis. Massive invasion may cause rupture, and livers containing *Clostridium novyi* may develop fatal lesions of black disease.

In chronic LFD, the parasites occupy the bile ducts, where they cause leakage of blood into the bile and thus into the intestine. This continuous loss of erythrocytes and albumin results in anemia and hypoalbuminemia, as well as chronic cholangitis.

Both stages of infection evoke host responses. Bone marrow produces significant and persistent eosinophilia. Following parasite migration, the parenchyma fibroses, and during parasite residence, ductal epithelium undergoes hyperplasia. Enzyme γ-glutamyl transpeptidase (γ-GT) leaks from injured epithelial cells into the blood and builds high plasma levels that form within 30 to 60 days after infection and persist for about 9 months.

The plasmacytes and lymphocytes synthesize antibodies, and the lymphocytes generate a cell-mediated response against complex antigens in parasite secretions and excretions. The parenchymal fibrosis mechanically impedes new migrations, and the antibodies and the cell-mediated response attach both young and adult flukes. Together these reactions may give sheep sufficient resistance to reject many adult flukes, thus converting heavy burdens to light burdens, and to reduce the fluke establishment rates for subsequent infections.

In endemic areas, snails, the intermediate hosts, profoundly influence the epidemiologic characteristics of fascioliasis. Large snail populations can support vast numbers of fluke larvae. Both snails and their fluke larvae favor soil habitats with water saturation from rainfall, streams, lakes, or swamps and temperatures that range from 18 to 26°C. In temperate zones with freezing winters, snails emerge from hibernation, mature, and lay first-generation eggs in early spring; these hatch and mature by midsummer. Second-generation eggs hatch, but because of low ambient temperatures, the immature snails often hibernate through the winter.

The important first-generation snails become parasitized by fluke larvae from eggs excreted by early grazing ruminants and give rise to a vast number of metacercariae—the summer infection. The lesser second-generation snails may be parasitized by fluke larvae that produce metacercariae (the winter infection) or larvae that hibernate with the snails. Lambs may enter feedlots with either summer or winter infections.

2. Fasciola gigantica. The giant liver fluke causes infections that closely simulate those of *F. hepatica.*

3. Fascioloides magna. The large American liver fluke is a natural parasite of deer and elk. Sheep are an abnormal host of the fluke. The preparasitic stages develop similarly to

Fasciola. In deer and elk the mature flukes become encapsulated in the liver parenchyma. Eggs produced by the mature fluke enter the bile ducts and are passed in the feces. In sheep, however, the larval stages continue to migrate in the liver parenchyma causing extensive destruction of hepatic tissue. Occasionally because of extensive hepatic destruction, the egg may enter the bile ducts and be excreted in the feces. In sheep most infections are fatal in 6 months.

4. *Dicrocoelium dendriticum.* The lancet fluke uses three hosts. The first intermediate host, the snail *Cionella lubrica,* extrudes clusters of cercariae, or slime balls, which are eaten by the second intermediate host, the ant *Formica fusca,* where metacercariae form in their body cavities. When the metacercariae are eaten by sheep, they undergo excystation in the small intestine, and the resulting young flukes move along the common bile duct into its branches, where individual flukes reside for several years and cause limited biliary fibrosis.

CLINICAL SIGNS AND POSTMORTEM LESIONS. Acute LFD affects sheep during infection weeks 6 to 8 when migration has severely traumatized the liver. Affected animals isolate from the flock, decline feed, are immobilized, and remain standing. The distended abdomen is painful upon manipulation. Death may occur after a few days of illness. In massive infections, mortality is high, and the nonfatal course is 10 to 14 days.

At necropsy, the swollen liver is pale, friable, tunneled and occasionally ruptured. The changes are concentrated in the ventral lobe. The straight or tortuous tunnels are dark red from blood content during the first week of infection and gray from leukocyte and fibrocyte content during infection weeks 2 through 5. Healed tunnels are scarred and depressed near the surface (Fig. 4-6). If the blood-filled tunnels are dissected, some young flukes 1 to 2 mm in length may be found and collected.

Chronic LFD results from prolonged residence of adult flukes in major bile ducts. Affected animals gradually lose weight and become unthrifty, anemic, weak, and edematous in the lips and intermandibular tissues.

Ascites may form. The wool loses luster, flexibility, and tensile strength. Some severely parasitized ewes shed their wool and abort their lambs. Blood analysis shows eosinophilia and elevated levels of γ-GT.

The morbidity varies directly with the degree of infestation in the grazing land, and mortality may reach 20%. The course may extend through several months. At necropsy, the carcass may be emaciated and pale. Bile ducts, especially those in the ventral lobe, are slightly enlarged, fibrous, and firm. The walls may be ulcerated and focally dilated. The lumina contain adult flukes and fluke excrement (Fig. 4-7). The ventral lobe may be atrophied and the dorsal lobe hypertrophied.

Fig. 4-6. Acute hepatitis from migrations by young flukes. Tunnels filled with leukocytes (a) and blood (b).

Fig. 4-7. Chronic cholangitis from mature flukes (a) in enlarged bile duct with thickened but not mineralized wall (b).

The lancet fluke is only slightly pathogenic since there is no migration of the fluke in the liver parenchyma. In heavy infections the liver is cirrhotic and the bile ducts are thickened.

The American liver fluke is highly pathogenic in sheep. Larvae migratory tracks filled with blood are found in the liver parenchyma. Large dark cysts several centimeters in diameter may project from the serosal surface of the liver. Two to three flukes may be fatal in sheep.

DIAGNOSIS. Veterinarians diagnose acute LFD on evidence from history of grazing endemic lands, clinical signs, and postmortem lesions, and they diagnose chronic LFD from typical signs, the presence of fluke eggs in feces, and postmortem lesions. It should be remembered, however, that eggs are absent during prepatent periods and, in some sheep infected with large American flukes, throughout the entire time of parasitism.

Fluke eggs are too heavy to recover with the fecal flotation procedures used to recover other helminth eggs. Eggs can be recovered using several sedimentation techniques. A relatively simple procedure is to mix 3 to 4 g of feces in 200 ml of water. This mixture is then poured through a tea strainer. The fluid is collected and let to stand for 15 to 20 minutes or centrifuged and the sediment is examined under a dissecting microscope. *Fasciola* eggs measure $140 \times 75 \mu$, are golden brown color and have an indistinct operculum on one end. Eggs are not distributed uniformly in the feces and one negative fecal examination does not always rule out an infection.

A serologic test (ELISA) has been developed which shows promise for the diagnosis of *Fasciola* infections in sheep. ELISA detecting antibodies to flukes are found 2 weeks post-infection, but do not reach diagnostic levels until 6 to 8 weeks post-infection.

PREVENTION AND TREATMENT. Control of fluke infections in sheep requires measures to destroy the intermediate host or preventing animals from grazing infected pastures along with the treatment of infected animals. In some areas molluscicides can be applied to destroy the snail population. The most commonly used molluscicide is N-tritylmorpholine applied at the rate of 0.45 kg/hectare to moist grazing areas during the spring. No molluscicides are approved for use in the United States. In some areas it is possible to fence off wet areas in the pastures and irrigation ditches where the snail population is high. Also some of these wet areas can be drained. Worldwide, several anthelmintics are approved for use in sheep to treat fascioliasis. Ideally the anthelmintic used should have efficacy for immature as well as adult flukes.

Albendazole is effective against adult stages of *Fasciola* and Fascioloides in sheep. It is not effective against immature (parenchymal) stages. The dose of albendazole is 10 to 20 mg/kg body weight. Albendazole was made available in the United States as an emergency Investigational New Animal Drug for a short period but has been recently withdrawn. It is still available in other countries.

Clorsulon, a sulfonamide, is the newest anthelmintic cleared for flukes. In the United

States clorsulon is the only product cleared and only for use in cattle. Clorsulon is effective against adult and 8-week-old immature flukes. The dose in sheep is 7 mg/kg body weight.

Closantel is highly effective in reducing *Fascioloides* burdens in sheep. The drug can be given orally or by intramuscular injection. The dose of closantel is 15 mg/kg orally or 7.5 mg/kg body weight intramuscularly. Closantel is also highly effective against *Haemonchus* and all larval stages of *Oestrus*.

Diamphenethide is probably the drug of choice for acute fasciolosis in sheep. It kills immature flukes as soon as they reach the liver parenchyma. The drug is only partially effective against adult flukes in the bile ducts. The dose of diamphenethide is 80 to 120 mg/kg for immature infections and 120 mg/kg body weight for adult flukes.

Niclofolan is a nitro substituted analog of hexochlorophene. It is effective against mature *Fasciola,* but higher doses are required for immature flukes. The dose in sheep for mature flukes is 2.7 mg/kg and for 6-week-old immature fluke 6.0 mg/kg and 8.0 mg/kg body weight for 4-week-old immature flukes. The dose required to remove immature flukes is close to the toxic dose in sheep.

Nitroxynil has been used in Europe since the late 1960s. It is highly effective against adult *Fasciola* but less effective against immature flukes. The dose in sheep is 10 mg/kg body weight and is given by subcutaneous injection.

Oxyclozanide has good efficacy against adult *Fasciola,* but negligible effects against immature stage. For this reason it should not be used for acute fascioliasis in sheep. The dose of oxyclozanide in sheep is 15 mg/kg body weight.

Rafoxanide is one of the most effective anthelmintics for mature and immature *Fasciola* infections in sheep. The dose in sheep is 7.5 mg/kg orally and 3.0 mg/kg body weight by injection. Rafoxanide also has high efficacy against adult and immature *Haemonchus* and all larval stages of *Oestrus*.

Triclalbendazole is a new benzimidazole anthelmintic with high efficacy against mature and immature *Fasciola* infections in sheep. Triclalbendazole is probably the anthelmintic of choice today for acute and chronic *Fasciola* infections. The dose of Triclalbendazole in sheep is 10 mg/kg body weight.

In moderate fluke infected areas, ewes and rams should be treated at the time they are placed on pastures in the spring. All the sheep should be treated again in the fall when they are removed from pastures. In areas of heavy fluke infections one or more additional treatments may be required during the grazing season.

Animal Health Yearbook. FAO-WHO-OIE (Italy), 1970.

Boray, J.C.: Fascioliasis in Australia. Adv. Parasitol., 7:95-210, 1969.

Boray, J.C., Jackson, R., and Strong, M.B.: Chemoprophylaxis of fascioliasis with Triclalbendazole. N.Z. Vet. J., 33:182-185, 19.

Boray, J.E., et al: Treatment of immature and mature *Fasciola hepatica* infections in sheep with Triclalbendazole. Vet. Rec., 113:315-317, 1983.

Corba, J.C.: Transfer of immunity to *F. Hepatica* infection by lymphoid cells. Res. Vet. Sci., 12:292-295, 1971.

Dargie, J.D., et al.: Proc. Sixth Congress World Assoc. Adv. Vet. Parasitol (Vienna), 1974.

Doyle, J.J.: Acquired immunity to experimental infection with *F. hepatica*. Res. Vet. Sci., 12:527-534, 1971.

Doyle, J.J.: Relationship between duration of primary infection and subsequent development of acquired resistance to infections. Res. Vet. Sci., 14:97-103, 1973.

Fetterer, R.H., Rew, R.S., Gasbarre, L.C., and Ostlind, D.A.: Prophylactic efficacy of clorsulon against *Fasciola hepatica* in calves and sheep. Vet. Parasitol., 18(1):21-27, 1985.

Flagstad, T. and Eriksen, L.: Hepatic immunoglobulin synthesis in *F. hepatica* infected calves. Res. Vet. Sci., 17:59-63, 1974.

Foreyt, W.S. and Hunter, R.J.: Clinical *Fascioloides magna* infection in sheep in Oregon on pastures shared by Columbian white-tailed deer. Am. J. Vet. Res., 41:1531-1532, 1980.

Foreyt, W.S. and Todd, A.C.: Development of large American liver fluke *Fascioloides magna* in white-tailed deer, cattle and sheep. J. Parasitol., 62:26-32, 1976.

Holmes, P.H., et al.: Anemia in fascioliasis. Vet. Rec., 80:285-286, 1967.

Holmes, P.H., Dargie, J.D., MacLean, J.M., and Mulligan, W.: Anemia in fascioliasis. J. Comp. Pathol., 78:415-420, 1968a.

Holmes, P.H., Dargie, J.D., MacLean, J.M., and Mulligan, W.: Albumen turnover in fascioliasis of sheep. Vet. Rec., 83:227-228, 1968b.

Krull, W.H.: Migratory route of metacercariae of *Dicrocoelium dendriticum*. Cornell Vet., 48:17-24, 1958.

Krull, W.H.: Biology of *Dicrocoelium dendriticum*. Cornell Vet., 43:389-410, 1953.

Krull, W.H. and Mapes, C.R.: Biology of *Dicrocoelium dendriticum*. Cornell Vet., 42:276-285; 339-351; 444-489; 603-604, 1952.

Leuckart, R.: Development of liver flukes. Zool. Anzeig., 5:524-528, 1882.

Mapes, C.R.: Biology of and infection with *D. dendriticum*. Cornell Vet., *41*:382-432, 1951.

Nansen, P., Eriksen, L., Siemesen, M.G., and Nielsen, K.: Metabolism of ^{131}I-labeled albumen. Nord. Vet. Med., *20*:638-650, 1968.

Roberson, E.L.: Anticostodal and antitrematodal drugs. In *Veterinary Pharmacology and Therapeutics*. 4th Edition. Edited by L.M. Jones, N.H. Booth, and L.E. McDonald, Iowa State University Press, 1977.

Sewell, M.M.H., Hammond, J.A., and Dinning, D.C.: Etiology of anemia in ovine fascioliasis. Br. Vet. J., *124*:160-170, 1968.

Siemesen, M.G., Nielsen, K., and Nansen, P.: Effects of *F. hepatica* infection in cattle on serum activities of γ-glutamyl transpeptidase and glutamic oxaloacetic transaminase. Res. Vet. Sci., *15*:32-36, 1973.

Smeal, M.G. and Hell, G.A.: The activity of Triclabendazole against immature and adult *Fasciola hepatica* infections in sheep. Aust. Vet. J., *60*:329-331, 1983.

Stromberg, B.E., Schlottbauer, J.C., and Conboi, G.A.: Efficacy of albendazole against *Fascioloides magna* in sheep. Am. J. Vet. Res., *45*(1):80-82, 1984.

Stromberg, B.E., et al.: Activity of closantel against experimentally induced *Fascioloides magna* infections in sheep. Am. J. Vet. Res., *46*(12):2527-2529, 1985.

Taylor, E.L.: Fascioliasis and liver fluke. FAO (Rome), 1964.

Thomas, A.P.: Liver fluke in sheep. Nature, *26*:606-608, 1882.

Wescott, R.B. and Foreyt, W.S.: Epidemiology and control of trematodes in small ruminants. In *Vet. Clin. N. Am.—Food Animal Practice, Parasites: Epidemiology and Control*. Edited by H.C. Gibbs, R.P. Herd, and K.D. Murrell. Philadelphia, W.B. Saunders Co., 1986.

Zimmerman, G.L., et al.: Diagnosis of *Fasciola hepatica* infections in sheep by an enzyme-linked immunosorbent assay. Am. J. Vet. Res., *43*:2097-2100, 1982.

DISEASES OF THE RESPIRATORY SYSTEM

Verminous Pneumonia

(*VP; lungworms*)

Verminous pneumonia, a chronic and prolonged infection of sheep and goats, is characterized clinically by respiratory distress and pathologically by bronchitis and bronchopneumonia and is caused by nematode parasites. Because the general disease occurs in all major sheep-producing countries and causes significant financial waste, it has importance to the entire sheep industry. Economic losses result from unthriftiness, retarded growth, reduced production of meat and wool, deaths, and diminished utility of infected pastures, and from the costs of preventive and treatment programs.

OCCURRENCE. Although the disease occurs in all breeds, sexes, and ages of sheep, animals 2 to 18 months old have higher incidence than do other age groups. Most outbreaks of VP occur during cool seasons, especially autumn and early winter, because the larval stages of the causative worms tolerate and prefer low temperatures.

Geographically, the disease is widespread in South America, Europe, Africa, the Middle East, USSR, and North America, and less prevalent in Australia and New Zealand. The malady prevails where moisture, either from precipitation or irrigation, is abundant. In the United States, therefore, farm flocks of the eastern, southern, and midwestern states have a much higher incidence than do range bands of the semiarid states of the west and southwest.

ETIOLOGY AND PATHOGENESIS. Three species of nematodes cause VP. Although mixed infections may occur, *Dictyocaulus filaria* predominates in most outbreaks.

1. *Dictyocaulus filaria*. These prevalent parasites, mixed with exudate, occupy the lumina of large bronchi and are the most pathogenic of ovine lungworms. Measuring 30 to 100 mm in length, they lay embryonated eggs that are expelled by coughing; they also escape occasionally through the nose, but usually through the alimentary tract. Hatching occurs in the intestine, and the larvae, along with feces, move to the exterior. Under favorable conditions, they molt twice and, after 6 to 7 days, become infective.

Following ingestion by a susceptible sheep, the larvae invade the intestinal mucosa and move through the lymphatics and venous blood into the lungs. By penetrating the capillary walls, they enter the alveoli and move into the bronchioles and bronchi. The migration from host mouth and intestine to bronchi and the development to maturity require about 5 weeks. The free-living larvae need both moisture and cool temperature for survival; they quickly succumb to desiccation and the heat of summer. During winter, many fifth-stage larvae are inhibited in their development, but resume the process in the spring.

In bronchi, the irritating worms cause epithelial hyperplasia and muscular hypertrophy. Ova, larvae, bacteria, and exudate are extruded from parasitized bronchi into alveoli and there provoke bronchopneumonia and atelectasis. The prepatent period is about 35 days, and patency persists for approximately 3 months. Recovered sheep resist reinfection.

2. *Protostrongylus rufescens.* These nematodes, the second most pathogenic species of ovine lungworms, inhabit the lumina of small bronchioles. Measuring 16 to 35 mm in length, the worms have a life cycle similar to that of *D. filaria* except that, after expulsion, the first-stage larvae require intermediate hosts—snails of the genus *Helicello*—in which they develop to the infective third stage.

Transmission occurs when a sheep consumes infected snails along with forage. From their definitive position in the bronchioles, the adult worms provoke chronic bronchiolitis and hyperplasia of peribronchiolar lymphoid tissue. Exudate may descend into alveoli and cause focal lobular pneumonia.

3. *Muellerius capillaris.* These worms inhabit the lungs but, because of minor pathogenicity, usually cause no clinical manifestations. Measuring 12 to 23 mm in length, they locate in subpleural alveoli and stimulate around themselves granulomatous reactions that become nodules. Following egg hatching in the lungs, first-stage larvae are expelled to the exterior where, like *Protostrongylus,* they require intermediate hosts—snails of the genera *Cepaea, Helicigona,* and others, or slugs—for further development.

When infected intermediate hosts are consumed by sheep, the larvae penetrate the intestinal mucosa and move through lymphatics and venous blood back to the lungs, where they develop into adults.

CLINICAL SIGNS AND POSTMORTEM LESIONS. The clinical manifestations of VP vary with the number of infecting worms. Young sheep heavily infected with *D. filaria* show febrile episodes, coughing, nasal discharge, rapid breathing, retarded growth, physical weakness, and emaciation. Some animals develop diarrhea. Deaths may result from accompanying bacterial infections. *Protostrongylus* infections cause few clinical signs and *Muellerius* none.

At necropsy, most lesions are found in the respiratory system. With infection by *D. filaria,* the bronchi, especially those of the diaphragmatic lobes, contain tangled masses of worms mixed with frothy exudate. Atelectatic and infected lobules often surround or extend ventrally from infected bronchi. Bronchioles infected with *P. rufescens* often are closed with worms and exudate and, consequently, affected lobules may be atelectatic and infected. Lungs infected with *M. capillaris* contain red, gray, or green nodules 1 to 20 mm in diameter (Fig. 4-8). These lesions, located in the subpleura of the diaphragmatic lobes, vary in consistency, number, and shape.

DIAGNOSIS.   Veterinarians diagnose VP on evidence of signs and lesions. Persistent coughing and nasal discharge in young sheep are suggestive signs of infection with *D. filaria,* and

Fig. 4-8. *Muellerius capillaris* in ovine lung. HE stain. × 170.

finding larvae in feces or adults in bronchi confirms the diagnosis. The differential diagnosis requires consideration of other types of pneumonia.

PREVENTION AND TREATMENT. Producers and veterinarians prevent LP by avoiding grazing susceptible sheep on infected pastures. Draining and resting pasture during dry summers kill many larvae that readily survive cold winters.

In some countries a radiation attenuated live larval vaccine is available to protect sheep against *D. filaria* infections. Variations in the efficacy of the vaccine have been observed between different strains of *D. filaria* used to make the vaccine.

Several benzimidazole anthelmintics are used to treat lungworm infections in sheep. At the present time more of these anthelmintics are cleared for use in sheep in the United States. Albendazole used at 2.5 to 10 mg/kg body weight is highly efficacious for immature and adult *D. filaria* infections. Fenbendazole at 5 mg/kg body weight has 100% efficacy for both immature and adult *D. filaria* infection. Oxfendazole at 5 mg/kg body weight is > 99% efficacious against 5th stage and adult *D. filaria* but less effective against 3rd and 4th stage larvae. In bighorn sheep fenbendazole and albendazole is used effectively to treat *Protostrongylus* spp and prevent deaths.

Levamisole is the only anthelmintic cleared in the United States for the treatment of lungworm infections in sheep. At 7.5 mg/kg body weight levamisole is 97 to 99% effective against immature and mature 5th stage *D. filaria* infections. Levamisole is also effective against *P. rufescens* but not *M. capillaris* infections in sheep.

Ivermectin is the newest anthelmintic to have efficacy against sheep lungworms. At 0.2 mg/kg body weight ivermectin has 80 to 100% efficacy against *D. filaria* and *P. rufescens* infections in sheep. Ivermectin is not effective against *M. capillaris* infections.

Al-Saadi, A.A., Al-Samarrac, S.A.G., and Altaif, K.I.: Effect of anthelmintic treatment on the development of resistance in sheep vaccinated or experimentally infected with *Dictyocaulus filaria*. Res. Vet. Sci., *36*: 144-146, 1984.

Animal Health Yearbook. FAO-WHO-OIE (Italy), 1970.

Ayalew, L., Frechett, J.L., Malo, R., and Beauregard, C.: Seasonal fluctuations and inhibited development of populations of *D. filaria* in ewes and lambs. Can. J. Comp. Med., *38*:448-456, 1974.

Berger, J.: Oxfendazole: Anthelmintic activity in sheep artificially infected with nematodes. Results of trials against nine species including benzimidazole resistant *Haemonchus contortus*. J. So. Afr. Vet. Asso., *51*: 51-58, 1980.

Casarosa, L., Macchioni, G., and Marconcini, A.: Vaccination of sheep against *Dictyocaulus filaria* with irradiated larvae. Arch. Vet. Ital., *19*:321-336, 1968.

Foreyt, W.J., Wescott, R.B., Rolfe, J., and Coggins, V.: Treatment for lungworms (*Protostrongylus* spp) in Rocky Mountain Bighorn Sheep. VMSAC, *78*:1435-1439, 1983.

Gibson, T.E. and Parfitt, J.W.: Tetramisole against *Dictyocaulus filaria* in lambs. Vet. Rec., *82*:238-239, 1968.

Jovanovic, M., Sokolic, A., Movsesijan, M., and Cuperlovic, K.: Immunization of sheep with irradiated larvae of *D. filaria*. Br. Vet. J., *121*:119-131, 1965.

Jovanovic, M.: Duration of immunity induced by application of an irradiated vaccine against *D. filaria*. Acta Vet., *33*(5/6):315-322, 1983.

Kutzer, E. and Prosl, H.: Control of sheep helminths with ivermectin. Inst. Parasitol., *72*(10):298-303, 1985.

Malan, F.S. and Roper, N.A.: The efficacy of fenbendazole at a dosage of 5 mg/kg against the third and fourth stage larvae of *Dictyocaulus filaria* in sheep. J. So. Afr. Vet. Asso., *54*(2):92, 1983.

Nilsson, O. and Sorelius, L.: Field trials with tetramisole in sheep. Nord. Vet. Med., *18*:314-322, 1966.

Ross, D.B., Eichler, D.A., and Cameron, D.: The efficacy of albendazole on nematode parasites in experimentally infected lambs. Vet. Rec., *102*:556-557, 1978.

Ross, D.B.: Efficacy of fenbendazole. Vet. Rec., *96*:357-359, 1975.

Schmidt, R.L., Hibler, C.P., Spraker, T.R.: An evaluation of drug treatment for lungworms in bighorn sheep. J. Wildlife Management, *43*(2):461-467, 1979.

Sedlmeier, H., Schiefer, B., and Menschel, E.: Differentiating lungworm infections in sheep. Zentralbl. Veterinaermed., *16B*:143-157, 1969.

Sokolic, A., Jovanovic, M., Cuperlovic, K., Movsesijan, M.: Vaccination against *Dictyocaulus filaria* with irradiated larvae. Br. Vet. J., *121*:212-222, 1965.

Soleman, K.N.: Bionomics of *Dictyocaulus filaria*. Br. Vet. J., *109*:364-381, 1953.

Swan, G.E., et al.: Efficacy of ivermectin against internal parasites of sheep. J. So. Afr. Vet. Asso., *54*(4):165-169, 1984.

Theodorides, V.J., Nawalinski, T., and Chang, J.: Efficacy of albendazole against *Haemonchus, Nematodirus, Dictyocaulus,* and *Moniezia* of sheep. Am. J. Vet. Res., *37*(12):1515-1516, 1976.

Turton, J.A.: Efficacy of levamisole against lungworm in lambs. Vet. Rec., *93*(4):108-109, 1973.

Van Schalkwyk, P.C., Geyser, T.L., Recio, M., and Erasmus, F.P.G.: The anthelmintic efficacy of albendazole against gastrointestinal roundworms, tapeworms, lungworms and liver flukes in sheep. J. So. Afr. Vet. Asso., *50*(1):31-35, 1979.

Yazwinski, T.A., et al.: Antiparasitic efficacy of ivermectin in naturally parasitized sheep. Am. J. Vet. Res., *44*(11):2186-2187, 1983.

DISEASES OF MUSCULAR AND SKELETAL SYSTEMS

Malignant Edema

(Gas gangrene)

Malignant edema, an acute infectious but noncontagious disease, is characterized by fever, depression, edematous swellings around wounds, and a short fatal course. It is caused by anaerobic bacteria residing in manure and soil. Because the disease is widely distributed, attacks all classes of sheep often with high incidence in parturient ewes, and thus causes extensive financial waste, it seriously concerns the entire sheep industry. Economic losses result from high mortality, costs of preventive programs, and market depreciation of heavily infected properties. The fact that it occurs in cattle, horses, goats, and people adds both economic importance and public health significance to the malady.

OCCURRENCE. Malignant edema occurs in all breeds, sexes, and ages of sheep: in lambs following docking, castrating, and earmarking, in adults after shearing, and in ewes following parturition. Most cases develop when these operations occur in habitually used and pathogen-seeded corrals. Since producers usually schedule these operations for spring, that is the season when malignant edema commonly develops. The disease probably exists in all sheep-producing countries.

ETIOLOGY AND PATHOGENESIS. The bacteria causing malignant edema include several species of anaerobes: Clostridium chauvoei and C. septicum commonly, and C. perfringens, C. novyi, and C. sordellii occasionally. Infections usually are mixed. The organisms normally inhabit soil and manure, where they endure as spores for prolonged periods and may germinate and grow in the presence of adequate organic material, moisture, and temperature.

C. chauvoei and C. septicum are motile, anaerobic, sporing rods that are gram-positive in young cultures and frequently gram-negative in old cultures. The vegetative rods measure 0.5 to 0.6 × 2 to 8 μm and develop oval subterminal spores. Table 6-1 presents their fermentation reactions. In smears from the surface of infected guinea pig liver, C. chauvoei forms single bacilli or short chains, whereas C. septicum forms mostly chains; this morphologic difference has diagnostic importance.

The vegetative forms are highly susceptible to prolonged drying, high temperatures, and chemical disinfectants, but the spores withstand temperatures of 120°C for 10 minutes and survive in soil for many years. The spores, however, are killed in 15 minutes in 3% formaldehyde.

Strains of C. chauvoei possess a single serologic type. Although exotoxin is produced in blood-enriched liquid media, its concentration is low. Different strains of C. septicum may be separated into four major antigenic groups; these produce two potent exotoxins: alpha exotoxin, which is necrotizing and lethal, and beta exotoxin, which is hemolytic deoxyribonuclease.

In the pathogenesis of malignant edema, a rapidly spreading mixed infection develops in and around a wound. Castrating, docking, shearing, and parturitional injuries favor the disease. At the time of or following injury, spores of C. chauvoei, C. septicum, as well as other anaerobes of clostridia-seeded soil, manure, and skin, are carried into the wound. Under anaerobic conditions, the spores vegetate, proliferate, and synthesize toxin. The necrotizing component of toxin increases the permeability of capillaries and necrotizes tissue; the hemolytic component hemolyzes erythrocytes. Some gas is generated by metabolism of the bacteria.

The infection spreads along loose connective tissue and fascial planes. Inflammatory edema and exudate accumulate in the affected region. Early in the process, affected tissues are viable and sensitive. In advanced stages, however, necrotic and gangrenous tissues become insensitive. Specific exotoxins and toxic substances from infected tissues enter the blood and cause severe systemic depression. The high mortality results from the toxic effects on the central nervous system.

CLINICAL SIGNS AND POSTMORTEM LESIONS.
Following an incubation period of 2 to 4 days
from the time of wound contamination, body
temperature often rises to 41 to 43°C, but in
some cases, body temperature remains normal.
The affected animal does not feed, breathes
rapidly, and is profoundly depressed.

An edematous and occasionally emphysematous swelling forms around the infected
wound. The swelling spreads rapidly and, when
extending over muscles of locomotion, causes
lameness. In early stages, the swollen tissue is
painful but later becomes insensitive. A serosanguineous, gaseous, and malodorous fluid
exudes from the wound and from incisions of
the swollen tissue. In advanced stages of the
disease, the animal is prostrated and often
disoriented. As the disease progresses, the
swelling gravitates to lower planes in the tissue.

Infection of the genitalia following normal
parturition or dystocia gravitates in the perineum ventrally along medial aspects of the
thighs; the swollen edematous mucosa is translucent. Infection from castration wounds gravitates anteroventrally along the abdominal wall
and laterally to the thighs; horn infection in
fighting rams gravitates ventrally over the eyelid, face, and neck of the infected side.

Death occurs after a course of 12 to 48
hours. Although the morbidity is usually low,
the mortality of affected animals is high.

At necropsy, the prominent lesion is the
swelling in and around a wound. The opened
affected tissue shows an extensive serosanguineous and occasionally gaseous transudate
in the loose connective tissue and fascia
around the wound (Fig. 4-9). The muscles,
usually intact, are invaded only slightly. Butyric and foul odors are detectable. Regional
lymph nodes are swollen and hemorrhagic.
During healing stages of nonfatal cases, the
gangrenous skin and subcutaneous tissues
may slough.

Histopathologically, the tissue shows peracute inflammation. Necrosis is widespread.
Hemorrhagic transudate with some leukocytes
fills the interstices of the loose connective tissue between muscles and along fascial planes.
In some cases, muscle cells are necrotic. Gas

Fig. 4-9. Malignant edema in abdominal wall. ×
2.0.

vacuoles, *C. chauvoei* and *C. septicum,* and
often other species of bacteria are discernible.

DIAGNOSIS. The clinical diagnosis of malignant edema is based on typical signs and lesions. A significant sign is the rapidly spreading,
crepitant, painful swelling around a wound in a
febrile animal. Additional evidence is the serosanguineous fluid in and around necrotic tissue revealed by incision of the swollen tissue at
necropsy.

Confirmatory evidence can be obtained in
the laboratory from study of affected tissues.
C. chauvoei and *C. septicum,* as well as *C.
novyi, C. perfringens,* and other bacteria, frequently can be isolated from the necrotic tissue and from the serosanguineous transudate.
The intramuscular inoculation of guinea pigs
with the affected tissue causes a hemorrhagic
necrotizing myositis. Following death of the
guinea pig, individual cells of *C. chauvoei* and
short chains of *C. septicum* can be demonstrated in smears from the surface of the liver.

The differential diagnosis requires consideration of blackleg and venomous snakebite.

PREVENTION AND TREATMENT. Malignant edema is a result of tissue damage with impairment of blood supply setting up an anaerobic condition favorable for the development of *C. chauveoi* and *C. septicum* organisms. It is therefore a basic management practice to have properly designed equipment and facilities and these in good repair to prevent injuries from nails, split boards, sharp corners, or other protrusions. Docking, vaccinating, castrating, and other surgical procedures should be done in a clean environment under as sanitary procedures as practical. Following these procedures the animals should be placed on clean pastures away from contaminated corrals or holding facilities. On premises that have an endemic problem a vaccination program should be designed using a multivalent bacterin toxoid including a minimum of *C. chauvoei* and *C. septicum*. Including the other strains of clostridia in the immunization program may be beneficial. The immunization program should be designed to give the greatest amount of protection during the period of highest risk. At the time of initiating a vaccination program, it is necessary to give two immunizations 2 to 4 weeks apart. This gives maximum antibody response in about 2 weeks following the last immunization. The level of protective immunity drops rapidly, requiring a booster annually and possibly more often under certain environments and management systems. Passive protection, via colostral antibodies, declines rapidly and is of little protection by 6 weeks of age. On premises where malignant edema is a problem in young lambs, it will require an immunization program designed to stimulate active antibody production following the decline of passive antibody protection. An initial immunization followed by a second in 2 to 4 weeks may be required. Malignant edema is a rapid and fatal disease syndrome, therefore satisfactory treatment is based on early detection and prompt treatment. Clinically ill animals should be isolated from the flock and treated with penicillin (20,000 units/kg daily for 3 to 5 days). Tetra-

cyclines may also be effective. Proper disposal of carcasses and contaminated bedding is necessary to prevent the buildup of the clostridial spores.

Erwin, B.: Clostridial bacteria and clostridial myositis. In *Current Vet. Therapy 2: Food Animal Practice.* Edited by J.L. Howard. Philadelphia, W.B. Saunders Co., 1986.
Miessner, H. and Albrecht: DTW, *33*:179, 1925.
Pasteur, L. and Joubert: Bull. Acad. Med. II Ser., 6:781, 1877.
Raebiger, H. and Spiegl, A.: Z. Infektr. Haust., 26:208, 1924.
Roberts, R.S. and McEwen, A.D.: Gas gangrene infection in sheep. J. Comp. Pathol., 44:180-191, 1931.
Sutherland, A.K. and Moule, G.R.: Malignant edema of lambs in Northwestern Queensland. Queensland J. Agric. Sci., 4:12-18, 1947.

White Muscle Disease (WMD)

(Nutritional Muscular Dystrophy (NMD)

Selenium Responsive Unthriftiness (SeRU). A complex syndrome in young lambs, caused by a deficiency of selenium during gestation and early life is manifested by: (1) an acute or subacute pathologic degeneration and necrosis of skeletal and cardiac muscle and is referred to as White Muscle Disease (WMD) or Nutritional Muscular Dystrophy (NMD), (2) a subclinical condition causing poor health and decreased productivity and referred to as Selenium Responsive Unthriftiness (SeRU). The condition has a worldwide distribution wherever soils are deficient in selenium. The economic impact to production is due to selenium responsive unthriftiness. Additional economic impact of the selenium deficiency syndrome is seen in selenium responsive infertility (SeRI) in ewes. The overall selenium responsive diseases of cattle and sheep (White Muscle Disease, retained placenta, abortions, stillbirths, neonatal weakness, diarrhea, unthriftiness, immunosuppression, myodegeneration, and infertility) add to the economic significance.

OCCURRENCE. WMD occurs in all breeds and sexes of lambs from birth to 3 months of age; 2 to 4 weeks are common ages, however, for lesion development. The disease usually occurs in lambs whose dams subsist during pregnancy on alfalfa or clover. Most cases develop during spring and summer, the usual seasons of scheduled lambing. Seasonal variations occur depending on the grazing of weaned lambs. Rarely do sheep of other ages develop the disease. Besides lambs, WMD seriously affects calves of the beef breeds.

Geographically, there are extensive areas in northwestern, northeastern and southeastern United States where selenium content of crops and forages are below 0.1 ppm (the minimum level for preventing deficiency). A level of 0.2 mg/kg diet DM may be necessary if legume forages are fed. There are localized areas in Colorado, Wyoming, Arizona, New Mexico, Missouri, Arkansas, and Oklahoma which have Se deficient crops and forages. Farms producing alfalfa and clover for supplemental feed may have an increased prevalence of NMD and SeRU. Selenium responsive diseases occur in Canada, Norway, Sweden, Italy, Yugoslavia, USSR, South Africa, Japan, New Zealand, and Australia and possibly other sheep rearing countries.

ETIOLOGY AND PATHOGENESIS. A deficiency of metabolizable selenium causes WMD. Two circumstances commonly lead to low intake of metabolizable selenium: (1) continuous consumption by pregnant ewes of a diet having a selenium content of less than 0.02 ppm DW, because (a) the forage plants grow on selenium-deficient soil, or (b) the forage plants, such as alfalfa and clover, have a low capacity to extract the element from normal soil, and (2) reduction by ruminal bacteria of selenium compounds, especially selenoproteins, to elemental selenium, a form having low biologic activity.

Under normal conditions, selenium moves from soil to plants to consuming animals. Plants absorb selenates and selenites from the soil and, with these compounds, biosynthesize selenium analogs of sulfur amino acids: selenocystine, selenocysteine, selenomethionine, and selenocystathionine. The plant tissues incorporate these forms into proteins, which are the dietary source of organic selenium for sheep and cattle.

Selenium is an essential component of glutathione peroxidase (GSH-PX) enzyme sys-

tem in erythrocytes. Presently, selenium's only verified biochemical role is in GSH-Px activity. The selenium dependent GSH-Px appears to play a major role in cellular oxidation reduction reactions. Glutathione peroxidase acts as a catalyst in reactions that aid in the destruction of hydrogen peroxide and fatty acid hydroperoxidases. GSH-Px along with superoxide dismutase (SOD), catalase, glutathione S-transferase (GSH-Tr), ascorbate, and vitamin E (-tocopherol) are believed to play an important role in protecting mammalian cells against oxidant damage. The probable cellular reactions involving GSH-Px are: (1) peroxides reduced via GSH-Px-catalyzed reactions, (2) glutathione reduced (regenerated for subsequent reactions) via a reaction involving glutathione reductase and a hydrogen donor. These reactions aid in controlling the peroxide levels in mammalian cells, as high levels of peroxide tend to oxidize proteins and lipids altering the normal function of these molecules within the cells. Vitamin E is believed to aid in eliminating peroxides and has been shown to protect against myopathies associated with diets high in polyunsaturated fats. Selenium and vitamin E are separate nutrients with similar biochemical roles.

CLINICAL SIGNS AND POSTMORTEM LESIONS. On the basis of lesion location, veterinarians recognize two clinical forms of WMD: skeletal and cardiac. Skeletal WMD may exist at birth or develop at 2 to 4 weeks of age. Affected lambs show locomotor weakness and unsteadiness. They rise with difficulty and stand with the limbs, especially the scapulae, abducted. Because of muscular weakness, the lambs prefer the reclining position.

If rising and/or standing are especially difficult, nursing ceases, weight declines, and death ensues. Cardiac WMD causes rapid and weak pulse, accelerated breathing, pulmonary edema, dyspnea, and death. The skeletal and cardiac forms may occur separately or together in the same flock or the same lamb. Body temperatures are normal unless pneumonia or some other infection supervenes. Serum glutamic oxaloacetic transaminase (SGOT), creatine phosphokinase (CPK), lactate dehydrogenase (LDH) and malate dehydrogenase (MDH) are elevated in lambs with clinical and subclinical nutritional muscular dystrophy (NMD).

The morbidity ranges up to 50% with an average near 15%, and the mortality of affected and untreated lambs may reach 70%. The course varies from 1 to 2 weeks.

At necropsy, lesions are limited to skeletal and cardiac muscles. Bilateral pairs of limb muscles, including intercostal muscles, usually are affected. The individual lesions are pale to white and may involve all or part of a muscle. Affected fiber bundles within a muscle cause linear white streaks (Fig. 4-10). Petechial hemorrhages and muscular edema may also occur. In cardiac WMD, the pale or white tissue, located in the subendocardial muscle of a ventricle, may extend into the septum and opposite ventricle. Lesion size ranges up to several centimeters in diameter. If death results from

Fig. 4-11. Muscle affected with white muscle disease. HE stain. × 550.

left ventricular failure, the lungs are congested and edematous.

In early lesions, the sarcoplasm is swollen, granular, and fragmented; later, after liquefaction of the injured sarcoplasm, the sarcolemmal tubes are empty. Phagocytes may have accumulated around the injured and regenerating muscle cells (Fig. 4-11).

DIAGNOSIS. Veterinarians diagnose WMD on evidence of typical signs and lesions. Locomotor weakness and/or sudden deaths with pulmonary edema, especially in endemic areas, are indicative signs. Identifying skeletal or cardiac muscle lesions confirms the diagnosis.

The selenium status in the body can be estimated by whole blood Se assay or red blood cell glutathione peroxidase (GSH-Px) assay. Measuring the level of GSH-Px in red blood cells gives a more accurate estimation of the selenium status as whole blood levels will fluctuate with variations in daily intake. Fresh or

Fig. 4-10. Lamb muscle affected with white muscle disease. × 1.3.

freshly refrigerated blood with anticoagulant (EDTA) is assayed for GSH-Px activity in the red blood cells. The assay is expressed in units per milligram of heme per minute. The whole blood Se (WBSe) assay is conducted on blood with anticoagulant (EDTA) for total Se content and expressed in parts per million. The established levels of cattle are:

	WBSe (PPM)	GSH-Px (units mg heme/min)
Deficient	0.01–0.04	0–15
Marginal	0.05–0.06	15–25
Toxicity	73.0	

Reports from New Zealand on whole blood assay from weaned lambs with severe selenium unthriftiness usually contain < 0.05 ppm Se. Mildly or moderately affected lambs have 0.05 to 0.10 ppm Se and selenium responsive infertility in ewes appears to be associated with whole blood levels below 0.10 ppm. Selenium responsive deficiency levels are variable under different conditions warranting a close monitoring and supplementation program for individual operations. A spot-test has been developed which allows rapid assessment of GSH-Px activity in whole blood and can therefore be used on a regular basis for monitoring the selenium status in grazing animals.

Differential diagnosis requires consideration of arthritis, omphalophlebitis (joint-ill) and vitamin E deficiency. A nutritional myodegeneration disease clinically indistinguishable from Se nutritional muscular dystrophy has been reported in lambs with adequate selenium and a deficiency in vitamin E (-tocopherol).

PREVENTION AND TREATMENT. Production and death losses due to Se or vitamin E deficiencies can be prevented. A preventive program is based on a thorough understanding of the selenium status in the flock during all seasons and a supplementation program designed to meet the required needs. It is essential to establish the degree of Se deficiency by the level of GSH-Ps activity followed by adequate supplementation and continuous monitoring. The method of supplementation varies from drenching, injectables, slow release, boluses, feed or salt supplementation to top dressing with other fertilizer applications.

Labor, cost of the product, control of intake, and ease of administering must be considered when selecting the program most suitable for each operation. Top dressing at the rate of 10 g/ha Se is effective and safe for 12 months. Although the cost is considerably more than the materials for drenching, at a rate of 0.124 mg/kg Se for young lambs or 25 mg/adult ewe, it is a convenient labor saving method of correcting a Se deficiency. Various schemes of pasture rotation and management can be used to maximize the benefits from top dressing. Injectable barium selenate preparations are a safe and effective means of providing adequate Se for about 6 months. In the U.S. the Food and Drug Administration has approved the use of selenium for ewes and ewes with lambs up to 8 weeks of age. Selenium can be added to a complete feed at a level not to exceed an 0.1 mg/kg diet. In a feed supplement selenium can be added to a level that, when consumed with the total ration, will not exceed an intake of 0.23 mg Se per sheep per day. Selenium is also approved for salt-mineral mixtures up to 30 mg Se/kg diet not to exceed an intake of 0.23 mg Se per sheep per day. Injectable preparations of Se-vitamin E are commercially available and maintain adequate Se levels for about 40 days. These products can be used for treating clinical cases of NMD. If vitamin E deficiency is diagnosed as the problem with adequate levels of selenium, it will be necessary to supplement ewes with (700 IV and lambs with 300 IU of vitamin E). Vitamin E is supplied as an injectable or can be added to the water. Monensin as a feed additive for controlling coccidia in lambs has been shown to elevate GSH-Px activity without an increase in dietary selenium.

Anderson, P., et al: Effect of monensin on the selenium status of sheep. Vet. Rec., *113*:498, 1983.
Cawley, G. and McPhee, I.: Trials with a long acting parenteral selenium preparation on ruminants: Sheep. Vet. Rec., *114*:565-566, 1984.
Chiatti, C.: Muscle dystrophy of lambs. Veterinaria, *13*: 159, 1964.
Gardiner, M.R.: White muscle disease of sheep in Australia. Aust. Vet. J., *38*:387-391, 1962.

Goto, M. and Fujimoto, Y.: Myocardial and skeletal muscle lesions in lambs. Jpn. J. Vet. Sci., *13*:13, 1951.

Hamdy, A.H., et al.: Effects on lambs of selenium administered to pregnant ewes. JAVMA, *143*:749-751, 1963.

Hopkins, L.L., Pope, A.L., and Bauman, C.A.: Contrasting nutritional responses to vitamin E and selenium in lambs. J. Anim. Sci., *23*:674, 1964.

Koller, L.: Influence of selenium on livestock. Modern Vet. Pract., *62*:25-27, 1981.

Lilleengen, K.: Muscle degeneration. Sversk. Vet. T., *49*:231, 1944.

Maas, J.: Diagnosis and management of selenium-responsive diseases in cattle. Comp. C.F. Pract. Vet., *5*: 5393-5399, 1983.

Maas, J., et al.: Nutritional myodegeneration associated with vitamin E deficiency and normal selenium status in lambs. JAVMA, *184*:201-204, 1984.

MacPherson, A. and Chalmers, J.: Methods of selenium supplementation of ruminants. Vet. Rec., *115*:544-546, 1984.

Muth, O.H.: White muscle disease in Oregon lambs. JAVMA, *126*:355-361, 1955.

Muth, O.H., Oldfield, J.E., Remmert, L.F., and Schubert, J.R.: Effects of selenium and vitamin E on WMD. Science, *128*:1090, 1958.

National Research Council. Nutrient Requirements of Sheep. 6th Edition. National Academy Press Washington, D.C., 1985.

Petr, D., Board, P., Palmer, M.: Selenium supplementation of grazing sheep. I. Effects of selenium drenching and other factors on plasma and erythrocyte glutathione peroxidase activities and blood selenium concentrations of lambs and ewes. Aust. J. Agric. Res., *31*:991-1004, 1980.

Petr, D.: Selenium supplementation of grazing sheep. II. Responses in plasma and erythrocyte activities of lambs and adult wethers. Aust. J. Agric. Res., *31*: 1005-1015, 1980.

Ribe, O.: Muscular dystrophy in lambs. Med. Vet. Foren., *4*:55, 1963.

Sheppard, A., Blom, L., and Grant, A.: Levels of selenium in blood and tissues associated with some selenium deficiency diseases. The New Zealand Sheep. N.Z. Vet. J., *32*:91-95, 1984.

Watkinson, J.: Prevention of selenium deficiency in grazing animals by annual top dressing of pasture with sodium selenate. N.Z. Vet. J., *31*:78-85, 1983.

Erysipelothritic Polyarthritis

(*EP*)

Erysipelothritic polyarthritis, a chronic infection of sheep limb joints, is characterized by prolonged lameness and stunted growth and is caused by a soil-borne pathogen. During the third and fourth decades of the twentieth century, EP developed among young sheep, often with high incidence. Since that time, the rate of flock attack has diminished. The decline

may be due to the pervasive practice of disinfecting the umbilici of newborn lambs and docking and castrating by elastration. Consequently, the disease has minor importance to the sheep industry, but individual enterprises occasionally encounter the disease and incur financial waste. Economic losses result from lamb deaths, slow growth, and the cost of preventive and treatment programs.

The occurrence of a similar condition among swine adds economic importance to the disease.

OCCURRENCE. EP occurs in all breeds of sheep from 1 to 6 weeks and even up to 3 months of age, but castrated and docked lambs have more wounds, thus more exposure to inoculation, and probably higher disease incidence than do other classes of lambs. Lambs born, docked, and castrated in habitually used and pathogen-contaminated buildings and corrals develop a high incidence. Animals born and processed on open ranges and pastures rarely develop EP. Most outbreaks occur during the spring because lambing and associated operations are scheduled for that season. EP develops among sheep of Australia, New Zealand, United States, Europe, and probably other sheep-producing countries.

ETIOLOGY AND PATHOGENESIS. *Erysipelothrix rhusiopathiae* causes EP. This bacterium, a straight or curved, nonmotile, nonsporing, noncapsulating, gram-positive rod, measures 1 to 2 μm in length. It resides in alkaline soil and manure and resists drying at 20°C for several months, but it is destroyed in 5 to 10 minutes at 70°C and by exposure to 1% mercuric chloride, 2% formalin, 3.5% cresol, or 5% phenol. It readily grows in laboratory media, especially when enriched with serum, and forms acid (but not gas) from glucose, galactose, fructose, and lactose. All strains possess a common antigen and are classified into three serologic types: A, B, and N.

The pathogenesis of EP begins with polluted soil and manure in buildings and corrals. The soil and bacteria accidentally contaminate fresh wounds, such as umbilical stumps, docked tails, and incised scrotums of lamb, and grow slowly. From the local primary infection, the bacteria enter the blood and are transported to many organs. In the limb joints they establish chronic proliferative arthritis. Severe infection leads to death from starvation and intercurrent diseases, such as pneumonia. The bacterial antigens stimulate the formation of agglutinins. The organisms return to the soil in infected secretions, exudates, and tissues.

CLINICAL SIGNS AND POSTMORTEM LESIONS. Following an incubation period of 1 to 5 weeks, the body temperature rises and fluctuates. Stiffness and lameness develop in one to four limbs. Affected lambs become depressed, lose their appetites, and either grow slowly or lose body weight. Affected joints are tender to pressure but not conspicuously enlarged. The morbidity commonly ranges from 1 to 10%, but may reach 30% in some flocks, and the eventual mortality varies up to 70% of affected lambs. The prolonged course may extend through many weeks, especially in lambs 1 to 2 months of age at the time of arthritis inception.

At necropsy, affected lambs are undersized and often emaciated. The stifle, hock, elbow, and carpal joints commonly are infected. In these articulations, the capsules are thickened and, on the inner surface, granular and rough. The articular cartilages may show erosions, each about 1 mm in diameter. Joint fluid is increased in amount but not purulent. Beyond the joints the primary wound infection may persist, and secondary focal infection may exist in the lungs, liver, and kidneys.

Histopathologically, the infected joint capsule is thickened from fibroplasia and infiltration with lymphocytes and mononuclear macrophages. Demonstrable bacteria are scarce.

DIAGNOSIS. Veterinarians diagnose EP on evidence of signs, lesions, and laboratory findings. Chronic stiffness and lameness in lambs 1 to 3 months of age with slight enlargement of one or more joints suggest the disease. Increased volume of flaky synovium without pus is additional supporting evidence. Finding a positive agglutination titer against *E. rhusiopathiae* and isolation of the organism from joints confirm the diagnosis.

The differential diagnosis requires consideration of chlamydial polyarthritis, colibacillary arthritis, caseous lymphadenitic arthritis, white muscle disease, and in some countries, contagious agalactia. The diagnosis of each arthritic disease requires isolation of the causative agent. White muscle disease presents characteristic muscle changes at necropsy.

PREVENTION AND TREATMENT. Producers prevent EP by avoiding wound contamination in lambs. The environment of young lambs should be kept free of *E. rhusiopathiae* by lambing at pasture or in clean disinfected buildings. Docking and castrating should be performed in new temporary pens on pasture or range. At the time of birth, umbilical stumps should be disinfected by submergence in tincture of iodine or a 2% aqueous solution of cresol. Tail docking and scrotal incisions should be performed with a hot iron; if a cold knife is used, a disinfecting solution should be applied to the incision.

Lambs in early stages of the disease should be treated with an antibiotic or sulfonamide that, in the laboratory, is effective against the specific infecting organism.

Cornell, Z. and Glover, R.E.: Joint ill in lambs. Vet. Rec., 5:833, 1925.

Gill, D.A.: Illness associated with lameness in sheep after dipping. Aust. Vet. J., 24:297-302, 1948.

Howarth, J.A.: Polyarthritis of sheep. North Am. Vet., 14:26-39, Sept., 1933.

Marsh, H.: Serological identity of strains of *Erysipelothrix rhusiopathiae* of ovine and porcine origin. JAVMA, 82:584-586, 1933a.

Marsh, H.: Experimental erysipelothritic arthritis in lambs. JAVMA, 82:753-766, 1933b.

Marsh, H.: Bacillus of swine erysipelas associated with arthritis in lambs. JAVMA, 78:57-63, 1931.

McLean, J.W.: Lameness in sheep following dipping in rotenone and BHC (Gammexane). Aust. Vet. J., 24:144-146, 1948.

Mohn, S.F. and Utklev, H.E.: Chronic polyarthritis in lambs caused by *Erysipelothrix insidiosa*. Nord. Vet. Med., 22:296-306, 1970.

Nurnane, D.: Arthritis in lambs. Aust. Vet. J., 14:23-26, 1938.

Poels, 1913, cited in Marsh, H.: JAVMA, 78:57-63, 1931.

Ray, J.D.: Arthritis in lambs and *Erysipelothrix rhusiopathiae*. JAVMA, 77:107-108, 1930.

Reinhardt, R.: Septicemic disease of sheep caused by swine erysipelas. Monatsschr. Prokt. Tierheilk., 34:155-158, 1923.

Whitten, L.K., Harbour, H.E., and Allen, W.S.: Cutaneous erysipelothrix infection in sheep. Aust. Vet. J., 24:157-163, 1948.

Cyclopian Malformation

(CM; monkey face; veratrum poisoning)

Cyclopian malformation, a developmental abnormality of lambs, is characterized by facial hypoplasia, by close, contiguous, or fused eyes, by prolonged gestation, and by embryonic deaths. It is caused by alkaloids of false hellebore, a common plant of western alpine meadows. Even though the disease has limited distribution and low regional incidence and hence causes minor concern to the sheep industry, it may result in serious financial waste to individual enterprises. Economic losses come from death of affected embryos and lambs, illnesses and deaths among ewes, and incomplete use of affected ranges.

Occurrence of the disease among goats and cattle, plus the horrifying organ dysgenesis from dietary intoxication, adds economic importance and scientific significance to the condition.

OCCURRENCE. CM occurs in newborn lambs of all breeds and sexes and in pregnant ewes of all breeds and ages. Embryos are most susceptible 14 days after conception. Although most cases of poisoning occur during August, some may also occur among nonbreeding sheep in July. Geographically, CM develops in alpine meadows of southwestern Idaho, but false hellebore grows at altitudes of 1500 to 3400 m in most western states and could cause the disease throughout its geographic range.

ETIOLOGY AND PATHOGENESIS. *Veratrum californicum* (false hellebore, skunk cabbage, corn-lily) is the cause of cyclopian malformation. This perennial nonbranching herb grows to 250 cm high. Leaves are glossy, alternately oval to elliptical, pleated with parallel veins and measure 15 to 30 cm long and 8 to 20 cm wide. The many flowers, greenish-white in color, are produced on a pancile up to 60 cm long.

The teratogenic compounds in *V. californicum* are complex steroidal alkaloids, the most toxic of which are cyclopamine, cycloposine, and jervine. The alkaloids occur in all plant parts, with highest concentration in the roots.

Fig. 4-12. False hellebore (*Veratrum californicum*). x 0.1.

The teratogenic dose ranges from 170 to 340 g of green plant per pregnant ewe. Over 50 glycoalkaloid compounds have been isolated from *Veratrum* spp and account for signs of acute poisoning of sheep and other animals.

Presumably, the toxic alkaloids adversely affect cephalic primordia, possibly by inhibiting glucose metabolism, and thereby result in developmental anomalies, especially of the face, eyes, and brain. Pregnant ewes consuming *V. californicum* during the 14th day of gestation develop lambs with cyclopian malformation. Consumption of the plant between the 28th to 30th days of gestation results in shortened metacarpal and metatarsal bones. Cleft palates and harelips may also be present. Ewes consuming *V. californicum* during days 31 to 33 of gestation develop lambs with complete tracheal stenosis that is usually fatal. The intoxication may affect all or one of the lambs in utero, and by unknown mechanisms, may delay parturition for 6 to 9 weeks.

CLINICAL SIGNS AND POSTMORTEM LESIONS. Adult sheep, after ingesting toxic amounts of *V. californicum,* become ill within a few hours and show acutely distressful salivation, incoordination, weakness, vomiting, accelerated pulse, and depressed respiration; severely poisoned animals progress into convulsions, coma, and death.

Embryos of poisoned ewes may die and be resorbed or survive and develop cephalic and limb abnormalities and prolonged gestation. Lambs with teratologic abnormalities survive for hours to days but eventually die from starvation and pneumonia.

At necropsy, the large newborn lambs show varying amounts of malformations: the domed head contains a supraocular protuberance; the maxillae, and consequently the face, are hypoplastic; the upturned mandible, incisor teeth and tongue prominently protrude; the eyes are close, contiguous, or fused; and the cerebral hemispheres are fused (Fig. 4-13). In addition, limb bones and joints may be deformed. Lambs that are stillborn or die shortly after birth should be examined for tracheal stenosis.

DIAGNOSIS. The occurrence of lambs with cyclopian deformity, shortened legs, or tracheal stenosis, and a history of the ewes having had access to *V. californicum* in early pregnancy will establish the diagnosis.

Although cyclopian malformation in lambs is highly suggestive of *V. californicum* poisoning, other range plants have teratogenic effects in sheep and should be considered in the differential diagnosis. Plants known to cause abnormalities in lambs include wild tree tobacco (*Nicotiana glauca*) causing limb, spine, and head deformities and locoweed (*Astragalus* and *Oxytropis* spp) causing limb and other anatomic malformations.

PREVENTION. Pregnant ewes should not be allowed access to *V. californicum* during the first 35 days of gestation or until after the first killing frost which destroys the plants. If exposure cannot be avoided, ample alternative feed should be provided to minimize consumption of the toxic plant.

Fig. 4-13. Face of lamb affected with congenital cyclopian malformation from poisoning with *Veratrum californicum*. x 0.9.

Binns, W., Anderson, W.A., and Sullivan, D.J.: Cyclopian-type malformation. JAVMA, *137*:515-521, 1960.

Binns, W., James, L.F., Shupe, J.L., and Everett, G.: Cyclopian malformation in lambs from feeding *Veratrum californicum*. AJVR, *24*:1164-1175, 1963.

Binns, W., Shupe, J.L., Keeler, R.F., and James, L.F.: Chronologic evaluation of teratogenicity in sheep of *V. californicum*. JAVMA, *147*:839-842, 1965.

Binns, W., Thacker, E.J., James, L.F., and Huffman, W.T.: Cyclopian lambs. JAVMA, *134*:180-183, 1959.

Binns, W., Keeler, R.F., and Balls, L.D.: Congenital deformities in lamb calves and goats resulting from maternal ingestion of *Veratrum californicum*: harelip, cleft palate, ataxia and hypoplasia of metacarpal bones. Clin. Toxicol., 5:524-261, 1972.

James, L.F., Shupe, J.L., Binns, W., and Keeler, R.F.: Abortive and teratogenic effects of locoweed in sheep and cattle. AJVR, *28*:1379-1388, 1967.

Keeler, R.F.: Toxins and teratogens of higher plants. Lloydia, *38*:56-86, 1975.

Keeler, R.F.: Known and suspected teratogenic hazards in range plants. Clin. Toxicol., 5:529-565, 1972.

Keeler, R.F.: Reducing incidence of plant-caused congenital deformities in livestock by grazing management. J. Management, *31*:355-360, 1978.

Keeler, R.F. and Binns, W.: Teratogenic compounds of *V. californicum*. Can. J. Biochem., *44*:819-828, 1966.

Keeler, R.F. and Crowe, M.W.: Teratogenicity and toxicity of wild tree tobacco *Nicotiana glauca* in sheep. Cornell Vet., *74*:50-59, 1984.

Keeler, R.F., Young, S., and Smart, R.: Congenital tracheal stenosis in lambs induced by maternal ingestion of *Veratrum californicum*. Teratology, *31*:83-88, 1985.

Smith, C. and Varma, M.: Louping ill. *CRC Handbook Series in Zoonosis: Viral Zoonosis*. Edited by J. Steel. Vol. I, Sec. D. Boca Raton, Fl., CRC Press, 1984, pp. 191-199.

Van Kampen, K.R., Binns, W., and Balls, L.D.: Embryonic deaths from *V. californicum*. AJVR, *30*:517-519, 1969.

DISEASES OF THE CENTRAL NERVOUS SYSTEM

Louping-ill

(LI; ovine encephalomyelitis; trembling; springkrankheit)

Louping-ill, an acute infectious but noncontagious encephalomyelitis, is characterized by diphasic fever, locomotor incoordination, trembling, salivation, coma, and death and is caused by an arbovirus transmitted by the sheep tick, *Ixodes ricinus*. Although geographically limited, the disease may cause severe financial waste to sheep enterprises of the endemic areas. Economic losses result from extra husbandry, deaths, disposal of carcasses, and market depreciation of affected land, and from the cost of expensive research and preventive programs. The susceptibility of people to the virus adds public health significance and extra human interest to the disease.

OCCURRENCE.   Louping-ill probably occurs in all breeds and sexes, but is especially common and virulent in rams raised in LI-free regions and introduced into endemic areas for genetic improvement of flocks. Lambs and yearlings are generally more susceptible than sheep in other age groups. In addition to sheep, LI occasionally occurs in people, cattle, horses, dogs, and swine and can be induced in laboratory mice. Seasonally, LI occurs during spring and early summer, and again in autumn when vectoring ticks are prevalent. Geographically, the disease occurs in Scotland, England, and Ireland. Veterinarians have also identified related viral diseases among sheep of Bulgaria and Poland.

ETIOLOGY AND PATHOGENESIS.   A virus of the RNA family Togaviridae causes LI. The spherical virion, consisting of capsid and nucleoid measuring 44 and 20 nm in diameter respectively, probably contains single-stranded RNA and multiplies in cytoplasm. The virus, when stored in infected tissue at 0°C, persists for several months and when lyophilized and stored at −70°C, for much longer periods. Antigenicity is probably homogenous.

The natural transmission of LI virus occurs through the bite of the vectoring tick, *Ixodes ricinus*. The tick has a three-host life cycle and becomes infected by feeding on viremic blood of febrile sheep and possibly wood mice and common shrews. Trans-stadial, but not trans-ovarial, passage of the virus readily occurs; consequently, virus ingested by tick larvae or nymphae can be transmitted during feeding of emerged nymphae or adults. Infected shrews, wood mice, and possibly some birds, such as the red grouse, may form a natural reservoir of virus.

Even though scientists have not extensively investigated the pathogenesis of LI, some aspects of disease development are known, and others are conjectural. During feeding of an infected tick, the LI virus, along with saliva, passes from the tick into the blood of the susceptible host sheep.

Within a short time, the viral particles presumably replicate in target cells and, in enhanced numbers, re-enter the plasma. The viremia provokes the first febrile reaction. In some sheep, the virus passes from the plasma through the blood-brain barrier into nerve tissue of the spinal cord, brain stem, cerebellum, and hippocampus, where the particles attack, injure, and kill neurons. Neuron damage and inflammation cause the second febrile reaction. Death probably results from neuronal dysfunction and shock.

The majority of infected sheep probably do not develop encephalomyelitis, but, within 5 to 10 days after inoculation, form protective neutralizing and hemagglutination-inhibiting antibodies; complement-fixing antibodies form later. Neutralizing antibodies persist for many months, pass into colostrum, and passively immunize newborn lambs. Clinically recovered sheep are immune.

CLINICAL SIGNS AND POSTMORTEM LESIONS. After the usual incubation period of 6 to 18 days, the body temperature of affected sheep rises to approximately 42°C. Sheep with LI develop one febrile phase from the initial viremia and, after 5 days, another from the subsequent encephalomyelitis. Most cases escape diagnosis because animals recover following the first febrile reaction.

During the second febrile phase, affected sheep become dull and may lower their heads towards the ground. Movements are incoordinated, and the hopping gait is characterized by simultaneous advancement of the hind limbs and then the fore limbs. Muscular tremors of the lips and neck are common. Profuse salivation and tongue protrusion occur and probably result from bulbar paralysis. The jaws chomp. After 1 to 2 days, the sheep become prostrated and comatose, and, while recumbent, violently kick with all limbs.

The regional incidence approximates 5%, but may be higher in individual flocks. About 50% of encephalomyelitic sheep die.

At necropsy, saliva soils the face, and one or more ticks inhabit the skin. Meningeal blood vessels may be congested. Characteristic histopathologic changes include perivascular inflammation, gliosis, and degeneration and necrosis of neurons. These lesions commonly occur in the lumbar ventral horns, vestibular nuclei, cervical ventral horns, basal ganglia, motor trigeminal nuclei, reticular formations, lateral cuneate nuclei, hippocampus, and cerebellar Purkinje's cells.

DIAGNOSIS. In endemic areas, veterinarians diagnose LI on evidence of typical signs and laboratory findings. The presence of potentially vectoring ticks, fever, and incoordinated movements are strong indicators. In the laboratory, scientists can confirm clinical diagnoses by testing paired serum samples for virus-neutralizing and hemagglutination-inhibiting antibodies, and later for complement-fixing antibodies. The specific virus can be isolated from infected blood, brain stem, and spinal cord in embryonating chicken eggs and sheep kidney-cell cultures.

PREVENTION. Louping-ill is prevented by immunizing all susceptible sheep with a commercially available (Moredum Type: Wellcome) vaccine. To achieve optimal immunity to natural infection, it is advisable to give two doses of vaccine 2 to 8 weeks apart. The last dose should be given about 3 weeks prior to the period of high risk. Toxoplasma infection acts as an immunosuppressant if concurrent with louping-ill infection or immunization. Since LI virus infection in people causes a serious, but not fatal, encephalitic syndrome, veterinarians, workers in laboratories and slaughterhouses, and flock managers should avoid vectoring tick bites and unnecessary exposure to the virus in infected sheep tissues. LI virus can also be transmitted in goat's milk.

Borysiewicz, J. and Potec, Z.: Studies on occurrence of arboviruses in Cracow Province. II. Antibodies in encephalitides viruses of groups A and B in sheep population of Nowy Targ district. Med. Welt, *24*: 101-104, 1968.
Brotherson, J.G. and Boyce, J.B.: Development of a non-infective protective antigen against louping-ill (arbovirus group B). Laboratory experiments. J. Comp. Pathol., *80*:377-388, 1970.

Brotherson, J.G. and Boyce, J.B.: A new vaccine against louping-ill. Vet. Rec., *84*:514-515, 1969.

Reid, H., Buxton, D., Pow, I., and Einlayson, J.: Transmission of louping-ill virus in goat milk. Vet. Rec., *114*:163-165, 1984.

Reid, H., et al.: Immunosuppression in toxoplasmosis: Studies in lambs and sheep infected with louping-ill virus. J. Comp. Path., *92*:181-190, 1982.

Shaw, B. and Reid, H.: Immune responses of sheep to louping-ill virus vaccine. Vet. Rec., *109*:529-531, 1981.

Tetanus

(*Lockjaw*)

Tetanus, an acute neurointoxication, is characterized by muscle spasms and is caused by noninvasive bacteria from manure and soil. Because of its low general frequency, this sporadic disease causes little concern to the sheep industry; however, it does cause economic losses to some individual enterprises from deaths and expensive treatments. Its occurrence in other species of domestic animals and people adds economic and public health significance to the ailment.

OCCURRENCE. A disease found in all sheep-producing countries, tetanus develops in all breeds, sexes, and ages, but more often in lambs up to age 6 months than in animals of older age groups. Farm flocks experience a higher incidence because the sheep occupy spore-seeded corrals during and following docking, castrating, tagging, shearing, and lambing. Range animals, however, may also become infected if similar facilities for the operations are used. Most cases develop during the spring and summer because the surgical operations preceding outbreak of the disease are performed during those seasons.

ETIOLOGY AND PATHOGENESIS. *Clostridium tetani,* the causative agent of tetanus, is a soil-bearing, gram-positive, anaerobic, motile, sporing, exotoxin-producing, slender rod with parallel sides and rounded ends. The vegetative cell measures 0.2 to 0.6 x 2 to 5 μm. The organism, occurring usually in tissue and culture as single cells, may also form short chains, which tend to separate into individual cells. The spores are terminal and spherical. The vegetative form is highly susceptible to drying, light, heat, and chemical disinfectants. Although the spore is highly resistant, enduring in soil and manure for many months and possibly years, aqueous phenol solution destroys most spores in 10 to 12 hours.

Surface colonies on solid media are flat, feathery, and elevated at the center. On agar, they hemolyze erythrocytes. Antigenically heterogenous, tetanus bacilli contain ten serotypes, all of which produce the same kind of exotoxin.

The toxin, a protein, contains two fractions: tetanospasmin, which attacks nervous tissue, and tetanolysin, which hemolyzes erythrocytes. Tetanus toxin is stable to freezing and thawing, is destroyed by direct sunshine in 15 hours at 40°C, and in solution is destroyed in 5 minutes at 65°C. The toxin is not absorbed from the lumen of the alimentary tract.

Although investigators do not agree fully on the pathogenesis of tetanus, the consensus is that the toxin acts primarily through the central nervous system. The spores, along with pyogenic bacteria from soil and manure, enter tissues through injuries such as foot punctures, parturition, shearing, castration, elastration, docking, tagging, nail and grass awn punctures, needle perforations, dog bites, and compound fractures. Professional surgical procedures, performed under acceptable hygienic standards, do not result in tetanus. In the anaerobic wound, the pyogenic bacteria produce exudate and kill tissue. The dead tissue, with a low oxygen-reduction potential, and the presence of calcium salts favor growth of the *C. tetani.*

Within these wound conditions, tetanus spores vegetate, and the bacilli synthesize tetanospasmin but remain localized to the wound. The tetanospasmin diffuses into surrounding muscle, enters nerve terminals, and moves within motor axons to the central nervous system. Some tetanospasmin, if a large amount is present, may enter lymph or blood and be transported to the central nervous system. In the cord and medulla, neurons are injured, and reciprocal synaptic inhibitions are abolished. Afferent stimuli are exaggerated, and both prime-moving and antagonistic muscles contract convulsively and more or less continuously. The muscle spasms may bring physical exhaustion. Deaths result from medullary neuron injury and respiratory failure. Nonfatal cases develop protective humoral antitoxin, which probably resides in IgM and IgG fractions. Adult sheep commonly have low titers of antitoxin, which may have formed as a result of toxin synthesized in and absorbed from the rumen.

CLINICAL SIGNS AND POSTMORTEM LESIONS. Following a usual incubation period of 4 to 10 days, clinical signs, all related to muscular spasticity, are initiated in animals with a history of recent injury. In early stages of tetanus, the ears are erect, the tail is stiff and elevated a few inches, the head is extended, the anxious eyes are immobile, and the nictitating membranes are prolapsed. The rigidity and extension of the limbs make walking difficult. The prehension of food and water is difficult, and bloating is common. The temperature rises to a range of 37 to 42°C. Sudden auditory and tactile stimuli provoke violent muscular contractions.

As the disease progresses, enhanced muscular rigidity and continuous extension of the limbs make walking and other coordinated movements impossible. Frequently, the reclining animal cannot rise. When assisted to the standing position, this posture can be maintained only temporarily. Respiration accelerates and anxiety increases. The jaws are firmly set, and nostrils are dilated. Death occurs after 3 to 10 days. In sheep, the mortality is approximately 100% of affected cases.

At necropsy, visible lesions are nonspecific and secondary to intoxication and muscular spasticity. The injury and point of infection are usually discernible. Commonly, purulent exudate from secondary infection is present. Petechial hemorrhages may be found in the voluntary muscles and on serosal surfaces, especially of the heart. Frequently, as a result of difficult breathing, the lungs show emphysema. Histopathologically, the wound shows inflammation and necrosis. *C. tetani* cells are demonstrated with difficulty because of the paucity of organisms.

DIAGNOSIS. Veterinarians diagnose tetanus on evidence of typical signs and a history of injuries within the previous 30 days. An important sign is muscular spasticity provoked by auditory and tactile stimuli. The differential diagnosis requires consideration of strychnine poisoning and hypomagnesemia. Although strychnine poisoning induces similar signs, its course is usually only a few hours. Hypomagnesemia can be evaluated by chemical analyses of sera and by determining the effect of administering aqueous solutions of magnesium salts to the symptomatic animal.

A diagnostic laboratory can provide technical assistance only by analyzing ingesta and sera for conditions considered in the differential diagnosis.

PREVENTION AND TREATMENT. Producers prevent tetanus by removing from pens all sources of potential puncture wounds, such as protruding nails, wood splinters, and traumatizing glass and stone; by removing or blunting horns; and by performing all surgical procedures, such as castrating, docking, tagging, vaccinating, and obstetrics, under hygienic conditions. Although both passive and active immunizations are possible, only passive immunization of exposed animals is practiced. At the time of treating puncture wounds, 500 units of tetanus antitoxin should be administered to an adult sheep. Animals with puncture wounds or parturitional injuries should receive doses of procaine penicillin.

On premises where tetanus is a major problem, the management procedures should be corrected. If tetanus is a result of elastorator bands for docking and castration, the procedure should be changed using a hot iron for docking and aseptic surgical techniques for castration. Following any of these procedures animals should be moved to a clean environment. If problems continue following managemental changes, an immunization program should be considered. *C. tetanus* is available in combination with other clostridial immunogens and can be incorporated into the clostridial immunization program with minimal added expense. Adequate passive immunity, via the colostrum, can be provided by immunizing the ewe with clostridium toxoid. The initial immunization program will require 2 doses of toxoid, the first dose at 8 weeks and the second at 4 weeks prior to lambing. An annual booster given 3 to 4 weeks prior to lambing will provide passive protection in subsequent years. To receive adequate passive protection from colostrum, the lamb must receive an adequate amount shortly after birth as described under Colibacillosis.

Treatment consists of cleaning wounds and administering antibiotics and tranquilizers. Affected animals should be placed in a quiet dark room and should receive chlorpromazine daily at the rate of 100 mg given in divided doses for several days. Puncture wounds should be opened, cleaned, and irrigated with hydrogen peroxide. Penicillin should be given to prevent further growth of *C. tetani*. Tetanus antitoxin, although of questionable value, may be given in large doses. In addition, supportive therapy, such as intravenous fluids with glucose and intragastric fluids and nutrients, should be given daily until normal feeding is resumed. Treatment may be needed for 30 days.

Able, J.J., Frior, W.M., and Chalian, W.: Bull. Johns Hopkins Hosp., *63*:373, 1938.

Behring, S. and Kitasato, S.: Zustandekommen der diphtherie immunitat und der tetanus immunitat bei thieren. Dtsch. Med. Wochenschr., *16*:1113, 1899.

Belschner, H.G.: Mortality among sheep due to tetanus following severe infestation with grass seed and subsequent dipping. Aust. Vet. J.: *1*:108-110, 1925.

Cameron, B., Van Biljon, B., Botha, W., and Knoetze, P.: Comparison of oil adjuvant and aluminum phosphate-absorbed toxoid for the passive immunization of lambs against tetanus. Onderstepoort J. Vet. Res., 30:229-231, 1983.

Kerrin, J.C.: The distribution of *B. tetani* in the intestines of animals. Br. J. Pathol., *10*:370-373, 1929.

McCulloch, E.C.: Tetanus in range lambs. JAVMA, *93*:40-41, 1938.

Noble, W.: Experimental study of the distribution and habitat of the tetanus bacillus. J. Infect. Dis., *16*:132, 1915.

Price, D.L., et al.: Tetanus toxin: direct evidence for retrograde intraaxonal transport. Science, *188*:945-948, 1975.

Ramon, G. and Descombey, P.: L'Anatoxine tetanique et la prophylaie du tetanos chez le cheval et les animaux domestiques. Ann. Inst. Pasteur, *41*:834-849, 1927.

Van Heyningen, W.E.: Tentative identification of the tetanus toxin receptor in nervous tissue. J. Gen. Microbiol., *20*:310-320, 1959.

Enzootic Ataxia

(EA; swayback)

Enzootic ataxia, a metabolic disease of lambs up to 3 months of age, is characterized clinically by progressive incoordination of the hind limbs and pathologically by disruption of neuron and myelin development in the central nervous system. It is caused by a nutritional deficiency during the last half of pregnancy.

Because the disease occurs among lambs of all continents, attacks successive lamb crops in endemic areas, and is manifested in a variety of complex interactions reducing total productivity, the malady has major concerns for the sheep industry. Economic losses result from the death of most affected lambs, the reduced growth rate of subclinically deficient lambs, ill thrift, the interaction with other pathologic diseases, and the cost of preventive programs.

OCCURRENCE. The rate of intestinal absorption of copper and accumulation in the liver varies among breeds of sheep and in family lines. The disease occurs in subsequent pregnancies more frequently in certain family lines and breeds that are continually subjected to copper deficient diets.

Geographically, the disorder occurs in Australia, New Zealand, Peru, Iceland, Britain, Sweden, the Netherlands, Germany, Greece, South Africa, USSR, India, and America. In the United States, the disease uncommonly occurs in California, Colorado, Nebraska, Utah, and possibly other western states.

ETIOLOGY AND PATHOGENESIS. The cause of EA is a deficiency of metabolizable copper in pregnant ewes. Primary deficiency begins in the soil, extends to forage plants, and continues into consuming animals. Conditioned deficiency results from ewes consuming copper antagonists—molybdenum, sulfate, and cadmium from high natural levels in soil and associated plants and from industrial fallout on forage—that cause excretion and finally depletion of copper stores. Copper levels below 80 mg/kg DW of liver and 50 μg/100 ml of plasma indicate low copper status and may lead to cases of EA.

TABLE 4-3. *Copper in Ovine Tissue*

Organ	Normal	Enzootic Ataxia
Liver (mg/kg DW)	120–1000	10–25
Brain (mg/kg DW)	7–20	2–6
Plasma (μg/100 ml)	70–120	20–30

Copper has important metabolic functions in hematopoiesis, osteogenesis, wool and hair pigmentation, and myelination. Secondarily, there are a number of diseases that owe their pathogenesis to copper deficiency and its molecular effect on the copper enzymes and copper dependent systems. Cytochromic oxidase, lysyl oxidase, and superoxidase dismutase control the phagocytosing efficiency of leukocytes, normal oxidative phosphorylation, effect in tissue and erythrocytes, control over inflammatory response, elastin and collagen maturation, and the clearance of cholesterol from plasma. The exact mechanisms causing decreased productivity and unthriftiness are not fully understood. High-energy compounds, biosynthesized by catalytic action of copper-containing cytochrome oxidase, are essential to the production of myelin. In lambs with incipient EA, therefore, the pathogenesis begins with copper deficiency, leads to depression of cytochrome-oxidase activity, and progresses to failure of myelin synthesis. In addition, neurons of the brain stem and spinal cord degenerate and ultimately necrose. In congenital cases, the cerebral white matter progressively gelatinizes, liquefies, and cavitates. In delayed forms, the alterations are limited to neurons in the brain stem and spinal cord and to motor tracts in the spinal cord.

Some changes may be arrested, but not reversed, by supplying copper to affected lambs during early stages of lesion development. Lambs surviving mild spinal cord and brain stem lesions suffer permanent ataxic paraplegias. Deaths at birth probably result from respiratory failure, and deaths in delayed cases from intercurrent diseases.

CLINICAL SIGNS AND POSTMORTEM LESIONS. In affected flocks, different classes and different animals may show different signs. Early signs of copper deficiency in ewes include crimpless wool and general unthrift, followed by anemia and depigmentation of black wool.

In congenital EA, severely affected lambs are dull and often prostrated. The limbs present variable amounts of flaccid paralysis, but may evince some reflex activity. Lambs less severely affected may be alert and show both ocular and limb reflexes. Developing in lambs 2 to 4 months of age, delayed EA produces posterior weakness, incoordination, and paralysis that slowly progresses forward to include the forelimbs. Early signs can be provoked by forced running and driving. The abnormal ambulation is accomplished by lateral oscillations and hopping movements of the hind limbs. Bones are brittle.

The flock morbidity ranges up to 90% of the lambs, with a high mortality among affected animals. The clinical course varies from a few days to several weeks.

At necropsy, gross lesions occur in the brain. Some congenital cases show variable amounts of thickening or thinning of gyri in intact brains and gelatinous degeneration and gross cavitation in white matter of cut brains (Fig. 4-14). Many delayed cases 2 to 4 months of age show no gross changes.

Distinctive histopathologic alterations occur in both the brain and spinal cord. Areas of gelatinous white matter consist of a loose mass of fluid, glial fibers and neuronal fibers. Many

Fig. 4-14. Amyelination of cerebrum in a lamb with enzootic ataxia. Cavitations (*a*) and lateral ventricles (*b*). × 0.8. (Courtesy of Professor Stuart Young)

axons are unmyelinated. Throughout the brain stem and spinal cord, some large neurons show chromatolysis, swelling peripheral nuclei, necrosis, and hyalinization. Dorsolateral, dorsal spinocerebellar, and ventral corticospinal tracts of the spinal cord may be bilaterally unmyelinated (Fig. 4-15).

DIAGNOSIS. Veterinarians diagnose EA on evidence of signs, lesions, and chemical analyses. Incoordinated movements of the posterior limbs of lambs, and uncrimped and depigmented wool in ewes are important signs. Gelatinous degeneration and cavitation in cerebral white matter, neuron degeneration in the brain stem and spinal cord, and unmyelinated tracts in the spinal cord are indicative lesions. Low copper levels in the blood, liver, and brain confirm the diagnosis. In nonspecific or subclinical copper deficiency, other biochemical criteria are required to support a diagnosis. Levels of erythrocyte superoxide dismutase (ESOD), a copper zinc containing enzyme in erythrocytes, and fleece copper may correlate more closely with clinical or

Fig. 4-15. Amyelination of dorsolateral, dorsal spinocerebellar, and ventral corticospinal tracts in the spinal cord of a lamb with enzootic ataxia. Weil's stain. × 11.

subclinical illness than the conventional liver and plasma copper, but need further study to be incorporated into a diagnostic and prevention scheme. The differential diagnosis requires consideration of Border disease, fetal injuries from blue tongue virus and, in some areas, louping-ill.

PREVENTION. A program for the control of clinical and subclinical copper deficiency is extremely complex and depends on a knowledge of the geographical distribution of copper deficient soils with insufficient copper in forages or excesses of molybdenum, sulfate, and cadmium which block the absorption of available copper. Genetic predispositions must be taken into account as certain breeds and family lines absorb and store copper at different rates making them more or less susceptible to toxicity from treatments. Time of the year and parasite damage to the abomasum may alter the requirements and absorption. The clinical markers of wool changes, unthriftiness and depigmentation coupled with the biochemical markers of liver and plasma levels, and erythrocyte superoxide dismutase activity reflect the range of severity and are the basis for a comprehensive preventive program. Commercially available preparations for injection include copper methionate, copper calcium edetate, and copper oxyquinoline sulphonate. Copper supplementation is provided by commercial firms in the form of copper oxide from oxidized copper wires administered orally or from a bolus of copper-containing controlled release glass. Commercially available products for parenteral administration contain either copper methionate, copper calcium edetate, or copper oxyquinoline sulphonate and must be given early in pregnancy to prevent teratogenic defects in the fetus. These products provide rapid restoration of copper levels, but must be considered as short term supplementation requiring repeated administration over the period of greatest demand. The milk from supplemented ewes will not provide adequate copper to the lamb; therefore, it is necessary to provide copper to the lamb at 3 to 5 weeks of age. Oxidized copper wire at the rate of 2 g/lamb or

4 g/ewe provides adequate copper without problems of toxicity for longer periods of time than the parenteral preparations. The duration and dosage is somewhat dependent on the levels of molybdenum and sulfate.

The oxidized copper wire is commercially available in Europe, Australia, and New Zealand. Slow release glass boluses have not been as effective in maintaining adequate copper levels as oxidized copper wire, needing further development into rate of release adjusted for a variety of copper depleting conditions.

Allen, W. and Mallinson, C.: Parenteral methods of supplementation with copper and selenium. Vet. Rec., 114:451-454, 1984.

Allen, W. and Sanson, B.: Methods of copper supplementation. Vet. Rec., 117:479-480, 1985.

Barlow, R.M.: Further observations on swayback pathology. J. Comp. Pathol., 73:51-60, 1963a.

Barlow, R.M.: Further observations on swayback histochemistry and cytochrome-oxidase activity in the central nervous system. J. Comp. Pathol., 73:61-67, 1963b.

Barlow, R.M. and Cancilla, P.A.: Structural changes of the central nervous system in swayback of lambs. Acta Neuropath., 6:175-180, 1966.

Barlow, R.M., Field, A.C., and Ganson, N.C.: Measurement of nerve cell damage in the spinal cord of lambs with swayback. J. Comp. Pathol., 74:530-541, 1964.

Barlow, R.M., Purves, D., Butler, E.J., and MacIntyre, I.J.: Swayback: II. Clinical, pathological, biochemical aspects. J. Comp. Pathol., 70:411-427, 1960.

Behrens, H. and Schulz, L.C.: Swayback in lambs. DTW, 66:502-506, 1959.

Bennetts, H. W. and Beck A.B.: Enzootic ataxia and copper deficiency of sheep in West Australia. CSIRO Bull., 147, 1942.

Bennetts, H.W.: Enzootic ataxia of lambs in western Australia. Aust. Vet. J., 8:137-183, 1932.

Bennetts, H.W. and Chapman, F.E.: Copper deficiency in sheep: a report on etiology of enzootic ataxia of lambs. Aust. Vet. J., 13:138-149, 1937.

Boyne, R. and Arthur, J.: Effects of selenium and copper deficiency on neutrophil function in cattle. J. Comp. Path., 91:271-276, 1981.

Britt, D. and Yeoman, G.: Susceptibility of North Ronaidsay sheep to copper from cupric oxide needles. Vet. Res. Comm., 9:57-65, 1985.

Cancilla, P.A. and Barlow, R.M.: Structural changes of the central nervous system in swayback lambs: White matter of spinal cord. Acta Neuropath., 11:294-300, 1968.

Cancilla, P.A. and Barlow, R.M.: Structural changes in the central nervous system in swayback. Acta Neuropath., 6:251-259, 1966.

Cordy, D.R. and Knight, H.D.: California goats with a disease resembling enzootic ataxia. Vet. Pathol., 15:179-185, 1978.

Cunningham, I.J.: Copper deficiency in cattle and sheep in New Zealand. N.Z. J. Agric., 69:559, 1944.

Dandamaev, S.G. and Abramova, S.M.: Symptoms and pathology of enzootic ataxia in lambs of Daghestan. Veterinariia (Moscow), No. 1, 38-42, 1956.

Dick, A.T.: Assimilation and storage of copper in sheep. Aust. J. Agric. Res., 5:511-544, 1954.

Fell, B.F., Mills, C.F., and Boyne, R.: Cytochrome-oxidase deficiency in copper-deficient lambs: histochemistry. Res. Vet. Sci., 6:170-177, 1965.

Howell, McC. and Davison, A.N.: Copper content and cytochrome-oxidase activity in swayback lambs. Biochem. J., 72:365-368, 1959.

Howell, McC., Davison, A.N., and Oxberry, J.: Biochemical and neurological changes in swayback. Res. Vet. Sci., 5:376, 1964.

Hurley, L.: Teratogenic aspects of manganese, zinc and copper nutrition. Physiology Reviews, 61:277-287, 1981.

Innes, J.R.M. and Shearer, G.D.: Swayback: a demyelinizing disease of lambs. J. Comp. Pathol., 53:1-35, 1940.

Jensen, R., Maag, D.D., and Flint, J.C.: Enzootic ataxia from cooper deficiency in sheep in Colorado. JAVMA, 133:336-340, 1958.

Judson, G., et al.: Oxidized copper wire particles for copper therapy in sheep. Aust. J. Agric. Res., 33:1073-1083, 1982.

Judson, G., et al.: Oxidized copper wire as a copper supplement: a study of some variables which may alter availability. Aust. Vet. J., 61:294-295, 1984.

Judson, G., Trengove, C., and Langman, M., Vandergraff, R.: Copper supplementation of sheep. Aust. Vet. J., 61:40-43, 1984.

MacPherson, A.: Methods of copper supplementation. Vet. Rec., 117:330-331, 1985.

McDonald, I.W.: Enzootic ataxia of lambs in Australia. Aust. Vet. J., 18:165, 1942.

McMurray, C.: Copper deficiency in ruminants. Excerpta medica (Ciba Foundation Symposium 79), 183-207, 1980.

Mills, C.F. and Fell, B.F.: Demyelination in lambs born of ewes maintained on high intake of sulphate and Mo. Nature, 150:20-22, 1960.

Mills, C.F. and Williams, R.B.: Copper concentrations and cytochrome oxidase activities in brains of copper-deficient lambs. Biochem. J. 85:629, 1962.

Schulz, K.C.A., Van der Merwe, P.K., Van Rensburg, P.J.J., and Swart, J.S.: Demyelinating diseases of copper deficient sheep. Onderstepoort J. Vet. Res., 25:35, 1951.

Stewart, W.L.: Swingback in lambs. Vet. J., 88:133-137, 1932.

Suttle, N.: Effectiveness of orally administered cupric oxide needles in alleviating hypocupraemia in sheep and cattle. Vet. Rec., 108:417-420, 1981.

Suttle, N.: Use of erythrocyte copper: zinc superoxide dismutase activity and hair or fleece copper concentrations in the diagnosis of hypocuprosis in ruminants. Res. Vet. Sci., 35:47-52, 1983.

Tabusso, M.E.: Paraplegia enzootica of sheep in Peru. Inst. Natl. Biol. Anim., 1:5-30, 1942.

Telfer, S., Zervas, G., and Carlos, E.: Curing or preventing deficiencies in copper, cobalt, and selenium in cattle and sheep using tracerglass. Can. J. Anim. Sci., 64:Suppl. 234-235, 1984.

Vanderberg, R., Levels, F., and Vanderschee, W.: Breed differences in sheep with respect to the accumulation of copper in the liver. Vet. Quarterly, 5:26-31, 1983.

Whitelaw, A., et al.: Studies in the prophylaxis of induced copper deficiency in sheep grazing reseeded hill pastures. Anim. Prod., 37:441-448, 1983.

Whitelaw, A., et al.: Use of cupric oxide needles in the prophylaxis of induced copper deficiency in lambs grazing improved pastures. Vet. Rec., 112:382-384, 1983.

Yeoman, G.: Copper in relation to lamb loss. Vet. Rec., 113:547, 1983.

Border Disease

(BD; hairy shaker disease)

Border disease (BD) is a congenital viral infection of sheep and goats, characterized by embryonic death with or without abortion, mummification, stillbirths, weak lambs with low viability, abnormal hairy birthcoat, and defective central nervous system with nervous symptoms. Because of increasing incidence and significant financial waste, the disease concerns all sheep breeders. Economic losses result from total reproductive performance (embryonic and fetal death and poor viability and production of live births). Cattle and goats can become infected adding to the epizootiologic significance of the disease.

OCCURRENCE. The virus of BD can infect sheep and goats and cattle from the embryonic stage of development to the adult animal. The pathologic insult varies with the time of viral encounter with early embryonic life being most susceptible to damage. This susceptibility to cellular damage gradually decreases with embryonic age and becomes insignificant as the animal matures. The disease was first reported in the late forties along the border between England and Wales, thus the term Border disease. The syndrome has subsequently been reported from Ireland, Scotland, Germany, Netherlands, Norway, Switzerland, Greece, New Zealand, Australia, Canada, and the United States.

ETIOLOGY. Border disease virus, Bovine viral diarrhea virus (BVDV) and Hagcholera virus (HCV) share an antigenic interrelationship and have been incorporated into the genus Pestivirus of the family Togaviridae. The genus Pestivirus constitutes a homogeneous group with a buoyant density in sucrose of 1.12 g/cm^3 and a sedimentation coefficient of 1.38 ± 115, irrespective of the virus strain or the host cell used for its propagation. The shape and size of BVD is at present unknown, but in view of its antigenic and structural similarities it may be assumed that the morphology will not differ from the BVDV. BVD can be grown in primary or secondary cell cultures of calf testis, calf kidney, sheep kidney, or in continuous lines of fetal lamb muscle, bovine turbinate, and pig kidney cells. Most isolates are non-cytopathogenic. Some strains may show cytopathogenic effects in fetal lamb kidney and lamb muscle cells.

BVD and BVDV have similar physical and biologic properties; their antigenic relationship, as determined by virus-specific neutralization tests and their heterogenicity both within and between strains, make BVD and BVDV indistinguishable in vitro. These properties and the ability to cross-infect the bovine and ovine species and cause comparable congenital defects are justification for considering the etiologic agents as a single viral entity with the terms BVD and BVDV referring to the host species of origin resulting in congenital hypomyelinogenesis. This is manifested clinically by varying degrees of tremor, and in smooth fleeced breeds a hairiness of the fleece. Thus the "hairy-shaker" syndrome. These lambs do not contain precolostral BD virus-neutralizing antibodies.

The tremor and hypomyelinogenesis gradually resolve (16 to 20 weeks post mortem), the colostral antibody wanes and the recovered hairy shaker lamb again becomes seronegative and excretes virus for life. However, an infection before the onset of immune competence does not necessarily produce fetal abnormalities, but the development of a seronegative, clinically normal lamb that may harbor and excrete the virus for life and thus be tolerant to the infecting strain of virus. Early fetal infections (70 to 80 days) may lead to an array of malformations including hydranencephaly, porencephaly, cerebellar hypo- or dysplasia, and severe skeletal abnormalities. The pathologic effects which retard the growth and production potential of the infected clinically normal individual are not clearly understood.

TRANSMISSION. In infected sheep, either congenitally or as adults, the virus can be isolated from the respiratory, digestive, urinary tract, and skin, which suggests that excretion of the virus is by these pathways. All uterine discharges at the time of delivery or abortion contain virus. The route of infection is unknown but the most probable mode of entry is via ingestion or inhalation. The infected adult may shed the virus for only a short period, but the congenitally infected lamb can shed the organism for a lifetime. The virus infects the fetus via the transplacental route. If the infection occurs prior to the development of fetal immunocompetence (70 to 90 days), the lamb will become a tolerant persistent excretor of the virus, rarely developing neutralizing antibodies, and can excrete the virus for a lifetime. Infected seronegative ewes may produce infected lambs with each consecutive lambing. The BD viral antigen is in almost all tissues of affected newborn lambs including primary oocysts of the ovaries and in the spermatogenic epithelium of the testicles. Upon maturing, the infected ram or ewe provides the opportunity for vertical transmission with the germ-cells to the embryo.

Transmission of BVDV from cattle to sheep occurs and can be responsible for a BD outbreak when the two species are commingled.

PATHOGENESIS. Following infection of a susceptible ewe and development of viremia, the virus is disseminated to the maternal placenta. The BVD replicates in the placentome and crosses the placental barrier to the fetus with or without placental lesions. Following viral access to the fetus, the virus can spread via the fetal blood stream from cell to cell. A favorable environment for replication of the virus is created by the active metabolism of fetal cells, therefore becoming established in almost all fetal tissues. The development age of the fetus at the time of viral insult as well as the virus strain-host genotype interaction determines the type and extent of placental and fetal damage. In general, the fetus is most

vulnerable prior to the onset of immunocompetence (70 to 90 days). Within about 10 days following infection, the ewe develops a focal or diffuse placentitis with caruncular necrosis which may contribute to the fetal death, resorption, mummification, or abortion. If the pregnancy is sustained, the placentitis heals in about 25 days.

Infection of the fetus after 80 to 90 days of gestation is followed in about 15 to 20 days by a disseminated nodular periarteritis particularly marked in the fetal CNS affecting mainly small distributing arteries and arterioles in meninges and brain substance. These lesions tend to disappear in a few months. This periarteritic form of BD is subclinical and produces precolostral antibodies. The capability to excrete infective virus is doubtful. Infections in the first 70 to 80 days of gestation results in interference with the process of myelination of the CNS.

CLINICAL SIGNS AND POSTMORTEM LESIONS. Among infected ewes, the prominent sign is abortion of macerated or mummified fetuses. Newborn lambs present characteristic signs varying from slight to severe in degree. The birthcoat contains excessive hair and long curly wool. Pigmented fibers, distributed throughout the fleece, concentrate over the neck. Muscular tremors are prominent in posterior limbs and are often evident in the head and neck. Severe muscular dysfunction may cause incoordinated movements and inability to stand and nurse. Affected lambs are unthrifty and grow slowly. The morbidity varies up to 35%, and the mortality of affected animals is high, especially during the first month of life. Both signs and effects abate with maturation.

Lesions are located in the placenta, skin, central nervous system, and joints. Some placentomes contain carunculitis with thrombosis and infarction, and some fetuses are mummified. Aborted fetuses, stillbirths, and lambs present the more characteristic lesions. Dermal follicles are enlarged, and primary fiber shafts are thickened and heavily medullated. In the central nervous system, hydranencephaly, microgyria, hydrocephalus and cerebellar hypoplasia may be present. Microscopic changes include focal microgliosis in the cerebrum and spinal cord, perivascular inflammation in ventral horns, and neuronal vacuolation, axon swelling, and dysmyelinogenesis in the spinal cord and brain stem. Some joints present arthrogryposis.

DIAGNOSIS.   Veterinarians diagnose BD on evidence of typical signs, lesions, and serologic studies. Abortions and hairy fleece, unthriftiness, and muscular tremors in young lambs strongly suggest the disease. Laboratory findings of hypomyelinogenesis and microgliosis in fetuses and lambs, and neutralizing antibodies specific to BD virus in sera of dams and lambs confirm the diagnosis.

The differential diagnosis requires consideration of genetic hairiness that is not associated with tremor of unthriftiness, and swayback that is caused by copper deficiency.

PREVENTION.   Principles and procedures for minimizing or avoiding BD include the following:

1. Separate breeding ewes from cattle.

2. Eliminate affected lambs and their placentas from herd access, and isolate affected dams until genital discharges cease.

3. Eliminate affected ewes that have produced infected offspring more than once.

4. Consider a vaccination program with BVD vaccine in flocks suffering annual BD outbreaks. Vaccine failures, however, may occur due to the existence of non-cross-protecting strains of BVD or BVDV. Regulations may prohibit use of BVDV vaccines in some countries. Two doses of an inactivated vaccine prior to breeding would provide protection for the vaccine strain and avoid complications associated with MLV vaccines.

Acland, H.M., Gard, G.P., and Plant, J.W.: Infection of sheep with mucosal disease virus. Aust. Vet. J., 48:70, 1972.
Bagley, C., Ross, S., and Thomas, J.: Prevention of Border disease in lambs. VM/SAC, 78:426–428, 1983.
Barlow, R.M.: Pathologic changes in ewes with Border disease. J. Comp. Pathol., 82:151-157, 1972.
Barlow, R.M. and Dickinson, A.G.: Neuropathology in Border disease of sheep. Res. Vet. Sci., 6:230, 1965.
Barlow, R.: Some interactions of virus and maternal/foetal immune mechanisms in border disease of sheep. Immunology of Nervous System Infections. Progress in Brain Research. Vol. 59. Edited by P.O. Behan, V. Meulen, and F. Rose. New York, Elsevier Science Publishers, Inc., 1983, pp. 255–268.
Done, J., et al.: Border disease of sheep: Spinal cord morphometry. J. Comp. Path., 95:325-333, 1985.
Gardiner, A. and Barlow, R.: Vertical transmission of Border disease infection. J. Comp. Path., 91:467-470, 1981.
Groverman, F. and Salsbury, D.: Passive antibody response in lambs after vaccination of pregnant ewes with modified live bovine virus diarrhea vaccine. VM/SAC, 78:1445-1449, 1983.
Hamilton, A. and Timoney, P.J.:B.V.D. virus and "border disease." Vet. Rec., 91:468, 1972.
Jackson, T.A., Osburn, B.I., and Crenshaw, G.L.: Reproduction of hairy fleece in California sheep. Vet. Rec., 91:223-224, 1972.
Manktelow, B.W., Porter, W.L., and Lewis, K.H.C.: Hairy shaker disease of lambs. N.Z. Vet. J., 17:245-248, 1969.
Osburn, B.I., Crenshaw, G.L., and Jackson, T.A.: Hairy fleece and tremors in lambs. JAVMA, 160:442-445, 1972.
Plant, J., Acland, H., Gard, G., and Waler, K.: Clinical variations of Border disease in sheep according to the source of the inoculum. Vet. Rec., 113:58-60, 1983.
Potts, B., Berry, L., Osburn, B., and Johnson, K.: Viral persistence and abnormalities of the central nervous system after congenital infection of sheep with Border disease. J. Infect. Dis., 151:337-343, 1985.
Roeder, P., Sweasey, D., and Terlecki, S.: Border disease virus infection of the newborn lamb. Br. Vet. J., 139:129-136, 1983.
Salsbury, D.: Control of respiratory disease and Border disease in sheep. Vet. Med., 79:401-404, 1984.
Shaw, I.G., Winkler, C.E., and Terlecki, S.: Reproduction of hypomyelinogenesis congenita in lambs. Vet. Rec., 81:115, 1967.
Shelton, M.: Relation of temperature to birth weight and mortality in lambs. J. Anim. Sci., 23:360-364, 1964.
Terpstra, C.: Border Disease. A congenital infection of small ruminants. Prog. Vet. Microbiol. Immu., 1:175-198, 1985.

DISEASES OF THE BLOOD AND BLOOD-FORMING SYSTEM

Tularemia

(Rabbit fever)

Tularemia, an acute septicemic zoonosis of range sheep, especially lambs, is characterized by fever, muscular stiffness, and lymph node enlargement and is caused by bacteria transmitted by wood ticks. Because of its limited geographic distribution, the disease has minor importance to the entire sheep industry, but in some individual enterprises within enzootic areas the malady may cause severe financial waste. Economic losses result from deaths of lambs and ewes, from abortions and stillbirths, from loss of live weight, unthriftiness, and wool damage among surviving animals, from the cost of expensive herd treatments, from restricted use of affected range lands, and from temporary incapacitation of infected workers. Occurrence of the disease among cattle and people of enzootic areas adds economic importance and public health significance to the malady.

OCCURRENCE. Tularemia occurs in all breeds, sexes, and ages of sheep, but nursing lambs and yearling ewes are more susceptible than other age groups. In addition to sheep, tularemia also occurs in cattle, rodents, rabbits, and people. Since ticks transmit the causative bacteria, the clinical disease occurs during spring months when vectoring ticks are abundant and active.

Geographically, tularemia occurs among sheep of the western states of America—especially Idaho and Montana—where numerous epizootics have developed since 1929. The malady also occurs in western Canada and the southern republics of the USSR. Despite limited distribution of the disease, the causative organism is widely distributed throughout the world.

ETIOLOGY AND PATHOGENESIS. *Francisella tularensis*, the specific cause of tularemia, is a pleomorphic, nonmotile, nonsporing, capsulated, aerobic, gram-negative bacillus, measuring 0.2 to 0.7 × 0.3 to 3.0 μm. It grows on blood-glucose-cystine agar at pH values near 7.0. Reduced oxygen tension enhances growth on solid media, where the translucent colonies develop a viscid consistency. The organisms produce no gas but some acid by fermenting glucose, glycerol, mannose, maltose, fructose, and dextrin.

F. tularensis possesses moderate resistance to inimical factors of the environment. In dried feces, it lives 25 to 30 days and in infected tissue preserved in glycerol at $-14°$C for several years, but a temperature of $58°$C kills the bacteria in 10 minutes and 1% tricresol in 2 minutes.

Strains of *F. tularensis* possess homogeneous antigens and stimulate the formation of agglutinins. The organisms can be isolated from infected ticks and from infected sheep viscera.

Tularemia, primarily an environmental disease of rodents and rabbits, is transmitted among those mammals by ticks and biting flies. Among American sheep, however, the wood tick, *Dermacentor andersoni,* is the vector, and in western epizootics, large numbers of this arthropod parasitize tularemic sheep. In enzootic areas, infected rodents on sheep-grazing ranges maintain a reservoir of pathogens. Larval and nymphal ticks acquire infection by feeding on infected rodents and rabbits; the trans-stadially infected adult ticks feed on susceptible sheep and, in the process, transmit *F. tularensis*. Large numbers of infective ticks in a range area attack and parasitize bands of grazing or marching sheep and thus initiate an epizootic of tularemia. People contract tularemia from infected tick bites and from handling infected sheep tissues.

The pathogenesis of tularemia begins with the hematophagous tick. While feeding on susceptible sheep, the infected ticks exsanguinate the host and simultaneously inject *F. tularensis*-containing saliva. In the sheep, the pathogens, moving through afferent lymphatics, enter the regional lymph nodes. Some organisms localize in the nodes, but others, moving through efferent lymphatics, eventually enter the blood and produce septicemia.

The organisms, transported by the blood to all tissues, may establish infection in other lymph nodes, spleen, liver, lungs, and joints. Nodal infection persists in some sheep for several months. During the course of an epizootic, infected sheep develop high titers of agglutinins, which gradually decline over 7 or more months. Recovered sheep are immune. In fatal cases, deaths probably result from shock and intoxication.

CLINICAL SIGNS AND POSTMORTEM LESIONS. Epizootic tularemia usually attacks range bands of ewes and lambs, but lambs are more seriously affected than the ewes. Sick lambs, lagging behind the moving flock, move stiffly, act depressed, incline to recumbency, and lose weight. When walking, they carry their heads high. The body temperature ranges from 41 to 42°C and the pulse is weak and rapid. Breathing and coughing accelerate.

Anemia and diarrhea develop. Peripheral nodes, especially the prescapular nodes, are noticeably swollen. Large numbers of wood ticks parasitize the skin in the axillae and around the ears. Affected ewes may abort or bear stillborn lambs. The morbidity ranges up to 40% and the mortality of affected sheep up to 38%. In 1958, Idaho scientists found a 9% mortality among 22,000 lambs of 16 infected bands of sheep. The course varies from 5 to 10 days.

At necropsy, attached ticks and anemic tissues are conspicuous. Numerous hemorrhages, especially around tick injuries, are distributed through the subcutaneous and subserosal tissues. Lymph nodes are enlarged and may contain foci of necrosis and suppuration. Pneumonia in some lambs affects the apical and cardiac lobes of the lungs.

DIAGNOSIS. Veterinarians diagnose tularemia from evidence of clinical signs and laboratory findings. Fever, stiffness, and tick parasitism in range lambs and yearling ewes are indicative signs. In the laboratory, the isolation of *F. tularensis* from attached ticks or from lymph nodes, spleen, and liver of sick and moribund sheep and/or finding a rising agglutination titer among convalescent animals confirms the diagnosis.

The differential diagnosis requires consideration of tick paralysis and other pneumonias.

PREVENTION AND TREATMENT. Producers avoid tularemia by preventing sheep from grazing or trailing ranges when large numbers of infected ticks are active. In some instances, however, this cannot be practiced. Because of human susceptibility to tularemia, herdsmen and caretakers should avoid opening dead sheep.

Treatment of affected sheep consists of removing and destroying the ticks by applying approved tickcides to the flock as recommended in the discussion of ticks. Individual lambs can be successfully treated with 7 to 11 mg of oxytetracycline per kg of body weight or with 400,000 units of penicillin combined with 0.5 g dihydrostreptomycin.

Frank, F.W. and Meinershagen, W.A.: Tularemia epizootic in sheep. Vet. Med., 56:374-378, 1961.
Gwatkin, R., Painter, R.H., and Moynihan, I.W.: Tularemia in sheep. Can. J. Comp. Med., 6:163-168, 1942.
Jellison, W., Jacobson, H., and Flora, S.: Tickborne tularemia and tick paralysis in cattle and sheep. Proc. 68th Ann. Meeting USLSA, 1965, pp. 60-64.
Jellison, W.L. and Kohls, G.M.: Persistence of agglutinins against *Pasteurella tularensis* in naturally infected sheep. JAVMA, 127:405-408, 1950.
Jellison, W.L. and Kohls, G.M.: Tularemia in sheep. Public Health Monograph No. 28, 1955, pp. 1-17.
Parker, R.R. and Dade, J.S.: Tularemia in sheep in nature. U.S. Public Health Reports, 44-1:126-130, 1929.
Pogosyan, A.A.: Clinical and hematological studies of experimental tularemia in sheep. Tr. Armyan. nauchnoissled. ser. Vet. No. 9, 1956, pp. 63-80.
Saitsev, A.A., Poprovskaya, E.V., and Belikov, M.N.: Persistence and localization of tularemia in experimentally infected sheep. Veterinariia (Moscow), No. 7, 26-27, 1965.

Cobalt Deficiency

(CD; pining; bush-sickness; coast disease; enzootic marasmus)

Cobalt deficiency, a chronic wasting disease of sheep and cattle, is characterized by anorexia, anemia, and loss of live weight and is caused by dietary deficiencies. In New Zealand, it has also been associated with white liver disease, a hepatic lipodystrophy.

Because the disease is codistributed with deficiencies in soils and plants, pervades most flocks in deficient regions, and causes extensive financial privation to sheep enterprises, CD concerns the entire sheep industry. Financial losses result from unthriftiness, inefficient use of feed, stunted growth, wool damage, and deaths, and from the cost of preventive and therapeutic programs. Occurrence of the disease with comparable severity and extent in cattle adds to the economic significance of the malady.

OCCURRENCE. Cobalt deficiency affects ruminants grazing forages low in cobalt content with a higher susceptibility and prevalence in sheep than in other ruminants, and in young more than adults. Weaned lambs are highly susceptible. A combination of high soil pH, and high magnesium associated with low salt cobalt yields cobalt deficient forages. Plants on improved lowland pastures that have been reclaimed by draining, liming and reseeding have a decreased cobalt uptake. The most severely deficient areas in the United States are portions of New England and the lower Atlantic costal plain. Areas of New England, northern New York, northern Michigan and parts of the central plains are moderately deficient. Cobalt deficiences occur in New Zealand, Australia, Scotland, Holland, Norway, Poland, and western Canada. A cobalt deficiency syndrome called white liver disease (WLD) occurs primarily in New Zealand and occasionally in the other countries mentioned except the United States. White liver disease occurs in areas with sandy or pumice soils which are deficient in cobalt, and is associated with periods of high rainfall, exuberant growth, and an abundance of dead forage from the previous years.

ETIOLOGY AND PATHOGENESIS. An inadequate dietary supply of cobalt causes clinical cobalt deficiency. Continuous and exclusive grazing on forage containing less than 0.07 ppm DW cobalt and an average daily intake of less than 0.08 mg gradually leads to clinical deficiency. For rapidly growing young lambs the requirement may be as much as 0.2 mg per day during the first few months. Cobalt supplementation at less than weekly intervals may also, after a few years, result in serious unthriftiness.

The only known function of cobalt (Co) in sheep nutrition is to promote vitamin B_{12} synthesis by the rumen microflora. A deficiency in dietary cobalt leads to inadequate production of vitamin B_{12} and ultimately a failure in enzyme systems. One important energy-related enzyme system is the metabolism of propionate via methylmalonyl co-enzyme A to succinate.

In the rumen, microorganisms assist the host animal. Gram-negative bacilli convert cellulosic and other carbohydrate feeds into propionic, acetic, and butyric acids. At the same time, nonfermentative bacteria, in the presence of adequate amounts of cobalt, daily synthesize 600 to 1000 μg of vitamin B_{12}, a cobalamin compound containing 4.0% cobalt. Approximately 3% of the ruminal vitamin B_{12} is absorbed and, in the liver, concentrations of 0.15 to 0.2 ppm DW essentially convert propionic acid to glucose and thereby supply required energy to the sheep.

Cobalt deficiency begins in the soil, continues into the plants, and extends into consuming ruminants. Inadequate concentrations of cobalt in ruminal contents depress the daily synthesis of vitamin B_{12} to less than 50 μg. With 3% absorption of this low level, the liver concentration of vitamin B_{12} is reduced to 0.02 to 0.06 ppm DW, a subcritical amount for converting propionic acid to glucose; consequently, cobalt deficiency essentially is a fatal energy starvation. In the case of white liver disease, in addition to a cobalt deficiency, it has been proposed that a plant toxin or mycotoxin may be involved.

CLINICAL SIGNS AND POSTMORTEM LESIONS. The signs of CD gradually develop after sheep consume deficient forage for a few months. In early stages, appetite wanes, listlessness supervenes, body weight declines, and anemia appears. As they endure these progressive changes, the affected sheep become weak, the skin and membranes, pale, and a profuse lacrimation stains the face. The hemoglobin level declines from normal values of 11 to 12 g/dl to pathologic values of 8 to 9 g/dl.

Some animals develop exacerbating diarrhea, and lambs born to deficient ewes are weak and unthrifty. The emaciation and anemia, unless treated with cobalt, progress to death. Subclinical manifestations are lack of thrift, reduced fertility, decreased estrous activity, and decreased milk and wool production. There is an increased neonatal mortality and resistance to other diseases is reduced. In white liver disease the above clinical signs are accompanied, in about 10% of the cases, with photosensitization.

In seriously deficient regions, the morbidity reaches 60% and the mortality of affected animals, 80%. The disease develops after sheep graze 4 to 6 months on deficient forage, and the disease course varies from several weeks to a few months.

At necropsy, the emaciated carcass contains little or no adipose tissue. The liver shows fatty degeneration; the spleen, hemosiderosis; and the bone marrow, atrophy.

DIAGNOSIS. Veterinarians diagnose CD on evidence of herd history, clinical signs, and chemical analyses. Diminished appetite, anemia, and loss of live weight, especially among sheep grazing in regions of known deficiency, strongly suggest the disease. Favorable response of test animals daily given 1 mg of dietary cobalt confirms the diagnosis. Measuring less than 0.07 ppm DW cobalt in the forage, less than 0.15 ppm DW cobalt in the liver, or less than 1.0 ng/ml of vitamin B_{12} in serum gives additional evidence.

Vitamin B_{12} levels in the feces is an indicator of the cobalt status of sheep. An equation for estimating oral intake of cobalt on the basis of the amount of vitamin B_{12} in the feces is:

$$Y = 0.0779 X - 0.0757$$

Y represents the oral intake of cobalt expressed as mg/kg in dry feed and X represents the concentration of vitamin B_{12} in the feces expressed as mg of vitamin B_{12} per g of dry feces. In trials a cobalt-adequate diet for lambs containing 0.09 mg/kg diet DM had a corresponding vitamin B_{12} level of 2.13 mg/g of dry feces. The measurement of vitamin B_{12} in the feces can be used to monitor the adequacy of dietary cobalt intake.

The differential diagnosis requires consideration of gastrointestinal parasitism.

PREVENTION AND TREATMENT. To prevent deficiencies cobalt should be ingested frequently. This can be accomplished by supplementing cobalt in: (1) the water, (2) feed, (3) salt, (4) pellets of cobalt oxide, (5) soluble glass containing cobalt, (6) as a spray on forage, and (7) top-dressed on the soil alone or with other fertilizer applications. Drenching and parenteral administration of cobalt are not practical

for a preventive program. Tablets for use in the watering trough which automatically release a regulated amount of cobalt are commercially available. Cobalt can be metered into the water at the rate of 0.2 to 0.4 mg Co/L. Supplementing cobalt via water is most suitable for intensive operations where the amount of water intake can be determined. Where animals are being fed, cobalt supplementation can be added to the concentrate part of the ration at the rate of 2 mg Co/kg DM. The National Research Council (NRC) recommends the addition of 2.5 g Co/100 kg salt using either cobalt chloride or cobalt sulfate. An intake of 10 g salt per day will provide 0.25 mg of cobalt. The use of commercially available cobalt pellets will provide adequate cobalt levels up to 3 years provided they stay in the rumen and are not regurgitated. A controlled release glass bolus containing cobalt and designed to release 0.15 mg Co per day will meet the minimum daily requirements. The annual application of 350 g of cobalt sulfate per ha to deficient soils will meet the requirements for most sheep for the 12 months. Heavier applications .5 to 3 kg hydrated cobalt sulfate will effectively increase the cobalt concentration in pastures for 3 to 5 years. High soil pH and magnesium tend to interfere with cobalt, making the results on these types of pastures unpredictable. Supplementation of cobalt via salt, cobalt oxide pellets, slow-release glass boluses and top dressing are especially useful when sheep are managed under grazing conditions. The National Research Council (1985) suggests 10 mg Co/kg diet dry matter as a maximum level for ruminants.

Treatment consists of a daily dietary supplement of 1 mg of cobalt per animal until improvement occurs.

Allen, W., et al.: Boluses of controlled release glass for supplementing ruminants with cobalt. Vet. Rec., *116*:175-177, 1985.
Andrews, E.D., Stephenson, B.J., Issacs, C.E., and Register, R.H.: Effects of large doses of soluble and insoluble forms of Co given at monthly intervals to Co-deficient lambs. N.Z. Vet. J., *14*:191-196, 1966.
Baxter, J.: Deficiencies of mineral nutrients. In *Current Veterinary Medicine 2—Food Animal Practice*. Edited by J.L. Howard. Philadelphia, W.B. Saunders Co., 1986.

Dewey, D.W., Lee, H.J., and Marston, H.R.: Efficacy of Co pellets for providing Co for penned sheep. Aust. J. Agric. Res., *20*:1109-1116, 1969.

Gawthorne, J.M.: Effect of Co intake on the cobamide and cobinamide composition of rumen contents and blood plasma of sheep. Aust. J. Exp. Biol. Med. Soc., *48*:285-293, 1970.

McLoughlin, M., Rice, D., and Taylor, S.: Liver lesions resembling ovine white liver disease in cobalt deficient lambs. Vet. Rec., *115*:325, 1984.

Marston, H.R.: Requirement of sheep for Co or for vitamin B$_{12}$. Br. J. Nutr., *24*:615-633, 1970.

Marston, H.R.: Primary metabolic defect supervening on vitamin B$_{12}$ deficiency in sheep. Nature, *190*:1085-1087, 1961.

Marston, H.R.: Problems associated with "coast disease" in South Australia. Aust. CSIRO, *8*:111-116, 1935.

Miller, K. and Albyt, A.: A comparison of vitamin B$_{12}$ levels in the liver and serum of sheep receiving treatments used to correct cobalt deficiency. N.Z. Vet. J., *32*: 105-107, 1984.

National Research Council. *Nutrient Requirements of Sheep*. Washington, D.C., National Academy Press, 1985, pp. 18-19.

Pope, A.L., Phillips, P.H., and Bohstedt, G.: Effects of Co on growth and blood constituents of sheep. J. Anim. Sci., *6*:334-342, 1947.

Richards, R. and Harrison, M.: White liver disease in lambs. Aust. Vet. J., *57*:565-568, 1981.

Rickes, E.L., et al.: Vitamin B$_{12}$ a cobalt complex. Science, *108*:134, 1948.

Sutherland, R.J., Cordes, D.O., and Carthew, G.C.: Ovine white liver disease—an hepatic dysfunction associated with vitamin B$_{12}$ deficiency. N.Z. Vet. J., *27*:227-232, 1979.

Underwood, E.J.: *Trace Elements in Human and Animal Nutrition*. New York, Academic Press, 1971, pp. 123-156.

Underwood, E.J. and Filmer, J.F.: Enzootic marasmus. Determination of the biologically potent element (cobalt) in limonite. Aust. Vet. J., *11*:84-92, 1935.

Underwood, E.J. and Harvey, R.J.: Enzootic marasmus: Cobalt content of soils, pastures and animal organs. Aust. Vet. J., *4*:183, 1938.

Zalewska, E., Klebowska, A., Luczycka, M., and Domanski, E.: A deficiency disease of ruminants in Poland. Pol. Arch. Weter., *9*:119-133, 1966.

Watery Mouth Syndrome

Watery mouth syndrome (WMS) is a condition of newborn lambs characterized by depression, inappetance, lethargy, and moistening of the hair around the mouth due to excessive salivation. The syndrome has only in recent years appeared in veterinary literature, although it has been a concern of the practicing veterinarian for some time. The prevalence, distribution, and epidemiology have not been well documented, but WMS is an economically important condition to the sheep industry wherever lambing is conducted under housed conditions in temperate climates.

Clinically WMS occurs most frequently within the first 12 to 72 hours. The lamb first separates itself in a corner of the mothering pen, refuses to nurse, and becomes lethargic and depressed with an attitude of abdominal discomfort. A decrease in gastrointestinal motility may result in an accumulation of gas in the small intestine and abomasum causing abdominal distension in a majority of the cases. The early phases of the syndrome may or may not be associated with diarrhea. As the condition persists, enteritis and diarrhea are frequent sequelae, although retained meconium may be observed. Rectal temperature ranges from 39 to 37°C or less. Epidemiologically the syndrome reaches its peak prevalence during the lambing seasons that are associated with inclement weather conditions. Castration and docking with rubber bands has been incriminated as a predisposing factor, although the incidence can be high in operations where these practices are not conducted at this time. Although a causative microbial agent or agents have not been identified, some operators reduce the incidence by the administration of antibiotics immediately following parturition. As the morbidity rate fluctuates on a daily basis, increasing on cold wet days and decreasing on warm dry summer days, the condition may be precipitated by hypothermia. The only consistent pathogenic factor is a decrease in gastrointestinal motility with increase in abomasal emptying time and an accumulation of gas in the abomasum and small intestine. The morbidity may reach 10% or greater with a high mortality of untreated cases. Oral administration of antibiotics at birth has been effective in reducing losses. Preventive measures include hygienic lambing practices, reduced crowding, adequate dry bedding, early and adequate colostrum intake, and measures to reduce stress and exposure at lambing time. Treatment consists of oral antibiotics as determined by culture and sensitivity. Supportive therapy with oral administration of electrolyte products, which contain electrolytes, an energy source and high quality protein, every 4 hours is beneficial. Treatment with additional colostrum or milk containing a high percentage of fat may not be beneficial as the fat further reduces intestinal motility.

Collins, R., Eales, F., and Small, J.: Observations on watery mouth in newborn lambs. Br. Vet. J., *141*: 135-140, 1985.

Collins, R.: Lamb survival. Vet. Rec., *109*:43-44, 1981.

Cottrell, D.: Watery mouth in lambs. Vet. Rec., *117*:418-419, 1985.

Eales, F., Small, J., and Murray, L. McBean: Abomasal size and emptying time in healthy lambs and in lambs affected by watery mouth. Vet. Rec., *117*:332-335, 1985.

Gilmour, J., Donachie, W., and Eales, F.: Pathological and microbiological findings in 38 lambs with watery mouth. Vet. Rec., *117*:335-337, 1985.

Haig, G.: Lamb survival. Vet. Rec., *108*:195, 1981.

Linklater, K. and Mitchell, G.: Differential diagnosis of scouring lambs. In Practice, 5:4-12, 1983.

Winkler, E.: Lamb survival. Vet. Rec., *108*:342, 1981.

Entropion

Entropion is characterized by the inversion of the eyelids causing irritation to the cornea with subsequent lacrimation usually occurring in the first days of life. As the condition is nonfatal the main economic impact is from culling of potential breeding animals and the necessity for treatment. Entropion occurs in all breeds and both sexes, most frequently involving the lower lid and may involve one or both eyes. The exact cause is unknown although the predisposing factors are thought to be genetic or environmental from extended exposure to heat lamps or ultraviolet irradiation. Some family lines of the white face breeds are more prone to the problem. Clinically, entropion may go unnoticed or misdiagnosed as a pink-eye conjunctivitis. The first clinical response is excessive lacrimation which moistens the hair of the face. If uncorrected, the inverted lower lid damages the cornea resulting in opacity and ulceration.

Diagnosis is by closely examining the eyelids of all lambs that have lacrimation soiling the hair on the side of the face. Shepherds correct the condition by surgically removing an elliptical portion of the skin under the lower lid with a sharp pocket knife. The ensuing scar formation draws the lower lid into proper placement. A more esthetic correction is made by injecting 1 ml of a long-acting, slowly absorbed antibiotic under the skin of the lower lid into proper position. Michelle surgery clips are also used to tighten the skin of the lower lid correcting the inversion. These procedures are most effective early in life while the skin is soft and pliable. Advanced cases may require surgical removal of an elliptical piece of skin with suturing. An ophthalmic ointment may also be indicated in cases of corneal damage.

Replacement and breeding stock should be selected from animals free of the condition.

Severin, G.A.: *Veterinary Ophthalmology Notes.* 2nd Edition. Fort Collins, Colorado State University, 1976.

PART II DISEASES OF FEEDLOT LAMBS

5

ADAPTING LAMBS TO FEEDLOTS

TABLE 5-1. *Schedule for Diets in Feedlots*

Preparation Options	Days in Feedlot	Diet
Pelleted feed		Lambs may graze fields before entering feedlot.
	1–7	Prestarter pellets containing: roughage 67%, concentrate 33%; present in self-feeders free choice. Whole alfalfa available free choice. Adequate fresh water.
	8–14	Starting pellets containing: roughage 45%, concentrate 55%; present in self-feeders free choice. Whole alfalfa available free choice.
	15–20	Intermediate pellets containing: roughage 40%, concentrate 60%; present in self-feeders free choice. Whole alfalfa available free choice.
	21–	Finishing pellets containing: roughage 10%, concentrate 90%; present in self-feeders free choice. Whole alfalfa available free choice. Continue diet until desired live weight is achieved.
Loose feed		Lambs may graze fields before entering feedlot.
	1–7	Ensilage 67%, concentrate 33%; mix and present in self-feeders free choice. Whole alfalfa available free choice. Adequate fresh water.
	8–14	Ensilage 45%, concentrate 55%; mix and present in self-feeders free choice. Whole alfalfa available free choice.
	15–20	Ensilage 40%, concentrate 60%; mix and present in self-feeders free choice. Whole alfalfa available free choice.
	21–	Ensilage 20%, concentrate 80%; mix and present in self-feeders free choice. Whole alfalfa available free choice. Continue diet until desired live weight is achieved.
Roughage and supplement with whole corn	1–3	Pelleted sun cure alfalfa 75%. Pelleted soybean base supplement 10%. Whole corn 12.5%.
	4–	Increase whole corn 10% and reduce sun cure 10% every 3rd day until the ration is 90% whole corn 10% supplement. Grass or whole alfalfa hay free choice adequate fresh water salt free choice.

Table 5-2. *Schedule of Health Treatments in Feedlots*

Days in Feedlot	Vaccinations and Other Treatments
1	—Sort, isolate, and treat all sick lambs. —Vaccinate for enterotoxemia and other clostridia as needed. —Monitor for internal and external parasites and treat accordingly.
1–14	—Monitor lambs closely for any sick individuals or ones not adjusting to the environment. —Provide a sick pen for lambs requiring treatment. —Provide a small pen with less competition for lambs which need help adjusting. —Provide electrolytes in the water (especially beneficial for stressed lambs). —Lasalocid in the feed aids in control of coccidiosis and acidosis.
14	—Revaccinate for enterotoxemia. —Vaccinate for other conditions as needed (e.g., sore mouth). —Shearing and tagging depends on the climate, staple length of wool and pelt credit. —Aureomycin can be added to the supplement to provide 50 mg/head/day although this is being discouraged due to the growing concern over harmful residues in meats.

Entering the feedlot weighing approximately 30 kg, healthy lambs daily consume an average of 1.0 to 1.2 kg of concentrate feed and daily gain an average of 225 to 270 g of live weight. Smaller lambs may adapt slower, daily consume less concentrate feed, and daily gain less live weight. Live weights of marketable lambs usually range from 45 to 50

Table 5-3. *Systems Summary of Diseases at Necropsy for Three Lamb Feedlots, 1974–1978**

Disease Site	Lambs Necropsied	Percent
Digestive system	770	54
Respiratory system	215	15
Urinary system	68	4.9
Nervous system	49	3.4
Metabolic disease	50	3.5
Miscellaneous	281	19.6
Total	1433	

* Pierson, R., Jensen, R., and Breen, H.

kg per lamb. Tables 5-1 and 5-2 present diet and vaccination schedules for use in adapting lambs to the new conditions of fattening.

Health Concerns

Tables 5-3 and 5-4 present a summary of the causes of lamb mortalities in three lamb feedlots of northern Colorado. Tables 5-5, 5-6

Table 5-4. *Causes of Death Involving the Digestive System, 1974–1978, for Three Lamb Feedlots**

Disease Site	Lambs Necropsied	Percent
Enterotoxemia type D	311	40
Acidosis	111	14
Salmonellosis	106	14
Prolapsed rectum	92	12
Septicemic pasteurellosis	70	9
Enterotoxemia type C	22	2.8
Coccidiosis	14	1.8
Others	44	5.7
Total	770	

* Pierson, R., Jensen, R., and Breen, H.

TABLE 5-5. *Health Related Death Losses in a Commercial Lamb Feeding Operation*

Condition*	Mar	Apr	May	June	July	Aug	Sept	Oct	Nov	Dec	Jan	Feb	#	%
Pneumonia	21	3	62	47	105	136	80	86	86	71	21	5	723	37.1
Enterotoxemia**	16	20	28	59	36	47	47	79	42	63	19	14	470	24.1
Acidosis	10	9	51	29	59	65	24	84	76	72	8	6	493	25.3
Enteritis	2		3	6		2	3	1				3	20	1.0
Salmonellosis								1					1	.05
Coccidiosis														
Prolapsed rectum		2		7	10	13	9	4	2	2			52	2.7
Bloat														
Choke														
Polio						1		1	1		1	1	5	0.26
Urinary calculi	4	1		1	1	2		3	3	46	13	1	75	3.9
Transport tetany			4	8	3	7	11	33					66	3.4
Predators			2		2	5	8	3	2	1			23	1.2
Miscellaneous	4	2		1	5	1		4	2				19	1.0
Total	57	37	150	158	221	279	182	299	214	255	62	30	1947	

Survey conducted by Kimberling, C., Reif, J., and Salman, M. with support from the U.S.D.A. National Animal Disease Surveillance program.
* Necropsies were conducted 1 day each week, all other diagnoses were based on clinical observations.
** All lambs were vaccinated with *C. perfringens* C and D toxoid on entry and with *C. perfringens* type D toxoid in 2 weeks.

TABLE 5-6. *The Economic Impact of Death Loss in a Commercial Lamb Feeding Operation Over a Twelve Month Period*

Month	Year	# Purchases	# Sales	# Death Loss	Total Value*	Average Value
Mar	85	11,885	7,404	57	$ 3,959	$69.46
Apr	85	6,646	9,130	37	2,575	69.59
May	85	14,891	7,330	153	11,074	72.38
June	85	8,296	7,066	158	11,077	70.11
July	85	9,143	7,867	221	15,925	72.06
Aug	85	7,912	8,553	279	19,753	70.80
Sept	85	10,640	7,287	182	12,494	68.65
Oct	85	14,668	8,779	299	19,483	65.16
Nov	85	1,457	6,791	214	13,634	63.71
Dec	85	1,357	8,588	255	15,165	59.47
Jan	86	1,598	9,950	62	3,728	60.13
Feb	86	3,972	2,577	30	1,866	62.20
Total		92,465	91,322	1947	$130,733	$67.15

Cost of death loss for each animal entering the feeding program = $1.41.
Death loss as a percentage of animals purchased = 2.1%.
Survey conducted by Kimberling, C., Reif, J., and Salman, M. with support from the U.S.D.A. National Animal Disease Surveillance program.
* Value was based on current market value on the day of the death loss.

TABLE 5-7. *Summary of the Economic Impact of Health Conditions by Systems Involved in a Commercial Lamb Feeding Operation Over a Twelve Month Period*

System	Economic Loss	Percent
Respiratory	$48,549	37.1
Digestive	66,076	50.5
Urinary	5,036	3.9
Prolapse	3,492	2.7
Nervous	4,768	3.6
Miscellaneous	1,276	1.0

and 5-7 present the health related death losses over a 12-month period in a commercial lamb

feeding operation and the economic impact of these conditions. Preventive health programs should be directed toward the most significant problems in each individual operation. As presented in the tables digestive problems cause the greatest economic loss followed by respiratory diseases. Each operation should attempt to diagnose all losses and concentrate the preventive health program on the major problems. As consumer demands for less fat impact the lamb feeding industry, a shift towards higher roughage diets will alter the dietary disease problems.

Pierson, R. and Kimberling, C.: Commercial lamb feedlot management. *Current Veterinary Therapy. 2. Food Animal Practice*. Edited by J. Howard. Philadelphia, W.B. Saunders, 1986, pp. 171-181.
Rench, R.: Personal communication on lamb feedlot management, 1987.

6

DISEASES OF THE DIGESTIVE SYSTEM

Contagious Ecthyma

(CE; contagious pustular dermatitis; sore mouth; scabby mouth; orf)

Contagious ecthyma, an acute eruptive dermatitis of sheep and goats, is characterized by sequential papules, vesicles, pustules, and scabs on the skin of the face, genitals, and feet, and on the mucosae of the mouth, rumen, and genitals. CE is caused by a virus. Because of near universal distribution, CE, as a major disease, prevails against the entire sheep industry. Even though loss to single enterprises is low, the total waste to the industry is high.

Economic losses result from unthriftiness, loss of physical condition, and occasional deaths among feedlot lambs; slow growth, abandonment, premature weaning, and some deaths among suckling lambs; and mastitis and lameness among ewes. Since CE sometimes affects people working directly with infected sheep, rural public health aspects of the disease add to its interest and significance.

OCCURRENCE. CE occurs in all sexes and breeds. Exceptionally resistant or susceptible breeds have not been identified. Although the virus attacks all ages of sheep, the disease more commonly develops among animals less than 1 year of age. Feedlot lambs 3 to 7 months of age typically contract the disease within 2 weeks after entering the fattening pens.

In addition, young lambs, born and temporarily maintained at central lambing buildings, may contract the disease, and some ewes may develop lesions especially on skin of the teats and udder. The probable cause of low incidence among adult sheep is the immunity acquired from exposure to the virus during the first 2 years of life. In addition to sheep, CE also occurs in goats, bighorn sheep and mountain goats, rarely in people and dogs, and possibly in cats.

Seasonally, CE occurs most commonly during the fall months of August, September, and October when lambs commonly enter the feedlot; during some years, nearly all fed lambs contract the disease. During early spring months, the disease incidence may be high among newborn lambs.

Geographically, CE occurs in all countries where the sheep industry has developed.

ETIOLOGY, PATHOGENESIS AND EPIZOOTIOLOGY. The CE virus, a member of the family poxviridae, genus parapoxvirus shares a common morphology, characteristic C + G content in their DNA and group-specific antigens with the viruses of sheep pox, vaccinia, and lumpy skin disease. The virus is a complex structure with the tubular surface of the viron being covered with a closely opposed structure 1.6 to 2 nm thick designated coats and a loosely opposed structure of variable thickness (9 to 18 nm) called envelopes with a total mass measuring 200 to 300 × 125 to 175 nm. Strains of the virus share similar polypeptide profiles

135

but differ in molecular weight from 37,000 to 44,000.

The virus is transmitted by both direct and indirect contact. In feedlots, it contaminates equipment, fences, manure, bedding, and feed. Crowding facilitates direct transmission. Contamination of operating vehicles and workers may disseminate the virus among animals of different pens and enterprises. Infected suckling lambs contaminate teats and udders of dams and, by this means, spread virus among siblings.

The virus will remain viable on the wool of recovered animals for extended periods. Persistent infections, especially subclinical, play an important role in propagating the disease. The clinical disease or vaccination provides variable and incomplete immune protection. Subsequent infections can occur in 1 to 3 months but are less severe and heal more rapidly. The protective response is probably associated with a cell mediated rather than humoral response as passively acquired antibodies from the dam do not play a role in protection. Cell culture-propagated CE virus preparations are less effective for vaccination purposes than are those propagated in sheep. Lambs vaccinated at 1 to 4 days of age will develop protective immunity provided the pre-inoculation passive antibody levels are low as occurs when lambs are born to naturally-infected ewes.

The pathogenesis of CE, usually direct and simple, may become complex from secondary bacterial infection. The virus causes a lesion sequence of papule, vesicle, pustule, and scab. In the feedlot, dried stemmy and spiny feed, such as alfalfa, grass, and awns, may abrade and puncture tissues of the lips, nostrils, mouth, and forestomachs. Through these superficial injuries, the virus penetrates the skin or mucosa and causes acanthosis, ballooning degeneration of spinose cells, hyperplasia of basal cells, and edema and granulomatous inflammation of the derma. Ballooning leads to vesication, and hyperplasia to nodulation.

Bacteria may penetrate the vesicle or pustule and cause secondary infection, extensive necrosis, and ulcers of lips, mouth, and forestomachs; these infections may lead to otitis media, liver abscesses, pneumonia, inanition, and occasionally death.

CLINICAL SIGNS AND POSTMORTEM LESIONS. Following an incubation period of 2 to 3 days, sequential papules, vesicles, pustules, and scabs form on the lips, nostrils, eyelids, mouth, gums, tongue, palate, and middle ears of feedlot lambs, on the feet, eyelids, and mouths of nursing lambs, and on skin and mucosae of genitals and skin of the feet of breeding ewes and rams. The vesicle endures for only a few hours and, consequently, seldom is detected. The fragile pustule, opaque-yellow in color, easily ruptures. By day 11, the scab begins to form and endures as a firm brown mass for 1 to 2 weeks. The pustules and scabs are nodules up to 5 mm in diameter and elevated 2 to 4 mm above the level of surrounding skin. The nodules, composed of exudate and proliferated epithelial cells, may be discrete or confluent and, when forcibly removed, leave a bleeding derma. On the oral and buccal surfaces, the lesions are morphologically similar to the ones on the skin (Fig. 6-1).

One or few lesions on the lips or nostrils cause little discomfort to the animal, but confluent lesions over both upper and lower lips and in the mouth and ears or on the eyes cause intense pain and anorexia; severely affected

Fig. 6-1. Lips (a) and mouth (b) of a feedlot lamb with contagious ecthyma. × 0.8.

lambs lose body weight and may be attacked by screwworms. Sheep with extensive lesions in the mouth and forestomachs may become prostrated and die from complications such as pneumonia. Nursing lambs with severe foot lesions and laminitis may slough their hooves, and ewes with teat lesions may develop mastitis and consequently wean and abandon young lambs.

Among feedlot lambs, the morbidity may reach 90% or more, but mortality is low and due to secondary bacterial infection. The course varies from 1 to 4 weeks.

At necropsy of fatal cases, both discrete and confluent pustules and crusts cover the areas of predilection. In some animals, necrotic tissue and ulcers may exist on the tongue, gums, palate, pharynx, rumen, or omasum and show evidence of spreading bacterial infection. As a result of gastric lesions, liver abscesses may be present. In terminal stages, pneumonia usually develops and causes death.

Histopathologic changes vary with the stage of lesion development. During early stages, the spinose epithelial cells show acanthosis, ballooning degeneration, vesication, pustulation or crusting, and epithelial hyperplasia. The derma is edematous, hyperemic, and infiltrated with leukocytes. Granulomatous reaction forms and then regresses at the time of healing.

DIAGNOSIS. Veterinarians and producers diagnose CE on evidence of characteristic lesions on the anatomic areas of predilection. Usually, the disease is readily diagnosed, but in early stages it may require expert attention. The differential diagnosis requires consideration of ulcerative dermatosis and sheep pox. Ulcerative dermatosis is characterized by ulcers and crusts on skin of the face, feet, and genitalia. The lesion is not elevated, except for some dried exudate, because epithelial hyperplasia is absent.

Sheep pox, a contagious and devastating disease, is characterized by elevated papules over much of the skin surface. The systemic reaction is profound and often fatal. The poxvirus can be isolated and identified by electron microscopy and structural analysis of the poly-

peptide by sodium dodecyl sulfate-polyacrylamide gel electrophoresis.

PREVENTION AND TREATMENT. Veterinarians prevent CE by vaccinating lambs with commercial vaccine prepared from sheep passaged virus. The vaccine is applied to scarified skin of nonwooled areas, such as the medial surface of thighs or the inner surface of the ear. Feedlot lambs should be vaccinated soon after entering the fattening facilities. Suckling lambs 1 to 3 days of age can be vaccinated whenever exposure to virus is anticipated. Annual vaccination of pregnant ewes may deposit enough antibodies in the colostrum to passively immunize nursing lambs for several weeks. Vaccine should not be used, however, in flocks free of the disease.

CE in feedlot lambs should be treated by vaccinating the flock during early stages of the outbreak; by this procedure, the disease course in the flock is shortened, and many complications are avoided. Infected lips, mouths, and nostrils should be softened by applying an ointment containing a broadsprectrum antibiotic to the lesions.

Animal Health Yearbook. FAO-WHO-OIE (Italy), 1970.
Aynaud, M.: La stomatite pustuleuse contagieuse des ovins (chancre du mouton). Ann. Inst. Pasteur, 37: 497-527, 1923.
Buddle, B., Dellers, R., and Schurig, G.: Heterogenecity of contagious ecthyma virus isolates. Am. J. Vet. Res., 45:75-79, 1984.
Buddle, B. and Pulford, H.: Effect of passively-acquired antibody and vaccination of the immune response to contagious ecthyma virus. Vet. Microb., 9:515-522, 1984.
Buddle, B., Dellers, R., and Schurig, G.: Contagious ecthyma virus-vaccination failures. Am. J. Vet. Res., 45:263-266, 1984.
Glover, R.E.: Contagious pustular dermatitis of the sheep. J. Comp. Pathol. Ther., 41:318-340, 1928.
Greig, A.S.: Contagious ecthyma of sheep. II. In vitro cultivation of the virus. Can. J. Comp. Med. Sci., 21:305-308, 1957.
Greig, A., Linklater, K., and Clark, W.: Persistent orf in a ram. Vet. Rec., 115:149, 1984.
Kadyrov, V.G.: Morphological changes in the hearing organs of sheep with pustular dermatitis. Veterinariia (Moscow), No. 11, 45-48, 1968.
Kerry, J.B. and Powell, D.G.: The vaccination of young lambs against contagious pustular dermatitis. Vet. Rec., 88:671-672, 1971.
Le, Jan C., et al.: Transfer of antibodies against the contagious ecthyma virus through colostrum and milk. Ann. Rech. Vet., 9:343-346, 1978.

McKeever, D.: Orf virus persistence. Vet. Rec., *114*:548, 1983.

McKeever, D.: Persistent orf. Vet. Rec., *115*:334-335, 1984.

Mitchner, M.B.: The envelope of vaccinia and orf viruses: An electron-cytochemical investigation. J. Gen. Virol., *5*:211-220, 1969.

Nagington, J., Newton, A.A., and Horne, R.W.: The structure of orf virus. Virology, *23*:461-472, 1964.

Plowright, W., Whitcomb, M.A., and Ferris, R.D.: Studies with a strain of contagious pustular dermatitis virus in tissue culture. Arch. Gesamte. Virusforsch., *9*:214-231, 1959.

Richter, J. and Jansen, J.: Active immunization of sheep against contagious ecthyma. A field trial with an unheated and heated autogenous vaccine. Tijdschr. Diergeneeskd., *93*:757-773, 1968.

Rosenbusch, R. and Reed, D.: Reaction of convalescent bovine antisera with strain-specific antigens of parapoxviruses. Am. J. Vet. Res., *44*:875-878, 1983.

Royer, J., Joubert, L., and Prave, M.: Grave ocular damage in man due to ovine contagious pustular dermatitis. Bull. Soc. Sci. Vet. (Lyon), *72*:93-104, 1970.

Sawhney, A.N.: Studies on viruses of ecthyma contagiosum. Izv. Mikrobiol. Inst. (Sofia), *18*:163-189, 1966.

Subba, M., Malik, B., and Sharama, S.: Antigenic relationships among sheep pox, goat pox and contagious pustular dermatitis viruses. Acta. Virol., *28*:380-387, 1984.

Bloat

(*Tympanites*)

Bloat, a retention of gas in the rumen, is characterized by increased intra-abdominal and intrathoracic pressures and is caused by complex interactions of plant, animal, and microbial factors. This common disease adversely affects the sheep and crop industries and causes vast agricultural waste. Economic losses result from deaths, unthriftiness of recovered animals, incomplete utilization of bloat-provoking feeds, premature marketing of repetitive bloaters, extra labor, costs of therapeutic and preventive programs, and the costs of research and extension plans. Occurrence of the condition also in cattle adds economic importance to the general malady.

Veterinarians classify bloat as:

1. Froth bloat, due either to
   (a) green legumes (GLB),
   (b) hay legumes (HLB), or
   (c) grain concentrate (GCB); and
2. Free-gas bloat (FGB)

OCCURRENCE. All categories of bloat occur as serious diseases in all breeds and sexes beyond weaning age. The incidence of GLB is high, however, among lambs 3 to 9 months of age shipped from range to agricultural pasture of succulent alfalfa or clover for growth and fattening. For preliminary growth, lambs commonly graze legume pasture for 1 to 4 weeks before entering feedlots to complete fattening. Hungry lambs, entering legume pasture, eat rapidly and excessively and become bloated. Farm flocks of ewes grazing legume pasture and range bands grazing lupine on forest or brush lands may engorge and become dangerously or fatally bloated. Seasonally, GLB occurs during plant growing seasons, and HLB occurs during all seasons. In feedlot lambs, GCB develops during late summer and early fall following weaning.

Geographically, bloat among feedlot lambs occurs in agricultural areas of western and midwestern states where lamb-fattening enterprises have developed. GLB from grazing lupine occurs on mountain ranges of western states. Bloat among sheep of farm flocks occurs in all sheep-raising countries.

ETIOLOGY AND PATHOGENESIS. Gas production in the rumen is a normal function of an aerobic fermentation and neutralization of salivary bicarbonate by volatile fatty acid and consists of CO_2 (45 to 75%) CH_4 (20 to 30%) and N_2, O_2, H_2 and H_2S (minor amounts). These gases are largely eliminated by the eructation mechanism. In the normal animal the reticuloruminal movements consist of a biphasic contraction of the reticulum followed by a monophasic contraction of the dorsal ruminal sac and then the ventral ruminal sac. This sequence constitutes the primary cycle which occurs about once a minute unless accelerated by feeding and rumination. A secondary cycle follows alternate primary cycles and consists of a monophasic contraction of the dorsal ruminal sac and then of the ventral ruminal sac. The frequency of secondary cycles are variable and related to the animal's need to eructate.

Gaseous distension of the reticulorumen reflexly elicits an increase in the force and frequency of secondary cycles, stimulates the opening of the caudal esophageal sphincter, and initiates the other respiratory, esophageal, pharyngeal, and buccal actions of the eructation sequence. A prerequisite for the caudal esophageal sphincter opening is that the region be clear of fluid and froth, otherwise an inhibitory reflex overrides the reflex opening. Normally the caudal esophageal sphincter is cleared when the dorsal ruminal sac contractions of the secondary cycles force the gas layer forward, thereby depressing the fluid level below the level of the caudal esophageal sphincter. This simplified version of eructation is under the influence of a complex system of sensors and receptors of the autonomic nervous system. Serotonin (5-hydroxytryptamine) a product of tryptophan biosynthesis in the rumen has an inhibitory effect on the reflex opening of the caudal esophageal sphincter.

GLB, a ruminal overdistension and cardial obstruction with stable froth, results from grazing agricultural pastures of growing alfalfa or clover and from eating chopped green alfalfa or clover, sometimes included as a part of summer diets. The gas derives from acidification of dissolved bicarbonates and from decarboxylation of organic acids, and the surface-active materials originate from dissolved leaf proteins, salivary mucoproteins, and protozoal proteins. The disbursed gas cannot escape.

HLB, also a ruminal overdistension by stable froth, frequently has some free gas overlaying the froth. It results from feeding whole, chopped, ground, or pelleted alfalfa or clover hay, which is especially conducive to bloat when highly leafy, recently cured, combined with barley, and constituting more than 10% of the ration. The source of gas and the surface-active agents are similar to those of GLB.

GCB also overdistends the rumen and obstructs the cardia with stable froth. It results from feeding bloat-producing concentrates, especially barley, corn, and soybean meal. Rations containing finely ground ingredients and less than 10% roughage favor development of the condition. The gas probably derives from acidification of dissolved bicar-

bonates and from microbial fermentation. The surface-active material appears to be bacterial capsular slime composed of nucleoproteins and polysaccharides. Quantitative deficiency of antifoaming mucin from saliva may facilitate the frothing.

FGB is ruminal overdistension with one or more pockets of gas overlying the ingesta. It results from impaired ability of the animal to eructate normally produced gas, and is commonly associated with systemic disease or conditions causing decreased rumen motility or rumen stasis. Cardial and esophageal obstructions, such as occlusive and compressive neoplasms, foreign bodies, expanding abscesses, inflammatory swelling, edematous allergic reactions, constrictive scars, enlarged thoracic nodes, diverticulae, and diphtheria, and dysfunctions, such as paralysis of the vagus nerve, atrophy of muscle, and disruption of reflexes, interfere with escape of gas and favor its accumulation. This form of bloat tends to be repeated in the same animal.

In both GLB and HLB, four essential intraruminal factors—acidity with a pH range of 6 to 5, vigorous gas production, adequate amount of surface-active soluble protein, and sufficient cations to bind protein molecules in a surface film—interact to produce the disease. The leaves of succulent legumes possess 14 to 19% soluble protein. During prehension and mastication, the ruptured and comminuted leaves release 65% of their soluble cytoplasmic protein and a considerable portion of their nonvolatile acids, especially citric, malonic, and succinic acids, into the ruminal fluid.

The plant-formed acids and the fermentation-formed acids immediately lower the pH to between 6 and 5, the bloat range. During this critical time, CO_2 is released from dissolved bicarbonate and from decarboxylated organic acids. The bloat pH range gives maximal strength to foam produced by the surface-active protein. The dissolved protein molecules are coiled, and those that rise to the gas-fluid interface unwind and, when joined by cations, form a strong surface film that traps and holds the bubbles.

As more gas generates, more foam forms and builds to produce an intraruminal pressure of 45 to 70 mm Hg. Foam plugs the cardia and prevents eructation. After variable time and agitation, the protein film folds and forms aggregates, and these changes allow the bubbles to coalesce, the foam to collapse, eructation to occur, and the pressure to subside.

In GCB, the biochemical and biophysical aspects of frothing have not been investigated, but the bacterial slime may have foaming properties similar to those of leaf-soluble proteins.

During the period of high intraruminal pressure, a series of pathophysiologic changes occur. The expanded rumen pushes the diaphragm forward, partially collapsing the lungs. The intra-abdominal and intrathoracic pressures force blood out of the viscera into peripheral blood vessels and cause more CO_2 to dissolve in the plasma and to produce acidosis. The interference with circulation and respiration and the plasma changes rapidly and alarmingly distress the animal and may cause death within a few minutes to a few hours. Following collapse of the foam, less severely affected animals recover.

CLINICAL SIGNS AND POSTMORTEM LESIONS. In frothy bloat, signs usually develop within a few hours after the animal ingests the bloat-producing feed; consequently, many fatal cases escape clinical observation. Intraruminal pressure bulges the left paralumbar fossa and tightly distends the entire abdomen, but this anatomic distortion in fat, heavily wooled sheep is inconspicuous and easily overlooked.

Affected animals, because of increasing discomfort, become uneasy, kick the abdomen, and may alternate between standing and reclining positions. Within a few minutes, the condition is exacerbated, and breathing becomes difficult, rapid, shallow, and oral. Nonpigmented membranes become cyanotic. During early stages, ruminal movements are prominent, but they are later suppressed. Passing a stomach tube into the dorsal part of the rumen removes any free gas that may have accumulated and in some cases provides limited relief. In animals with FGB, the tube allows escape of most of the gas and gives complete relief to the animal. The FGB may recur.

Morbidity varies up to 25% and mortality of affected animals up to 50%. At necropsy, the rumens of animals with frothy bloat are distended with foam and viscous ingesta, but the foam gradually collapses after death. Abdominal and thoracic organs contain little blood, but the rumen often has ecchymotic hemorrhages from ruptured blood vessels. Cervical vessels and nodes are congested, and the tissues are edematous and hemorrhagic. The esophagus is congested and cyanotic throughout the cervical part and blanched in the thoracic portion. Postmortem changes may include rupture of the rumen, diaphragm, or abdominal wall. Differentiation between antemortem and postmortem changes requires evaluation of all available information. Postmortem bloat does not empty the heart chambers as does antemortem bloat.

DIAGNOSIS. Veterinarians diagnose frothy bloat on the basis of evidence of typical signs and lesions and from history of access to bloat-producing diets. Necropsy lesions alone often are inconclusive because of gradual collapse of ruminal foam after death. A stomach tube should be passed into the rumen to differentiate frothy bloat from free-gas bloat. FGB is diagnosed from complete relief of pressure through a stomach tube and from history of previous attacks. The differential diagnosis requires consideration of rupture of the urinary bladder from calculosis, gaseous peritonitis, clostridial infections of the neck, and esophageal choke.

PREVENTION AND TREATMENT. Producers reduce or prevent GLB by judicious management and medicinal regimens in feeding. They cultivate alfalfa or clover with 50% grass for early grazing or for feeding as chopped green roughage; they may also provide poloxalene at the rate of 2 g per animal, either mixed with the feed or in molasses salt block. HLB may be prevented by providing grass as part of the mixed hay and by avoiding grinding the hay and other ration components too finely. Feeding poloxalene may be useful, or monensin (Rumensin) at the rate of 30 to 40 g per ton of dry, high-roughage feed. Poloxalene is not effective against GCB.

Treatment varies with the type of animal affected. Bloat in intractable and ungentled sheep may fatally exacerbate the condition owing to the excitement of restraint; for this reason, such animals should not be disturbed. In manageable and restrainable sheep, however, a stomach tube should be passed into the dorsal part of the rumen to remove any free gas and to administer 0.5 to 1.0 L of mineral oil or vegetable oil, and antiferments. In cases of frothy bloat poloxalene will aid in coalescence of the small gas bubbles trapped in the ingesta. Critically bloated animals should be pierced with a trocar or surgically opened in the left paralumbar fossa for immediate release of pressure. In case of FGB the use of a 5-HT$_2$ receptor antagonist (ritanserin) provides control of bloat for periods up to 2 hours. Ritanserin given at 0.1 mg/kg subcutaneously prevents bloat and increases the volume of eructated gas during ruminal stasis. Treatment of secondary bloat usually depends on removal of the primary cause. If this is not possible, animals with recurrent bloat should be slaughtered to avoid the risk of continuous expense or fatal attack.

Dougherty, R.W.: The continuing quest for the cause of bloat in ruminants. JAVMA, *122*:345-352, 1953.

Dougherty, R.W., Meredith, C.D., and Barrett, R.B.: Physiological effects of insufflation of the stomach of sheep. AJVR, *16*:79-90, 1955.

Fioramonti, J., Bueno, L., Ooms, L., and Ruckebusch, Y.: Effects of ketanserine on rumino-reticular motility and eructation in sheep: a possible application as an anti-bloating substance. J. Vet. Pharmacol. Therap., *5*:213-215, 1982.

Leek, B.: Clinical diseases of the rumen: A physiologist's view. Vet. Rec., *113*:10-14, 1983.

Lippke, H., Vetter, R.L., and Jacobson, N.L.: Effect of poloxalene on performance of calves and lambs. J. Anim. Sci., *31*:1195-1198, 1970.

Lippke, H., Vetter, R.L., and Jacobson, N.L.: Poloxalene for bloat prevention in lambs. J. Anim. Sci., *28*:819-821, 1969.

Mangan, J.L.: Bloat in cattle, XI. The foaming properties of proteins, saponins, and rumen liquor. N.Z. J. Agric. Res., *2*:47-61, 1959.

McArthur, J.M. and Miltimore, J.E.: Bloat investigations. The pH of rumen contents and its role in legume bloat. Can. J. Anim. Sci., *49*:59-67, 1969a.

McArthur, J.M. and Miltimore, J.E.: Bloat investigations. Studies on soluble proteins and nucleic acids in bloating and non-bloating forages. Can. J. Anim. Sci., *49*:69-75, 1969b.

McArthur, J.M., Miltimore, J.E., and Pratt, M.J.: Bloat investigations. The foam stabilizing protein in alfalfa. Can. J. Anim. Sci., *44*:200-206, 1964.

Miltimore, J.E., McArthur, J.M., Mason, J.L., and Ashby, D.L.: Bloat investigations. The threshold fraction 1 (18-S) protein concentration for bloat and relationships between bloat and lipid, tannin, Ca, Mg, and Zn concentrations in alfalfa. Can. J. Anim. Sci., *50*:61-68, 1970.

Reid, C.S.W., Littleton, J.W., and Mangan, J.L.: Bloat in cattle. XXIV. A method for measuring the effectiveness of chewing in the release of plant cell contents from ingested feed. N.Z. J. Agric. Res., *5*:237-248, 1962.

Rosen, W.G., Fassel, H., and Nichols, R.E.: The etiology of legume bloat–non-volatile acids. AJVR, *22*:117-121, 1961.

Ruckebusch, Y., Ooms, L., Degryse, A., and Allal, C.: Alleviation of excessive gas accumulation in the ruminant stomach by ritanserin. Am. J. Vet. Res., *46*:434-437, 1985.

Ruckebusch, Y.: Pharmacology of reticuloruminal motor function. J. Vet. Pharmacol. Therap., *6*:245-272, 1983.

Lactic Acidosis

(LA; ruminal acidosis; grain engorgement; grain overload; acute indigestion; founder)

Lactic acidosis, an acute metabolic disease of sheep, is characterized by inappetence, depression, lameness, and coma, by hyperacidity and rumenitis, and by acidemia and hemoconcentration. It is caused by sudden engorgement on grain and other easily fermentable substances by animals not accustomed to such amounts of these feeds. This prevalent disease commonly leads to other conditions and causes significant economic losses to producers through deaths, wasted feed, and delayed marketing, and to packers through condemnation of rumens and livers. The development of LA also in cattle adds economic importance to the malady.

OCCURRENCE. LA occurs in all breeds, sexes, and ages, but more commonly in farm flocks than in range and pasture bands, and more often in lambs 3 to 9 months of age than in other age groups. It develops accidentally in farm flocks of all sheep-producing countries of temperate climatic zones. It commonly occurs in animals transported from ranges during summer and fall to agricultural pastures and feedlots for fattening. In the United States, the incidence may be high in western, midwestern, and southwestern states where the lamb-fattening industry has developed. LA is often encountered following storms when animals have been unable to feed for a period of time followed by access to unlimited quantities of high concentrate feeds. In addition, LA often occurs among sheep being conditioned for public exhibitions and sales.

ETIOLOGY AND PATHOGENESIS. LA is caused by engorgement on barley, wheat, corn, rye, green whole corn, sugar beets, molasses, sugar cane, mangoes, potatoes, and fruits by animals not accustomed to large amounts of such crops. Access to these feeds results from too rapid a rate of dietary change from a diet of 100% roughage to 90% concentrate, from miscalculating excessive amounts of dietary concentrate, from resuming the same concentrate ration after periods of anorexia or accidental periods of thirst or fast, from mistaken distribution of feed among pens in different stages of adaptation, from accidental ingress to fields or stores, from individual animals separating concentrate from roughage in poorly mixed rations, and from changing ration ingredients, especially to incompletely cured grains.

The pathogenesis of acidosis is a series of biochemical changes in the rumen and blood. Excessive ruminal microbial production and subsequent absorption of lactic acid are responsible for the lactic acid syndrome. Lactate is normally present at low concentrations in blood but rises with excess production from highly fermentable feeds in the rumen. The metabolism of lactate is involved with maintenance of blood pH and glucose concentrations are high in an attempt to maintain a normal acid-base balance in the blood. Sheep accustomed to eating grass, hay, or other cellulosic feeds possess a ruminal microflora of cellulolytic gram-negative bacteria. Following engorgement on starch-rich feed, amylolytic gram-positive streptococci and lactobacilli rapidly multiply and replace the gram-negative bacilli. The new microflora swiftly ferment the

carbohydrates to form D- and L-lactic acid. The lactate, superimposed on other solutes, enhances the osmolality of ruminal fluid relative to plasma and causes a net water flow from blood into the rumen. Prolonged exposure to the acidity severely injures the ruminal mucosa and provokes acute ruminitis. Inflamed papillae clump; necrotic papillae slough. Hemorrhage into both mucosa and submucosa darkens the tissues. The acidosis may result in acute laminitis and polioencephalomalacia.

Concomitant hematologic changes also take place. The net flow of water into the rumen concentrates the blood and dehydrates the tissues. Because of acute and profound metabolic disturbances, the spleen releases its stored erythrocytes; these two changes—concentration and release—cause hematocrit percentages to rise. Blood levels of absorbed lactate increase beyond the absorptive ability of the liver and muscles resulting in systemic acidosis. Stimulated hyperpnea and acidified urine gradually compensate for the acidosis. Urine volume diminishes because of anhydremia. Death probably results from hypovolemic shock and respiratory failure. Sheep with nonfatal LA slowly recover and belatedly resume feeding, growing, and fattening. Nonfatal acidosis may lead to perforating ulcers and liver abscesses.

CLINICAL SIGNS AND POSTMORTEM LESIONS. Within 1 to 3 days after engorgement, the affected sheep develop inappetence, depression, and weakness. Body temperatures remain normal or are slightly elevated. Respirations and pulse accelerate, but the rumen becomes immobilized and the skin dehydrated. As the disease progresses, mucoid diarrhea and abdominal pains augment. Physical weakness causes incoordination and slows the movements, while acute laminitis lames and impedes the walk. Finally, the reclining animal passes into coma, possibly from polioencephalomalacia, and dies. Rumen samples have a pH range from 6.0 to 3.8, a lactate level of 220 to 320 μmol/L, and a rumen fluid-plasma difference of up to 100 mOsm. Urine is acidic and reduced in volume. The blood shows a hematocrit percentage rise from 27 to 33% (normal sheep values) to 40 to 55%. Blood levels of lactate may be as high as 10 μmol/L with pH as low as 7.1. The mortality of affected sheep is high, and the course ranges from 2 to 6 days.

At necropsy, the eyes are sunken, and the skin is inelastic from dehydration. Ruminal contents are fluid and acidic and include large amounts of grain. The mucous membrane in some areas is hemorrhagic and blackened. Many papillae are swollen and darkened, and some have sloughed (Fig. 6-2). Fragile patches of loosened epithelium are easily detached and expose a congested and hemorrhagic submucosa. The abomasal mucosa may contain hemorrhages (Fig. 6-3). Histologically, ruminal epithelium shows ballooning, microvesication, and bacterial invasion. Brains may show polioencephalomalacia, and the feet, acute laminitis.

DIAGNOSIS. Veterinarians clinically diagnose LA on the basis of evidence of circumstance, signs, lesions, and laboratory findings.

Fig. 6-3. Hemorrhagic abomasitis from lactic acidosis. × 1.0.

A history of unadapted animals having free access to grain or other fermentable substances and later developing typical signs strongly suggests acidosis. The diagnosis is confirmed at necropsy and in a laboratory by finding a urine pH of 6 to 5, a blood hematocrit value above 35%, and a pH below 7.4. For technical assistance from a diagnostic laboratory, practitioners should submit urine, blood, rumen fluid, brain, and feet. The differential diagnosis requires consideration of urea poisoning, polioencephalomalacia, urinary calculosis, perforating ulcers, bloat, and foot rot.

PREVENTION. Producers prevent LA by appropriate management. They avoid accidental access of sheep to excessive grain and other fermentable feeds. If storms or other conditions have dictated a temporary drop in feed

Fig. 6-2. Swollen, hemorrhagic, and necrotic ruminal papillae of lamb with lactic acidosis. × 1.0.

consumption, measures must be taken to prevent overloading when feed becomes available. In feedlots, they employ a gradual and stepwise change from a ration of 100% roughage to 90% concentrate over at least 10 days. The addition of monensin or lasalocid to the concentrate ration of feeder lambs aids in preventing LA during the adjustment and while on high concentrate rations.

TREATMENT. (1) At the earliest suspicion of LA sort all sheep or lambs showing any signs of anorexia or depression (the first signs of LA) or ones known to have ingested excess quantities, and treat individually by drenching with an antacid preparation such as magnesium hydroxide in water including 1,000,000 units of penicillin orally. Place these animals on a roughage diet and in a suitable area for close observation and retreatment as needed. After all signs of LA have subsided gradually increase the concentrates to the desired level. (2) Case which are down or comatose, in addition to the above drench, may require intravenous therapy of bicarbonate solutions to restore the acid base balance. (3) For the balance of the individuals not showing clinical signs, in an LA outbreak, removal of the source of the problem is essential. Treatment of this group with 0.3 to 1.0 g of tetracycline plus electrolytes in the water may prevent the development of clinical cases and reduce problems with rumenitis. (4) In cases of valuable animals, with accidental grain overload, showing advanced signs, an emergency rumenotomy to remove all the contents may be indicated. This should be accompanied with intravenous fluid therapy using bicarbonate solutions.

Allison, M.J., Bucklin, J.A., and Dougherty, R.W.: Ruminal changes after overfeeding with wheat and the effect of intraruminal inoculation on adaptation to a ration containing wheat. J. Anim. Sci., 23:1164-1170, 1964.
Bond, H.E.: A study on the pathogenesis of acute acid indigestion in the sheep. Dissertation Abstracts, 20:2354-2355, 1959.
Dain, J.A., Neal, A.L., and Dougherty, R.W.: Histamine in rumen ingesta of overfed sheep. J. Anim. Sci., 14:930-935, 1955.
Dunlop, R.H. and Hammond, P.B.: D-lactic acidosis of ruminants. Ann. N.Y. Acad. Sci., 119:1109-1130, 1965.
Huber, T.L.: Effect of acute indigestion on compartmental water volume and osmolality in sheep. AJVR, 32:887-890, 1971.
Huber, T., Wilson, R., and McGarity, S.: Hepatic metabolite concentration in lactic acidotic sheep. Am. J. Vet. Res., 45:1209-1211, 1984.
Hungate, R.E., Dougherty, R.W., Bryant, M.P., and Cello, R.M.: Microbiological and physiological changes associated with indigestion in sheep. Cornell Vet., 42:423-449, 1952.
Jensen, R., et al.: The rumenitis-liver abscess complex in beef cattle. AJVR, 15:202, 1954.
Juhasz, B. and Szegedi, B.: Pathogenesis of ruminal digestive disorders caused by easily digestible carbohydrates. Magy. Allatorv. Lap., 23:60-68, 1968.
Krogh, N.: Clinical and microbiological studies on spontaneous cases of acute indigestion in ruminants. Acta. Vet. Scand., 4:27-40, 1963.
Kutas, F., Galfi, P., and Neogrady, S.: Effect of monensin on development of ruminal parakeratosis in fattening lambs. Zbl. Vet. Med. A., 30:506-510, 1983.
Lusby, K.S. and Brent, B.E.: Model for polioencephalomalacia. J. Anim. Sci., 35:270, 1972.
Malchevski, M., Tsvetkov, A., Tsockev, I., and Uzunov, G.: Prevention of ruminal acidosis in intensively reared lambs. Veterinarnomeditsinski Nauki, 22:50-58, 1985.
Morrow, L.L., et al.: Laminitis in sheep injected with lactic acid. AJVR, 34:1305-1307, 1973.
Naylor, J., Kronfeld, D., Freeman, D., and Richardson, D.: Hepatic and extrahepatic lactate metabolism in sheep: effects of lactate loading and pH. Am. J. Physiol., 247:E747-E755, 1984.
Phillipson, A.T.: The fluctuation of pH and organic acids in the rumen of sheep. J. Exp. Biol., 19:186, 1942.
Scarisbrick, R.: Acid indigestion in a sheep fed on mangolds. Vet. Rec., 66:131-132, 1954.
Telle, P.P. and Preston, R.E.: Ovine lactic acidosis: intraruminal and systemic. J. Anim. Sci., 33:698-705, 1971.
Turner, A.W. and Hodgetts, V.E.: The dynamic red cell storage function of the spleen in sheep. I. Relationship to fluctuations of the jugular hematocrit. Aust. J. Exp. Biol., 37:399, 1959.

Ruminal Parakeratosis

Ruminal parakeratosis, a nutritional degenerative change in the mucosa, is characterized grossly by browning, hardening, thickening, and clumping of papillae, and microscopically by accumulation of excessive layers of keratinized squamous epithelial cells on the papillary surfaces, and is caused by diets of finely ground feed. This uncommon condition is limited to fattening lambs and has minor importance to the sheep industry. Some losses, however, result to producers from reduced efficiency in utilization of feed and to packers from condemnation of uncleanable rumens.

OCCURRENCE. Parakeratosis occurs in all breeds and sexes of fattening lambs. Although all ages probably are susceptible, only animals 3 to 9 months of age normally are fattened on ground feed for the fat-lamb market. In addition to fat lambs, the condition occurs in fat cattle.

Seasonally, parakeratosis commonly occurs during winter because that is the time of lamb fattening. The condition develops among lambs of the United States and other countries where animals are fattened on cereal feeds.

ETIOLOGY AND PATHOGENESIS. The continuous and exclusive feeding for prolonged periods on finely ground feed with or without pelleting, especially with less than 10% roughage, causes ruminal parakeratosis.

As dietary concentrate levels increase and roughage decreases, rumen microflora and products of fermentation change. The rumen pH lowers and the proportion of ruminal volatile fatty acids are altered with increases in butyrate and lactate. Butyrate in ruminal cell cultures causes morphologic indications of abnormal keratinization such as the appearance of refractive granules, an increase in the number of filamentous bundles, the formation of keratohyolin-like granules, and a thickening of the cell membrane. High butyrate levels may, either by itself or in association with other factors, be the chemical stimulus responsible for the induction of ruminal parakeratosis. The physical abrasive action of roughage on the rumen papillae is thought to play a beneficial role on preventing abnormal keratinization.

The normal stratified, keratinized epithelium of the rumen mucosa acts as a protective barrier and plays an important role in ruminal transport and metabolism. Abnormal keratinization of the rumen epithelium adversely affects the metabolism and absorptive efficiency of the mucosa.

CLINICAL SIGNS AND POSTMORTEM LESIONS. Ruminal parakeratosis, except for subjectively slow rates of gain, is asymptomatic. At necropsy, following fatal intercurrent disease, or at slaughter, the clumps of papillae may appear as dark areas, measuring about 10 mm², through the unopened rumen. After opening and washing the rumen, the parakeratotic papillae—hard, dark, thick, rough, and often clumped—are unevenly distributed over the surface of the anteroventral and anterodorsal sacs (Fig. 6-4). Clumped papillae are easily separated. Individual papillae may show change over all or part of their surface; often the distal part or tip is parakeratinized. The detachment of affected papillae may significantly reduce the number on a mucosal surface.

Histopathologically, the surface of the mucosa contains excessive layers of keratinized cell. On the surface and occasionally among the layers are fragments of feed and colonies of bacteria.

DIAGNOSIS. Ruminal parakeratosis is never clinically diagnosed. Veterinarians identify the condition at necropsy following fatal intercurrent disease or at inspection after slaughter.

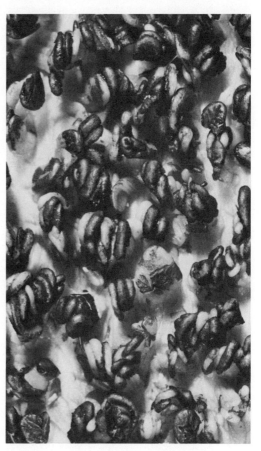

Fig. 6-4. Parakeratosis of ruminal papillae. × 3.0.

After opening and cleaning the rumen, the parakeratosis becomes evident. Laboratory confirmation is based on typical histopathologic changes. The differential diagnosis requires consideration of hypovitaminosis A.

PREVENTION AND TREATMENT. Veterinarians and producers both avoid and correct ruminal parakeratosis by providing as part of the diet 0.22 kg of unground roughage, such as alfalfa, per animal daily. The roughage should be available on a free-choice basis to the fattening lambs.

Monensin and lasalocid (ionophore antibiotics) decrease the production of acetate and butyrate, while increasing proprionate, and are effective in preventing parakeratosis.

Galfi, P., Neogrady, S., Kutas, F., and Veresegygazy, T.: Keratinization of cultured ruminal epithelial cells treated with butyrate and lactate. Zbl. Vet. Med. A., 30:775-781, 1983.

Hinders, R.G. and Owen, F.G.: Relation of ruminal parakeratosis development to fatty acid absorption. J. Dairy Sci., 48:1069-1073, 1965.

Jensen, R., et al.: Parakeratosis of rumens of lambs fattened on pelleted feed. AJVR, 19:277-282, 1958.

Jensen, R., et al.: The rumenitis-liver abscess complex in beef cattle. AJVR, 15:202-216, 1954.

Kutas, F., Galfi, P., and Neogrady, S.: Effect of monensin on development of ruminal parakeratosis in fattening lambs. Zbl. Vet. Med. A., 30:509-510, 1983.

Semjen, G., Galfi, P., and Kutas, F.: Effect of parakeratosis on bacterial adherence to ruminal epithelium. Zbl. Vet. Med. B., 29:317-319, 1982.

Tamate, H., et al.: Rumen parakeratosis in cattle fed a high-concentrate ration. Jpn. J. Zootech. Sci., 38:148-153, 1967.

Rumenitis

Rumenitis, an acute or chronic focal inflammation, is caused by endogenous irritants, microbial pathogens, and exogenous irritants. Even though the extent of the disease has not been measured or its effects assessed, hidden costs to the sheep industry are high. Economic losses accrue to producers from reduced efficiency in feed conversions and delayed marketing, and to packers from condemnation of rumens and livers at slaughter. The United States annually slaughters and inspects about 10 million sheep, and from these animals, an estimated 3% of the rumens and livers are condemned.

OCCURRENCE. Rumenitis occurs in all breeds, sexes, and ages, but more commonly in feedlot lambs 4 to 9 months of age than in animals of other age groups. The disease usually develops during the early stages of fattening. Most cases occur during late summer and early fall when lambs move into feedlots. Geographically, it occurs in western, southwestern, and midwestern regions of the United States where the lamb-fattening industry has developed.

ETIOLOGY AND PATHOGENESIS. Rumenitis is caused commonly by fermented lactic acid, occasionally by viruses such as the one causing contagious ecthyma, and rarely by poisons such as heavy metals. Because of discriminatory eating habits, sheep, unlike cattle, rarely ingest feed-contaminating fragments of wire and nails and consequently do not develop traumatic rumenitis and reticulitis.

The pathogenesis begins with action of the irritants—lactic acid (see section on lactic acidosis), viruses, and ingested poisons—on the mucosa. Concentrated irritants, in addition to specific changes, generally inflame and necrotize the epithelium and, in some cases, the lamina propria. Necrotic tissues slough and thus create ulcers. Continued movement of ruminal contents erodes the ulcers, stimulates production of granulation tissue, and impedes re-epithelialization. Eventually, however, healing occurs, often with contraction of cicatricial tissue.

Bacteria of the ruminal contents, especially ubiquitous *Fusobacterium necrophorum,* can penetrate early-formed necrotic tissue (but not late-formed granulation tissue), enter capillaries of the portal system, be transported to the liver, and there induce abscesses.

CLINICAL SIGNS AND POSTMORTEM LESIONS. Rumenitis of small to modest extent produces no signs, but extensive lesions, especially when associated with extraruminal changes such as stomatitis or hepatic abscesses, result in anorexia, depression, ruminal immobility, and loss of weight. Morbidity varies up to 10%, and mortality of affected animals up to 20%. The disease course is about 10 days.

At necropsy, ruminal lesions, usually located in the anteroventral sac, are subsumed acute inflammation and chronic ulcers. Either one or both forms may exist in an individual animal. The acute form shows hyperemia, edema, and necrosis, often with sloughing, especially papillae, of necrotic tissue (Fig. 6-5). The chronic form, however, shows depapillation, smooth granulation tissue surrounded by hyperplastic epithelium, and healed scars, often with stellate disfigurements from contractions of fibrous tissue (Fig. 6-6). Liver abscesses may also be present.

DIAGNOSIS. Rumenitis is seldom, if ever, clinically diagnosed. At necropsy of dead sheep and at inspection of slaughtered sheep, veterinarians diagnose the disease on evidence of acute necrosis, chronic ulcers, and/or scars on the mucosa of the cleaned rumen.

PREVENTION. Producers prevent rumenitis resulting from lactic acid irritation by systematically controlling the diet of lambs newly ar-

Fig. 6-6. Chronic ruminal ulcers from earlier lactic acidosis. × 1.0.

rived at the feedlot. A period of at least 10 days should be used for gradually changing the ration of all roughage to a ration of 90% concentrate. Vaccination of lambs soon after arrival at the feedlot prevents contagious ecthyma.

Some feeders incorporate oxytetracycline in the ration of a level of 50 mg per head per day to prevent rumenitis and liver abscesses.

Jensen, R., Connell, W.E., and Deem, A.W.: Rumenitis and its relation to rate of change of ration and the proportion of concentrate in the ration of cattle. AJVR, 15:425-428, 1954a.

Jensen, R., et al.: The rumenitis-liver abscess complex in beef cattle. AJVR, 15:202-216, 1954b.

Jensen, R., Flint, J.C., and Griner, L.A.: Experimental hepatic necrobacillosis in beef cattle. AJVR, 15:5-14, 1954c.

Madin, S.H.: A bacteriologic study of bovine liver abscesses. Vet. Med., 44:248-251, 1949.

Newsom, I.E.: A bacteriologic study of liver abscesses in cattle. J. Infect. Dis., 63:232-233, 1938.

Newsom, I.E. and Cross, F.: Lamb diseases in Colorado feedlots. Colorado Agric. Exp. Stat. Bull. 474, 1943.

Pounden, W.D., Bell, D.S., Edgington, B.H., and Thomas, D.L.: Disease conditions observed in lambs at slaughter. JAVMA, 128:298-301, 1956.

Fig. 6-5. Acute necrotic rumenitis from lactic acidosis. × 1.0.

Abomasal and Duodenal Ulcers

Gastric ulcers, focal disruptions of the mucous membranes, frequently are complications secondary to acute diseases such as blue-tongue, salmonellosis, and lactic acidosis. In addition, primary ulcers occasionally develop in the abomasum and duodenum, the category discussed here. Primary ulcers are uncommon and cause little concern to the industry, but they do cause waste in some enterprises. Economic losses to producers result from diminished weight gains, delayed marketing, and deaths.

OCCURRENCE.   Ulcers probably occur in all breeds, cross breeds, and sexes of feedlot lambs 3 to 6 months of age. They develop in late summer and early fall during the first few weeks of fattening, and they probably affect lambs in all geographic areas where the fattening industry has developed.

ETIOLOGY AND PATHOGENESIS.   The causes of primary ulcers are not known; however, we consider them to be gastric hypersecretion acting on areas of mucosa with lowered resistance. Factors that may contribute to the devitalization include (1) hemorrhage into the lamina propria, (2) mucositis, (3) penetration of nematode larvae, (4) inadequate or defective covering mucus, and (5) systemic stress from recent shipments and rapid changes from diets of roughage to concentrate.

The gastric secretions gradually digest the devitalized epithelial cells. Once the covering tissue is lost, the secretion directly contacts, kills, and digests the even more vulnerable mesodermal cells. This destructive process deepens the ulcer, which may eventually extend into and through the lamina propria, submucosa, muscularis, and peritoneum. The erosion and opening of arteries may cause fatal hemorrhage, and the perforation of the wall may cause spillage into the peritoneal cavity and fatal peritonitis.

CLINICAL SIGNS AND POSTMORTEM LESIONS. Many ulcers do not hemorrhage and are not perforating. Animals so affected may present anorexia and possibly pain with kicking of the abdomen. Lambs with hemorrhaging ulcers

Fig. 6-7.   A perforating duodenal ulcer (*a*).

may also show hematochezia, anemia, and weakness, whereas those with perforating ulcers show peritonitis with fever and abdominal distension from gas in the abdominal cavity. The incidence of uncomplicated cases of ulcer may reach 40%, but these are seldom diagnosed. Complicated fatal cases, however, may involve 4% of some individual pens.

At necropsy, abomasal ulcers are usually in the pylorus, single or multiple and measuring up to 20 mm in diameter, while duodenal ulcers are in the cephalad 5 cm of the duodenum, single or multiple and measuring up to 10 mm in diameter (Fig. 6-7). Hemorrhaging ulcers show gross amounts of blood in the abomasum and/or duodenum; perforating ulcers show peritonitis and ingesta in the peritoneal cavity. Either form may be infected with the *Phycomycetes*.

DIAGNOSIS.   Veterinarians diagnose complicated ulcers by finding the specific lesions at necropsy. Effective prevention and treatment have not been developed.

Shirley, A.G.H.: Two cases of phycomycotic ulceration in sheep. Vet. Rec., 77:675-677, 1965.

Enterotoxemia

(ET; infectious enterotoxemia; overeating disease)

An acute infectious but noncontagious disease of feedlot lambs, enterotoxemia is characterized by sudden deaths, convulsions, and hyperglycemia and is caused by anaerobic bacteria commonly found in soil, manure, and ruminant intestines. Prior to the development of commercial vaccine for protection against the disease, enterotoxemia probably caused more economic losses among feedlot and pasture-fattening lambs than the sum of all other diseases; even now, with an effective and easily available vaccine, the infection probably kills 0.1 to 0.5% of feedlot lambs, as noted in Tables 5-5, 5-6, 5-7.

Losses result from death of most affected sheep and from the costs of preventive and disposal programs. The name "enterotoxemia" accurately suggests an intoxication originating in the intestine, and the term "overeating disease" appropriately describes a circumstance under which the disease occurs.

OCCURRENCE. ET occurs in all breeds and sexes of sheep, but is more common in animals 1 to 12 months of age. Sheep fattening in feedlots suffer a high incidence, and the disease usually starts 2 to 3 weeks after fattening begins. The malady also affects sheep fattening in cornfields, pea fields, and succulent pasture.

Geographically, ET probably occurs in all countries where sheep fattening for the lamb market has developed, but cases have been diagnosed and reported from Australia, Britain, Canada, France, Germany, Iran, New Zealand, USSR, Yugoslavia, and South Africa. In the United States, the disease has economic importance in California, Colorado, Kansas, Montana, Oregon and Texas. ET may occur at any season, but the high incidence comes during the months following weaning, when fattening takes place. The disease may also occur in goats.

ETIOLOGY AND PATHOGENESIS. *Clostridium perfringens* type D, the cause of ovine ET, lives in soil, manure, and the alimentary tracts of animals. *C. perfringens* type D is recognized as the main agent of enterotoxemia, however, other clostridia may be involved: *C. perfringens, A, B, C, and E, C. septicum, C. sordelli* and *C. bifermentans. C. perfringens* is a gram-positive, anaerobic, non-motile, encapsulated, sporing bacillus that measures 4 to 8 by 0.8 to 1.5 μm. Except for mannitol, it ferments most sugars and produces both acid and gas. In wound infections, it ferments muscle glycogen and generates gas.

On the basis of toxin-antitoxin neutralization tests, the species is subdivided into 6 types: A, B, C, D, E, and F. The species produces 12 exotoxins, which are named with Greek letters. Each type produces one major toxin and may produce one or more minor toxins. The major toxin of type D is innocuous epsilon prototoxin, which is converted to lethal epsilon toxin by trypsin. Table 6-1 presents the types, toxins, and diseases.

TABLE 6-1. *Clostridium perfringens*

Types	Toxins Major	Toxins Minor	Action of Major Toxins	Diseases
A	α	—	lethal, necrotizing, hemolytic, leukocidal	1. Yellow lamb 2. Gas gangrene
B	β	α, ϵ	lethal, necrotizing	1. Lamb dysentery 2. Hemorrhagic enterotoxemia (ET) of lambs, kids, foals
C	β	α	lethal, necrotizing	1. Struck of young adult sheep 2. Hemorrhagic ET in lambs, calves, piglets
D	ϵ	α	lethal, necrotizing, enhances permeability of gut and capillaries	1. ET of young feedlot sheep, young lush-pasture sheep, nursing lambs
E	ι	α, κ	lethal, necrotizing	1. ET of calves

Overeating on grain, especially barley or corn, or succulent and highly nutritious forage is a secondary but important factor in the cause. Although some aspects of the disease are unknown, sufficient information exists for a reasonable hypothesis on pathogenesis.

Spores of *C. perfringens* type D reside in soil and manure for prolonged periods, and because of continuous excretion from sheep, they concentrate numerically in areas of feedlots, corrals, bedgrounds, and watering facilities. The spores enter the alimentary tracts along with contaminated feed and water. Some organisms perish in the acid of the abomasum, but small numbers survive and eventually enter the small intestine and finally the colon.

Under normal circumstances, the bacteria slowly multiply and form small amounts of epsilon toxin, but peristaltic movements propel intestinal contents to the exterior and prevent high concentrations of bacteria and toxin from accumulating. In the feedlot and other fattening facilities, however, some lambs consume excessive amounts of grain. Under this ruminal circumstance, some granules of starch pass through the abomasum into the small intestine.

In the ileum, the vegetative cells of *C. perfringens* type D, acting on the starch substrate, multiply rapidly and form as many as one billion organisms per gram, and swiftly synthesize epsilon prototoxin. Trypsin converts prototoxin into epsilon toxin, which may reach concentrations of 10,000 mouse-minimal-lethal doses per gram. These high concentrations of toxin slow intestinal motility, increase the permeability of the intestinal wall to toxins and similar substances, and aid passage of toxin into the blood.

In the blood, the toxin produces generalized toxemia and causes release of liver glycogen and the development of hyperglycemia. Glucosuria results from the passage of sugar from the plasma into the urine. In most affected sheep, injury to vital neurons and shock cause death. Sublethal doses of toxin stimulate the production of specific antitoxin in the surviving host. Along with infected feces and decomposing tissues, bacteria pass to the exterior, form spores, and re-enter the soil.

CLINICAL SIGNS AND POSTMORTEM LESIONS. Sudden and unexpected deaths characterize ET. Commonly, on early morning inspection, the husbandman finds the best-conditioned lambs dead. Sick lambs, however, often tremble in the muscles of the back and limbs and may violently jump with incoordinated movements. When disturbed, they usually convulse and fall to the ground with head, neck, and limbs rigidly extended, eyes oscillating, mouths salivating, and muscles jerking. Each convulsion lasts 5 to 15 seconds.

The animals may rise to the standing position between early repetitive attacks. Some lambs do not convulse, but push their heads against solid objects. Shallow, rapid breathing and, in some cases, diarrhea develop. Body temperature rises during violent actions. Finally, the infected animals collapse in coma, lose corneal reflexes, and, while recumbent, perform paddling movements with the limbs. Death usually occurs after a disease course of 30 to 90 minutes.

Fig. 6-8. Fluid-distended pericardium from a sheep with enterotoxemia. × 0.6.

At the onset of signs, hyperglycemia begins to develop, and by the time of death, glucosuria also exists. Among nonvaccinated lambs, mortality often reaches 5 to 10%, but among properly vaccinated lambs, it is reduced to 0.1 to 0.5%.

At necropsy, lesions are usually confined to the digestive, respiratory, and cardiovascular systems. The abomasum contains whole grain and particles of grain. The ileum may be acutely reddened in local areas. The pericardial sac often is distended with 50 to 60 ml of pale yellow fluid and clumps of fibrin (Fig. 6-8), and the subepicardium, subendocardium, intestinal subserosa (Fig. 6-9), and thymus contain small hemorrhages. The heavy lungs contain edematous fluid and congested blood. The sugar content of the blood increases from the normal level of 40 to 65 mg/dl to as much as 360 mg/dl, and of the urine from 1 to 6%.

DIAGNOSIS. Veterinarians diagnose ET among feedlot lambs on the basis of typical signs and lesions. Sudden deaths among lambs fattening on barley, corn grain, corn in the field, peas in the field, or lush pasture grass suggest this disease. The first deaths in an outbreak usually occur 2 to 3 weeks after fattening begins and when each lamb consumes an average of 0.5 to 1.0 kg of grain daily.

Since sick lambs usually are not available for study, postmortem lesions assume crucial importance. Fluid in the pericardial sac, congested and edematous lungs, hemorrhages in the thymus, and glucosuria indicate ET. In the laboratory, scientists confirm or establish the diagnosis by isolating and identifying epsilon toxin from contents of the ileum or the blood by counterimmunoelectrophoresis.

The differential diagnosis requires consideration of blackleg, black disease, bloat, anthrax, and acute poisoning. For technical assistance from a diagnostic laboratory, practitioners should submit cooled urine and cooled fluid contents from the ileum.

PREVENTION. All lambs entering the feeding program should be vaccinated immediately with *C. perfringens* C and D toxoid. A second shot should be administered in about 14 days.

Fig. 6-9. Multiple subserosal hemorrhages on cecum of a feedlot lamb with enterotoxemia.

In cases where the concentrate ration is high and death losses from enterotoxemia continue a third shot may be helpful keeping in mind the withdrawal period prior to slaughter. The adjustment onto high concentrate rations should be gradual over a 2- to 3-week period avoiding any interruptions or sudden changes. If an enterotoxemia problem continues, other clostridial causes should be investigated and the handling and administration techniques of the current immunization program fully reviewed.

Al-Mashat, R. and Taylor, D.: *Clostridium sordellii* in enteritis in an adult sheep. Vet. Rec., *112*:19, 1983.

Baldwin, E.M., Frederick, L.D., and Ray, J.D.: The control of ovine enterotoxemia by the use of *Clostridium perfringens* type D bacterin. AJVR, *9*:296-303, 1948.

Bennetts, H.W.: Infectious enterotoxemia of sheep in Western Australia. CSIRO Bull. 57, 1932.

Boughton, I.B. and Hardy, W.T.: Infectious enterotoxemia (milk colic) of lambs and kids. Tex. Agric. Exp. Stat. Bull. 598, 1941.

Bullen, J.J.: Enterotoxemia of sheep: *Clostridium welchii* type D in the alimentary tract of normal animals. J. Pathol. Bacteriol., *64*:201-206, 1952a.

Bullen, J.J. and Batty, I.: Experimental enterotoxemia of sheep: the effect on permeability of the intestine. J. Pathol. Bacteriol., *73*:511-518, 1957b.

Bullen, J.J. and Scarisbrick, R.: Enterotoxemia of sheep: experimental reproduction of the disease. J. Pathol. Bacteriol., *73*:495-509, 1957c.

Ellis, T., Rowe, J., and Lloyd, J.: Acute abomasitis due to *Clostridium septicum* infection in experimental sheep. Aust. Vet. J., *60*:308-309, 1983.

Gordon, W.S., Stewart, J., Holman, H.H., and Taylor, A.W.: Blood changes and postmortem findings following i/v inoculation of sheep with culture filtrates of *C. welchii* types A, C and D. J. Pathol. Bacteriol., *50*:251-269, 1940.

Harshfield, G.S., Cross, F., and Hoerlein, A.B.: Further studies on overeating (enterotoxemia) of feedlot lambs. AJVR, *3*·86, 1942.

Henderson, T.: The detection of *Clostridium perfringens* type D enterotoxin in the intestinal contents of animals by counter immunoelectrophoresis. N.Z. J. Sci., *27*:423-426, 1984.

Hungate, R.E., Dougherty, R.W., Bryant, M.P., and Cello, R.M.: Microbiological and physiological changes associated with indigestion in sheep. Cornell Vet., *42*:433-449, 1952.

McDonel, J.L.: *C. perfringens* toxins (A, B, C, D, E). Pharmacol. Ther., *10*:617-655, 1980.

Newsom, I.E. and Cross, F.: Lamb diseases in Colorado feedlots. Colorado Agric. Exp. Stat. Bull., 474, 1943.

Newsom, I.E. and Cross, F.: Diseases of Colorado feeding lambs. Colorado Agric. Exp. Stat. Bull., 305, 1925.

Popoff, M.: Bacterial examination in enterotoxemia of sheep and lambs. Vet. Rec., *114*:324, 1984.

Richards, S. and Hunt, B.: *Clostridium sordellii* in lambs. Vet. Rec., *22*, 1982.

Roberts, R.S.: Braxy-like diseases of sheep. Vet. Rec., *50*:591-604, 1938.

Tengerdy, R., et al.: Vitamin E-enhanced humoral antibody response to *Clostridium perfringens* type D in sheep. Br. Vet. J., *139*:147-152, 1983.

Turner, A.W. and Rodwell, A.W.: The epsilon toxins of *C. welchii* type D. 1-Proteolytic conversion of prototoxin into epsilon toxin by trypsin and other proteases. Aust. J. Exp. Biol. Med. Sci., *21*:17-25, 1943a.

Turner, A.W. and Rodwell, A.W.: The epsilon toxin of *C. welchii* type D. 2-Mechanism of its development in cultures through action of extracellular proteinases upon prototoxin. Aust. J. Exp. Biol. Med. Sci., *21*:27-36, 1943b.

Webster, A. and Frank, C.: Comparison of immune response stimulated in sheep, rabbits and guinea pigs by the administration of multi-component clostridial vaccines. Aust. Vet. J., *62*:112-114, 1985.

Yellow Lamb Disease

(*YLD; enterotoxemic jaundice; enterotoxemia type A*)

Yellow lamb disease, a highly lethal bacterial intoxication, is characterized by fever, hemolysis, and high mortality and is caused by a clostridial exotoxin formed in the intestine. Although the disease has low incidence for the entire industry and therefore attracts little research investment, it kills many animals and thus inflicts high losses in some enterprises.

OCCURRENCE. The disease probably develops in all breeds, sexes, and ages, but is most common in thrifty lambs 2 to 6 months of age and occasionally afflicts thrifty sheep over 12 months of age. It occurs during periods of high rainfall in all seasons and is recognized especially in lambs in the western United States and in adult sheep in Australia.

ETIOLOGY AND PATHOGENESIS. *Clostridium perfringens* type A, a producer of alpha toxin, causes YLD. This gram-positive, nonmotile, sporing rod commonly inhabits soil, manure, and alimentary tracts. Alpha toxin is proteinaceous, enzymatic, and antigenic (Table 6-1).

Spores from soil enter the ovine gastrointestinal tracts as contaminants in feed and water. They pass into the small intestine, and the vegetative forms, acting on substrate of dietary carbohydrate and protein, synthesize alpha toxin, which enters portal capillaries and produces toxemia. The normal indigenous intestinal flora have a definite barrier effect against colonization of newly introduced *C. perfringens*. Alteration of the intestinal mucosa by change in diet or other actions is therefore necessary for establishment of the organism. In the blood, the toxin hydrolyzes cellular lecithin and thus hemolyzes erythrocytes, injures and kills some tissue cells, and finally kills the host. The bacteria return to the soil in feces and autolyzed dead tissues.

It is hypothesized that a carrier state for enteropathogenic *C. perfringens* could result from neonatal exposure to the organism when the intestinal bacterial flora is being formed.

CLINICAL SIGNS AND POSTMORTEM LESIONS. Affected animals develop body temperatures of about 41°C and become physically weak and mentally depressed. Forced driving of the flock may cause animals in early stages to manifest their conditions. Anemia, icterus, and hemoglobinuria are prominent. Respirations are accelerated. Animals in advanced stages separate from the flock, remain recumbent, and die. Many are found dead without caretakers having observed signs.

At necropsy, petechial and ecchymotic hemorrhages may be found on serosal surfaces and transudate in body cavities. The small intestine is hyperemic. Histologic examinations reveal hemoglobin casts in kidneys and centrolobular necrosis in liver.

The course in acute disease ranges from 6 to 12 hours, but some cases become subacute or chronic. Morbidity in lambs is about 5%; in adults it may reach 50%. Mortality is high.

DIAGNOSIS. Veterinarians suspect YLD on the basis of evidence of typical signs and lesions and confirm the diagnosis in the laboratory by identifying the toxin from intestinal contents. The differential diagnosis requires consideration of leptospirosis, babesiosis, and copper poisoning.

For technical assistance from a diagnostic laboratory, practitioners should submit (1) contents from the small intestine collected and cooled in glass containers, (2) fresh liver and kidney, (3) intestine, liver, and kidney fixed in 10% formalin, and (4) unclotted blood.

An enzyme-linked immunosorbent assay (ELISA) provides a specific and highly sensitive serologic test for the detection of *C. perfringens* antienterotoxin in sheep and cattle.

PREVENTION AND TREATMENT. Sheep in endemic areas should be immunized in advance of exposure with toxoid vaccine, if available. Treatment is usually impractical and ineffective.

McDonel, J.L.: *C. perfringens* toxins (A,B,C,D,E). Pharmacol. Ther., *10*:617-655, 1980.

McGowan, B., Moulton, J.E., and Rood, S.E.: Lamb losses associated with *C. perfringens* type A. JAVMA, *133*:219-221, 1958.

Niilo, L. and Cho, H.: Clinical and antibody responses to *Clostridium perfringens* type A enterotoxin in experimental sheep and calves. Can. J. Comp. Med., *49*:145-148, 1985.

Rose, A.L. and Edgar, G.: Enterotoxemic jaundice of sheep and cattle. Aust. Vet. J., *12*:212-220, 1936.

Salmonellal Dysentery

(SD; salmonellosis)

An acute contagious disease of sheep, cattle, and people, SD is characterized by gastroenteritis, diarrhea, septicemia, and recovery of carriers and is commonly caused by *Salmonella enteritidis ser typhimurium, Salmonella enteritidis ser Bovis morbificans, Salmonella enteritidis ser Havana* and others with *S. typhimurium* being the most frequent pathogen. These bacteria commonly live in alimentary tracts and contaminate feed and water. Because of near universal distribution and high incidence within infected flocks, the disease has major economic importance to the entire sheep industry. Economic losses result from deaths and damaged wool and from the costs of expensive treatment, prevention, extra labor, and disposal of dead sheep. Additional losses come from incapacitation, discomfort, and treatment of infected people.

OCCURRENCE. SD occurs in all breeds, sexes, and ages, but more commonly in animals of weaning age and older than in younger age groups. Among feedlot lambs, the disease commonly develops after prolonged shipment and fasting. Although SD is common during summer and early fall, it may develop during other seasons. The geographic distribution probably includes all countries where the sheep industry is prominent. The disease has been observed and reported in the United States where lambs are fattened, and in Germany, Hungary, Yugoslavia, Rumania, Italy, Cyprus, USSR, New Zealand, and Australia.

ETIOLOGY AND PATHOGENESIS. *Salmonella enteritidis ser typhimurium,* a usual cause of SD, is widely distributed and commonly found in alimentary tracts of sheep and cattle and occasionally in contaminated feed and water. This gram-negative, motile, aerobic, nonsporing bacillus measures 0.5 to 0.8 × 1 to 3 μm. It grows readily on many laboratory media and ferments xylose, arabinose, trehalose, inositol, and maltose to form both acid and gas, but not lactose, sucrose, or salicin. It produces H_2S, but does not form indole or reduce nitrates. The antigenic structure consists of somatic

O-antigens 1,4,5, and 12 and H-antigens of specific phase ι and of nonspecific phases 1 and 2.

Factors increasing susceptibility to SD include several debilitating situations. Shipment by rail or truck for up to 7 days and fasting over much of the travel time often initiates an outbreak. Inclement weather adds to the ill effects of shipping and fasting. Crowding and inadequate feeding during times of shearing, weaning, and dipping may predispose the animals to infection.

Since the pathogenesis of SD has received little scientific study, the details on mechanism of disease development are largely conjectural. The causative organisms inhabit the alimentary tract, including the gallbladder, of some normal but carrier sheep. Slowly growing and multiplying, the bacteria mix with the feces and are discharged to the exterior. In the external environment, the bacteria are susceptible to the lethal effects of drying and sunshine, but survive in moist soil, manure, feed, and water for many weeks. From these media, they enter the alimentary tracts of susceptible sheep along with ingested feed.

In the unfilled rumen, the ingested pathogens rapidly grow, multiply, and pass into the small intestine. The disintegration of some *S. typhimurium* cells releases toxic lipopolysaccharides, which irritate the mucosa, accelerate peristaltic movements, and initiate diarrhea. The fluid feces contain bacteria, water, Na^+, Cl^-, K^+, and HCO_3^-. After a few days, the infected sheep lose as much as 12% of their body water; approximately 50% of the lost water probably comes from the plasma. The loss of water results in tissue dehydration and the loss of HCO_3^- in acidosis.

In the small intestine, living, virulent *S. typhimurium* cells penetrate the mucous membrane. On invasion of the lymphatics, the bacteria enter Peyer's patches, mesenteric lymph nodes and, finally the systemic blood, which transports them to all organs. Colonization may occur in lymph nodes, spleen, and liver. Death results from shock, septicemia, endotoxemia, dehydration, and acidosis. Of the surviving sheep, some animals may harbor the *S. typhimurium* and become carriers and excretors of the organisms for variable periods; others develop antibodies and become immune.

TRANSMISSION. Many animals, birds, and even people can carry and excrete Salmonellae without clinical signs of the disease. These carriers are instrumental in propagation and outbreaks of the disease. The healthy animal and the normal microflora of the intestine prohibit the establishment of infection when the animal is exposed to small numbers of the salmonella organism. Most outbreaks of salmonellosis in sheep are associated with a combination of crowding transportation, and food deprivation over an extended period of time resulting in stress plus exposure to large numbers of salmonella organisms. Stress produces a variety of unknown alterations in normal body functions causing: (1) the carrier animal to eliminate vast numbers of the salmonella organism, (2) changes in the intestinal microflora allowing for multiplication and colonization of salmonella, (3) suppression of the immune system from the release of corticosteroids allowing an infection to become established.

The disease spreads geographically by migration of carrier and excretor animals—sheep, cattle, horses, poultry, birds, and rodents—and by transporting contaminated feed. During shipment of lambs or adults, unavoidable delays may extend transit time for up to 7 days, and necessary unloading for resting and feeding at public stockyards or other public assemblage facilities may expose the animals to contaminated feed or water. In this event, the animals may be overtly sick on arrival at destination.

CLINICAL SIGNS AND POSTMORTEM LESIONS. At the time of arrival at the feedlot, some lambs may be sick and some dead, and within a few days, other sheep become ill. In the sick lambs, the body temperatures rise to a range of 41 to 42°C, and the animals decline feed. Diarrhea develops, and the fluid feces are mucoid, blood-flecked, and malodorous. Affected sheep become depressed, physically weak, and gaunt. With hanging heads, drooping ears, and arching backs, the lambs isolate themselves, recline, and gradually prostrate. Death may occur after a disease course of 1 to 5 days. Nonfatal cases recover after about 2 weeks. The morbidity varies up to 30% of the flock and the mortality up to 25% of affected sheep.

At necropsy, the perineal wool and skin are stained and soiled with fluid feces, and most tissues are dehydrated. During early stages, the abomasum and intestines are often filled with fluid and are locally congested and inflamed. In the intestines, mucus adheres to the mucous membranes and may contain flecks of blood. The mucous membranes of both intestine and gallbladder may be swollen and edematous. Small hemorrhages commonly discolor the subendocardial and subepicardial surface. *S. typhimurium* can be isolated from feces, bile, liver, spleen, mesenteric nodes, and heart blood. Mesenteric nodes, especially the caudal ones, are swollen, congested, and edematous.

DIAGNOSIS. Veterinarians diagnose SD on evidence of typical signs and lesions. In feedlot lambs, a history of shipping and fasting for 4 to 7 days in depressed, debilitated, and diarrheic animals is significant indication of salmonellosis. At necropsy, the congested and inflamed abomasum and intestines give further substantiating information. In the laboratory, scientists confirm or establish a diagnosis by isolating one or more species of *Salmonella* from affected organs. The differential diagnosis requires consideration of pneumonia, coccidiosis, acute septicemic pasteurellosis, and dietary diarrheas.

For technical assistance from a diagnostic laboratory, practitioners should submit suspect feces, swollen mesenteric and hepatic nodes, gallbladder, liver, spleen, and samples of pen water from fountains and puddles.

PREVENTION AND TREATMENT. Management is the most effective means of preventing salmonellosis. Avoiding undue stress or minimizing stressful situations is most important. SD can be prevented or at least reduced by executing collaborative programs by producer, shipper, and feeder. Before shipping, lambs should be weaned and adjusted to fibrous feed, such as grass or alfalfa hay. Immediately before loading for shipment, the animals should be given a full feed of hay and fresh water. Shipment should be expedited to avoid long fatiguing periods of travel and hunger. If transit requires more than 48 hours, the lambs should be unloaded, rested, fed, and watered in sanitary and disease-free yards. The feed should be bulky hay kept in troughs and protected against fecal contamination.

On arrival at destination, all sick lambs should be immediately isolated from the flock. Healthy sheep should receive high quality grass or alfalfa hay and fresh water. Pools of water should be drained from pens. Feed should be provided in sanitary bunks and water in sanitary fountains protected against fecal contamination. Rodent populations should be controlled and excluded from feed stores. Medicating the water with nitrofurazone (Furacin) or furazolidone may avoid some new cases. Dead animals and contaminated litter should be incinerated or buried in quicklime.

Pens of sheep should be treated by adding to the drinking water antibiotics that, in the laboratory, have inhibiting effects on the specific infecting bacteria. Electrolytes added to the water aid in preventing metabolic acidosis and maintenance of the acid-base balance.

New vaccines are being investigated and hold promise for those areas of the world where salmonellosis is an endemic problem.

Aserkoff, B., Schroeder, S.A., and Brachman, P.S.: Salmonellosis in the United States—a five-year review. Am. J. Epidemiol. *92*:13-24, 1970.

Bruns, H. and Gasters: Paratyphusepidemie einer hammelherde. Zeut. Hyg. Infections-krankheit., *90*:263-280, 1920.

Grau, F.H. and Brownlee, L.E.: Effect of some preslaughter treatments on Salmonella populations in the bovine rumen and feces. J. Appl. Bacteriol., *31*:157-163, 1968.

Grau, F.H., Brownlee, L.E., and Smith, M.G.: Effects of food intake on numbers of salmonellae and *Escherichia coli* in rumen and feces of sheep. J. Appl. Bacteriol., *32*:112-117, 1969.

Hemmingsen, P., Montgomery, R., Ward, C., and Henderson, T.: A fatal disease outbreak in sheep associated with *Salmonella enteritidis ser Havana*. N.Z. Vet. J., *30*:98, 1982.

Hindmarsh, W.L.: Dysentery in sheep due to Salmonella infection. Aust. Vet. J., *16*:112-117, 1940.

Jebson, J.L.: Salmonellosis in sheep. Aust. Vet. J., *26:* 256-258, 1950.

Jelinek, P., Robertson, G., and Millar, C.: Vaccination of sheep with a live gale mutant of *Salmonella typhimurium.* Aust. Vet. J., *59:*31-32, 1982.

Josland, S.W.: The immunogenic properties of *Salmonella typhimurium* in sheep. N.Z. Vet. J., *2:*2-7, 1954.

Langham, R.F., Feldman, H.F., and Thorp, F.: Paratyphoid dysentery in feeder lambs. Michigan State Coll. Vet., *45:*42-43, 1951.

Moule, G.R. and Young, R.B.: Salmonellosis in transported rams. Queensland Agric. J., *73:*84-86, 1951.

Newsom, I.E. and Cross, F.: An outbreak of paratyphoid dysentery in lambs. JAVMA, *66:*289-300, 1924.

Newsom, I.E. and Cross, F.: Paratyphoid dysentery in lambs again. JAVMA, *76:*91-92, 1930.

Robertson, G.: A new weapon against salmonellosis. J. Agr. West. Aust., *23:*61-62, 1982.

Salisbury, R.M.: Salmonella infections in animals and birds in New Zealand. N.Z. Vet. J., *6:*76-86, 1958.

Stewart, D.F.: Two mortalities among sheep due to infection with species of Salmonella group of bacteria. Aust. Vet. J., *16:*169-172, 1940.

Watts, P.S. and Wall, M.: The 1951 *Salmonella typhimurium* epidemic in sheep in South Australia. Aust. Vet. J.: *28:*165-168, 1952.

Septicemic Pasteurellosis

(*SP*)

Septicemic pasteurellosis, an acute contagious disease of feedlot lambs and yearlings, is characterized clinically by respiratory distress and sudden deaths, and pathologically by focal hepatitis and pulmonitis. It is caused by bacteria and environmental stresses. Because the malady attacks robust and thrifty animals and causes considerable financial waste, it concerns the entire lamb-feeding industry. Economic losses result from deaths of marketable animals and from the cost of preventive and treatment programs.

OCCURRENCE. SP occurs in all sexes and breeds of lambs 2 to 12 months of age, but lambs recently weaned and transported from range or pasture to fields and feedlots have a higher incidence than other age groups. Most outbreaks develop during late summer and early autumn, during or following inclement weather.

Geographically, SP probably occurs in all countries where sheep are produced. *Pasteurella haemolytica* has been isolated from sheep wherever surveys have been conducted. The prevalence of SP is especially high in California, Colorado, Iowa, and mid-western states where the feeding industry depends on lambs transported for distances.

ETIOLOGY AND PATHOGENESIS. An interaction between *Pasteurella haemolytica* and environmental stress causes SP. Based on their biochemical characteristics *P. haemolytica* strains are classified as A or T biotypes. On the bases of specific antisera and using the indirect hemoagglutination (IHA) test or the rapid counterimmunoelectrophoresis test, 15 serotypes have been identified. *P. haemolytica* biotype A (1, 2, 5, 6, 7, 8, 9, 11, 12, 13, 14) is a common inhabitant of the nasopharyngeal mucosa of healthy sheep and can be recovered at any age. The untypable *P. haemolytica* are more frequently isolated from the nasopharynx of the neonatal lamb. Strains of biotype T (T3, T4, T10, T15) are a normal inhabitant of the tonsil in lambs over 3 weeks of age and increase in frequency with age. One

Fig. 6-10. Primary intestinal ulcer in feedlot lamb with SP.

Fig. 6-11. Secondary metastatic foci of infection in liver of feedlot lamb with SP.

the diet rapidly from roughage to high-carbo-hydrate feeds. Stress on lambs produces increased levels of serum hydrocortisone. The stress produced elevation in hydrocortisone suppress PS to immune system by inhibiting blastogenic response of peripheral blood lymphocytes to phytohemagglutinin and conca-navalin A mitogens with a resultant suppression of T lymphocytes. The change from roughage to concentrate feed along with high serum hydrocortisone levels insult or injure the intestinal tract (Fig. 6-10) allowing the passage of the organism through the intestinal wall and into the portal circulation. The suppression of the immune system by the stress induced high serum hydrocortisone levels allows development of SP. The organisms invade branches of the portal vein causing hemorrhage, necrosis, and thrombosis. Infective microemboli transport in portal blood to the liver (Fig. 6-11), some transverse the liver, enter venous blood and transport to the lungs (Fig. 6-12). Thus the

or more strains may be isolated from a healthy sheep. Biotypes A and the untypable strains are associated with pneumonia of all ages or with septicemia in the neonatal lamb (less than 2 months). Biotypes T (3, 4, 10, 15) are associated with septicemic pasteurellosis in lambs 3 to 12 months old which are subjected to intensive management. The specific properties causing T3, T4, T10, and T15 to have a predilect for tissues other than the lung is unknown, possibly a difference in virulence. It is virtually impossible to infect a sheep either respiratory or systemic without a stress factor caused by weaning, transportation, changes in feed or severe weather accompanied by a temporary interruption of feed intake or concurrent viral infection. The exact pathogenesis of how the resident or recently transmitted *P. haemolytica* organism becomes virulent and establishes disease. To produce experimental septicemic pasteurellosis (SP), it is necessary to give lambs hydrocortisone and to change

Fig. 6-12. Tertiary metastatic foci of infection in lung of feedlot lamb with SP.

intestine, liver, and lungs can be considered primary, secondary and tertiary foci of infection respectively. The role of the tonsil in the pathogenesis of septicemic pasteurellosis is unclear. Based on the presence of tonsilar enlargement and necrosis and necrotic erosions in the esophagus, some investigators suggest the upper alimentary tract as the primary site of entry with multiplication in the lung and spread to other organs.

The genesis of necrotic foci within the liver, lungs, and other organs, increased vascular permeability and ultimate death is probably due to toxemia from bacterial endotoxins.

Transmission among sheep probably is by direct and indirect contact. The common practice of crowding lambs during shipping, driving, and confining provides opportunity for face-to-face contact, inhalation of infected aerosols, and consumption of organisms in contaminated feed and water.

CLINICAL SIGNS AND POSTMORTEM LESIONS. In outbreaks of SP, herdsmen usually find dead lambs without previously being aware of the animals' sickness. Careful inspection then reveals other affected sheep. These animals separate from the flock, decline feed, breathe rapidly, and become immobilized. Body temperature rises to 41 to 42°C, and depression becomes profound. Nasal discharges of mucus, foam, and blood may develop. Although the morbidity may be high, mortality seldom exceeds 5%.

At necropsy, the small intestine, and occasionally the cecum, has one or more ulcers with necrosis and hemorrhage. The liver and lungs each contain numerous, perhaps several hundred, gray, randomly distributed foci, each 0.1 to 1.0 mm in diameter. Histologically, portal branches in the intestine are infected and thrombosed, and capillaries in the hepatic and pulmonary foci are filled with colonies of bacteria.

DIAGNOSIS. Veterinarians suspect SP on the basis of typical signs and lesions, and they confirm the diagnosis by isolating *P. haemolytica* from the liver and lungs. The differential diagnosis requires consideration of enterotoxemia and acute pneumonia.

PREVENTION AND TREATMENT. Due to the sporadic nature of SP and the lack of cross protection among the strains of *P. haemolytica*, immunization programs have not gained general acceptance in the large commercial feeding operations. If SP is an endemic problem to an area, a bacterin including the identified serotypes can be used in a preventive program. Stress factors accompanying extreme dietary changes are known to precipitate problems with SP. Therefore, management strategies should be developed to reduce the traumatic insult of these on the lambs.

As the disease is sporadic in nature and the first signs of SP may be dead or terminally ill lambs, treatment may be difficult. Following a diagnosis of SP careful inspection of the other lambs for early signs, such as separation from the flock and rapid breathing, isolation and prompt treatment of SP is difficult due to the sporadic nature of the disease and the first indication may be dead or terminally ill lambs. At this point close observation of the others in the flock may reveal early cases which separate themselves, refuse food, show some degree of depression and have a rapid respiration. Early isolation and treatment of these individuals with oxytetracycline (3 mg/kg) and sulfonamides (1 mg/kg) plus oral electrolytes will reduce losses. Depending on the severity of the problem, it may be advisable to administer sulfonamides (1 mg/kg) and electrolytes in the drinking water for 4 to 6 days. Oxytetracyclines (12 mg/kg) can be added to the feed for 4 to 6 days. Close observation must be maintained for the individual animal which isolates themselves from the flock and does not accept the medicated feed or water.

Al-Sultan, I. and Aitken, I.: The tonsillar carriage of *Pasteurella haemolytica* in lambs. J. Comp. Path., *95*:193-201, 1985.

Biberstein, E.L. and Kennedy, P.C.: Septicemic pasteurellosis in lambs. AJVR, *20*:94-101, 1959.

Bosworth, T.J. and Lovell, R.: Hemolytic coccobacilli in the nose of normal sheep. J. Comp. Pathol., *54*:168-171, 1944.

Chengapa, M., Carter, G., and Baile, W.: Comparison of indirect hemagglutination and rapid plate agglutination tests with counterelectrophoresis for typing *Pasteurella haemolytica*. J. Clin. Microbiol., *20*:660-663, 1984.

Collins, M. and Suarez-Guemes, F.: Effect of hydrocortisone on circulating lymphocyte numbers and their mitogen-induced blastogenesis in lambs. Am. J. Vet. Res., 46:836-840, 1985.

Cowan, S. and McBeath, D.: Passive protection of lambs against septic pasteurellosis. Vet. Rec., 111:185-186, 1982.

Dungal, N.: Contagious pneumonia in sheep. J. Comp. Pathol., 44:126, 1931.

Ellis, J.: Pasteurella haemolytica infections in sheep. The Compendium on C.E., 6:5360-5366, 1984.

Fodor, L., Varga, J., Hajtos, I., and Szemeredi, G.: Serotypes of Pasteurella haemolytica isolated from sheep, goats and calves. Zbl. Vet. Med. B., 31:466-469, 1984.

Frank, G.: Serotypes of Pasteurella haemolytica in sheep in the midwestern United States. Am. J. Vet. Res., 43:2035-2037, 1982.

Marsh, H.: Pasteurella in sheep diseases. JAVMA. 123: 205-208, 1953.

Newsom, I.E. and Cross, F.: Bipolar organisms in pneumonia of sheep. JAVMA, 80:711-719, 1932.

Stamp, J.T., Watt, J.A.A., and Thomlinson, J.R.: Pasteurella haemolytica septicemia of lambs. J. Comp. Pathol., 65:183-196, 1955.

Suarez-Guemes, F., Collins, M., and Whiteman, C.: Experimental reproduction of septicemic pasteurellosis in feedlot lambs: Bacteriologic and pathologic examinations., 46:193-201, 1985.

Coccidiosis

(Hemorrhagic diarrhea; coccidial dysentery)

Coccidiosis, an acute contagious disease of feedlot lambs, is characterized by hemorrhagic diarrhea, depression, weakness, loss of live weight, and the presence of fecal oocysts. It is caused by numerous species of coccidia. Although coccidiosis is primarily a disease of feedlot lambs, the malady also affects nursing lambs of farm flocks. Because coccidiosis has worldwide distribution and causes extensive financial waste, it has major importance to the sheep industry. Economic losses result from deaths, loss of live weight, delayed marketing, damaged wool, extra labor, and costly treatment. Coccidiosis of cattle and wild ruminants, although similar to the ovine disease, is not transmissible to sheep.

OCCURRENCE. Coccidiosis occurs in all breeds and sexes of sheep, but feedlot lambs 3 to 5 months of age and, less commonly, nursing lambs 1 to 3 months old have high incidence. Older sheep carry the parasites but rarely develop the disease. The malady develops within 1 to 3 weeks after lambs enter fattening pens or succulent alfalfa or beet-top pastures during late summer and early fall. Nursing lambs usually contract the disease in pens or pastures during the summer.

As a major endemic disease, coccidiosis primarily occurs in feedlot enterprises of the western and midwestern states where the lamb-fattening industry has developed. Among nursing lambs sporadic or widespread coccidiosis occurs throughout the United States and all other sheep-producing countries.

ETIOLOGY. At least 12 species of Eimeria occur in sheep. Several species of Eimeria once thought to be parasites of sheep are now considered to occur only in goats. Eimeria ahsata, E. ovina, and E. ovinoidalis are the most pathogenic species of coccidia to occur in sheep. Other species occurring in sheep are E. crandallis, E. faurei, E. gonzalezi, E. granulosa, E. intricata, E. pallida, E. parva, E. punctata, and E. weybridgensis. Eimeria arlongi and E. ninakohlyakimovae once thought to be coccidia of sheep are now considered goat parasites. In most outbreaks of coccidiosis several species of coccidia are found, but one of the pathogenic species is always present. The oocyst of the three pathogenic species are morphologic differentiated by features presented in Table 6-2.

In general, oocysts are highly resistant to adverse environmental factors. Sporulation is not inhibited by 0.1 M solutions of barium chloride, calcium chloride, cobalt chloride, cadmium chloride, by 1 M solution of copper sulfate, or by 0.01 M solution of phenol. In contrast, however, sporulation does not occur in 10^{-6} M solution of mercuric chloride, 0.05 M solution of phenol, or 0.025 M solution of formaldehyde.

Exposure of oocysts to direct sunlight for 8 hours at 30°C, or to a relative humidity of 25% or less for 10 days, prevents most sporulation. Drying at 40°C not only inhibits sporulation, but eventually destroys the oocysts. At environmental temperatures of −19 to −25°C, oocysts endure for prolonged periods and retain the ability to sporulate and infect sheep.

Table 6-2. *Comparison of Pathogenic Oocysts from Sheep*

| Species | Size in Microns | | Morphologic Features | Color | Anatomic Location | |
	Range	Mean			Schizonts	Sporonts
E. ovinoidalis	16–27 × 13–22	23 × 18	ovoid to spherical; micropyle and cap absent	colorless to pale brown	ileum, cecum, colon	cecum, colon
E. ovina	17–42 × 13–27	27 × 18	elongate to ellipsoidal; micropyle and cap present	faint yellow to brown	small intestine lacteals	small intestine as white nodules
E. ahsata	29–37 × 17–28	33 × 23	ellipsoidal; micropyle and cap present	faint pink	unknown	unknown

Although oocysts may endure in feedlots through the winter, they probably are killed by the low humidity and high temperature of summer. Consequently, cleaned feedlots become sterilized during summer months of rest and are reinfected with oocyst-containing feces from the first fall occupants.

The coccidial life history consists of exogenous and endogenous phases. The exogenous phase begins with the discharge of oocysts in feces to the exterior. In the presence of sufficient oxygen and moisture and at favorable temperatures of 20 to 25°C, the oocysts sporulate and become infective in 24 to 48 hours. In the process, the single cell in the oocyst discards a polar body and becomes haploid in chromosomal formula. Division of the cell forms four sporoblasts, each of which, through maturation, forms a sporocyst. Each of the latter, from division of the cell within the sporoblast, contains two sporozoites. At this stage of development, the parasite becomes infective.

The endogenous phase of the life cycle begins with ingestion of the sporulated oocyst in contaminated feed and water. In the lumen of the small intestine, excystation releases the sporozoites, which penetrate the mucosa. The sporozoites of *E. ovinoidalis* form first-generation schizonts in epithelial cells of the ileum and second-generation schizonts in epithelial cells of the crypts of the cecum and colon. The sporozoites of *E. ovina,* in contrast, penetrate the small intestine wall and form schizonts in endothelial cells of lacteals. At the end of the process of schizogony, some merozoites, after penetrating epithelial cells, differentiate into female macrogametes, which enlarge and mature, while others form male microgametocytes which, on maturation, form many biflagellated microgametes. Following release from the cell, the microgametes fertilize the macrogametes to form zygotes, which have the diploid chromosomal formula. Gamonts, the sexual forms of *E. ovinoidalis,* form in epithelial cells of the crypts of the cecum and colon, and of *E. ovina* in epithelial cells of small intestinal villi.

TRANSMISSION. Coccidiosis is transmitted through ingestion with feed or water of large numbers of sporulated oocysts. All adult sheep and most range and pasture lambs carry small numbers of coccidia, but not sufficient in number to produce immunity, and they continuously excrete small numbers of oocysts.

In crowded feedlots and pastures, feed and water may become contaminated with oocyst-containing feces. Continuous contamination, as in open feed troughs and in succulent pastures, rapidly increases the number of oocysts in the feed. The succulent feed provides the required moisture for sporulation.

PATHOGENESIS. During the first month of pen fattening, the number of fecal oocysts rapidly increases to a normal peak. In clinical coccidiosis many epithelial cells in the mucosa are destroyed. Although epithelial cells are destroyed by the developing asexual stages, sporozoite schizonts and merozoite, the greater destruction of the mucosa occurs with the development of the sexual stage, macrogametocytes, microgametocytes, and oocysts. Capillaries of denuded lamina propria hemorrhage into tissues and into the intestinal lumen; the hemorrhage causes anemia and hypoproteinemia. Bacteria in the colon, especially *Fusobacterium necrophorum,* penetrate the coccidia-injured mucosa and thrombose small blood vessels.

Bacterial growth and circulatory disturbance cause local necrosis, which begins at the surface and extends to variable depths. Serous and fibrinous exudates suffuse the necrotic tissue. Sloughing of small, medium, and large amounts of necrotic mucosa produces ulcers of corresponding size that are partially filled with exudate. These tissue changes accelerate peristalsis and result in diarrhea. The fluid feces contain water, Na^+, K^+, Cl^-, and HCO_3^-. During the first few days of diarrhea, affected animals may lose 12% of body water. The loss of water results in tissue dehydration, and the loss of HCO_3^- results in acidosis.

Dehydration, acidosis, anemia, hypoproteinemia, and shock cause death; in some sheep, secondary bacterial infection also contributes to the cause of death. The injuries from severe coccidiosis may permanently impair the capacity of recovered lambs for efficient use of feed and for economic gains in body weight. Recovered sheep continue to carry and excrete small numbers of oocysts.

CLINICAL SIGNS AND POSTMORTEM LESIONS. Ovine coccidiosis begins within 1 to 3 weeks after the lambs enter fattening pens or succulent alfalfa or beet-top pastures. The first sign is softness of unpelleted feces, followed by fluid feces. Wool of the tail, perineum, and medial aspects of the hind limbs becomes soiled and may attract fly strike and screwworm attacks. The feces of some, but not all, animals in all outbreaks contain variable amounts of blood. The blood may be bright from rectal ulcers or dark and mixed with feces from cecal ulcers.

Affected sheep strain, and some may develop rectal prolapses. After a few days of diarrhea, lambs lose their appetites, become gaunt, dehydrated, and weak, and lose 5 to 15% of live weights. Body temperatures may rise to 42 to 43°C during early stages, but soon become normal to subnormal from diarrhea. Depression, inactivity, and recumbency are prominent. Recovering lambs gradually resume fattening; some, however, slowly grow and fatten and reach a state of marketability after a longer-than-average feeding time.

Among affected flocks, the morbidity ranges from 10 to 50% and the mortality of affected sheep up to 10%. The course varies from 1 to 2 weeks; some deaths, however, occur after 3 to 4 days of sickness.

At necropsy, most lesions are located in the alimentary tract. The posterior wool, soiled with fluid feces and possibly blood, emits malodors and may contain maggots. Most tissues are dehydrated. Enteritis and colitis are prominent. Infection from *E. ovina* produces white nodules, especially in the ileum, 1 to 3 mm in diameter; these foci, concentrations of fat-containing macrogametocytes in epithelial cells of villi, are visible from either serosal or mucosal surfaces.

Infection from *E. ovinoidalis* causes diffuse ileitis, cecitis, and colitis (Figs. 6-13 and 6-14). The ileocecal valve, cecum, colon, and rectum may show erosions and ulcers from 1 to 10 mm in diameter and hemorrhage into affected tissue and the lumen. Mucosal scrapings usually contain oocysts and blood, but tissue sections often show some stages of schizogony or gametogony. Necrosis, ulceration, and hemorrhage may extend into the submucosa. As a result of infection from *E. ovina,* schizonts, detached from lacteals, may occur in regional lymph nodes.

DIAGNOSIS. Veterinarians diagnose coccidiosis on evidence of history, signs, lesions, and laboratory findings. High incidence of diarrhea developing 1 to 3 weeks after sheep enter the feedlot or pasture, necropsy lesions

Fig. 6-13. Cecal coccidiosis from *Eimeria ovinoidalis.* × 1.0.

Fig. 6-14. Colonic coccidiosis with expansive necrosis and ulceration of the mucosa from primary infection with *E. ovinoidalis* and secondary infection with *Fusobacterium necrophorum.* × 1.2.

of ileitis, cecitis, and colitis, and the presence of significant numbers of oocysts in feces or mucosal scrapings firmly establish the diagnosis. Finding the lesions and the oocysts may require several necropsies and several fecal examinations of lambs in different stages of disease. For technical assistance from a diagnostic laboratory, practitioners should submit feces from each of several sheep, as well as ileum, cecum, and colon.

The differential diagnosis requires consideration of acute salmonellosis.

PREVENTION AND TREATMENT. In the feedlot proper sanitation is important in preventing clinical outbreaks of coccidiosis. Newly arriving lambs should be fed a good quality native or alfalfa hay for several days upon entering to help the lambs to adapt and prevent digestive disorders. The hay should be fed in such a way as to avoid fecal contamination. The pens should be kept as dry as possible and standing water should be drained from the pens. In most cases it is preferable not to use bedding in pens of newly arrived lambs, as it becomes contaminated with fecal material and the lambs have a tendency to eat the bedding.

Several drugs are available which aid in prevention of coccidiosis. Amproline can be given to feedlot lambs in the feed or drinking water. It should be used at 50 mg/kg body weight for the first 21 days. Dequonate is another coccidiostat which can be given to lambs. It should be fed for the first week at 2 mg/kg body weight and reduced to 0.5 to 1.0 mg/kg body weight for the next 3 weeks the lambs are in the feedlot.

Two ionophores used in ruminants to improve feed efficiency are also good coccidiostats. Lasalocid is the only one approved for use in sheep in the United States. It should be fed to sheep from the time they arrive in the feedlot through the entire feeding period. The dose of lasalocid is 0.5 to 1 mg/kg body weight which is the dose (30 g/ton) recommended to improve feed efficiency. Monensin another ionophore can be fed to feedlot lambs to prevent coccidiosis. It is mixed in the salt at 0.75%.

Clinical cases of coccidiosis in sheep should be treated with one of the sulfa drugs (sulfathiazole, sulfamerazine, sulfamethazine, sulfaquanidine) in the drinking water. In an outbreak in the feedlot all animals in the pen should receive the medicated drinking water. Electrolytes and vitamins can be added to the medicated drinking water to replace those lost in the diarrhetic animal. Combination of sulfas, electrolytes, and vitamins are commercially available.

Animal Health Yearbook. FAO-WHO-OIE (Italy), 1970.
Baker, N.F., Walters, G.T., and Fisk, R.A.: Amprolium for control of coccidiosis in feedlot lambs. AJVR, 33:83-85, 1972.
Bergstrom, R.C. and Maki, L.R.: Coccidiostatic action of monensin fed to lambs, body weight gains and feed conversions efficacy. Am. J. Vet. Res., 37(1):79-81, 1976.
Christensen, J.F.: The source and availability of infective oocysts in an outbreak of coccidiosis in lambs in Nebraska feedlots. AJVR, 1:27-35, 1940.
Christensen, J.F.: Sporulation and viability of oocysts of Eimeria arloingi from the domestic sheep. J. Agric. Res., 59:527-534, 1939.
Christensen, J.F.: Species differentiation in the coccidia from the domestic sheep. J. Parasitol., 24:453-465, 1938.
Deem, A.W. and Thorp, F.: Coccidia and coccidiosis in feeder lambs. JAVMA, 96:733-735, 1940.
Foreyt, W.J., Parish, S.M., and Foreyt, K.M.: Lasalocid for improved weight gains and control of coccidiosis in lambs. Am. J. Vet. Res., 42(1):57-60, 1981.
Foreyt, W.J., Gates, N.L., and Rich, J.E.: Evaluation of lasalocid salt against ovine coccidia. Am. J. Vet. Res., 42(1):54-56, 1981.
Foreyt, W.J.: Epidemiology and control of coccidia in sheep. In The Veterinary Clinics of North America, Food Animal Practice, Parasites: Epidemiology and Control. Edited by H.C. Gibbs, R.P. Herd, and K.D. Murrell. Philadelphia, W.B. Saunders Co., 1986.
Horton, G.M.J. and Stockdale, P.H.B.: Effects of amprolium and monensin on oocyst discharge, feed utilization and rumen metabolism of lambs with coccidiosis. Am. J. Vet. Res., 40(7):966-970, 1979.
Landers, E.J.: The effect of low temperatures upon the viability of unsporulated oocysts in ovine coccidia. J. Parasitol., 39:547-552, 1953.
Levine, N.D.: Taxonomy and life cycles of coccidia. In The Biology of the Coccidia. Edited by P.L. Long, Baltimore, University Park Press, 1982.
Mahrt, J.L. and Sherrick, G.W.: Coccidiosis due to Eimeria ahsata in feedlot lambs in Illinois. JAVMA, 146:1415-1416, 1965.
McCougald, L.R. and Dunn, W.J.: Efficacy of monensin against coccidiosis in lambs. Am. J. Vet. Res., 39(9):1459-1462, 1978.
Newsom, I.E. and Cross, F.: Coccidial dysentery in Colorado feeder lambs in 1930. Vet. Med., 26:140-142, 1931.
Newsom, I.E. and Cross, F.: An outbreak of coccidiosis in lambs. JAVMA, 77:232-235, 1930.
Smith, W.N., Davis, L.R., and Bowman, G.W.: The pathogenicity of Ah-sa-ta, a coccidium of sheep. J. Protozool., 7:8 abstracts, 1960.

Cryptosporidiosis

Cryptosporidiosis has only been recognized as a cause of clinical disease in animals during the past 4 to 5 years. The organism has been reported from several hosts including calves, lambs, foals, swine, dogs, man, bird, and reptiles. Since the organism is easily transmitted between different hosts, it is generally considered as a single species. In lambs, as other hosts, clinical infection occurs at 1 to 3 weeks of age with clinical signs varying from a mild enteritis to severe diarrhea.

ETIOLOGY AND PATHOGENESIS. The causative agent of cryptosporidiosis is a small protozoan organism (2 to 6 μm) classified with the coccidia. Unlike other members of enteric coccidia which develop within intestinal cell Cryptosporidia organisms adhere to the microvillous border of enterocytes. The life cycle of the organism is similar to coccidia including asexual or schizogonic cycle with 2 generations of schizonts and merozoites and a sexual or gametogonic cycle, with macrogametes, microgametes, zygotes, and oocysts. The oocysts sporulate within the host and are infective when passed in the feces. Some oocysts do not develop the two layered oocyst wall and rupture within the host and are capable of reinitiating the development cycle in the same host. Infection of new host occurs following ingestion of oocysts.

In experimentally infected lambs both the small and large intestine are infected, with the heaviest infections occurring in the terminal ileum. The organism attached to the microvilli produces villous atrophy with fusion and epithelial cross-bridging between villi.

CLINICAL SIGNS AND POSTMORTEM LESIONS. Clinical infections occur in lambs under 3 weeks of age, with the most severe infection occurring in lambs during the first week of life. Lambs are depressed, anorectic and have varying degrees of diarrhea. At necropsy the small and large intestine is congested, the mesenteric lymph nodes are large and edematous.

DIAGNOSIS. Most cases of cryptosporidiosis are diagnosed by finding oocysts in the feces. Oocysts can be separated from the feces by standard flotation procedures. Staining the fecal smear or flotation with Giemsa or an acid fast stain aids in identifying the small oocyst. Giemsa stained oocysts have blue staining cytoplasm with 2 or more red granules in the cytoplasm. The organism must be differentiated from yeast found in fecal smears.

TREATMENT AND CONTROL. Although various drugs used to treat and prevent coccidiosis in animals have been tried with cryptosporidiosis, they do not alter the course of the disease. Since most infections are mild and transient, it is recommended that only conservative and supportive therapy be used.

Angus, K., Tzipori, S., and Gray, E.: Intestinal lesions in specific-pathogen-free lambs associated with a cryptosporidium from calves with diarrhea. Vet. Pathol., 19:67-78, 1982.

Anderson, B.C.: Patterns of shedding of cryptosporidial oocyst in Idaho calves. JAVMA, 178(9):982-984, 1981.

Anderson, B.C. and Bulgin, M.S.: Enteritis caused by cryptosporidium in calves. VM/SAC, 76:865-868, 1981.

Anderson, B.C.: Cryptosporidiosis. A review. JAVMA, 180(12):1455-1457, 1982.

Anderson, B.C.: Location of cryptosporidia. Review of the literature and experimental infections in calves. Am. J. Vet. Res., 45(7):1474-1477, 1984.

Berg, I.E. and Peterson, A.C.: Ovine cryptosporidiosis. JAVMA, 173(12):1586-1587, 1978.

Current, W.L.: Cryptosporidiosis. JAVMA, 187(12): 1334-1338, 1985.

Gajadhar, A.A., Caron, J.P., and Allen, J.R.: Cryptosporidiosis in two foals. Can. Vet. J., 26:132-134, 1985.

Gardiner, C.H. and Imes, G.D.: Cryptosporidiosis sp in the kidneys of a black-throated finch. JAVMA, 185(11):1401-1408, 1984.

Pohjola, S.: Negative staining method with nigrosin for the detection of cryptosporidial oocyst: A comparative study. Res. Vet. Sci., 36:217-219, 1984.

Sisk, D.B., Gosser, H.S., Styer, E.L.: Intestinal cryptosporidiosis in two pups. JAVMA, 184(7):835-836, 1984.

Szabo, J.R. and Moore, K.: Cryptosporidiosis in a snake. VM/SAC, 79:96-98, 1984.

Tzipori, S., Angus, K.W., Campbell, I., and Gray, E.W.: Cryptosporidium: Evidence for a single-species genus. Inf. & Imm., 30(3):884-886, 1980.

Tzipori, S., et al.: Diarrhea in lambs experimentally infected with cryptosporidium isolated from calves. Am. J. Vet. Res., 42(8):1400-1404, 1981.

Willson, P.J. and Acres, S.P.: A comparison of dichromate solution flotation and fecal smears for diagnosis of cryptosporidiosis in calves. Can. Vet. J., 23:240-246, 1982.

Thysanosomiasis

(Fringed tapeworm livers)

Thysanosomiasis, a commensal relationship between parasitic tapeworms and domestic sheep, is characterized by innocuous residence of the parasites in the duodenum, bile ducts, and pancreatic ducts and is caused by the fringed tapeworm, an anoplocephaline cestode. Because the condition is limited to North and South America and does not impair production, it causes little concern to the sheep industry of the world, but in the United States it annually results in the condemnation of approximately 1.1 million kg of liver from slaughtered sheep. But as American production emphasis shifts from range bands where the incidence is high to pasture flocks where the incidence is low, the economic importance will decline. The occurrence of fringed tapeworms in goats, mountain sheep, antelope, deer, moose, and elk also adds scientific interest to the condition.

OCCURRENCE. Thysanosomiasis occurs in all breeds, sexes, and ages of sheep that graze noncultivated ranges. The condition is commonly encountered, however, among fattened range lambs because inspectors specifically examine the livers of slaughtered animals for parasites. Sheep acquire the infection during August and September grazing, and the worms become discernible upon inspection of livers within 4 to 5 months. Consequently, lambs slaughtered between January and May have a high infection rate.

Geographically, fringed tapeworms occur in Argentina, Chile, Peru, Mexico, Canada, and the United States; in the United States, incidence is high in states west of the Mississippi River and in North Dakota, Minnesota, Wisconsin, and Illinois.

ETIOLOGY. The causative fringed tapeworm, *Thysanosoma actinioides,* is of the family Anoplocephalidae. Adult worms, measuring 250 to 300 × 5 to 7 mm, contain scoleces 1 to 1.5 mm wide and hermaphroditic segments with fringed posterior borders. Occupying the duodenum, bile ducts, and pancreatic ducts as their definitive positions, the parasites, because of unesthetic appearance, cause liver condemnations of slaughtered sheep.

Only some features of the life cycle are known. Terminal segments, while still nongravid, detach from the parent worm and complete development in the intestinal lumen. At the time of expulsion, the gravid segments, 1.5 to 3.0 mm wide, conspicuously adhere to fecal pellets. On exposure to light, the segments disseminate capsules containing 5 to 12 hexacanths through an anterior uterine aperture.

From this point on, the cycle is conjectural. Even though the intermediate host is unknown, one presumably exists and sustains acystic cysticercoids which, when eaten by grazing sheep, develop through a prepatent period of several months into mature tapeworms. The worms do not provoke immunity in sheep.

CLINICAL SIGNS AND POSTMORTEM LESIONS. Even though thysanosomiasis causes no clinical manifestations, affected sheep feces during patent periods contain white gravid segments. The incidence ranges up to 75% of fattened lambs. At necropsy of dead sheep or at inspection of slaughtered sheep, the duodenum, bile ducts, and pancreatic ducts contain from 1 to 25 tapeworms (Fig. 6-15). When numerous, the contorted worms are packed into the thickened and dilated ducts. Duct

Fig. 6-15. *Thysanosoma actinioides* (a) in bile duct (b). × 1.0.

walls may show uneven fibrosis and epithelial hyperplasia.

DIAGNOSIS. Veterinarians diagnose thysanosomiasis by observing the characteristic segments on fecal pellets and by finding the worms in the duodenum, bile ducts, and pancreatic ducts. Other tapeworms must be considered in the identification.

TREATMENT. Treatment of sheep for thysanosomiasis is usually necessary and in most cases uneconomical. Two of the new benzimidazole anthelmintics have shown efficacy for *Thysanosoma.* Albendazole at 3.8 mg/kg body weight is not effective, but at 7.5 mg/kg to 11.5 mg/kg body weight, it has better than 90% efficacy. Cambendazole at 100 mg/kg body weight is 100% efficacious against *Thysanosoma* in range ewes.

Allen, R.W.: Biology of *Thysanosoma actinioides*. New Mexico Agric. Exp. Stat. Bull. 604, 1973.

Allen, R.W.: Preliminary evaluation of levamisole, parabendazole, cambendazole as thysanosomicide in sheep. Am. J. Vet. Res., *34*(1):61-63, 1973.

Allen, R.W.: Larval development of the fringed tapeworm of sheep in psocids. J. Parasitol, *45*:537-538, 1959.

Becklund, W.W.: Parasites in the United States and Canada. AJVR, *25*:1380-1416, 1964.

Bergstrom, R.C., Armstrong, D.A., and Hancock, H.A.: Evaluation of albendazole as a thysanosomicide in sheep. VM/SAC, *74*(4):549-551, 1979.

Cowan, I.M.: Parasites of black-tailed deer. Can. J. Res., *24*:71-103, 1946.

Craig, T.M. and Shephard, E.: Efficacy of albendazole and levamisole in sheep against *Thysanosoma actinioides* and *Haemonchus contortus* from Edwards Plateau, Texas. Am. J. Vet. Res., *41*(2): 525-526, 1980.

Curtice, C.: The tapeworm in sheep. Science, *11*:261-262, 1888.

Freire, J.J.: Mais um presente exotico par os nossos ovinos *Thysanosoma actinioides*. Bol. Ag. Indust. Com. Porte Alegre, *11*:3-7, Feb., 1955.

Fridkin, A.: *Thysanosoma actinioides*. Gac. Vet. (Buenos Aires), *9*:227-243, 1947.

Gassner, F.X. and Thorpe, F.: *Thysanosoma actinioides*. JAVMA, *96*:410-411, 1940a.

Gassner, F.X. and Thorpe, F.: *Thysanosoma actinioides*. AJVR, *1*:36-43, 1940b.

Hall, M.C.: Discharge eggs from segments of *Thysanosoma actinioides*. Proc. Helminthol. Soc. Wash., *1*: 6-7, 1934.

Led, J.E., Yannarella, F.G., Manazza, J.A., and Denegri, G.M.: Further trial of the action of albendazole on *Thysanosoma actinioides* a cestode of sheep. Gaceta Veterinaria, *42*(349):202-204, 1980.

Monieziasis

Monieziasis, a commensal relationship between the host sheep and the tapeworm *Moniezia expansa*, is characterized only by the presence of these cestode parasites, sometimes in alarming numbers, in young sheep. Infection also develops in goats and cattle. *M. expansa* occupies the small intestine, but 50 worms per lamb produce no measurable injury or interference with economic performance of the sheep; intestine-occluding numbers, however, conceivably could mechanically impede normal alimentation.

M. expansa, measuring 600 x 1.6 cm, possesses a four-suckered scolex with dimensions of 0.4 × 0.8 mm. Segments are broader than they are long, and each contains ovaries and testes, and, along the posterior border, a row of interproglottidal glands.

Research has established many factual details of the life cycle. As terminal proglottids mature and fill with triangular eggs, they detach from the parent worm and, along with host feces, pass to the exterior. Following disintegration of the gravid segment and release of their contents, soil mites, such as genera *Galumna* and *Oribatula* of the family Oribatidae eat the larvae and become the intermediate host. During a period of 6 to 16 weeks, one or more cysticercoids form in a mite, and these larvae, when eaten along with forage by grazing sheep, pass into the small intestine, mature, and live for about 3 months. Infected sheep develop resistance to reinfection.

CLINICAL SIGNS AND POSTMORTEM LESIONS. It is doubtful that *Moniezia* infections in lambs are pathogenic, although this opinion is not universally accepted. In the west (United States, Europe and Australia) it is generally thought that the parasite is not pathogenic. In the east (USSR), however, they consider the parasite an important pathogen causing depressed wool growth, decreased meat production, and even deaths. They also report an increase of enterotoxaemia in lambs infected with *Moniezia* spp.

DIAGNOSIS. Veterinarians diagnose monieziasis by identifying the white gravid proglotted in sheep feces and by finding adult worms in the small intestine at necropsy. The eggs of *Moniezia* can be recovered by routine fecal flotation procedures.

TREATMENT. It is doubtful that treatment of lambs for monieziasis is economically beneficial. However, several of the new benzimidazole anthelmintic have good efficacy for *Moniezia* spp. At 5 mg/kg body weight oxfendazole is 100% efficacious. Cambendazole at 20 mg/kg body weight is also 100% effective in eliminating infections. Fenbendazole at 5 to 15 mg/kg body weight eliminates greater than 95% of adult parasites. Albendazole at 3.8 mg/kg body weight is 100% effective in eliminating infections. None of these anthelmintics are approved for use in sheep in the United States, but fenbendazole is widely used.

Campbell, W.C. and Butler, R.W.: Efficacy of cambenda-zole against tapeworm and roundworm infections in lambs. Aust. Vet. J., 49(11):517-519, 1973.

Chalmers, K.: The efficacy of oxfenbendazole against natural infections of nematodes and cestodes in sheep. N.Z. Vet. J., 25(10):266-269, 1977.

Corba, J., Lietava, P., Duwell, D., and Reisenleiter, R.: Efficacy of fenbendazole against the most important trematodes and cestodes of ruminants. Br. Vet. J., 135(4):318-328, 1979.

Czipri, D.A., Nunns, V.J., and Shearer, G.C.: Bunamidine hydroxynaphthoate activity against Moniezia expansa in sheep. Vet. Rec., 82:505-506, 1968.

Deuell, D. and Tiefenbach, B.: Treatment of Moniezia infections in sheep with panacur (fenbendazole). Tiearztliche Umschau., 33(5):254-255, 1978.

Elliott, D.C.: Tapeworm (Moniezia expansa) in sheep: anthelmintic treatment studies to assess possible pathogenic effects and production loss in young infected animals in the field. N.Z. Vet. J., 32:185-188, 1984.

Freeborne, S.B. and Berry, L.J.: Sheep tapeworm, Moniezia expansa. JAVMA, 85:611-616, 1934.

Hawkins, P.A.: Moniezia expansa infections. J. Parasitol., 32:Suppl. 14, 1946.

Horak, I.G. and Snyders, A.J.: The efficacy of cambenda-zole against cestodes infections in lambs. J. So. Afr. Vet. Asso., 46(3):271-272, 1975.

Kates, K.C. and Goldberg, A.: Pathogenicity of Moniezia expansa for sheep. Proc. Helminthol. Soc. Wash., 18:87-101, 1951.

Krull, W.H.: Life cycle of Moniezia expansa. Proc. Helminthol. Soc. Wash., 6:10-11, 1939.

Led, J.E., Vannarella, F.G., Manazza, J.A., and Denegri, G.M.: Effect of albendazole on Moniezia expansa and Thysanosoma actinioides in sheep. Gaceta Veterinaria, 41(341):363-366, 1979.

McBeath, D.G., Best, J.M.J., Preston, N.K.: Efficacy of fenbendazole against naturally acquired Moniezia expansa infections in lambs. Vet. Rec., 101(20):408-409, 1977.

Soulsby, E.J.L.: Helminths, Arthropods, and Protozoa of Domestic Animals. 7th Edition. Philadelphia, Lea & Febiger, 1982.

Stunkard, H.W.: Life cycle of Moniezia expansa. Science, 86:312, 1937.

Visceral Cysticercosis

(VC; Taenia hydatigena infection)

Abdominal cysticercosis, a subacute or chronic parasitism of young sheep, is characterized by hepatitis and the formation of bladderworms in the abdominal organs and is caused by the larvae of a common tapeworm of dogs and coyotes. The disease has worldwide distribution and frequently high incidence. It causes occasional clinical manifestations and often subclinical effects.

Economic losses, although not high, result from occasional deaths and vague unthrifti-ness and from condemnation of infected organs at slaughter and devaluation of trimmed food carcasses. In the United States, both incidence and losses probably will increase as the population of coyotes and other wild canines increases on western rangelands. Besides sheep, the malady affects mountain sheep, goats, cattle, deer, moose, and pigs.

OCCURRENCE. VC occurs in all breeds and sexes of sheep, but animals 2 to 18 months old have higher susceptibility than those of other age groups. Feedlot lambs commonly show mild to heavy infestations at necropsy following death from intercurrent diseases and at inspection following slaughter. Sheep acquire infection during summer and autumn grazing and the bladderworms persist for several months.

Geographically, the condition occurs in most countries where sheep and dogs associate closely.

ETIOLOGY AND PATHOGENESIS. A tapeworm causes VC. The adult worm, Taenia hydatigena, inhabits the small intestine of dogs, coyotes, and other canids, and the larvae, Cysticercus tenuicollis, reside as bladderworms in the abdomen and other anatomic areas of sheep. The adult worm, 0.5 to 3.0 m in length, bears gravid segments measuring 10 to 14 × 4 to 7 mm and a rostellum with 26 to 46 hooks. The globular bladderworm, measuring 8 to 12 mm in diameter, contains clear fluid and a single invaginated scolex with an attenuated neck. Most of them are located on the omentum, mesentery, and pelvic organs; some, however, are in the thorax.

The life cycle begins with expulsion of gravid segments. The oncospheres contaminate feed and water, and when eaten by a young sheep, the larvae penetrate villi of the small intestine, especially the ileum, move to the villar bases, enter venules, and are transported to the liver, where they migrate in parenchyma and thus create bore channels with necrosis and hemorrhage. Eventually they leave the liver and move through the peritoneal cavity to a point of attachment, where they mature and then slowly degenerate. Rostellar hooks develop in 30 to 50 days.

Following ingestion of the viable cysticerci by a dog or other definitive hosts, the scoleces evaginate, attach to the small intestine, and mature into a tapeworm through a prepatent period of 50 to 70 days. Development of the bladderworms in sheep progresses through stages: 1 to 3 weeks in the liver, 18 to 20 days in peritoneal fluid, and 1 to 9 months in their attached positions.

Damage to the host occurs primarily in the liver and peritoneal cavity. In the peritoneal cavity, the larvae, along with mechanically conveyed bacteria, incite peritonitis. The degree of damage varies directly with the number of migrating larvae. Several dozen may inflict serious and fatal hepatitis and peritonitis. Recovered sheep strongly resist new attacks with homologous parasites. *Clostridium novyi,* the cause of black disease, may proliferate in the necrotic liver tissue.

CLINICAL SIGNS AND POSTMORTEM LESIONS. Small numbers of cysticerci cause no clinical signs, but large numbers migrating through the liver and peritoneal cavity elicit depression, anorexia, fever, weakness, and loss of live weight. Severely affected animals may die. The infection rate may reach 25%, but mortality of affected sheep is low. The bladderworms, once formed, cause no damage and evoke no signs.

At necropsy of sheep in the invasive stages, the swollen liver contains bore channels, which are red from blood content during infection days 10 to 20 and yellow from leukocyte infiltration during infection days 25 to 35 (Figs. 6-16 and 6-17). Most channels measure 1 to 2 mm in diameter. Peritonitis may be present. In later stages, the globular bladderworms are found on the omentum, mysentery, pelvic organs, portal fissure, and other anatomic areas (Fig. 6-18). After several months in position, the scoleces may show mineralization, and the vesicles may show collapse and fibrosis.

DIAGNOSIS. Because the signs are vague and not disease-specific, veterinarians seldom diagnose VC from clinical signs alone. Most diagnoses, therefore, are established at necropsy of fatal or sacrificed cases by finding bore channels in the liver, and in some cases,

Fig. 6-16. Blood-filled channel caused by migrating larvae of *T. hydatigena* in lamb liver. (By permission from Jensen, R., and Pierson, R.E.: Cysticercosis from *Taenia hydatigena* in feedlot lambs. JAVMA, *166*:1183, 1975.)

peritonitis. Newly recovered sheep contain the conspicuous bladderworms.

The differential diagnosis requires consideration of hepatitis from tunneling by young flukes of *Fasciola hepatica* and black disease.

PREVENTION. Producers and veterinarians prevent VC by interrupting the life cycle of the tapeworm; this break should be achieved by the following measures:

1. Inactivate bladderworms by heating or burying sheep offal to prevent infecting dogs and coyotes.

2. Treat work dogs at 3-month intervals with either:

Fig. 6-17. Leukocyte-filled channel caused by migrating larvae of *T. hydatigena* in lamb liver. During an earlier stage it resembled Fig. 6-16.

Fig. 6-18. Two larvae of *T. hydatigena* in omentum. × 1.5.

(a) oral yomesan at a rate of 50 mg/kg of body weight, or

(b) bunamidine hydrochloride at a rate of 25 to 30 mg/kg of body weight to remove adult tapeworms.

3. Constrain dogs, especially unowned animals, from frequenting and thus contaminating sheep pastures and other feeds with tapeworm eggs.

Featherston, D.W.: *Taenia hydatigena.* I. Growth and development of adult stage in the dog. Exp. Parasitol., 25:329-338, 1969.

Gemmell, M.A.: Induced resistance to cysticerci. Aust. Vet. J., 46:366-369, 1970.

Gemmell, M.A.: Acquired resistance to cysticerci. Aust. Vet. J., 45:521-524, 1969.

Gemmell, M.A.: Immunological response of sheep to hexacanth embryos of *Taenia hydatigena.* Immunology, 7:489-499, 1964.

Jensen, R. and Pierson, R.E.: Cysticercosis from *Taenia hydatigena* in feedlot lambs. JAVMA, *166*:1183-1186, 1975.

Orekhov, M.D.: Pathogenesis of *Cysticercus Tenuicollis* infection in sheep. Veterinariia (Moscow), No. 8, 67-69, 1970.

Sharma Deorani, V.P.: Histopathology of hepatitis—cysticercosa lesions in sheep liver. Indian Vet. J., *44*:939-942, 1967.

Sweatman, G.K. and Plummer, P.J.G.: Biology and pathology of *Taenia hydatigena.* Can. J. Zool., 35:93-109, 1957.

Rectal Prolapse

Rectal prolapse, a mechanical eversion of the rectum through the anus, is characterized by tenesmus, anorexia, and loss of weight. In some cases, visceral complications develop. Because the condition is sporadic and long-accepted, it causes little concern to the sheep industry. Despite this apathy, the disease results in some financial waste to feedlot enterprises from weight losses and eventual deaths of affected lambs. Salvage slaughter in early stages minimizes the losses.

To facilitate consideration of this complex subject, we recognize two forms: (1) eversion of the rectum and (2) evisceration of the intestines. Evisceration, however, usually is a complication of eversion.

OCCURRENCE. Although prolapse occurs in all breeds and sexes beyond weaning age, the condition is most prevalent among feedlot lambs 6 to 12 months of age. Most cases develop after the animals have adapted to the fattening ration and occur during all seasons, with highest incidence in summer, thus coinciding with the peak incidence of pneumonia and coughing. Evisceration develops during summer in lambs born during the previous winter.

ETIOLOGY AND PATHOGENESIS. Even though the full cause of prolapse is not known, several contributing factors are recognized. These include: (1) straining from coughing, proctitis, and cystitis, (2) intra-abdominal crowding from constant overfilling of the rumen, heavy deposits of fat, pregnancies, and prolonged recumbency, and (3) miscellaneous causes such as loose mesenteric attachment of the rectum, distensions of the rectum, weak anal sphincter, and possible over-stimulation from sequential anabolic implants.

Combinations of these causative factors create a pressure gradient, the axis of which extends from the abdomen into the pelvis and through the anus. An eversion may result from the exertion of equilateral pressures that force a cranial part of the rectum into a contiguous caudal part as an intussusception. Continued pressures and forceful peristalsis add successive increments to the intussusception until the point of fold and all parts of the rectum caudal to the fold are exteriorized through the anus. There, environmental adversities such as dessication, radiation, cooling, and abrasion irritate the delicate mucosa and reflexly stimulate persistent straining. Constrictive pressure at the anus closes veins but not arteries and causes congestion, edema, and eventually necrosis in the everted mass. Affected animals eventually die from exhaustion.

Evisceration commonly develops as a complication after rectal eversion has developed. High pressure jams the mobile intestinal mass—small intestine, large intestine, and cecum—into the rectogenital pouch. Pressure from these organs against the rectal floor indents that part of the wall in the caudal direction. The pressure locally closes some veins and ruptures others. These circulatory changes weaken the tissues, and continued pressure splits the wall. Once a tear is made, the pressurized mobile viscera pass through the rent into the rectal lumen and slide caudally through the anus to the exterior. In this process, the tear extends either longitudinally or vertically.

The anatomic relation of the tear to the previous eversion determines the point at which viscera emerge to the exterior: (1) If the tear is caudal to the mural fold, the viscera emerge between the anal mucosa and the eversion. (2) If the tear is cranial to the fold, they emerge through the lumen of the eversion. (3) If the viscera wedge in between layers of the rectum at the point of fold, they enter the pouch of peritoneum in the eversion, and then tear either through the external layer and emerge to the exterior, or through the inner layer and

emerge through the lumen of the eversion (Fig. 6-19). Eviscerated animals die promptly from shock. In some animals, however, evisceration develops independently of eversion by rupture of the rectal wall and passage of the mobile viscera into the rectal lumen.

CLINICAL SIGNS AND POSTMORTEM LESIONS. Animals with simple eversion refuse feed, separate from the flock, and frequently or continuously strain. After a few days, they become gaunt and rapidly lose weight. The length of extruded intestine varies up to 50 cm. The bulk of the tissue is congested, edematous, and necrotic; in summer it dehydrates and in winter it freezes. The morbidity is about 0.1%, but during summer it may reach 1.5% in some pens. All affected lambs die from inanition and

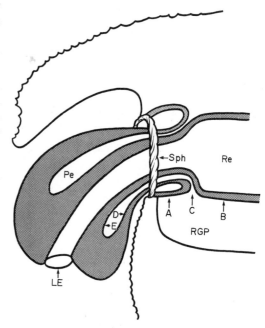

Fig. 6-19. Scheme of a rectal prolapse and the locations of rectal tears that result in evisceration. *Sph* = anal sphincter; *Re* = rectal lumen; *Pe* = peritoneum; *RGP* = rectogenital pouch of the peritoneal cavity; *LE* = lumen of the eversion. With a tear at (*A*), the viscera emerge between the eversion and the anal mucosa. With a tear at (*B*), the viscera emerge through the lumen of the eversion; with intrusion of viscera at (*C*) and a tear at (*D*), the viscera emerge through the external layer of the eversion. With intrusion of viscera at (*C*) and a tear at (*E*), the viscera emerge through the lumen of the eversion.

exhaustion after a usual course of 10 to 12 days.

Lambs with evisceration present extrusion of small intestine (except the duodenum), ansa spiralis, cecum, and colon, or variable combinations thereof. Usually such cases have a short course and are found dead.

At necropsy, cases of simple eversion are dehydrated and emaciated, and the prolapsed rectum protrudes from the anus. The tissue may be dehydrated, edematous, necrotic, or frozen. The fold in the rectal wall usually is within 10 cm anterior to the sphincter. Carcasses with evisceration present complex anatomic changes. Rectal eversion is usually present, and the expelled viscera emerge at one of three points: (1) between the anal mucosa and the eversion, (2) through the lumen of the eversion, or (3) through the outer layer of the eversion.

The rectal tear through which the viscera pass may be located caudal to the fold, cranial to the fold, or in the outer or inner layer of the everted rectum. Tears may be longitudinal up to 15 cm (Fig. 6-20) or circumferential (either partial or complete). The point of tear shows the predisposing hemorrhage and degeneration. If the rectum is severed transversely, the caudal stump is everted along with the viscera. In some ewe lambs, the tear is at the mucosa-skin junction of the vulva rather than in the rectum.

DIAGNOSIS.   Producers as well as veterinarians readily identify prolapse from the gross lesions. Interpretation of the pathogenesis, however, requires careful dissection.

PREVENTION AND TREATMENT.   Since coughing may be a factor in the cause of prolapse, preventing pneumonia through proper management and medications should reduce the incidence of prolapse. Surgical correction in feedlot lambs, as practiced in cattle, is economically prohibitive. Producers should slaughter affected lambs on the day prolapse develops for recovery of investment.

If rectal prolapse repair is elected, a nonsurgical approach can be applied using a counterirritant injected into the fascia surrounding the rectum. Scar tissue in the area where the

Fig. 6-20. Longitudinal tear (*a*) in rectal wall through which small intestines entered rectal lumen (*b*) and emerged through the anus. Caudal direction is to the right.

counterirritant is placed forms adhesions and permanently fixes the rectum within the pelvic cavity. To perform the operation tranquilization of the animal is helpful to prevent straining. The prolapsed portion of the rectum is cleaned and if the mucosal surface is inflamed or irritated, a mild antibiotic ointment, such as one containing furican, should be applied. Replace the prolapsed portion with two fingers making certain the intussusception is completely reduced. With the two fingers in the rectum to guide the needle, a counterirritant (7% iodine in alcohol solution or a commercially available product Hypodermin by Haver-Lockhart) is injected perirectally. Depending on the size of lamb a 2- to 3-inch 18 gauge needle is appropriate. Two ml of the counterirritant should be placed along the rectum of all four quadrants. A pursestring suture is placed about ½ inch from the mucocutaneous junction and tightened snugly to accommodate two fingers. This will prevent reprolapse until adhesions have formed. The suture can be removed in about 5 days. The animal should be given about 100 to 120 ml of mineral oil orally and feed withheld for 24 to 48 hours followed by a reduced portion of a soft bland diet for the next 3 to 4 days.

Gates, N.: Rectal Prolapse. *A Practical Guide to Sheep Disease Management.* Moscow, ID, News-Review Publishing, 1985, p. 130.

7

DISEASES OF THE RESPIRATORY SYSTEM

Pneumonia

(Enzootic pneumonia;
pasteurellosis; shipping fever;
hemorrhagic septicemia)

Ovine pneumonia, an acute infectious disease of sheep affecting all ages with especially high prevalence in nursing and feedlot lambs, is characterized clinically by signs of respiratory distress, mucopurulent, often blood tinged, oculonasal discharge, depression, anorexia and pyrexia, and pathologically by pneumonitis and pleuritis. Pneumonia is caused by a complex interaction of environmental factors producing stress, a variety of microorganisms working synergistically to damage the cells lining the respiratory tract allowing colonization and invasion of other organisms and a compensated host response. Irrespective of the management system, whether intensive, extensive, nomadic herds or sophisticated confinement operations pneumonia probably ranks the number one disease affecting the world's sheep population. The obvious economic impact is from deaths, but a substantial economic drain results from reduced gains, feed efficiency, general unthriftiness with reduced resistance to subsequent infections, loss of expensive treatments, and extra labor. Tremendous investment of time, labor, and talent has been expended on research into understanding of the pathogenesis and host response. Although advancements have been

made in these areas, pneumonia remains an uncontrolled drain on the worldwide sheep industry.

OCCURRENCE. Pneumonia commonly occurs in all breeds and ages of sheep throughout the world. The prevalence varies from region to region and is influenced by environmental factors and management practices. Although any age group is susceptible, the highest prevalence is among nursing and weaned lambs confined for feeding. As the intensity of management practices increase, there becomes a proportionate increase in the risk of predisposing factors to pneumonia. Extensive management systems encounter a different set of risk factors, primarily those associated with environmental stresses. Confinement or semiconfinement operations cover a spectrum from the highly sophisticated facilities in the United States and European countries to the small holder with only a few head, confined to a small facility with other classes of livestock, in the developing countries with environmental conditions varying from the subtropic in Africa to the high Andes of South America. Irrespective of geography, intensive and confinement operations have some common risk factors: (1) Those of close contact allowing for easy transmission of infective agents, (2) A build-up of potential pathogens in the environment, (3) The production of noxious gases such as ammonia, H_2S and CO_2 which irritate or damage the respiratory mucosa or alter the phagocytic properties of macrophages, (4) The small dust

173

particles from the dry feedlot carry pathogens deep into the respiratory tract. Seasonal variations of pneumonia vary with the enterprise, climatic conditions, and management procedures. In shed or semi-confinement lambing operations, the peak incidence will probably occur near the end of the lambing period. In extensive operations, the peak incidence may be associated with shearing, lambing, and concomitant inclement weather. The peak incidence of pneumonia in feedlot lambs occurs 1 to 3 weeks after arrival in the feedlot after being predisposed by the stress of weaning, transportation, change in feed, and comingled with lambs of different origins. In Colorado's lamb feeding operations, during the hot dry summer months the period of highest incidence is associated with dry dusty corrals.

TRANSMISSION. The proclivity of sheep, especially lambs, to crowd together and managerially imposed crowding in transport vehicles and feedlots facilitate transmission by contact of the infectious causes of pneumonia. Some normal sheep carry chlamydiae in their intestines and excrete them in feces; some carry pasteurellas and mycoplasmas in their upper respiratory systems and excrete them in nasal secretions. During crowding, the organisms contaminate equipment, feed, water, and air and probably are transmitted from carrier sheep to susceptible sheep by inhalation into the respiratory system and by ingestion into the digestive system.

ETIOLOGY AND PATHOGENESIS. In acute outbreaks of pneumonia, *Pasteurella haemolytica* is the organism most frequently isolated from the affected lung tissue but is probably the primary organism only in rare instances. *P. haemolytica* is a common inhabitant of the nasopharyngeal mucosa and tonsils of normal healthy sheep. *P. haemolytica* has been classified according to its carbohydrate fermentation characteristics into biotypes A and T and on the basis of specific antisera into 15 serotypes plus an untypable group. The A biotype includes serotypes 1, 2, 5, 6, 7, 8, 9, 11, 12, 13 and 14. These commonly inhabit the mucosa of the nasopharynx and are associated with pneumonia or septicemia in the very young

lamb. Biotype T includes serotypes 3, 4, 10 and 15. These commonly inhabit the tonsil and are associated with septicemic pasteurellosis affecting the 3- to 12-month-old lamb on high concentrate rations in a feeding program. Although serotype A2 is frequently isolated from the nares and pneumonic lesions, other serotypes may be involved simultaneously or separately.

The respiratory system is extremely vulnerable to pathologic insult and infection. Inhalation, during the normal respiratory cycle (12 to 20 times per minute), exposes the delicate mucosal surfaces to irritating gases, and pathogenic microorganisms carried on minute dust particles or droplet nuclei. The respiratory system has, therefore, developed a series of effective defense mechanisms. The nasal passage is lined with pseudostratified epithelial cells containing goblet cells and cilia. The anatomic structure of the turbinates warms the incoming air and produces a turbulence which physically aids in setting of larger dust particles (more than 10 μm) onto the mucous produced by the goblet cells which is in turn cleared from the respiratory system by the mucociliary action. Chemical properties of cell secretion also inhibit establishment of microorganisms. The trachea, bronchi, and bronchioles are lined with columnar ciliated cells which aid in clearing of particles and microorganisms reaching that area. Small particulate matter (1 to 2 μm) containing microorganisms may reach the lung alveoli and be inactivated by the bronchoalveolar macrophages or other agents of the immune system. Any of these areas are potential sights for the establishment of infection depending on the host-agent interactions. It is virtually impossible to infect the normal animal with massive numbers of *P. haemolytic* due to the clearing action of the normal respiratory system. Therefore, the disease process depends on a combination of events. Most respiratory viruses damage the lining epithelium by causing inflammation, edema, and necrosis thus destroying ciliary action and mucous protection allowing bacteria and mycoplasma to colonize on these damaged areas. Once established they multiply, produce toxins, and invade causing further damage. Besides damage to the epithelial cells, viral infections suppress the function of bronchoalveolar macrophages. The more common viral agents associated with damage to the respiratory epithelium are: (1) Parainfluenza Type 3, (2) Respiratory Syncytial Virus, (3) Adenoviruses, and (4) Reoviruses. Infection by these agents produce damage ranging from a mild upper respiratory tract disease to a proliferative bronchiolitis and interstitial pneumonitis. Although parainfluenza type 3 virus is the most prevalent virus associated with the enzootic pneumonia syndrome, this may vary in different ecologic systems. The viral infections by themselves may be noticed as only a transient respiratory discomfort or may go totally undetected. Severe acute exudative pneumonia and pleuritis usually follows the viral insult in a few days. Stress factors play an undetermined but potentially major role in the host response. A multitude of stress factors, whether environmental or management induced, elevate the serum cortisol levels with a resultant immunosuppression, a decrease in lymphocyte blastogenesis and a decrease in circulating leukocyte counts. In the case of *P. haemolytica* proliferation, there is evidence of a cytotoxic virulence factor which has a debilitating effect on bronchoalveolar macrophages. The bronchoalveolar macrophage activity is the major means of particle clearance from the alveolar areas of the lung. Therefore, viral suppression and bacterial cytotoxic debility of the bronchoalveolar macrophage activity are factors related to establishment of disease. The pathogenesis, a complex etiology is further confounded by the presence of other bacteria, *Mycoplasma* sp and *Chlamydia* sp. Their role as primary, secondary, or synergistic organisms is unclear. The appearance of these organisms in the pneumonic lesion is probably associated with the prevalence and high exposure rate of that particular organism in the environment. The agent-host interaction to all of these factors determines the acuteness and severity of the pathologic damage.

The disease probably begins with acute rhinitis and pharyngitis, and from this nidus, infection descends the respiratory tract. Early in the pathogenesis, the ventral parts of the pulmonary lobes develop congestion and edema. Viruses penetrate and multiply in the cytoplasm of septal and epithelial cells and thus initiate acute pneumonitis.

As a result of these changes, pasteurellas and mycoplasmas proliferate, and the three pathogens provoke the formation of serofibrinous exudate, which fills and incapacitates some alveoli. Leukocytes infiltrate the fibrin and, on their death, release fibrinolytic enzymes, which eventually bring about resolution. Infection spreads dorsally and by day 7 may affect 30% or more of the lung parenchyma. Contiguous spread of infection carries infection into the pleural and pericardial cavities, and hematogenous spread extends infection, especially of mycoplasmas, into joints.

Resolution and healing may occur by days 13 to 20. Complications of healing include the formation of fibrous adhesions between lobes, between lobes and ribs, and between visceral and parietal layers of the pericardial sac. Deaths during acute stages result from hypoxia, intoxication, and shock.

Infection in the nose and pharynx may also or exclusively enter one or both auditive tubes and progress into the tympanic cavities. In these locations, the space may fill with swollen lining membranes and exudate (Fig. 7-1). Some infections penetrate the fenestrae. From 25 to 35% of feedlot lambs with fatal pneumonia have otitis media as a complication.

CLINICAL SIGNS AND POSTMORTEM LESIONS. Pneumonia usually begins within 1 to 3 weeks after arrival of lambs at the feedlot or agricultural pasture. The first sign may be sudden deaths without noticeable prodromal symptoms. During the first 5 to 6 days of an outbreak, the daily number of new cases rapidly increases. Affected lambs show fever of 41 to 42°C. With drooping ears and lowered head, the sick lambs refuse to eat, become gaunt, and lose live weight.

Mucopurulent exudate is discharged from the nostrils, and lacrimal secretions escape from the eyes. Respirations are accelerated, difficult, and often accompanied by coughing.

Fig. 7-1. Otitis media showing ossicles in the epitympanic recess of the tympanic cavity (a), intact tympanic membrane with attached handle of the malleus (b), exudate in the ventral recess of the tympanic cavity (c), paramastoid process (d), and cranial cavity (e).

Weakened lambs isolate from the flock and recline. Because of arthritis, some lambs are lame. Auscultation of the thorax reveals consolidation of the anteroventral parts of both lungs, bronchitis, and pleuritis.

The morbidity ranges up to 50%, and the mortality approximates 10%. The course of early fatal cases is 2 to 3 days, but nonfatal cases recover after 14 to 20 days, and efficient fattening is resumed. The flock infection may extend over an entire month.

At necropsy, significant gross lesions are limited to the respiratory system and joints (Fig. 7-2). Ventral parts of the lobes, especially apical and cardiac, are consolidated to variable degrees. The gross appearance varies with the stage of pneumonia development: (1) during the initial stage, the affected lung is congested, cyanotic, and heavy with serum and small amounts of fibrin in the pleural cavities; (2) during red and gray consolidation, the affected lung is red or purple-gray, firm, and rigid, with abundant serum and fibrin in the pleural and pericardial cavities; and (3) during resolution,

lung tissue is pink, flexible, and moderately aerated and has lesser amounts of serum and fibrin in the cavities. All stages may exist simultaneously in different parts of the lungs.

At the junction of normal and pneumonic tissue, both atelectasis and emphysema may be evident. Bronchial and mediastinal lymph nodes are swollen and hyperemic, and petechial and ecchymotic hemorrhages are widely distributed over serosal surfaces, especially of the lungs and heart. In sheep with complications, extensive adhesions unite lobe to lobe, lobes to ribs, and pericardium to epicardium. The bronchi, trachea, larynx, pharynx, nasal cavity, and paranasal sinuses usually reveal acute catarrhal inflammation. Infected joints, especially those of limbs, contain increased synovial fluid and flakes of fibrin. Animals with severe fibrinous pleuritis usually show some icterus.

Histopathologic changes also vary with stage of disease development: (1) during the

Fig. 7-2. Chlamydial pneumonia and atelectasis in anteroventral part of left lung of a feedlot lamb.

initial stage, congestion, edema and proliferation of septal and epithelial cells predominate; (2) during red consolidation, fibrinous exudate fills some alveoli, and during gray consolidation, leukocytes obscure the fibrin, thrombi form in lymphatics, cuboidal epithelial cells line some alveoli, and lymphocytes accumulate around bronchioles and blood vessels; and (3) during resolution partially or fully lysed fibrin is replaced with macrophages. During early stages, chlamydiae and pasteurellas are discernible in Giemsa-stained smears and sections.

DIAGNOSIS. Veterinarians diagnose pneumonia on evidence of characteristic signs and lesions with laboratory assistance. The development of febrile disease, with nasal discharge, difficult breathing, and depression, within 1 to 3 weeks after lambs enter the feedlots or agricultural pasture strongly suggests pneumonia.

The necropsy finding of consolidation in the ventral planes of lungs accompanied by pleuritis and pericarditis provides sufficient additional evidence for a clinical diagnosis. Laboratory confirmation comes from isolating and identifying pasteurellas and chlamydiae from infected lungs.

The differential diagnosis requires consideration of septicemic pasteurellosis, polyarthritis of lambs, enterotoxemia, and in some areas, contagious agalactia.

PREVENTION AND TREATMENT. Due to the diversity of stress factors, primary and secondary etiologic agents and the complexity of the pathogenic process, a cookbook preventive program is impossible. Each operation, even in the same locality, is a completely independent ecologic system and therefore must be approached accordingly. To develop a preventive program, all factors predisposing the lambs to stress, etiologic agents, their transmission and the effectiveness of immunogens and medications must be fully understood. Preventive measures must then be analyzed on a cost-benefit basis applying those measures which will be most cost effective. Management practices to minimize the stress of transportation and adaptation of the lamb to its new

environment are usually not expensive and the returns are rewarding. Adherence to sanitary feed and watering facilities is always a good investment. Comingling of lambs from various sources is a potential risk factor which should be avoided. Immunization for the primary or secondary etiologic agent should be considered along with the cost benefits. The timing and number of immunizations required for protection is important in the decision analysis.

Treatment on an individual basis is difficult as the additional stress of identifying, isolating, and restraining the animal may be as detrimental as the beneficial effect of the treatment. The long-acting tetracycline and sulfas are preferable as a therapeutic drug level can be maintained for about 3 days eliminating the stress of daily treatment. In outbreaks of pneumonia total flock therapy via the water or feed with sulfonamides (1 mg/kg) or oxytetracycline (12 mg/kg) should be considered. Continual monitoring of the pneumonia problem with appropriate alterations in management and application of cost effective preventive medicine will effectively reduce death and economic losses.

Biberstein, E.L. and Kennedy, P.C.: Septicemic pasteurellosis in lambs. AJVR, *20*:94-101, 1959.
Boidin, A.G., Cordy, D.R., and Adler, H.E.: A pleuropneumonia-like organism and a virus in ovine pneumonia of California. Cornell Vet., *48*:410-430, 1958.
Bosworth, T.J. and Lovell, R.: The occurrence of hemolytic coccobacilli in the nose of normal sheep and cattle. J. Comp. Pathol. Ther., *54*:168-171, 1944.
Cameron, C. and Bester, F.: Formulation of an effective *Pasteurella multocida* vaccine for sheep. Onderst. J. Vet. Res., *51*:189-191, 194.
Collins, M. and Suarez-Guemes, F.: Effect of hydrocortisone on circulating lymphocyte numbers and their mitogen-induced blastogenesis in lambs. Am. J. Vet. Res., *46*:836-840, 1985.
Davies, D., Herceg, M., and Thurley, D.: Experimental infection of lambs with an adenovirus followed by *Pasteurella haemolytica*. Vet. Microbiol., 7:369-381, 1982.
Ellis, J.: *Pasteurella haemolytica* infection in sheep. Compendium on Continuing Ed., *6*:5360-5366, 1984.
Fodor, L., Varga, J., Hajtos, I., and Szemeredi, G.: Serotypes of *Pasteurella haemolytica* isolated from sheep, goats and calves. Zbl. Vet. Med. B., *31*:466-469, 1984.
Gilmour, N., Sharp, J., and Gilmour, J.: Effect of oxytetracycline therapy on experimentally induced pneumonic pasteurellosis in lambs. Vet. Rec., *111*:97-99, 1982.

Gilmour, N., et al.: Experimental immunization of lambs against pneumonic pasteurellosis. Res. Vet. Sci., *35*:80-86, 1983.

Jensen, R. and Mackey, D.R.: *Diseases of Feedlot Cattle.* 2nd Edition. Philadelphia, Lea & Febiger, 1971, pp. 38-47.

Jensen, R., et al.: Middle ear infection in feedlot lambs. JAVMA, *181*:805-807, 1982.

Jones, G.E., Buxton, D., and Harker, D.B.: Respiratory infections in housed sheep, with particular reference to mycoplasmas. Vet. Micro., *4*:47-59, 1979.

Lehmkuhl, H. and Cutlip, R.: Experimental infection of lambs with ovine adenovirus isolate RTS: Clinical, microbiological, and serologic responses. Am. J. Vet. Res., *45*:260-262, 1984.

Lehmkuhl, H. and Cutlip, R.: Characterization of two serotypes of adenovirus isolated from sheep in central United States. Am. J. Vet. Res., *45*:562-566, 1984.

McGowan, B., Moulton, J.E., and Shultz, G.: Pneumonia in California lambs. JAVMA, *131*:318-323, 1957.

McKercher, D.G.: A virus possibly related to psittacosis-lymphogranuloma-pneumonitis group causing pneumonia in sheep. Science, *115*:543, 1952.

Marsh, H.: The role of *Pasteurella* in sheep diseases. JAVMA, *123*:205-208, 1953.

Montgomery, R.F., Bostworth, T.J., and Glover, R.E.: Enzootic pneumonia in sheep. J. Comp. Pathol., *51*:87, 1938.

Mukkur, T., Blanck, J., and Barnes, A.: Prevention of experimental pneumonia in rams by immunization. Agri-Prac., *4*:16-20, 1983.

Newsom, I.E. and Cross, F.: An outbreak of hemorrhagic septicemia in sheep. JAVMA, *62*:759-762, 1923.

Newsom, I.E. and Cross, F.: Some bipolar organisms found in pneumonia in sheep. JAVMA, *80*:711-719, 1932.

Palfi, V., Vetesi, F., Belak, S., and Papp, L. Adenovirus infection in lambs. III. Studies on chronic infection. Zbl. Vet. Med. B., *29*(3):231-241, 1982.

Pavlov, N.: Histopathology of neorickettsial pneumonias in sheep. Zentralbl. Veterinaermed., *14B*:343-355, 1967.

Payla, V., Belak, S., and Palfi, V.: Adenovirus infection in lambs. II. Experimental infection of lambs. Zbl. Vet. Med. B., *24*:529-541, 1977.

Pierson, R.E.: Unpublished records. Veterinary Hospital, Colorado State University, 1971.

Robinson, R.: Respiratory disease of sheep and goats. Vet. Clin. N. Am., LA Pract., *5*:539-555, 1983.

Salisbury, R.M.: Enzootic pneumonia of sheep in New Zealand. N.Z. Vet. J., *6*:124-127, 1957.

Sharp, J.M., Gilmour, N.S.L., Thompson, B.A., and Rushton, B.: Experimental infection of specific pathogen free lambs with parainfluenza types and *Pasteurella haemolytica*. J. Comp. Pathol., *88*:237-243, 1978.

Stevenson, R.G. and Robinson, G.: The pathology of pneumonia in young lambs inoculated with Bedsonia. Res. Vet. Sci., *11*:469-474, 1970.

Sutherland, A., Gray, E., and Wells, P.: Cytotoxic effect of *Pasteurella haemolytica* on ovine bronchoalveolar macrophages *in vitro*. Vet. Microb., *8*:3-15, 1983.

Wells, P., et al.: Development of a combined clostridial and *Pasteurella haemolytica* vaccine for sheep. Vet. Rec., *114*:266-269, 1984.

Viral, Mycoplasma and Chlamydia Respiratory Infections

The adenoviruses, respiratory syncytial virus, parainfluenza type 3, mycoplasmas, and chlamydia are often referred to as the primary infective agent in enzootic pneumonia and are of economic significance as they are associated with subclinical and chronic pneumonia causing loss due to inefficiency of production and ill thrift of the affected animal.

Adenovirus

(OAV)

On the basis of morphology, physiochemical characteristics and the possession of the adenovirus group antigen 6 ovine adenovirus have been isolated from sheep in the United Kingdom, Sweden, New Zealand, Australia, the United States, Hungary and Turkey and probably have a far greater distribution. OAV infections are characterized by a serous nasal discharge, coughing and forced respiration frequently accompanied by diarrhea. The acute process is often followed by a chronic phase of the disease involving mainly the lungs and kidneys. Lambs from 2 to 4 months of age and those weaned lambs confined during the feeding period are at highest risk, but outbreaks can occur under extensive management systems. The initial clinical signs are depression and anorexia followed by conjunctivitis, lacrimation, and swelling of the retropharyngeal and submandibular lymph nodes. Serous nasal discharge, sneezing, spontaneous recurring cough, and forced respiration are common symptoms. The disease is frequently accompanied by diarrhea of 1- to 2-weeks' duration. A mucopurulent nasal discharge, spontaneous cough, persistent nephritis, and weak body condition characterize the chronic phase of the disease.

Gross pathologic lesions in the acute phase are rhinitis, enlarged retropharyngeal and mediastinal lymph nodes, acute catarrhal pneumonia and in some cases enteritis. In chronic cases the pneumonic lesions become more pronounced and interstitial nephritis develops. The predominant feature is a chronic intralobular interstitial pneumonia with peri-bronchitis and proliferation of the peribronchial lymphoid follicles. An acute exudative pneumonia develops in the presence of *P. haemolytica* and chronic changes may be observed late in the course of some outbreaks in association with *M. ovipneumoniae*. A carrier state of adenovirus infection does exist. Specific control measures have not been developed. Diagnosis has been by virus isolation and identification. Vaccines are available in some countries for protection against adenovirus infections. Treatment is directed towards preventing secondary bacterial pneumonia. The long acting tetracyclines and sulfas are the drugs of choice.

Adair, B., McFerran, J., and McKillop, E.: A sixth species of ovine adenovirus isolated from lambs in New Zealand. Arch. Virol., 74:269-275, 1982.

Belak, S., Palfi, V., and Palya, P.: Adenovirus infection in lambs. I. Epizootiology of the disease. Zbl. Vet. Med. B., 23:320-330, 1976.

Belak, S., Thunegard, E., and Rusvae, M.: Occurrence of adenoviral pneumoenteritis among sheep kept under extensive conditions in Sweden. Nord. Vet. Med., 37:219-250, 1985.

Al-Darraji, A., Cutlip, R., Lehmkuhl, H., and Graham, D.: Experimental infection of lambs with bovine respiratory syncytial virus and *Pasteurella haemolytica*: Pathologic studies. Am. J. Vet. Res., 42:224-229, 1982.

Al-Darraji, A., Cutlip, R., and Lehmkuhl, H.: Experimental infection of lambs with bovine respiratory syncytial virus and *Pasteurella haemolytica*: Immunofluorescent and electron microscopy studies. Am. J. Vet. Res., 42:230-235, 1982.

Elazhary, M., Silim, A., and Dea, S.: Prevalence of antibodies to bovine respiratory syncytial virus, bovine viral diarrhea virus, bovine herpesvirus-1, and bovine parainfluenza-3 virus in sheep and goats in Quebec. Am. J. Vet. Res., 45:1660-1662, 1984.

Evermann, J., et al.: Properties of a respiratory syncytial virus isolated from a sheep with rhinitis. Am. J. Vet. Res., 46:947-951, 1985.

LeaMaster, B., et al.: Serologic and virologic studies on naturally occurring respiratory syncytial virus and *haemophilus somnus* infections in sheep. Amer. Assn. Veterinary Laboratory Diagnosticians 26th Annual Proceedings, 256-276, 1983.

Trigo, F., Breeze, R., Evermann, J., and Gallina, A.: Pathogenesis of experimental bovine respiratory syncytial virus infection in sheep. Am. J. Vet. Res., 45:1663-1670, 1984.

Trigo, F., et al.: Interaction of bovine respiratory syncytial virus and *Pasteurella haemolytica* in the ovine lung. Am. J. Vet. Res., 4:1671-1678, 1984.

Parainfluenza Virus Type 3

(*PI3*)

Parainfluenza type 3 virus belongs to the genus *Paramyxovirus* of the family Paramyxoviridae and is the most common viral agent associated with enzootic pneumonia. The viral infection by itself may cause only a slight febrile response, listlessness, anorexia, and a mild respiratory distress with a cough and rapid breathing followed by forced expiration. The pathologic changes are generally confined to the anterior lobes of the lung where focal areas of atelectasis may be found. There may be more extensive areas of consolidation near the tips of the lungs. Histologically, there is a mild bronchiolar epithelial destruction and regenerative hyperplasia of the remaining epithelium. The most significant histologic findings is the hyperplastic and desquamative changes in the epithelium with the denuded cells occluding the small bronchioles and alveolar ducts. The bronchioles and alveolar ducts may be devoid of epithelium and in the parenchyma there is engorgement of capillaries with widespread interstitial and alveolar edema with formation of hyaline membranes in the alveoli. This damage to the epithelial lining makes an ideal environment for the establishment of secondary bacterial invaders. Enzootic pneumonia is readily produced in lambs by intranasal and intratracheal inoculation with PI3 virus followed in 4 to 7 days by a challenge with *P. haemolytica*. Establishment of the natural disease probably follows a similar pattern of events; it is therefore important to protect the lambs against the primary insulting virus. Intramuscular and intranasal PI3 vaccines give protection against PI3 infections and reduce the incidence of enzootic pneumonia. Other viral and mycotic agents may act as the primary agent so complete protection with PI3 vaccines cannot be expected.

Cutlip, R. and Lehmkuhl, H.: Experimentally induced parainfluenza type 3 virus infection in young lambs: Pathologic response. Am. J. Vet. Res., 43:2101-2107, 1982.

Davies, D., Davis, G., McSporran, K., and Price, M.: Vaccination against ovine pneumonia: A progress report. N.Z. Vet. J., 31:87-90, 1983.

Davies, D., Herceg, M., Jones, B., and Thurley, D.: The pathogenesis of sequential infection with parainfluenza virus type 3 and *Pasteurella haemolytica* in sheep. Vet. Microbiol., 6:173-182, 1981.

Hore, D. and Stevenson, R.: Respiratory infection of lambs with an ovine strain of parainfluenza type 3. Res. Vet. Sci., 10:342-350, 1969.

Hore, D., et al.: Isolation of parainfluenza virus from the lungs and nasal passages of sheep showing respiratory disease. J. Comp. Path., 78:259-265, 1968.

Lehmkuhl, H. and Cutlip, R.: Experimental parainfluenza type 3 infection in young lambs: Clinical, microbiological and serological response. Vet. Microbiol., 8:437-442 1983.

Lehmkuhl, H. and Cutlip, R.: Characterization of parainfluenza type 3 virus isolated from the lung of a lamb with pneumonia. Am. J. Vet. Res., 43:626-628, 1982.

Morein, B., Sharp, M., Sundquist, B., and Simons, K.: Protein subunit vaccines of parainfluenza type 3 virus: Immunogenic effect in lambs and mice. J. Gen. Virol., 64:1557-1569, 1983.

Sharp, J., Gilmour, N., Thompson, D., and Rushton, B.: Experimental infection of specific pathogen-free lambs with parainfluenza virus type 3 and *Pasteurella haemolytica*. J. Comp. Path., 88:237-243, 1978.

Wells, P., et al.: The assessment in sheep of an inactivated vaccine of parainfluenza 3 virus incorporating double stranded RNA (BRL 5907*) as adjuvant. J. Hyg. Comb., 77:255-261, 1976.

Wells, P., et al.: The effect of vaccination with a parainfluenza type 3 virus on pneumonia resulting from infection with parainfluenza type 3 virus and *Pasteurella haemolytica*. J. Comp. Path., 88:253-259, 1978.

Respiratory Syncytial Virus

(*RSV*)

The respiratory syncytial virus (RSV) has been isolated from natural cases of sheep with rhinitis, but its pathogenesis and role as a primary agent of disease is not fully understood. Respiratory syncytial virus is an important pathogen in calves in many countries. It causes respiratory disease in man and other animals. Serologic surveys conducted in Iowa, Idaho, Washington and Canada indicate that sheep have encountered the RSV with a prevalence ranging from 31% in Canada to 57% in Idaho. The sheep isolates are related to the bovine RSV and are considered as a sheep isolate of RSV. The viral infection alone produces mild clinical signs characterized by a conjunctivitis and multifocal intra-alveolar inflammatory response. Experimental infections produce evidence that the virus concentrates mainly in individual cells in alveolar walls, some alveolar macrophages, and bronchiolar epithelial cells with a resultant mild bronchiolitis and alveolitis. RSV is considered pathogenic for lambs with the potential of facilitating *P. haemolytica* pneumonia and depress the activity of bronchoalveolar macrophages. The RSV has been associated with *Haemophilus somnus* pneumonia in some field studies. Although serologic evidence indicates a high prevalence of both organisms, in some sheep populations the significance requires further investigation.

Al-Darraji, A., Cutlip, R., Lehmkuhl, H., and Graham, D.: Experimental infection of lambs with bovine respiratory syncytial virus and *Pasteurella haemolytica*: Pathologic studies. Am. J. Vet. Res., 42:224-229, 1982.

Al-Darraji, A., Cutlip, R., and Lehmkuhl, H.: Experimental infection of lambs with bovine respiratory syncytial virus and *Pasteurella haemolytica*: Immunofluorescent and electron microscopy studies. Am. J. Vet. Res., 42:230-235, 1982.

Elazhary, M., Silim, A., and Dea, S.: Prevalence of antibodies to bovine respiratory syncytial virus, bovine viral diarrhea virus, bovine herpesvirus-1, and bovine parainfluenza-3 virus in sheep and goats in Quebec. Am. J. Vet. Res., 45:1660-1662, 1984.

Evermann, J., et al.: Properties of a respiratory syncytial virus isolated from a sheep with rhinitis. Am. J. Vet. Res., 46:947-951, 1985.

LeaMaster, B., et al.: Serologic and virologic studies on naturally occurring respiratory syncytial virus and *haemophilus somnus* infections in sheep. Amer. Assn. Veterinary Laboratory Diagnosticians 26th Annual Proceedings, 256-276, 1983.

Trigo, F., Breeze, R., Evermann, J., and Gallina, A.: Pathogenesis of experimental bovine respiratory syncytial virus infection in sheep. Am. J. Vet Res., 45:1663-1670, 1984.

Trigo, F., et al.: Interaction of bovine respiratory syncytial virus and *Pasteurella haemolytica* in the ovine lung. Am. J. Vet. Res., 4:1671-1678, 1984.

Reoviruses

Reoviruses have been isolated from man and domestic animals (pigs, cattle and sheep) with a wide distribution as indicated by serologic response. On the basis of morphologic, chemical and serologic characteristics they have been classified into types 1, 2 and 3. All three types have been isolated from sheep, but only type 1 has been shown to produce a disease syndrome. The condition is characterized by an early acute phase with a rhinitis, conjunctivitis, diarrhea, and slight increase in body temperature. Pathologic lesions of the early phase include acute catarrhal pneumonia and catarrh of upper respiratory and intestinal tracts. The chronic phase is characterized by a purulent nasal discharge, cough and dyspnea with pleuritis, pericarditis, and catarrhal-purulent pneumonia. Although serologic surveys indicate a wide distribution, the significance as a primary agent for either pneumonia or enteritis is unknown.

Belak, S. and Palfi, V.: Isolation of reovirus type 1 from lambs showing respiratory and intestinal symptoms. Arch. Ges. Virus for Sch., 44:177-183, 1974.
McFerran, J., Nelson, R., and Clarke, J.: Isolation and characterization of reovirus isolated from sheep. Arch. Ges. Virus for Sch., 40:72-81, 1973.
Snodgrass, D., Burrells, C., and Wells, P.: Isolation of reovirus type 2 from respiratory tract of sheep. Arch Virol., 52:143-149, 1976.

Mycoplasma Pneumonia

M. ovipneumonia has been isolated from the lungs of healthy and pneumonic sheep, often in combination with other microorganisms. However, the role of mycoplasma in the etiology of pneumonia has not been established.

Buddle, B., Herceg, M., and Davies, D.: Experimental infection of sheep with *Mycoplasma ovipneumoniae* and *Pasteurella haemolytica*. Vet. Microbiol., 9:543-548, 1984.
Jones, G., Gilmour, J., and Rae, A.: Investigations into the possible role of *Mycoplasma arginini* in ovine respiratory disease. Res. Vet. Sci., 38:368-372, 1985.
Stalheim, O.: Mycoplasmal respiratory diseases of ruminants: A review and update. JAVMA, 182:403-406, 1983.

Chlamydial Pneumonia

Chlamydia psittaci is considered by some investigators to be a primary agent of ovine pneumonia. In addition to pneumonia the chlamydia organism causes polyarthritis, conjunctivitis, and abortions. The isolates of these conditions will produce similar pneumonic lesions. Clinical pneumonia may not be manifested until late in the disease when proliferative changes resemble those of atypical pneumonia. Gross pathologic lesions range from small areas of consolidation scattered throughout the anterior lobes of the lung to atelectasis of the anteroventral parts, involving up to 80% of the lung.

Early histologic changes are characterized by foci of necrosis and a sero-cellular exudate in the alveoli and small bronchioles. As these changes subside, hyperplasia of bronchiolar epithelium, epithelialization and pseudoepithelialization of alveoli, infiltration of alveolar septa by mononuclear cells, and lymphoid hyperplasia around bronchioles and blood vessels become the prominent features. Although chlamydial vaccines are utilized to prevent abortions, the economic significance of chlamydial pneumonias has not warranted a commercial vaccine. There is no therapy specifically outlined for chlamydial pneumonia as the customary treatments of penicillin, tetracyclines, and sulfas are effective against chlamydia.

Davies, D.: An etiology of pneumonias of young sheep. Prog. Vet. Microbiol. Immun., 1:229-248, 1985.
Storz, J.: *Current Veterinary Therapy. 2. Food Animal Practice*. Edited by J. Howard. Philadelphia, W.B. Saunders Co., 1986, pp. 532-533.

8

DISEASES OF THE EYE

Follicular Conjunctivitis

(FC; pinkeye, ophthalmia; infectious keratitis; keratoconjunctivitis)

Follicular conjunctivitis, an acute contagious, and usually epizootic disease, is characterized by conjunctival hyperemia and corneal opacity and by lymphoid follicle formation on the nictitating membrane and eyelids. It is caused by a chlamydial organism related to the cause of polyarthritis. Because FC occurs in sheep of most countries where animal agriculture has developed, and because the incidence may reach 90% in infected flocks, the disease is of major importance to the sheep industry, especially feedlot enterprises. Economic losses result from reduced mobility of affected sheep, diminished capacity to seek and find feed, lowered live weight, and the cost of labor and drugs for treatment.

OCCURRENCE. FC occurs in all breeds, sexes, and ages of sheep, but feedlot and nursing lambs have a higher incidence than do other age groups. Feedlot lambs usually develop the disease during the late summer and early fall, but nursing lambs are affected during the spring. Although FC probably occurs in all countries where the sheep industry has developed, known endemic areas include Algeria, Tunisia, Kenya, Union of South Africa, Argentina, Chile, Peru, United Kingdom, Iceland, Norway, Italy, Pakistan, Iran, India, New Zealand, Australia, and North America. In the United States, the disease is prevalent in feedlots of western and midwestern states.

ETIOLOGY, PATHOGENESIS AND EPIZOOTIOLOGY. *Chlamydia psittaci*, a gram-negative, nonmotile, obligate parasite, inhabits cytoplasmic vacuoles of host cells, where latency is prolonged. The infectious particle, consisting of cell membrane and nucleoid, measures 0.3 nm in diameter and contains both DNA and RNA. Mature particles, or elementary bodies, color purple with Giemsa's stain and red with Macchiavello's stain. Chlamydiae, in general, are inactivated in about 10 minutes at 60°C and in 30 minutes, 24 hours, and 24 hours when exposed to ether, 0.1% formalin, or 0.5% phenol, respectively; however, they maintain infectivity for many months or years when lyophilized and stored at −50 to −70°C.

Like other chlamydiae, the organism of FC possesses two antigens—group and specific—associated with the cell wall. The group antigen, common to all chlamydiae, resists heat, nucleases, and proteases, but is inactivated from treatment with lecithinase. The specific antigen is shared by a limited group of related chlamydiae, is detectable with immunofluorescence, and is neutralized by specific antibodies. The specific antigens separate the chlamydiae into the immunotypes 1 and 2. Immunotype 1 is associated with abortions, pneumonia, and intestinal infections, whereas immunotype 2 is associated with kerato conjunctivitis and polyarthritis with its associated intestinal phase of the infection. Chlamydiae

183

of FC inhabit ovine conjunctival sacs and nasal secretions and are antigenically related to chlamydiae of polyarthritis of lambs. The infectious chain is maintained directly in the sheep population by the intestinal infections which persist over long periods with continued shedding.

FC spreads easily and rapidly and probably by direct contact, vectoring flies, and aerial sprays. In crowded feedlots, the faces, including nostrils and eyes, often directly contact and may transfer infection. Coughing, blowing, and sneezing forcefully expel infected droplets into air and susceptible eyes. During warm months, house flies and possibly face flies feed on ocular secretions and often move from face to face and eye to eye and, in the process of feeding and moving, mechanically transfer pathogens from infected to susceptible eyes.

The pathogenesis of FC begins with entrance of the chlamydiae into susceptible eyes. There the organisms enter conjunctival epithelial cells where, in cytoplasmic vacuoles, they replicate by forming initial bodies and elementary bodies. The latter escape into the lacrimal environment and infect new cells. Injury to the cells provokes acute inflammation and the formation of purulent exudate. The conjunctiva becomes hyperemic and edematous, and lymphoid follicles later form. The cornea may pass through sequential changes of edema, opacity, pannus, erosion, ulcer, and perforation.

Usually the eye interrupts the sequence and heals. In some cases, the chlamydiae invade the blood and migrate to the opposite eye and to joints. Cases of chlamydiosis develop complement-fixing antibodies. Most eyes clear the infection within 6 to 10 days, but about 40% retain organisms for 3 months and a few for 20 months. Following recovery, most eyes resist reinfection for 3 months, and 30% resist for 8 months.

CLINICAL SIGNS AND LESIONS.   FC spreads rapidly among both feedlot and nursing lambs, and the disease may affect one or both eyes. Animals with severe bilateral lesions are blind and unable to find feed and water. During the first day of infection, eyes show hyperemia and edema of the conjunctiva and profuse lacrimation with epiphora. Throughout the next 2 days, the cornea may develop variable amounts of opacity, pannus, erosion, ulcer, and perforation.

Opacity and vascularization begin from the dorsal limbus and later from the ventral limbus and both move toward the corneal center. Healing usually begins within 2 to 4 days and prevents the formation of severe lesions. After several days, lymphoid follicles, 1 to 10 mm in diameter, form on the nictitating membrane and mucosa of the eyelids. Some sheep may be lame from arthritis.

Among feedlot lambs, the morbidity reaches 90%, and 80% of the ocular lesions may be bilateral. No animals die. The usual course ranges from 6 to 10 days, but in case of complications from corneal ulceration, it may extend to several weeks. Remissions, with less severity, are common.

Histopathologic changes are limited to the conjunctival sac and cornea. During the early stages of disease, some epithelial cells of the conjunctiva contain cytoplasmic initial bodies and later elementary bodies. Hyperemia and edema are prominent. Follicles show hyperplasia of lymphocytes. Corneal edema, erosions, and ulcers may be present.

DIAGNOSIS.   Veterinarians diagnose FC on evidence of characteristic signs and lesions and laboratory findings. Rapidly spreading diseases, showing lacrimation, conjunctival hyperemia, corneal opacity, and follicular hypertrophy, are highly suggestive and significant. In the laboratory, initial bodies and/or elementary bodies may be identified in epithelial cells from stained scrapings of the conjunctival sac. The use of immunofluorescent techniques increases the accuracy.

The differential diagnosis requires consideration, in some areas, of contagious agalactia; in this disease, affected ewes show keratitis, arthritis, and mastitis. The causative *Mycoplasma agalactiae* can be isolated from the diseased organs. Entropion, if not corrected, produces lacrimation and corneal opacity.

TREATMENT.   Most infected eyes require no treatment. Severe infections can be effectively treated by daily applying 0.5% tetracycline ointment to the conjunctival sac. Veterinarians may use subconjunctival injections of antibiotics and steroids for the treatment of individual animals.

Animal Health Yearbook. FAO-WHO-OIE (Italy), 1970.

Beveridge, W.I.B.: Investigations on contagious ophthalmia of sheep, with special attention to the epidemiology of infection by *Rickettsia conjunctivae*. Aust. Vet. J., *18*:155-164, 1942.

Blackmore, F.: Conjunctivitis and keratitis of cattle and sheep associated with the presence of "cell-inclusion bodies." J. Comp. Pathol. Ther., *57*:223-231, 1947.

Coles, J.D.W.A.: A Rickettsia-like organism in the conjunctiva of sheep. 17th Rep. Dir. Vet. Serv. Anim. Ind. Union of South Africa. 1931, pp. 175-186.

Dickenson, Lois and Cooper, B.S.: Contagious conjunctivo-keratitis of sheep. J. Pathol. Bacteriol., *78*: 257-266, 1959.

Donatiens, A. and Lestoquard, F.: Occurrence of conjunctivitis of sheep in Algiers due to *Rickettsia conjunctivae*. Bull. Soc. Pathol. Exot., *30*:18, 1937.

Johnson, L.V.: A pannus-forming infection of sheep eyes. Proc. Soc. Exp. Biol. Med., *38*:42-43, 1938.

Mitscherlich, E.: Infectious keratoconjunctivitis of sheep in Germany, and its relationship to infectious keratoconjunctivitis of cattle. Arch. Wiss. Prokt. Tierheilk., *78*:241-244, 1943.

Norton, W.L. and Storz, J.: Observations on sheep with polyarthritis produced by an agent of the psittacosis-lymphogranuloma-venereum-trachoma group. Arthritis Rheum., *10*:1-10, 1967.

Stephenson, E.H., Storz, J., and Hopkins, J.B.: Properties and frequency of isolation of chlamydia from eyes of lambs with conjunctivitis and polyarthritis. AJVR, *35*:177-180, 1974.

Storz, J.: Chlamydia-induced disease of sheep and goats. In *Current Veterinary Therapy 2. Food Animal Practice*. Edited by J. Howard. Philadelphia, W.B. Saunders Co., 1986, pp. 532-533.

Storz, J., Pierson, R.E., Marriott, M.E., and Chow, T.L.: Isolation of psittacosis agents from follicular conjunctivitis of sheep. Proc. Soc. Exp. Biol. Med., *125*:857-862, 1967.

Storz, J., Shupe, J.L., Marriott, M.E., and Thornley, W.R.: Polyarthritis of lambs induced experimentally by a psittacosis agent. J. Infect. Dis., *115*:9-18, 1965.

9

DISEASES OF THE MUSCULAR AND SKELETAL SYSTEMS

Muscular Sarcocystosis

(*Eosinophilic Myositis*)

Eosinophilic myositis (EM) is a collective term used by the meat inspection service to designate a condition of clinically healthy animals that have focal, green, muscular lesions. Under this broad category there is no differentiation as to the magnitude or dissemination of the lesions. The economic impact of EM involves the loss of the value of the edible portion of the carcass to the meat-producing and meat packing industry. The condemned carcass represents a loss of the total production cost, investment, and interest on that investment. From 1966 through 1983 the U.S. Meat Inspection Service annually condemned an average of 43 (or 1/190,458) ovine and 3619 (or 1/8768) bovine for EM. Research observations of the multiple, small disseminated lesions in the tongue, esophagus, heart, diaphragm, or skeletal muscle indicate that under the broad category of eosinophilic myositis that over 90% of the bovine cases and all ovine cases should be classified as muscular sarcocystosis. It has been suggested that carcasses having a single or a few large (5 to 15 cm in diameter) irregular globular, firm and fibrous lesions located in muscles of the thigh or other anatomic areas that are pale yellow with variable amounts of green and red be classified as eosinophilic myositis.

In view of these findings the etiologic agent, pathogenesis, and prevention can be described.

OCCURRENCE. Muscular sarcocystosis can occur in all ages and classes of sheep in temperate and warm climates whose feed source is contaminated with cat or dog feces containing the infective form of sarcocysts. As the condition is usually diagnosed only at slaughter, the highest prevalence is recorded in 10 to 12 month old lambs. Slaughter plants dealing in old ewes report a high prevalence from certain localities in southwestern Colorado and southeastern Utah. Other localities may also be involved.

ETIOLOGIC AGENT AND LIFE CYCLE. The genus sarcocystis is in the family Sarcocystidae which belongs to the order Eimeriorina and is related to toxoplasma and other protozoa. Sarcocystis is common in many species of domestic and wild animals throughout the world. Sarcocystis is heteroxenous. The asexual stages occur in sheep (intermediate host), the sexual stage in cats, dogs, coyotes, and red fox (definitive or final host). Oocysts develop in the lamina propria of the small intestine of the cat and other animals. They sporulate at this sight forming 2 sporocysts each with 4 sporozoites. The sporocysts generally break out of the oocysts in the intestine of the definitive host so that sporulated sporocysts and a few sporulated oocysts are passed in the feces. No meronts (sarcocysts) or merozoites are produced in the definitive host. The intermediate

Fig. 9-1. Eosinophilic myositis in the diaphragm. The discrete small foci are gray to green to yellow.

host can be infected by ingesting feed contaminated with sporocysts. There appears to be one or two generations of meront (sarcocyst) in the endothelial cells of small blood vessels that produce a variable number of tachyzoites that later enter the striated muscle and form the last meront (sarcocyst) generation. The sarcocyst has a definitive wall and forms metrocytes within itself; these divide repeatedly by endodyogeny to form intermediate stages and then bradyzoites which live in compartments divided by septa in the mature sarcocyst. The tachyzoites are able to infect other intermediate hosts, but bradyzoites are not infective. The definitive host becomes infected by ingesting mature sarcocysts containing bradyzoites. Definitive hosts do not appear to develop an immunity and can become reinfected repeatedly.

Three sarcocystis have been identified in sheep: 1. *Sarcocystis gigantea* (*S. ovifelis*) is common throughout most of the world. The intermediate hosts are the domestic sheep and

Rocky Mountain bighorn sheep with the cat and red fox the definitive host. The sarcocysts are large (up to 1 cm long) and compartmented. The prepatent period in cats is 10–14 days with a 4–43 day patent period. The pathogenicity for lambs or cats is extremely low. 2. *Sarcocystis medusiformis* has been found so far only in New Zealand. The intermediate host is the domestic sheep while the definitive host is the cat with a prepatent period in cats of 11–20 days. 3. *Sarcocystis tenella* (*S. ovicanis*) is common throughout the world. The intermediate host is the domestic sheep while the definitive hosts are the dog, coyote, red fox and probably dingo. The prepatent period in dogs or coyotes is about 8–14 days but may extend to 36 days. This species is highly pathogenic for lambs, mildly pathogenic for the dog and not pathogenic for the red fox. The disease can cause fever, inappetance, anemia, and death in lambs.

Macro- and Microscopic Lesions. Numerous, small lesions are located in the tongue, esophagus, heart, diaphragm (Fig. 9-1), and skeletal muscles. The discrete lesions are mostly fusiform and 0.5 to 5 × 0.5 to 2 mm with the long axes parallel to muscle fasciculi. New lesions are green, and older lesions tend toward gray with green blended in at the peripheries. Damaged areas form scars of gray and yellow often with green foci and occasionally with movable brown nodules 0.1 to 0.5 mm in diameter. Variations in lesions occur with ones having a gray center surrounded by concentric color zones, first red and then green. Coalesced units may form firm masses 1 to 4 mm in diameter. Progressively narrowing lines of green tissue radiate along perimysial tissue away from the main lesion for 5 to 30 mm. Lesions in different stages of development may be seen in the same carcass. The regional lymph nodes are enlarged and green, especially with advanced and generalized lesions. Microscopically, granulomas are the central feature of these small disseminated lesions varying in size and shape and each often involving the entire width of a fasciculus. Although granuloma formation is a continuous process, they may be divided into 3 stages—

early, intermediate, and late for purpose of description. The early stage consists of a mass of necrotic tissue, including segments of myocytes, endomycium, and perimycium. Skeletal myocytes have segmental necrosis and hyaline degeneration. Some fragments of sarcoplasm separate from the muscle fiber with empty sarcolemmal tubes. Cardiac myocytes shrink and some fragment. The necrotic tissue contains many eosinophils and few macrophages which concentrate at the peripheries of large lesions throughout entire small lesions. Pyknosis and chromatolysis is evident indicating cellular degradation.

The intermediate-stage granulomas are characterized by more degraded central contents than in early granulomas. Myocyte fragments lose all nuclei and all striations with some being phagocytized by multinucleated giant cells. There is an increase of dead eosinophils having a more neutral staining cytoplasmic droplets plus an increase of eosinophils at the peripheries of the degraded masses. Some areas may be partially calcified with many unidentifiable cells. The granuloma wall has prominent palisades of epithelioid cells with their pale staining cytoplasm oriented toward the granulomas center. The zone between the granuloma and viable muscle contains large numbers of lymphocytes and eosinophils, small numbers of macrophages, degranulated mast cells, and extravasated erythrocytes in a fine stroma of fibrocytes and capillaries.

The late stage granulomas are characterized by severely degenerated tissues. The granuloma centers contain fragments of sarcoplasm, dead leukocytes, and granules of disintegrated cells. The centers of some granulomas consist of mostly amorphous granules, containing a diffuse brown nonferrous pigment. The granuloma wall has multinucleated giant cells, lymphocytes, and fibrous tissue. Areas around and within the granulomatous space contain fibrous tissue, few myocytes, and scars composed of fibrous tissue, fat cells, aggregates of lymphocytes, and degraded eosinophils. Muscle cells surrounding the lesions show severe fatty change with some atrophied cells. These changes diminish with distance from the gran-

uloma. Many granulomas contain central sarcocysts. The sarcocysts form a regression series. In early stages the sarcocyst wall is opened but otherwise normal. After the sarcocyst ruptures, the bradyzoites generally remain within the cyst cavity. In the intermediate stage, some sarcocyst walls may be seen, others fragmented or dislocated, and others may be absent. The bradyzoites are dead with some being lysed. In the late stages, the sarcocysts may not be seen.

DIAGNOSIS. As muscular sarcocystosis causes no recognizable clinical signs, the infection is diagnosed only at slaughter or necropsy, usually for some other condition. Muscular sarcocystosis can be tentatively diagnosed by typical disseminated lesions in tongue, esophagus, heart, diaphragm, and skeletal muscles. Histologic examination is required for a definitive diagnosis.

PREVENTION. Sheep acquire sarcocystis infections by ingesting the sporocysts during grazing or from contaminated feed sources. Hence, prevention depends on keeping sheep away from areas where the definitive hosts have defecated or keeping those feces from contaminating feed sources. In many management systems this may be impossible. Prevention of infecting the definitive host may be more practical by proper disposal of all dead animals or raw meat, and not allowing domestic dogs and cats to feed on raw meat. In cases of coyote and fox, it is impossible to eliminate the preditor-prey transmission.

Jensen, R., et al.: Eosinophilic myositis and muscular sarcocystosis in the carcasses of slaughtered cattle and lambs. Am. J. Vet. Res., 47:587-593, 1986.

Johnson, A., Hildebrandt, P., and Fayer, R.: Experimentally induced sarcocystis infection in calves: Pathology. Am. J. Vet. Res., 36:995-999, 1975.

Leek, R., Fayer, R., and Johnson, A.: Sheep experimentally infected with sarcocystis from dogs. I. Disease in young lambs. J. Parasitol., 63:644-650, 1977.

Leek, R. and Fayer, R.: Sheep experimentally infected with sarcocystis from dogs. II. Abortion and disease in ewes. Cornell Vet., 68:108-123, 1978.

Levine, N.: Veterinary Protozoology. 2nd Edition. Ames, Iowa, Iowa State University Press, 1985, pp. 233-260.

Muscular Cysticercosis

(*MC; Taenia ovis infection; measles*)

Muscular cysticercosis is an invasion of sheep muscles by the larvae of a tapeworm of dogs and foxes. Although the disease has wide geographic distribution, its incidence is generally low, and the clinical effect is usually insignificant. For these reasons, MC causes minor concern to sheep producers. At slaughter, however, infected carcasses are condemned and trimmed because of unesthetic appearance, and these actions cause direct and indirect losses to meat packers and sheep producers. Between 1967 and 1971, the United States annually slaughtered and inspected an average of 10.6 million sheep; of these carcasses, 380 (0.004%) were condemned and 15,860 (0.15%) were trimmed because of cysticercosis.

OCCURRENCE. MC occurs in all breeds and sexes of sheep, but young animals generally are more susceptible than adults. Geographically, the condition occurs in most sheep-producing countries. In America, sheep of the western states are infected, and in some areas, the incidence reaches 2%.

ETIOLOGY AND PATHOGENESIS. A tapeworm causes MC. The adult worm, *Taenia ovis*, inhabits the small intestines of dogs and foxes, and the larvae, *Cysticercus ovis*, reside as bladderworms in the cardiac and skeletal muscles of sheep and goats. The adult worm, measuring 0.5 to 1.0 m in length, bears a prominent rostellum with 24 to 36 hooks and gravid segments filled with oval eggs, measuring 24 × 24 to 28 μm. The mature bladderworm measures up to 10 × 20 mm and contains clear fluid and a single invaginated scolex.

The life cycle begins with expulsion of gravid segments to the exterior. When the eggs are eaten by a sheep, the released oncospheres enter the small intestine, penetrate the tips of ileal villi, move to villar bases, enter venules, traverse the liver and lungs, and are transported via systemic blood to cardiac and skeletal muscles, where they locate and, in 10 to 12 weeks, form mature bladderworms. The

bladderworms, when ingested by dogs, develop into tapeworms.

Most bladderworm infections are innocuous, but heavy cardiac parasitism may cause failure. Presumably, recovered sheep resist infection. Experimentally, susceptible lambs inoculated intraperitoneally with activated *Taenia ovis* embryos resist oral challenge with *T. ovis* eggs. Lambs are also protected against infection with *T. ovis* eggs by means of colostral antibody for a period of 9 weeks.

CLINICAL SIGNS AND POSTMORTEM LESIONS. The usual infection with *C. ovis* causes no signs. Extraordinarily heavy infection, however, may cause muscular weakness and heart failure. At necropsy of dead sheep or at inspection of slaughtered sheep the bladderworms are discernible. They usually are located in myocardium (Fig. 9-2), diaphragmatic crura (Fig. 9-3), masseter muscles, and tongue, but other skeletal muscles may be affected. The epicardium, pleura and peritoneum form surface elevations over submesothelial bladderworms. At slaughter, carcasses with one to five

Fig. 9-2. Degenerating cysticercus (*A*) from *Taenia ovis* in heart muscle of a fattened lamb.

Fig. 9-3. Three cysticerci (*A*) from *Taenia ovis* in the diaphragm of a fattened lamb.

cysticerci are trimmed, and those with more are condemned.

DIAGNOSIS.   Veterinarians diagnose MC by finding the characteristic bladderworms at necropsy of dead sheep or at inspection of slaughtered animals. For technical assistance from a diagnostic laboratory, practitioners should submit suspect muscle in 10% formalin.

PREVENTION.   Producers and veterinarians prevent MC by the same procedures as they use for preventing visceral cysticercosis.

Gemmell, M.A.: Distribution of *Cysticercus ovis* in sheep. Aust. Vet. J., *46*:22-24, 1970.
Jensen, R., Pierson, R.E., and Schubach, R.D.: Muscular cysticercosis from *T. ovis* in feedlot lambs. JAVMA, *167*:742-745, 1975.
Ransom, B.H.: *Cysticercus ovis* in mutton. J. Agric. Res., *1*:15-58, 1913.
Rickard, M.D. and Arundel, J.H.: Passive protection of lambs against infection with *Taenia ovis* via colostrum. Aust. Vet. J., *50*:22-24, 1974.
Rickard, M.D. and Bell, K.J.: Induction of immunity of lambs to a larval cestode by diffusable antigens. Nature, *232*:120, 1971.

Chlamydial Polyarthritis

(CPA; polyarthritis of lambs; stiff lamb disease)

Chlamydial polyarthritis of lambs, an acute contagious but nonfatal disease of feedlot and nursing lambs, is characterized by fever, lameness, arthritis, serositis, conjunctivitis, and emaciation and is caused by a chlamydial organism. Because of high prevalence among feedlot lambs and increasing sporadic outbreaks in nursing lambs of range flocks, the disease has major importance to the United States sheep industry. Economic losses result from reduction in live weight, prolonged fattening time, inefficient use of feed, extra labor for care of sick and convalescent animals, and the cost of treatment, and from protein deficiencies among sheep-dependent people of the southwestern region of the United States. The existence of a similar or identical disease among calves gives additional importance to the malady; and the occurrence of analogous arthritis, venereal disease, and conjunctivitis in people adds public health significance and human interest.

OCCURRENCE.   CPA occurs in all breeds and sexes of sheep and in lambs 1 to 8 months of age. Although nursing lambs 1 to 2 months old often contract the disease, weaned lambs 3 to 5 months of age and lambs recently transported from range or pasture to feedlots suffer an especially high incidence. Some range bands especially those in the high mountain areas have reported a high incidence in nursing lambs. CPA develops among feedlot lambs during July, August, September, October, and November, and in nursing lambs during July and August. In feedlots, the disease begins 4 to 8 weeks after entrance when feed consumption rate is high and the fattening rate is rapid.

Geographically, the malady primarily occurs in North America, but it also occurs in Spain. In the United States, western regional sheep contract the disease: nursing lambs on range and pasture and feedlot lambs in enterprises of both western and midwestern states.

ETIOLOGY AND PATHOGENESIS.   *Chlamydia psittaci* causes CPA. This gram-negative, nonmotile, obligate parasite inhabits cytoplasmic vacuoles of host cells, where it may form prolonged and possibly lifetime latency. The infectious particle, consisting of a cell membrane and nucleoid, measures 0.3 nm in diameter and contains both DNA and RNA. The cell contains lipid and mucopeptide, and like some bacteria, its growth is inhibited by penicillin, tetracycline, and cycloserine. Mature particles, or elementary bodies, color purple with Giemsa's stain and red with Macchiavello's stain. Chlamydiae in general are inactivated in about 10 minutes at 60°C, and in 30 minutes, 24 hours, and 24 hours when exposed to ether, 0.1% formalin, or 0.5% phenol, respectively, but they maintain infectivity for many months or years when lyophilized and stored at −50 to −70°C. Nutritional disorders have been suspected as factors predisposing to infection.

Like other chlamydiae, the agent of CPA possesses two antigens—group and specific—associated with the cell wall. The group antigen, common to all chlamydiae, resists heat, nucleases, and proteases, but is inactivated by the action of lecithinase. The specific antigen is shared by a limited group of related chlamydiae, is detectable with immunofluorescence and gel-diffusion reactions and is neutralized by specific antibodies.

The specific antigens separate the chlamydia into immunotypes 1 and 2. Strains isolated from abortions, pneumonia, and intestinal infections and from cases of epizootic bovine abortion are classified into immunotype 1. Whereas those isolated from keratoconjunctivitis and polyarthritis with the associated intestinal phase of infection are immunotype 2.

The natural method of CPA transmission is uncertain and conjectural. The circumstances of disease development, however, suggest direct contact as a strong possibility: the causative organism is excreted in feces, urine, tears, and nasal secretions; disease frequently begins following excessive crowding during transit from range and pasture to feedlots; during transit, feeding may be on the ground where contamination with infective excretions is easy; and in crowded feedlots, watering and feeding facilities inevitably become contaminated. These conditions facilitate transfer of chlamydiae from infected sheep to the alimentary tracts of susceptible animals. Whether or not carriers initiate flock infection is not known.

Information on the pathogenesis of CPA has been obtained from parenteral inoculations, followed by serial slaughter, of experimental sheep. After intramuscular or intra-articular inoculation, chlamydemia develops by days 3 or 4, maximal joint and visceral infection by days 7 to 14, and clearance of joint infection by day 28. After intra-articular inoculation, the lesions occur in three stages: serous synovitis and tenosynovitis 2 to 14 hours after inoculation, fibrinopurulent inflammation after 24 to 96 hours, and finally, changes of resolution after 6 to 24 days.

Healing usually occurs without morphologic alterations in the articular cartilages. Complement-fixing antibodies form within 7 to 10 days and maintain significant titers for a few months; serum-neutralizing antibodies develop later and persist longer, and recovered lambs probably are immune.

Within individual lambs, follicular conjunctivitis usually develops in conjunction with arthritis. After natural transmission, probably through the alimentary tract or conjunctivae, the period of chlamydemia may be longer than after inoculation. Chlamydiae are discharged to the external environment through ocular fluids, nasal secretions, feces, and urine.

CLINICAL SIGNS AND POSTMORTEM LESIONS. During early stages of CPA, affected lambs develop body temperatures ranging from 41 to 42°C, lose appetite, and separate from the flock. Muscular movements are stiff and painful, and lameness may exist in one to four limbs; usually all limbs are affected to some degree, but the limb with most pain shows the greatest incapacitation. The major limb joints—shoulder, elbow, hip, stifle, and hock—are painful to palpation, but enlargement is difficult to assess except for the skilled clinician.

As the disease progresses, lameness increases, and the gaunt, immobilized lamb stands with humped back and the lamest of the limbs out of function. Some animals assume lateral recumbency for prolonged periods. Deterioration of physical condition causes an average live weight loss of 10%. Nearly all arthritic lambs also contract bilateral conjunctivitis, but conjunctivitis can exist without arthritis. Affected eyes are, to variable degrees, hyperemic and the conjunctivae folliculated over the lower and third eyelids; the individual elevations measure up to 10 mm in height and diameter.

In severe cases, vascularization of the cornea and edema of the conjunctivae develop.

Ocular secretions discharge over facial skin, and photophobia may be prominent. In infected flocks, the morbidity commonly reaches 30% and may reach 80% or more, but if arthritic lambs are isolated where feed and water are easily available, the mortality is low. Mortality may be higher under range conditions where lambs are unable to keep up with the flock, become separated, and are subject to predation. The disease course ranges from 2 to 4 weeks. Most recovered lambs fatten to marketable quality.

At necropsy, gross changes are found in and around joints, tendon sheaths, eyes, and lungs (Fig. 9-4). The large limb joints and the atlantooccipital articulation commonly show dis-

Fig. 9-4. Chlamydial arthritis in a sagittal gross slice of stifle joint showing patella (*a*), femur (*b*), tibia, (*c*), infected ulcer in articular cartilage of femoral condyle (*d*), and capsular pouches filled with exudate (*e*).

tension of the articular capsule with increased volume of amber-colored fluid. The synovium contains flakes and plaques of loose or attached fibrin. Edema, hyperemia, and petechial hemorrhages extend, in varying degrees, through the fibrous layer into adjacent muscles. Usually, articular cartilages appear normal.

In joints infected for several weeks, the synovial layer may be roughened from villous proliferations. Tendon sheaths show changes similar to those of joints, but with lesser amounts of fibrin. Lungs may contain pink areas of atelectasis and modest consolidation.

Histopathologic changes, although qualitatively similar in most animals, vary in extent and degree. Synovial fluid contains an increased number of mononuclear cells and detached synovial cells. Synovial cells of the joint capsule are hyperplastic and enlarged. In advanced stages, villous proliferations project into the cavity.

The synovial layer contains granulomas, and the fibrous layer contains perivascular accumulations of mononuclear leukocytes. Synovial cells, either intact or detached, endothelial cells, and mononuclear leukocytes contain cytoplasmic masses of chlamydiae. Affected lobules of lungs show atelectasis of some alveoli, thickening of alveolar walls, and accumulations of leukocytes. Mononuclear leukocytes may contain cytoplasmic inclusion bodies.

Ultrastructural changes are characterized by focal necrosis of synovial lining cells, edema, fibrin deposition, and cellular infiltration.

DIAGNOSIS. Veterinarians diagnose CPA on evidence of typical signs and lesions. The development among feedlot lambs of a high incidence of febrile lameness and stiffness a few weeks after entering the feedlot strongly indicates the disease. The additional necropsy evidence of arthritis in the shoulder, elbow, hip, stifle, and hock joints, and tendon sheaths with plaques of fibrin in the synovial fluid are sufficient reason, in endemic areas, for a clinical diagnosis.

In the laboratory, confirmation can be obtained by finding an ascending titer for complement-fixing antibodies on paired serum samples or the enzyme-linked immunosorbent assay or by double immunodiffusion; for this test, blood samples should be collected early in the disease course and again 2 weeks later. Smears and sections of infected synovial layers may be examined for inclusion bodies. The strongest diagnostic evidence, however, is the isolation of chlamydiae from infected joints and/or tendon sheaths in inoculated yolk sacs of embryonating chicken eggs. In some cases, several blind egg passages may be necessary for activation of the organisms. Isolation can be made in cultured cells using infectivity enhancing methods (centrifugation) and is more sensitive and less time consuming.

The differential diagnosis requires the consideration of founder, navel ill, colibacillosis, erysipelas and, in south European countries, contagious agalactia.

PREVENTION AND TREATMENT. In the feedlot, lambs affected with CPA should be isolated to avoid excessive exposure of susceptible animals to excreted chlamydiae and to enable affected lambs to obtain feed and water easily. Vaccine for immunizing against the disease has not been developed, although trials using the vaccine for chlamydial abortions lessens the number and severity of cases of polyarthritis.

Chlamydia are susceptible to tetracyclines, chlortetracycline, erythromycin, and penicillin. Individual treatment with long acting tetracyclines (LA200) at the rate of 20 mg/kg is an effective treatment. A second treatment in 3 to 4 days may be necessary depending on the response. Tetracyclines may be added to the feed at the rate of 10 to 20 mg/kg.

The use of long acting tetracyclines (LA200) should be considered for mass medication. Although the labor for such treatment is intensive, all animals are assured of receiving adequate dosage as the severely affected animal may not be consuming feed.

Blanco Loizelier, A.: Polyarthritis and keratoconjunctivitis in sheep and goats. Rev. Patron. Biol. Anim., *13*: 201-213, 1969.

Cutlip, R.C.: Ultrastructure of the synovial membrane of lambs affected with chlamydial polyarthritis. AJVR, *35*:171-176, 1974.

Cutlip, R.C. and Ramsey, R.K.: Ovine chlamydial polyarthritis: Sequential development of articular lesions in lambs after intraarticular exposure. AJVR, *34*: 71-75, 1973.

Delong, W. and Bulgin, M.: Chlamydial polyarthritis of lambs. Station Bull. U. Idaho, 1986.

Hopkins, J.B., Stephenson, E.H., Storz, J., and Pierson, R.E.: Conjunctivitis associated with chylamydial polyarthritis in lambs. JAVMA, *163*:1157-1160, 1973.

Kawakami, Y., et al.: Miyagawanella: psittacosis-lymphogranuloma group of viruses, isolation of a virus from feces of naturally infected sheep. Bull. Natl. Inst. Anim. Health, No. 36, 1958.

Livingston, C.W., Moore, R.W., Redmond, H.E., and Hardy, W.T.: Polyarthritis virus—a cause of "stiff lambs" in Texas. South West. Vet., *18*:279-281, 1965.

Mendlowski, B. and Segre, D.: Polyarthritis of sheep. I. Description of the disease and experimental transmission. AJVR. *21*:68-73. 1960a.

Mendlowski, B., Kraybill, W.H., and Segre, D.: Polyarthritis in sheep. II. Characterization of the virus. AJVR, *21*:74-80, 1960b.

Norton, W.L. and Storz, J.: Observations on sheep with polyarthritis produced by an agent of the psittacosis-lymphogranuloma-venereum-trachoma group. Arthritis Rheum., *10*:1-10, 1967.

Page, L.A. and Cutlip, R.C.: Chlamydial polyarthritis in Iowa lambs. Iowa Vet., *39*:10-11; 14-18, 1968.

Pierson, R.E.: Polyarthritis in Colorado feedlot lambs. JAVMA, *150*:1487-1492, 1967.

Schachter, J., et al.: Isolation of bedsoniae from joints of patients with Reiter's syndrome. Proc. Soc. Exp. Biol. Med. *122*:283-285, 1966.

Shupe, J.L. and Storz, J.: Pathologic study of psittacosis-lymphogranuloma polyarthritis of lambs. AJVR, *25*: 943-951, 1964.

Stamp, J.T., McEwen, A.D., Watt, J.A.A., and Nisbet, D.I.: Enzootic abortion in ewes. Vet. Rec., *62*:251-254, 1950.

Storz, J.: *Chlamydia and Chlamydia-induced Diseases.* Springfield, Ill., Charles C Thomas, 1971.

Storz, J.: Chlamydia-induced diseases of sheep and goats. *Current Veterinary Therapy. 2. Food Animal Practice.* Edited by J. Howard. Philadelphia, W.B. Saunders Co., 1986, pp. 532-533.

Storz, J.: Psittacosis agents as cause of polyarthritis in cattle and sheep. Vet. Med. Rev., *2/3*:125-139, 1967.

Storz, J.: Psittacosis-lymphogranuloma infection of sheep. Antigenic structure and interrelationships. J. Comp. Pathol., *76*:351-362, 1966.

Storz, J. and McKercher, M.G.: Etiological studies of epizootic bovine abortion. Zentralbl. Veterinaermed., *9*:411-427, 1962.

Storz, J., Pierson, R.E., Marriott, M.E., and Chow, T.L.: Isolation of psittacosis agents from follicular conjunctivitis of sheep. Proc. Soc. Exp. Biol. Med., *125*: 857-860, 1967.

Storz, J., Shupe, J.L., James, L.F., and Smart, R.A.: Polyarthritis of sheep in the intermountain region caused by a psittacosis-lymphogranuloma agent. AJVR, *24*: 1201-1206, 1963.

Storz, J., Shupe, J.L., Marriott, M.E., and Thornley, W.R.: Polyarthritis of lambs induced experimentally by a psittacosis agent. J. Infect. Dis., *115*:9-18, 1965.

Storz, J., Smart, R.A., and Shupe, J.L.: Virus-bededingte polyarthritis bei kalbern. Nord. Vet. Med., *16*: 109-115, 1964.

Storz, J. and Thornley, W.R.: Serologische und aetiologische studien uber die intestinale psittacosis-lymphogranuloma-infektion der schafe. Zentralbl. Veterinaermed., *13*:14-24, 1966.

10

DISEASES OF THE CENTRAL NERVOUS SYSTEM

Listeriosis

(Circling disease)

Listeriosis, an acute infectious but non-contagious disease of sheep and other domestic mammals and poultry, is characterized by neurologic disturbances, such as circling movements, facial paralysis, and abortions and is caused by soil- and silage-residing bacteria. On the basis of clinical manifestations, the disease is usually classified into three forms: (1) encephalitis with neurologic disturbance, (2) placentitis with abortions occurring in the last trimester of gestation, and (3) gastrointestinal septicemia with acute hepatitis, splenitis, and pneumonitis. Encephalitis is the common form diagnosed in sheep.

Because of its near-universal distribution and its several clinical forms, listeriosis has major importance to the sheep industry. Economic losses result from deaths, loss of live weight, costly treatments, and delayed marketing among feedlot lambs, septicemia in young lambs, and from abortions and some deaths among farm flocks. Development of the disease among cattle, swine, poultry, and people adds both economic importance and public health significance to the malady.

OCCURRENCE. Listeriosis occurs in all breeds, sexes, and ages of sheep. The prevalent form will depend on the management and class of sheep being maintained. Lambs as young as 5 weeks may develop the septicemic form. Feedlot lambs from 4 to 8 months most commonly encounter the encephalitic form, although the septicemic form may go undiagnosed. All three forms, septicemia, abortions, and encephalitis, may affect the pregnant ewe. Although worldwide in distribution, it is more prevalent in temperate and cold climates. The disease does not necessarily recur in the same facilities on successive seasons, however. Furthermore, confined sheep, especially those consuming silage, have a higher incidence than do range flocks. Most cases develop during late autumn, winter, and early spring when animals are maintained in crowded pens. Geographically, listeriosis occurs as sporadic or widespread disease among sheep of New Zealand, Australia, United States, Canada, Mexico, Iceland, Britain, Scandinavia, Belgium, France, Germany, Italy, Bulgaria, Rumania, USSR, and Japan.

ETIOLOGY. There are currently four recognized species of *Listeria*: *L. monocytogenesis,* *L. grayi, L. murrayi* and *L. denitrificans.* *L. monocytogenesis* is the common species causing listeriosis in animals. *L. monocytogenes* is a small (0.4 to 0.5 $\times$ 0.2 to 0.2 μm), motile, pleomorphic gram-positive nonsporing coccobacilli. Listeria grows under a wide range of temperature (4 to 44°C) which is important diagnostically for the "cold enrichment" technique of primary isolation of listeria from suspected cases of encephalitis. Brain suspensions are refrigerated at 4°C and cultured at weekly intervals. The large number of listeria organisms present in aborted materials does not require this procedure for primary isolation.

On the basis of antigenic determination *L. monocytogenes* has been classified into at least 6 serovars with a number of subtypes. Serovars 1/2a and 4b account for most of the isolates from animal and humans. Serovar 5 causes sporadic abortions in sheep. The organisms may be found in the brain stem of sheep and other animals affected with listeric encephalitis; in liver, spleen, and lungs from animals suffering from septicemia; and in placentas and fetuses of sheep contracting the uterine form of listeriosis. *L. monocytogenes* is an inhabitant of the soil and the mammalian (including birds) intestinal tract. Healthy animals and humans may shed the organism via the intestinal tract. Human infections are not necessarily direct animal contact. Indications are that the majority of animal and human cases are subclinical or latent and go undiagnosed. The ability of the listeria organism to survive for extended periods of time (2 years) in cool moist organic conditions and its ability to multiply in the soil at 18 to 20°C aid in its propagation and establishment in an ecologic system. Grazing animals pick up the organism from grass and associated soil particles, become subclinically infected, and may become inapparent carriers passing the organism in their feces and secretions, further contaminating the environment. Most outbreaks of listeriosis are associated with poor quality ensilage (pH 5.6 or greater) which has been prepared from grass or other plants containing soil both of which are from a highly contaminated environment. Improperly prepared pH silage with inadequate acid production allows multiplication of the listeria organisms. Outbreaks are often associated with feeding the spoiled ensilage from the edges where oxygen has inhibited proper fermentation and acid production. Pit or bunker type silos are more often involved than the upright tank type as there is a greater opportunity for soil contamination during the filling and packing process. All sheep in an outbreak are exposed to the same contaminated feed source indicating a low pathogenicity and high infectivity as a total

population may be infected with only 5 to 10% manifesting clinical signs. Stress factors, sudden changes in feed, concurrent disease, and physical or viral damage to the epithelial lining of the digestive tract are factors involved in pathogenesis.

Available information now indicates that encephalitis, the important and common form in feedlot lambs, develops as a local infection. Susceptible sheep are exposed to the organism in contaminated feed, especially silage, contaminated water, and possibly infected secretions and excretions from diseased animals, including domestic and wild mammals and birds.

Feeding on diets containing grass and grain awns results in abrasions and small puncture wounds in the mucosa of the mouth and lips, and in the skin of the lips, muzzle, and nose. These anatomic areas may also be injured by viruses, such as contagious ecthyma, caustic irritants, and photosensitization. The loss and eruption of the deciduous and permanent teeth interrupts the protective mucosal lining. Through areas of injury in the mouth, lips and face, the causative bacteria, especially those in feed, penetrate tissues innervated by the trigeminal and hypoglossal cranial nerves. The organisms enter branches of these nerves, grow and move along lymphatics of the trunks, and enter the brain stem, where they grow and spread into much of the medulla and pons. Throughout the infected nerves and brain stem, an inflammatory reaction is provoked, and neurons and fibers are damaged or destroyed. Clinical signs vary according to functions of damaged neurons. In severe cases, death probably comes from respiratory failure. Nonfatal cases slowly recover.

The mode of entry plays a role in the clinical manifestations of the disease. Entry via abrasions or lesions of the baccal mucosa, lips and nostrils, inhalation or conjunctival contamination leads to encephalitis. The septicemic, visceral, or latent infections develop from ingestion and inhalation. Following entry *L. monocytogenes* has a predilection to localize in the intestinal wall, placenta, and medulla oblongata. In septicemic or visceral listeriosis the organism causes focal lesions in liver, spleen, lungs, mammary glands, kidney, and placenta. If the organism invades via the alimentary tract, it may localize in the intestinal wall, especially in Peyer's patches, resulting in subclinical infections with persistent shedding of *L. monocytogenes*. These localized foci of infection lead to excretion of the organism into the external environment in feces, tears, milk, nasal secretions, urine, and uterine discharges perpetuating the listeric cycle.

The pregnant uterus is highly susceptible to listeric infection causing placentitis with a resultant fetal death, abortion, stillbirths, and neonatal deaths. Metritis follows abortion and is rarely complicated when the fetus and membranes are quickly and completely expelled. Future reproduction is not affected, although the organism may be shed in uterine discharges for a month or more.

CLINICAL SIGNS AND POSTMORTEM LESIONS. Following an incubation period of 2 to 3 weeks, sheep with listeric encephalitis become depressed, disoriented, and mildly febrile. Feeding is erratic and finally discontinued. The nose discharges mucus, and the eyes may show conjunctivitis. Walking may be in circles and, in some cases, pivoted around one hind limb. Facial paralysis—with drooping ear, dilated nostril, and lowered eyelid on the affected side—often develops. The head and neck often laterally flex away from the paralyzed side (Fig. 10-1).

Prostration, followed by coma and death, sometimes rapidly develops. During recumbency, even in coma, the affected animal constantly lies on one side only and, when forcibly changed to the opposite side, attempts resumption of the original position. The cerebrospinal fluid is opaque and increased in volume. Ewes with listeric placentitis abort during the last trimester of pregnancy. Following abortion, most ewes fully recover. The morbidity ranges from 1 to 20% and averages about 10%. The mortality of affected sheep is high, and the course varies from 1 to 3 days.

Intravenous inoculation of pregnant ewes in the second half of gestation is followed by abortion in 10 to 18 days. A blood-tinged vaginal discharge precedes abortion, and listeria are recovered from aborted fetuses. Microscopic changes include thrombosis, vasculitis, and neutrophil accumulation in the allantochorion. Focal hepatic necrosis, focal lung necrosis, and bronchopneumonia are microscopically evident in aborted fetuses. Lesions observed in natural cases of abortion are similar to those experimentally induced. This similarity indicates that listeria enter the maternal circulation and are carried to the uterus causing placentitis. The fetus becomes infected secondary to the placentitis uterine dysfunction.

Septicemia in lambs is characterized by dullness, inappetance, pyrexia, and diarrhea. Death may follow in 24 hours. In adults the

Fig. 10-1. Torticollis in a feedlot sheep with encephalitic listeriosis.

septicemic form causes listlessness, depression, a slight elevation in temperature (39 to 41.5°C), and diarrhea.

At necropsy, sheep with listeric encephalitis show no significant gross lesions, and ewes with listeric placentitis show edema and necrosis of cotyledons and brown discoloration of fluid around the placentomes. Microscopically, the trigeminal nerve shows neuritis, and the medulla and pons show foci of inflammation. Neutrophils, mononuclear macrophages, and lymphocytes predominate in each focus. Neurons in the reactive tissue may be degenerated and necrotic.

DIAGNOSIS.   Veterinarians diagnose listeric encephalitis from typical signs and laboratory findings. Circling movements, lateral inclination of the head and facial paralysis, especially in lambs feeding on silage, suggest the disease. Confirmation of both encephalitic and metritic listeriosis requires isolation and identification of *L. monocytogenes* from infected tissues. Isolations from ground brain stem may require prior storage at 4°C for several days.

The differential diagnosis of listeric encephalitis requires consideration of central nervous system diseases, such as polioencephalomalacia, rabies, pregnancy toxemia, focal symmetrical encephalomalacia, brain abscesses, and gid.

PREVENTION AND TREATMENT.   Listeriosis outbreaks are associated with a contaminated and stressful environment and most often in conjunction with the feeding of poor quality silage. Prevention is based, therefore, on reducing contamination of feed sources and the environment. Extreme care should be taken to prevent soil contamination of the grass or forages being ensiled. Adequate packing of the silage to exclude oxygen is necessary for fermentation and production of a low pH (below 5) to prevent multiplication of the organism. Dispose of moldy or poor quality silage. Do not feed silage to sheep if the pH exceeds 5, or ash content exceeds 70 mg/kg dry matter which is an indicator of high soil contamination. Strict adherence to sanitary feeding and watering practices will aid in preventing contamination. Feed and watering troughs should be constructed to prevent contamination. Excess or moldy silage should be removed from feed troughs daily. Affected animals should be isolated, and carcasses of fatal cases should be burned or buried in unslaked lime with disinfection of the contaminated liter.

The protection provided by the immune system is largely dependent on macrophages. Stress increases serum cortisol levels which in turn depresses macrophage activity; therefore elimination of a stressful environment will aid in preventing the disease. The humoral antibody protection has been of questionable benefit in protecting against listeric infections, although Bulgarian researchers have reported an efficacious attenuated vaccine containing strains of *L. monocytogenes*, serovar 1/2 and 4b.

L. monocytogenes is sensitive to ampicillin, erythromycin, gentamicin, penicillin, neomycin, and tetracycline. Penicillin in high doses is the most economical drug for use in large animals, although accounting for labor and the stress of daily restraining and treating the long acting forms of penicillin or tetracycline may be considered. The essentials of effective treatment are an early diagnosis with prompt and adequate treatment continued over a sufficient time period. Cases of advanced encephalitis do not respond, therefore early detection of the slightest nervous disorder with prompt treatment is essential. The response to treatment is directly proportional to the development of the infection. Treatment of clinically evident septicemic or visceral cases will rarely prevent abortions.

Penicillin G intramuscularly (44,000 units/kg, BID) for 7 to 14 days with a reduced level (22,000 units BID or SID) for an additional 7 to 14 days has been effective in cattle, even those in the recumbent state. Dehydration, acid-base imbalances and electrolyte disturbances must also be corrected. Although specific treatment regimens have not been studied, long acting antibiotics in high therapeutic dosages should provide satisfactory results without excess labor and handling.

Asahi, O.: Present situation of *Listeria* vaccine for animal use. In *Second Symposium on Listeric Infection.* Bozeman, Montana, Artcraft Printers, 1963a, pp. 49-56.

Asahi, O.: Pathogenesis of listeric encephalitis: invasion of nerve fibers by *Listeria monocytogenes.* In *Second Symposium on Listeric Infection.* Bozeman, Montana, Artcraft Printers, 1963b, pp. 99-108.

Barlow, R. and McGorum, B.: Ovine listerial encephalitis: Analysis, hypothesis and synthesis. Vet. Rec., *116*: 233-236, 1985.

Charlton, K.M. and Garcia, M.M.: Spontaneous listeric encephalitis and neuritis in sheep. Light microscope studies. Vet. Pathol., *14*:297-313, 1977.

Dennis, S.: Listeriosis. *Current Veterinary Therapy. 2. Food Animal Practice.* Edited by J. Howard. Philadelphia, W.B. Saunders Co., 1986, pp. 562-565.

Diplock, P.T.: Ovine listerel abortion. Aust. Vet. J., *33*:68-70, 1957.

Gill, D.A.: Ovine bacterial encephalitis (circling disease) and the bacterial genus *Listerella.* Aust. Vet. J., *13*:46, 1937.

Gill, D.A.: "Circling disease" of sheep in New Zealand. N.Z. Vet. J., *87*:60-74, 1931.

Govet, P., Girardeau, J.P., and Riou, Y.: Inhibition of *Listeria monocytogenes* by defined lactic microflora in gnotobiotic silages of lucerne, fescue, ryegrass and maize-influence of dry matter and temperature. Anim. Feed. Sci., *2*:297-305, 1977.

Graham, R., Levine, N.D., and Morrill, C.C.: Listerellosis in domestic animals. Univ. Illinois Agric. Exp. Stat. Bull. 499, 1943.

Gray, M.L.: Isolation of *Listeria monocytogenes* from oat silage. Science, *132*:1767-1768, 1960.

Gudding, R., Gronstol, H., and Larsen, H.: Vaccination against listeriosis in sheep. Vet. Rec., *117*:89-90, 1985.

Irvin, A.D.: The effect of pH on the multiplication of *Listeria monocytogenes* in grass silage media. Vet. Rec., *82*:115-116, 1968.

Low, C. and Linklater, K.: Listeriosis in sheep. In Pract., *7*:66-67, 1985.

Low, J. and Renton, C.: Septicemia, encephalitis and abortions in a housed flock of sheep caused by *Listeria monocytogenes* type 1/2. Vet. Rec., *116*: 147-150, 1985.

Meredith, C. and Schneider, D.: An outbreak of ovine listeriosis associated with poor flock management practices. J. S. Afr. Vet. Med. Assoc., *55*:55-56, 1984.

Molello, J.A. and Jensen, R.: Placental pathology. IV. Placental lesions of sheep experimentally infected with *Listeria monocytogenes.* AJVR, *25*:441-449, 1964.

Murray, E.G.D., Webb, R.A., and Swann, M.B.R.: A disease of rabbits characterized by a large mononuclear leucocytosis, caused by a hitherto undescribed bacillus *Bacterium monocytogenes.* J. Pathol. Bacteriol., *29*:407-439, 1926.

Njoku, C.O. and Dennis, S.M.: Listeric abortion studies in sheep. II. Fetoplacental changes. Cornell Vet., *63*: 171-192, 1973.

Njoku, C. and Dennis, S.M.: Listeric abortion studies in sheep. IV. Histopathological comparison of natural and experimental infection. Cornell Vet., *63*:211-219, 1973.

Njoku, C.O., Dennis, S.M., and Cooper, R.F.: Listeric abortion studies in sheep. I. Materno-fetal changes. Cornell Vet., *62*:608-627, 1972.

Njoku, C.O., Dennis, S.M., and Noordsy, J.L.: Listeric abortion studies in sheep. III. Fetoplacentalmyometrial interaction. Cornell Vet., *63*:193-210, 1973.

Ohara, R., et al.: Ontogeny of macrophage-mediated protection against *Listeria monocytogenes.* Infection and Immunity, *48*:763-768, 1985.

Palsson, P.A.: Relation of silage feeding to listeric infection in sheep. In *Second Symposium on Listeric Infection.* Bozeman, Montana, Artcraft Printers, 1963, pp. 74-84.

Paterson, J.S.: Studies on organisms of the genus *Listerella.* IV. An outbreak of abortion associated with the recovery of *Listerella* from the aborted fetuses. Vet. J., *96*:327-332, 1940.

Potel, J.: Active immunization against listeriosis with avirulent *Listeria monocytogenes.* In *Second Symposium on Listeric Infection.* Bozeman, Montana, Artcraft Printers, 1963, pp. 57-59.

Rebhun, W. and deLahunta, A.: Diagnosis and treatment of bovine listeriosis. JAVMA, *180*:395-398, 1982.

Sandvik, O., Molmen, K., and Kvaal, M.: Septicemic listeriosis in newborn lambs. Nord. Vet. Med., *10*:17-20, 1958.

Schleicher, J., Gunther, H., and Potel, K.: Experimental listeriosis in domestic and laboratory animals. XIV. Experimental infection of the hypoglossal nerve and in the ramification area of other cerebral nerves of sheep. Arch. Exp. Vet. Med., *22*:1027-1050, 1968.

Schleicher, J. and Urbaneck, D.: Experimental listeriosis in domestic and laboratory animals. X. Reproduction of cerebral listeriosis in sheep. Arch. Exp. Vet. Med., *20*:23-48, 1966.

Urbaneck, D.: Experimental listeriosis of domestic and laboratory animals. Arch. Exp. Vet. Med., *17*:35-53, 1963.

Volgin, I.P.: Survival of listeria outside the host. Veterinariia (Moscow), No. 10, *43*:14-17, 1966.

Wardrope, D. and Macleoid, N.: Outbreak of listeria meningoencephalitis in young lambs. Vet. Rec., *113*: 213-214.

Focal Symmetrical Encephalomalacia

(FSE)

Focal symmetrical encephalomalacia, a subacute noncontagious disease of sheep, is characterized clinically by incoordination, blindness, and prostration and pathologically by bilateral necrosis in the striatum and midbrain. It is suspected to be caused by sublethal amounts of toxin from *Clostridium perfringens* type D. Because FSE is sporadic and uncommon, it has minor importance to the sheep industry.

OCCURRENCE. FSE probably occurs in all breeds and sexes of nursing lambs 2 to 10 weeks of age and feedlot lambs 3 to 6 months of age. Nursing lambs develop the disease during late spring and early summer, and feedlot lambs during fall and winter. Most cases occur during outbreaks of enterotoxemia or as isolated instances among flock vaccinated against enterotoxemia.

Geographically, the disease occurs in New Zealand, Britain, South Africa, and the United States.

ETIOLOGY.   The cause of FSE is not known for certain. Development of the disease, however, during and following outbreaks of enterotoxemia, and the identification, in some cases of FSE, of epsilon toxin in the ileum, and the production of lesions by injecting the toxin have led investigators to suspect sublethal amounts of toxin from *C. perfringens* type D as the cause; however, scientists have not produced the disease by intravenous administration of sublethal doses of toxin.

CLINICAL SIGNS AND POSTMORTEM LESIONS. During an outbreak of enterotoxemia, some sheep may develop FSE. Some affected animals become prostrated, and others, with assistance, stand and move about. Recumbent animals, usually comatose, make paddling limb movements and extend the head in opisthotonos. Standing cases, dull and often blind, walk in circles and press their heads against firm objects.

The morbidity for FSE ranges up to 5% of animals with enterotoxemia, and the mortality of affected sheep exceeds 90%. Among sheep immunized against enterotoxemia, only sporadic cases of FSE develop. The course usually ranges from 2 to 6 days.

At necropsy, lesions are confined to the brain. Areas of necrosis, 1 to 15 mm in diameter, occur in the striatum (Fig. 10-2), thalami, midbrain, and cerebellar peduncles. The soft and often hemorrhagic lesions tend towards bilateral symmetry. In brains from clinically recovered cases, cavities replace the necrotic tissue.

Microscopically, the necrotic tissue usually contains hemorrhage. In lesions 3 to 4 days of age, compound granular cells infiltrate, and later, at the periphery of the lesions, astrocytes and capillaries proliferate.

Fig. 10-2.   Bilateral necrosis and hemorrhage (*A*) in corpus striatum of feedlot lamb with FSE.

DIAGNOSIS.   Veterinarians diagnose FSE on evidence of typical signs and lesions. Blindness, incoordination, prostration, paddling, and coma suggest the disease; finding gross brain lesions in fatal or sacrificed cases confirms the diagnosis.

The differential diagnosis requires consideration of polioencephalomalacia, brain abscesses, and tetanus. Polioencephalomalacia and FSE produce similar signs. At necropsy, however, the former shows multiple areas of necrosis in the cerebral cortex with, in some cases, areas of necrosis in the thalami. Brain abscesses are readily identified at necropsy. Tetanus produces general rigidity of voluntary muscles, and is associated with recent surgical procedures or injury.

PREVENTION AND TREATMENT.   If FSE is caused by clostridial exotoxin, immunization against enterotoxemia should prevent the disease, except for isolated animals that fail to acquire immunity. Treatment consists of isolating affected sheep, assisting them to stand, administering fluids and glucose, and providing accessible feed and water. Recovered animals, however, may not possess economic value.

Donnelley, W.J.C.: Focal symmetrical encephalomalacia of sheep in Ireland. Irish Vet. J., *25*:7-10, 1971.

Gill, D.A.: Report on pulpy kidney disease of lambs. Res. Rep. N.Z. Dep. Agric., 1933.

Griner, L.A.: Effects of *C. perfringens* type D toxin on sheep brain. AJVR, *22*:429, 1961.

Hartley, W.J.: A focal symmetrical encephalomalacia of lambs. N.Z. Vet. J., *4*:129-135, 1956.

Pienaar, J.G. and Thornton, D.J.: Focal symmetrical encephalomalacia in sheep in South Africa. J. S. Afr. Vet. Med. Assoc., 35:351-358, 1964.

Pierson, R.E.: Unpublished clinical records. Veterinary Hospital, Colorado State University, 1972.

Robertson, J.M. and Wilson, A.L.: Focal symmetrical encephalomalacia in lambs. Vet. Rec., 70:1201-1202, 1958.

Polioencephalomalacia

(PEM; polio; cerebrocortical necrosis)

Polioencephalomalacia, a noninfectious disease of sheep and cattle, is characterized clinically by blindness, depression, and incoordination and pathologically by necrosis of the cerebral cortex. It is caused by a deficiency or possibly by a poisoning.

Because of high incidence among feedlot lambs and wide distribution among pasture and farm flocks, the disease is of concern to the entire sheep industry and has major importance to feedlot enterprises. Economic losses result from deaths, loss of live weight, delayed marketing, extra labor, and the cost of treatment. Occurrence of the disease among pasture and feedlot cattle adds economic importance to the malady.

OCCURRENCE. PEM occurs in all breeds, sexes, and ages of sheep, but feedlot lambs 5 to 8 months of age have a higher incidence than do other ages and classes. Most feedlot cases develop during late autumn and early winter, and episodes often begin during and following periods of freezing temperatures. Outbreaks of PEM also develop in farm flocks following changes from overgrazed to lush pasture. In addition to sheep, PEM occurs in both pasture and feedlot cattle and goats.

Geographically, the disease occurs as an important problem in Australia, New Zealand, Britain, France, Germany, USSR, and America. In the United States, most cases occur in western states where feedlot enterprises have developed.

ETIOLOGY AND PATHOGENESIS. Although the specific and certain cause of PEM is not known, one hypothesis with considerable substantiation is that acute thiamine deficiency is an important factor in the cause. Although it is largely empiric and clinical, supporting evidence for the hypothesis is the successful treatment of affected sheep and cattle; even some moribund cases favorably respond to treatment. The high and prolonged blood levels of pyruvate following the intravenous administration of glucose and the rapid fall of pyruvate after injecting thiamine add validity.

The mechanism by which the thiamine deficiency develops is obscure because the dietary intake of thiamine appears to be more than adequate. Within the rumen, abnormally high concentrations of thiaminase from unusual microflora may destroy the vitamin before absorption can take place. Because thiamine has a central role in metabolizing carbohydrate, a deficiency of this compound results in blood accumulations of pyruvate and reduced transketolase and causes cerebral edema and neuronal degeneration and necrosis. These cellular changes in the region of the calcarine sulcus, an area of visual cortex, result in impaired vision.

During clinical recovery, necrotic tissue is removed by lysis and phagocytosis. A second hypothesis relates to the excessive intake of salt together with restricted intake of water. Presumably, recovered animals are fully susceptible to recurrence. This major neurologic disease of sheep and cattle merits intensive research to determine its full cause and pathogenesis.

CLINICAL SIGNS AND POSTMORTEM LESIONS. Feedlot sheep with PEM show two degrees of severity—acute and subacute. In the acute form, sheep may be found dead or prostrated. Live animals, even though comatose, may have hyperesthesia and develop involuntary contractions of some muscles, limb movements, and convulsive seizures. Death occurs after 1 to 2 days.

In subacute PEM, affected sheep are blind, incoordinated, and weak. Some early cases become isolated from the flock, and others are unable to walk or run with the herd. When disturbed, they may develop muscle contractions and tremors and fall to recumbency. Some obviously blind sheep move aimlessly, sometimes in circles, and hold their heads high as if staring above the horizon. Such animals, after 6 to 12 hours, usually become prostrated, develop opisthotonos (Fig. 10-3), and rise only with assistance. The body temperature and eye reflexes are normal, but saliva, presumably because of paralysis of deglutitive muscles, drips from the mouth.

The morbidity ranges from sporadic cases up to 10% of large flocks, and 50% of affected animals die. The course varies from 2 to 6 days.

At necropsy, primary lesions are limited to the central nervous system. The gray matter of the cerebral cortex contains necrotic foci that measure 1 to 20 mm in diameter; these areas are soft and usually faintly yellow (Fig. 10-4). In some cases, noncortical tissues, such as the thalamus, are involved. Fixing the entire brain in 10% formalin before sectioning facilitates evaluation of the lesions. Brains from recovered animals contain cavities or tissue disruptions from removal of necrotic cells.

Microscopic changes in diseased tissue are most obvious in nerve cells. Neurons show pericellular edema, shrinkage, chromatolysis, hyperchromatism, and eosinophilic cytoplasm. Lesions of 4 to 6 days' duration often contain compound granular cells, foci of gliosis, and areas of capillary proliferation. In recovered brains, the dead cells have been removed. Electron microscopic studies revealed three

Fig. 10-4. Soft, swollen, yellowish cerebral gyri in brain of a feedlot lamb with PEM.

basic types of lesions: compact necrosis, edema necrosis, and edema alone.

DIAGNOSIS.   Veterinarians diagnose PEM on evidence of signs and lesions. Blindness, normal temperature, and locomotor disturbances are suggestive signs. Cerebrospinal fluid (CSF) may aid in diagnosis. In acute cases the protein level of the CSF may be normal (<40 mg/100 ml) to slightly elevated with normal (<5 WBC/mm^3) numbers of cells. As the case progresses there is a mild to moderate increase in protein and white blood cell count. Thiamine diphosphate is essential in the formation of the enzyme transketolase. Therefore, in cases of PEM the blood transketolase activity declines before the onset of clinical signs and remains low unless treated. Although blood pyruvate and lactate levels may be elevated, the most consistent indications are a decrease in transketolase activity and an increase in fecal thiaminase activity. The response to treatment with thiamine may also be an aid in a tentative

Fig. 10-3. A feedlot lamb with PEM showing opisthotonos.

diagnosis. Finding gross and/or histopathologic foci of necrosis in gray matter of the cerebral cortex confirms the diagnosis.

The differential diagnosis requires consideration of focal symmetrical encephalomalacia, listeriosis, enterotoxemia, and tetanus.

PREVENTION AND TREATMENT. Affected sheep should be isolated and provided appropriate nursing care during treatment and convalescence. Parenteral administration of 10 mg/kg of thiamine hydrochloride twice daily for 2 to 3 days is an effective treatment. Other therapeutic agents may be beneficial in reducing cerebral edema and inflammation such as: (1) Dexamethazone (1 to 2 mg/kg) or prednisolone (1 to 4 mg/kg) intravenously as anti-inflammatory agents and, (2) Furosemide (0.5 to 1.0 mg/kg) as an anti-edema agent. During recovery feed and water are essential and easy access without competition should be provided. It may be necessary to correct dehydration and provide nutrients for anorectic animals. Fluids, electrolytes, and nutrients can be administered intravenously or via a stomach tube. For oral administration, electrolyte mixtures used for calf scours treatments, such as life-guard, provide both energy and electrolytes. These can be supplemented with 1 to 2 cups of corn syrup for added energy. Care must be taken to assure proper placement of the stomach tube to prevent inhalation pneumonia. Those cases which recover may take one to several days. Complete remission of depression, ataxia, and blindness depends on the extent of cerebral damage. Antibiotic support may be beneficial in severely depressed recumbent animals.

Bestetti, G. and Fonkhauser, R.: Comparative light and electron microscopic investigations on cerebrocortical necrosis in ruminants. Schweiz. Arch. Tierheilk. *121*:457-477, 1979.

Daly, F.J.: Polioencephalomalacia: Response to thiamine treatment in sheep and a cow. Aust. Vet. J., *44*:394, 1968.

Davies, E.T., et al.: Cerebrocortical necrosis. Vet. Rec., *77*:290, 1965.

Dill, S.: Polioencephalomalacia in ruminants. *Current Veterinary Therapy. 2. Food Animal Practice.* Edited by J. Howard. Philadelphia, W.B. Saunders Co., 1986, pp. 68-72.

Edwin, E.E., Lewis, G., and Allcroft, R.: Cerebrocortical necrosis. A hypothesis for the possible role of thiaminases in the pathogenesis. Vet. Rec., *83*:176-178, 1968a.

Edwin, E.E., Spence, J.B., and Woods, A.J.: Thiaminases and cerebrocortical necrosis. Vet. Rec., *83*:417, 1968b.

Espinasse, J., Redon, P., and Sinha, R.P.: Experimental induction of cerebrocortical necrosis in sheep. Rev. Med. Vet., *122*:529-545, 1971.

Hartley, W.J. and Kater, J.C.: Polio-encephalomalacia of sheep. N.Z. Vet. J., 7:75-80, 1959.

Jensen, R., Griner, L.A., and Adams, O.R.: Polioencephalomalacia of cattle and sheep. JAVMA, *129*:311-321, 1956.

Jubb, K.F.V. and Kennedy, P.C.: *Pathology of Domestic Animals.* Vol. 2. New York, Academic Press, 1970.

Lewis, G., et al.: Thiamine status of lambs in relation to cerebrocortical necrosis. Proc. Nutr. Soc., *26*:8-14, 1967.

Little, P.B. and Sorenson, D.K.: Bovine polioencephalomalacia, thrombolic meningoencephalitis and acute lead poisoning. JAVMA, *155*:1892-1903, 1969.

Loew, F.M. and Dunlop, R.H.: Induction of thiamine inadequacy and polioencephalomalacia in sheep. AJVR, *33*:2195-2205, 1972.

Loew, F.M. and Dunlop, R.H.: Blood thiamine concentrations in bovine polioencephalomalacia. Can. J. Comp. Med., *36*:345-347, 1972.

Pierson, R.E. and Jensen, R.: Polioencephalomalacia in feedlot lambs. JAVMA, *166*:257-259, 1975.

Pill, A.H.: Evidence of thiamine deficiency in calves with cerebrocortical necrosis. Vet. Rec., *81*:178-180, 1967.

Pill, A.H., Davies, E.T., Collings, D.F., and Venn, J.A.J.: Experimental reproduction of lesions of cerebrocortical necrosis. Vet. Rec., *78*:737-738, 1966.

Potel, K. and Seffner, W.: Cerebrocortical necrosis in sheep. Arch. Exp. Vet. Med., *21*:141-148, 1967.

Skrypnik, T.T.: A nervous disease of sheep (assoc. with thiamine deficiency). Veterinariia (Moscow), No. 4, 73-74, 1971.

Terlecki, S. and Markson, L.M.: Cerebrocortical necrosis in cattle and sheep. Vet. Rec., *73*:23-27, 1960.

Tournut, N., Labie, C., and Espinasse, J.: Identification of cerebrocortical necrosis in species of ruminants. Rev. Med. Vet., *118*:883-896, 1967.

11

DISEASES OF THE URINARY SYSTEM

Calculosis

(Urinary calculi; urolithiasis; waterbelly)

Calculosis, a metabolic disease of male sheep and cattle, is characterized by the formation within the urinary tract of struvitic concretions composed of matrix and minerals, by occlusion of the urethra, by retention of urine, and by rupture of the bladder or urethra. It is caused by dietary mineral imbalance and other factors. Because the disease occurs, often at high incidence, among feedlot wether lambs, it is of major economic importance to the lamb-fattening industry, and as lamb meat production is emphasized over wool production, calculosis will acquire major importance for the entire sheep industry. Financial waste results from death of affected sheep and condemnation of carcasses at emergency slaughter. The occurrence of calculosis in cattle and people adds both economic importance and public health significance to the condition.

OCCURRENCE. Although urinary calculi form in all breeds and sexes of sheep, calculosis, the disease, occurs only in males, usually feedlot wethers, 3 to 6 months of age. Most cases develop during autumn and winter, particularly following periods of inclement weather.

Geographically, calculosis occurs in most major sheep-producing countries, especially Australia, South Africa, and North America. In the United States, the disease has high incidence in arid and semiarid southwestern, western, and midwestern states where feedlot enterprises operate.

ETIOLOGY AND PATHOGENESIS. An interaction of dietary, hormonal, and environmental factors causes calculosis. Feedlot economics require operators to fatten and market lambs in minimum time; consequently, the fattening ration contains from 70 to 90% concentrate. The grains, especially sorghum or wheat, often have high phosphorus contents and a calcium-to-phosphorus ratio near 1. This dietary imbalance creates high serum and urine levels of phosphate and magnesium, and high urine levels of low-molecular-weight peptides.

Ureaplasma infections may contribute to the production of uroliths by increasing the urine pH thus providing an environment in which magnesium and phosphate ions are less soluble and ammonium ions are more available.

Animals on high grain diets with poorly balanced mineral composition (high in phosphorous and low in calcium) produce calculi for phosphatic (struvite) type containing calcium, magnesium, and ammonium phosphates. The pathogenesis of these struvite calculi is due to high concentrations of peptides, magnesium cations, and phosphate anions. The ammonium phosphate ion forms a nucleation center for binding repeating structural units. Mucoproteins, cell cast, or epithelial cells may contribute to the initiation of calculus formation, depending on the diet and environment of the animal.

205

In arid regions where grass or cereal hays are the main dietary components, silicate (SiO_2H_2O) calculi are commonly formed. Animals grazing subterranean clover, which is high in calcium, have calcite ($CaCO_3$) calculi. Plants high in oxalates, such as *Halogeton*, may contribute to calcite or weddelite ($CaC_2O_34 2H_2O$) calculi formation. Water deprivation has been incriminated as being conducive to calculogenesis, although research has failed to support this conclusion. Low ambient temperature and inclement weather probably contribute more to calculosis by increasing the urinary excretion of peptides and by reflexly contracting the penis and urethra.

Castration at an early age further aggravates the problem of urolithiasis when calculi are formed. Maturation of the urethra and urethral process is dependent upon testosterone, size, and maturity. The urethral process in the intact immature male is small in caliber, adhered to the wall of the prepuce, and remains so in the lamb until body weight reaches about 70 lb, irrespective of age. Early castration removes the hormonal influence on development of the penis, urethra, and urethral process, causing these structures to remain hypoplastic during the entire growing and fattening period.

In ewe lambs, all calculi easily discharge through the expansive urethra, but in wethers, descending calculi 1 to 2 mm in diameter may traumatize the delicate tissues and lodge either at the sigmoid flexure or at the urethral process of the hormonally hypoplastic and environmentally contracted urethra. Irritation and swelling at the point of lodgment tightly seal the calculus and occlude the urethra.

Gradually accumulating urine eventually ruptures the bladder or urethra. Following bladder rupture, urine spills into the peritoneal cavity, and reabsorption leads to uremia and finally death. Rupture of the urethra discharges urine into subcutaneous tissues of the abdomen and finally, through sinuses, to the exterior. Urine-infiltrated tissues may slough or become secondarily infected.

Some of the highest incidences of urolithiasis occurs in housed lambs in controlled environment not subjected to the inclement weather and adverse low temperatures. The fact remains that urolithiasis is a complex interaction of dietary, hormonal, and environmental factors.

CLINICAL SIGNS AND POSTMORTEM LESIONS. Calculosis begins with uneasiness, straining, and attempts to urinate, accompanied by rapid side-to-side movements of the tail. In some wethers, small amounts of urine leak from the prepuce and, after evaporating, leave deposits of crystals on preputial hairs. Later, affected animals refuse food and water, isolate from the flock, and kick at the abdomen. After rupture of the bladder, the abdomen distends noticeably. Following rupture of the urethra, the subcutaneous tissues of the abdomen thicken and devitalize; eventually, urine leaks through one or more sinuses of the skin. Most cases develop 4 to 6 weeks after animals enter the fattening pens. Among feedlot wethers, the morbidity ranges up to 20%, and most affected animals die unless successfully treated. The course varies from 1 to 2 weeks.

At necropsy of an animal with a ruptured bladder, the abdominal cavity contains several liters of urine, and the bladder shows a rent, which may be sealed with fibrin. Beginning hydronephrosis may be evident. In cases with rupture of the urethra, urine infiltrates the abdominal wall. Dissection of the bladder and urethra reveals one or more calculi in the urethra at the sigmoid flexure or at the urethral process (Figs. 11-1 and 11-2). Proximal to the occlusion, the urethra is necrotic and hemorrhagic. Additional calculi may be found in the bladder. Urinous odors emanate from the tissues.

DIAGNOSIS. Veterinarians diagnose calculosis on evidence of typical signs and lesions. Uneasiness, kicking the abdomen, and abdominal distention are indicative signs. Finding urine in the abdominal cavity or tissues and an occluding calculus in the urethra confirms the diagnosis.

The differential diagnosis requires consideration of bloat, perforating ulcers, and acidosis.

PREVENTION. Knowledge of the type and composition of crystals involved is necessary

Fig. 11-1. Dissected urethra plugged with crystalline calculi containing 16% Mg, 12% P, 3.6% Ca, and 2% protein. × 1.1.

Fig. 11-2. Dissected urethral process filled with crystalline calculi (a). × 1.6.

for establishing a preventive program. The most common calculi in the United States are those associated with grain rations high in dietary phosphorous. Prevention of this type of urolithiasis is by nutritional and management alterations.

1. Provide a 2:1 calcium-to-phosphorous ratio in the total ration. Calcium chloride should be added to the diet to adjust the calcium-to-phosphorous ratio.

2. Add common salt (NaCl) to the ration, 1 to 4% is usually adequate. Up to 9% NaCl can be added to the ration before feed consumption or rate of gain is affected. Prevention is attributed to an ionic action rather than diuresis from increased water intake.

3. Provide an ample supply of fresh potable water.

4. The addition of ammonium chloride (2% of the concentrate ration) will aid in preventing calculosis. Ammonium chloride has been incriminated in initiating excessive coughing, which contributes to rectal prolapse.

5. A well-balanced diet that includes adequate amounts of vitamin A.

TREATMENT. Economic considerations usually restrict surgical treatment of urolithiasis. Some simple procedures can be accomplished without expenditure of much money or time. If the calculus is located in the urethral process, simply cut off the process with scissors. Calculi that lodge at the sigmoid flexure require exteriorization of the penis at the proximal part of the sigmoid flexure. In early cases, the calculi may be palpated and removed by an incision into the urethra at the sight of the calculus.

If the urethra is patent, as determined by a saline flush, the urethra can be sutured and returned to its normal position with a simple skin closure. In more complicated cases, it may be necessary to exteriorize the penis and amputate it at the proximal portion of the sigmoid flexure or the perineal area. The amputated portion is sutured to the exterior with the skin closure around the amputated stump. A more cosmetically acceptable perineal urethrostomy may be performed on pet wethers. Satisfactory regional anesthesia is attained by injecting 1 to 2 ml of 2% lidocaine into the epidural space at the lumbosacral junction.

Struvite crystals associated with high-grain rations are soluble at pH of less than 6.8. Prior to complete obstruction, withholding feed for 24 hours in conjunction with oral dosing of ammonium chloride (7 to 10 mg per head per day for a 30-kg lamb) is a satisfactory method of acidifying the urine. Ammonium chloride should also be administered for 7 to 10 days following surgical treatment of urolithiasis, as it is common for reobstruction to occur as a result of the presence of multiple calculi in the bladder. Smooth muscle relaxants to relieve the spasm around the calculi and allow its passage have limited success. If treatment is to be effective, an early diagnosis and immediate initiation of therapy must be accomplished early in the course of the disease. Owing to the complexity of the condition, many treatments are of limited value. Knowledge of the chemical composition of the urolith, nutritional and environmental factors which influence initiation of urolith formation is important in developing a prevention program or subsequent treatment.

Belonje, P.C.: I. An investigation into a problem of urinary calculi in Merino wethers. J. S. Afr. Vet. Med. Assoc., 36:377-379, 1965.

Bushman, D.H., Emrick, R.J., and Embry, L.B.: Experimentally induced ovine plastic urolithiasis: relationships involving dietary calcium, phosphorus and magnesium. J. Nutr., 87:499-504, 1965.

Chow, F.H.C., Hamar, D.W., and Udall, R.H.: Studies on urolithiasis. XI. Interaction of urine polyelectrolytes and inorganic ions. Invest. Urol., 5:557-567, 1968.

Chow, F.H.C., Hamar, D.W., and Udall, R.H.: Studies on urolithiasis. XII. Association of urine polyelectrolytes. Biochem. Med., 2:337-344, 1969.

Crookshank, H.R., Robbins, J.D., and Kunkel, H.O.: Relationship of dietary mineral intake to serum mineral level and the incidence of urinary calculi in lambs. J. Anim. Sci., 26:1179-1185, 1967.

Elam, C.J., Ham, W.E., and Schneider, B.H.: Influence of dietary sodium chloride on incidence of urinary calculi in sheep. Proc. Soc. Exp. Biol. Med., 95:769-772, 1957.

Emrick, R.J. and Embry, L.B.: Effects of calcium and phosphorus levels and diethylstilbestrol on urinary calculi incidence and feedlot performance in lambs. J. Anim. Sci., 23:1079-1083, 1964.

Godwin, I. and Williams, V.: Urinary calculi formation in sheep on high wheat grain diets. Aust. J. Agric. Res., 33:843-855, 1982.

Gohar, H. and Shokry, M.: Efficacy of sodium chloride in prevention of sheep urolithiasis. Bull. Anim. Hlth. Prod. Afr., 29:321-324, 1981.

Hoar, D.W., Emerick, R.J., and Embry, L.B.: Influence of calcium source, phosphorus level and acid-base-forming effects of diet on feedlot performance and urinary calculi formation in lambs. J. Anim. Sci., 31:118-125, 1970a.

Hoar, D.W., Emerick, R.J., and Embry, L.B.: Potassium, phosphorus and calcium interrelationships influencing feedlot performance and phosphatic urolithiasis in lambs. J. Anim. Sci., 30:597-600, 1970b.

Kimberling, C. and Arnold, K.: Diseases of the urinary system of sheep and goats. Vet. Clin. N. Am.: Large Animal Practice, 5:637-655, 1983.

Livingston, C., Calhoun, M., Gauer, B., and Baldwin, B.: Effect of experimental infections with ovine ureaplasma upon the development of uroliths in feedlot lambs. Israel J. Med. Sci., 20:958-961, 1984.

McIntosh, G.H.: Urolithiasis in animals. Aust. Vet. J., 54:267-271, 1978.

Mia, A.S. and Cornelius, C.E.: Ruminal urolithiasis. VI. Fractionation of ovine urinary biocolloids by gel filtration. Invest. Urol., 1:439-445, 1964.

Newsom, I.E., Tobiska, J.W., and Osland, H.B.: The effect of rations on the production of urinary calculi in sheep. Colorado Agric. Exp. Stat. Tech. Bull. 31, 1943.

Packett, L.V. and Coburn S.P.: Urine proteins in nutritionally induced ovine urolithiasis. AJVR, 26:112-119, 1965.

Packett, L.V. and Hauschild, J.P.: Phosphorus, calcium and magnesium relationships in ovine urolithiasis. J. Nutr., 84:185-190, 1964.

Packett, L.V., Lineberger, R.O., and Jackson, H.D.: Mineral studies in ovine phosphatic urolithiasis. J. Anim. Sci., 27:1716-1721, 1968.

Udall, R.H.: Studies on urolithiasis. III. The control by force feeding sodium chloride. AJVR, 20:423-425, 1959a.

Udall, R.H.: Studies on urolithiasis. IV. The effects of the ration on the predisposition as measured by the urinary mucoproteins. AJVR, 20:426-429, 1959b.

Udall, R.H. and Chow, F.H.C.: The etiology and control of urolithiasis. Adv. Vet. Sci., 13:29-57, 1969.

Udall, R.H. and Chow, F.H.C.: Studies on urolithiasis. VII. The effects of sodium, potassium and chloride ions in the control of urinary calculi. Cornell Vet., 55:538-544, 1965a.

Udall, R.H., Seger, C.L., and Chow, F.H.C.: Mechanism of action of sodium chloride in the control of urinary calculi. Cornell Vet., 60:198-203, 1965b.

PART III DISEASES OF ADULT SHEEP

12

DISEASES OF THE DIGESTIVE SYSTEM

Dental Attrition

(Tooth wear)

Dental attrition, a rapid and excessive wear of teeth, is characterized by inefficient prehension, mastication, and utilization of feed and by unthriftiness, unprofitability, and unmarketability, and is caused by abrasion of soft teeth by diets. This variable condition exists to some extent in most grazing sheep and therefore causes variable amounts of financial waste and industrial concern. Economic losses result from inefficient use of feed, lowered production of meat and wool, and premature culling of affected animals. Because of dental attrition, range sheep probably average 2 years less in productivity than do farm-fed sheep. Occurrence of the condition also among grazing goats and cattle adds economic importance and agricultural interest to the general problem.

OCCURRENCE. Dental attrition occurs in all types of sheep, but breeding ewes 5 years of age and older manifest a higher incidence than do other categories of sheep. Ewes usually show the condition after grazing forage-deficient pastures and ranges throughout several successive winters. Geographically, the condition occurs at a high rate among grazing sheep of arid and semiarid ranges of the western and southwestern United States and other countries, and among sheep grazing sandy pastures of New Zealand, Australia, Scotland, and other sheep-producing countries.

ETIOLOGY AND PATHOGENESIS. Masticating soil and sand along with prehended forage causes dental attrition. Calcium deficiencies with softness of tooth enamel and dentine accelerate the rate of wear, and malalignment may predispose individual teeth to excessive wear.

The pathogenesis of dental attrition relates to both tooth and diet quality. Sheep subsisting on calcium-deficient diets or calcium/phosphorus-unbalanced diets during their first 18 months develop defective tooth enamel and dentine, and ewes supporting annual pregnancies lose dental calcium; tooth softness varies directly with the degree of early deficiency and with the extent of gestational decalcification.

While grazing, especially during winters when grass and other forage are short, sheep ingest and masticate soil and sand along with grass. Prehension and mastication abrade and wear the incisor and molar teeth. The rate of wear varies directly with the volume of ingested soil and sand and with tooth softness. Continuation of the process gradually shortens the crowns and dulls the cutting and grinding surfaces. Eventually, producers cull and market affected animals because of their inability to graze. If not culled, such sheep become malnourished and die from exhaustion or intercurrent diseases.

CLINICAL SIGNS AND LESIONS. Sheep with dental attrition fastidiously graze and slowly masticate feed, and, because of tooth sensitivity, they inadequately consume cold water. Consequently, they gradually lose live weight, become weak, and develop anemia. Emaciation supervenes, accelerated by pregnancy, and death occurs from starvation, pneumonia, pregnancy disease, or carnivorous predation. Examination of the mouth reveals worn, loosened, fractured, or missing teeth (Fig. 12-1). Uneven wear may erode into gum and bone.

DIAGNOSIS. Veterinarians and producers diagnose dental attrition from typical signs and lesions. Unthriftiness in grazing sheep 5 years of age and older strongly suggests dental diseases, including attrition. Finding worn incisor and molar teeth at oral examination confirms the diagnosis. The differential diagnosis requires consideration of periodontal disease and chronic progressive pneumonia.

PREVENTION. Producers prevent dental attrition by judicious herd management. Calcium deficiencies in growing sheep should be avoided by providing balanced diets; the inclusion of 1% ground limestone in the ration supplies adequate calcium. Sufficient feed, by supplement if necessary, should be provided on winter ranges and pastures; this practice reduces the amount of ingested soil and thus decelerates tooth attrition. During autumn, all grazing sheep should be examined for unsound teeth, and all animals showing excessive dental wear should be culled and marketed or maintained on preground feed.

Fig. 12-1. Attrition of incisor teeth from an adult ewe. × 1.7.

Arnold, G.W., McManus, W.R., and Bush, I.G.: Teeth wear. Aust. J. Agric. Anim. Husb., 6:101-107, 1966.

Franklin, M.C.: Influence of diet on dental development in sheep. Aust. CSIRO Bull., 1950, p. 252.

Healey, W.B., Cutress, T.W., and Michie, C.: Reduction of soil ingestion and tooth wear by supplemental feeding. N.Z. J. Agric. Res., 10:201-209, 1967.

Healey, W.B. and Ludwig, T.G.: Wear of sheep's teeth. I. Role of ingested soil. N.Z. J. Agric. Res., 8:737-752, 1965.

McRoberts, M.R., Hill, R., and Dalgarno, A.C.: Effects of deficient diets on teeth of growing sheep. J. Agric. Sci. (Cambridge), 65:1-27, 1965.

Periodontal Disease

(PD; periodontitis; periodontosis)

Periodontal disease, a chronic infection in the sockets of mandibular teeth, is characterized clinically by loosening, lengthening, wearing, spreading, malocclusion, and expulsion of individual teeth and pathologically by destruction of the periodontal ligament and osteopathy. The disease is probably caused by nutritional deficiencies and oral bacteria. Because the disease distributes widely, attacks continuously, and frequently incapacitates affected animals, it concerns the entire sheep industry. Economic losses result from unthriftiness, inefficient use of feed, premature culling, and reduced production of meat and wool. Because its development is insidious and its attack rate low, the malady attracts little research investment and scientific attention. Occurrence also in cattle adds economic importance to the disease.

OCCURRENCE. PD probably occurs in all breeds and sexes of sheep, but ewes 3 years of age and older have a higher incidence than do other age groups. Sheep from some enterprises consistently experience a higher incidence than do sheep from others; these variances, however, may relate to differences in management practices. The disease probably begins in, and certainly continues through, all seasons. Geographically, PD is prominent in New Zealand, Scotland, the United States, and possibly other sheep-producing countries.

ETIOLOGY AND PATHOGENESIS. Mineral deficiencies, such as calcium inadequacies, may degenerate and predispose the periodontal tissues, and oral bacteria, such as diphtheroids, may infect and destroy these tissues.

The periodontal tissues (periodontium) consist of the epithelium of the gum, cementum of the tooth, fibers of the periodontal ligament, and bone of the alveolus. At the gingival sulcus, epithelium normally attaches to the enamel or cementum and protectively covers the subjacent tissues. Fibers of the ligament, attached centrally to the cementum and peripherally to the bone, suspend the tooth in its socket and absorb energy from occlusal pressures.

Initial pathologic changes probably begin with degeneration of cementum, periodontal fibers, and bone, or possibly with gingivitis. A small calculus then attaches to the enamel at the gingival sulcus. Movements of the tooth and calculus erode and ulcerate the epithelium. Bacteria enter through the ulcer and destroy periodontal fibers. Epithelium proliferates and, more apically, reattaches to the cementum. Again, new calculus precipitates on the cementum, movements of the tooth and calculus ulcerate the epithelium, infection destroys more ligamental fibers, and epithelium proliferates and, still more apically, reattaches to cementum.

Repetitions of this process move the point of epithelial attachment apically and thus create a periodontal pocket 1 to 2 mm deep around all or part of the circumference of the affected tooth. Bacteria, exudate, and feed accumulate in the pocket and accelerate the ulceration and apical advancement of the point of epithelial attachment. Eventually, the pocket reaches the tooth apex. The large pocket then consists of a cavity with cementum as an inner wall and epithelium-covered connective tissue as an outer wall. During the entire time of tissue destruction and pocket formation, alveolar bone, especially at its crest, gradually resorbs and thereby widens the distance between cementum and bone. Granulation tissue, in some areas covered with epithelium, forms in this space and exerts ejective force on the loosened tooth.

The pathologic changes may affect either of several complications. The tooth may move upward and outward, or it may retain normal position, held by opposing teeth, and jam into its socket because of occlusal pressure. The invading microorganisms may form an abscess at the apex with a tract to the exterior or cause infection in the marrow. Following expulsion of the tooth, the socket fills with granulation tissue and is covered over with epithelium. The disease usually does not spread to other teeth.

CLINICAL SIGNS AND POSTMORTEM LESIONS. Clinical signs vary directly with the number of teeth affected and the extent of disease development. Incisor and/or cheek teeth may be affected. In early stages, prehension and mastication may be nearly normal. Examination of the mouth, however, may reveal lengthening of affected teeth, beginning of malocclusion, recession of gums, and periodontal pockets. Digital pressure may express exudate around the tooth. In advanced stages, prehension and

Fig. 12-2. Heavy calculosis and beginning gingival recession (a) in molar teeth. × 1.5.

mastication, as well as drinking cold water, are quantitatively reduced because these functions inflict pain. During idle chewing movements, drops of saliva and fragments of food dribble from the mouth. The animal may fail to gain and may lose weight. Palpation of the maxilla and mandible may disclose bony enlargements.

Oral examination shows incisors that are lengthened beyond the front of the dental pad, widely spread, loose, and sometimes missing. Gums may be receded or focally hypertrophied, and the mandibular body may be thickened and disfigured. Affected cheek teeth may also show deposits of calculus, periodontal pockets containing feed and exudate, loosenings, displacements, and partial or complete expulsions (Fig. 12-2). Incidence varies up to 10%, and the course extends through many months.

At necropsy, dissection may show apical abscesses with tracts to the surface (Fig. 12-3), bone enlargements, and dentigerous cysts.

DIAGNOSIS. Veterinarians diagnose PD on evidence of typical signs and lesions. A detailed oral examination is essential. The differential diagnosis requires consideration of (1) uneven dental wear, fractures, foreign bodies, and infections, (2) oral infections, injuries, and neoplasm, (3) pharyngeal ulcers, infections,

injuries, and paralyses, and (4) esophageal chokes.

PREVENTION AND TREATMENT. Producers prevent PD by providing adequate and balanced diets and by culling affected animals at least once annually. Treatment consists of extraction of loose teeth and provision of chopped or ground feed.

Armstrong, M.C.: Paradontal disease of sheep in South Canterbury. N.Z. J. Agric., *100*:429-431, 1960.
Bruère, A.N., et al.: Syndrome of dental abnormalities of sheep. I. Clinical aspects. N.Z. Vet. J. 27:152-158, 1979.
Dalgarno, A.C. and Hill, R.: Histological appearance of periodontal tissues associated with loss of incisor teeth in sheep. Res. Vet. Sci., 2:107-110, 1961.
Hart, E.K. and MacKinnon, M.M.: Enzootic paradontal disease in adult sheep. N.Z. Vet. J., 6:118-123, 1958.
MacKinnon, M.M.: Pathology of enzootic paradontal disease of mature sheep. N.Z. Vet. J., 7:18-26, 1959.
Orr, M.B., et al.: Syndrome of dental abnormalities of sheep. II. Pathology and radiology. N.Z. Vet. J., 27:276-278, 1979.
Salisbury, R.M., Armstrong, M.C., and Gray, K.G.: Ulceromembranous gingivitis in sheep. N.Z. Vet. J., 1:51-52, 1953.

Actinobacillosis

Actinobacillosis, a chronic infectious but noncontagious disease of sheep and cattle, is characterized by purulent granulomas in soft tissues of the head and, rarely, other organs and is caused by *Actinobacillus lignieresii*. Because the general incidence of this disease is sporadic and low, it is of little economic importance to the sheep industry, but some individual enterprises encounter high incidence and significant waste. Losses result from incapacitation of breeding rams and ultimate death of most infected sheep. Occurrence of the disease more often among cattle and occasionally in people adds both economic importance and public health significance to the malady.

OCCURRENCE. Actinobacillosis occurs in all breeds and sexes of sheep beyond weaning age. The incidence is higher among breeding rams and ewes than among other classes of sheep. Most cases develop during summer, autumn, and winter when grass awns commonly occur in grazed feed and fed hay. Geographically, the disease sporadically occurs

Fig. 12-3. Lingual surface of right dissected mandible, showing periodontal disease around a partially ejected molar (*a*) and granulation tissue (*b*) deep to the tooth.

in sheep of the western United States, Australia, Britain, USSR, Europe, South Africa, North Africa, Iceland, Bolivia, Peru, and New Zealand.

ETIOLOGY AND PATHOGENESIS. The causative organism, *Actinobacillus lignieresii,* is a pleomorphic, nonmotile, nonspore-forming, nontoxin-forming, gram-negative rod. In cultures, coccoid and rod forms measures 1 to 15 × 0.4 μm. Although aerobic, the organisms grow better in an atmosphere of 10% carbon dioxide. Even though the pathogens contain six antigenic types, most ovine strains belong to types 2, 3, and 4, and bovine strains to type 1. In infected tissues, the bacteria form rosettes, which are bosselated colonies measuring less than 1 mm in diameter. The organisms are demonstrable in stained smears of crushed rosettes. These small granules are similar to those formed by *Actinomyces.* The difference being that in the center of the granule the filamentous mycelium of *Actinobacillus ligniersi* are gram-negative. The organism is killed by heating to 62°C for 10 minutes and rapidly succumbs to drying. It remains virulent for a month or two in pus. *Actinobacillus ligniersi* is susceptible to chloramphenical and variable susceptibility to streptomycin, chlortetracycline, and oxytetracycline with weak susceptibility to sulfathiazole and resistant to penicillin.

Probably, *A. lignierseii* is widely distributed in soil and manure. In many healthy cattle and possibly in sheep, it resides on the mucous membranes of the mouth, forestomachs, abomasum, intestines, nose, larynx, and skin, but is unable to invade healthy intact mucosa and skin. Tissue penetration probably takes place through points of injury from grass awns and other foreign bodies.

In deep noncovering tissues, the organism produces a chronic inflammation, known as infectious granuloma. Exudate accumulates and fibrous connective tissue proliferates around each of many infected loci. Sinus tracts often develop and intermittently discharge pus to the surface. Frequently, the infection spreads through afferent lymphatics to regional lymph nodes, where secondary infection develops. From here, spread may continue through the lymphatic chain and eventually enter the blood. Hematogenous dissemination establishes infection in the lungs and many other organs. The disease is progressive and fatal unless properly treated.

CLINICAL SIGNS AND POSTMORTEM LESIONS. Affected sheep contain one or more firm nodules, up to 5 cm in diameter, in thickened subcutaneous tissues of the lower lip and other parts of the face. Sinus tracts, extending from some nodules, discharge purulent exudate to the surface. Sheep in advanced stages of the disease are unable to eat and consequently become emaciated, weak, and often affected with intercurrent diseases, such as pneumonia.

The morbidity in infected flocks ranges up to 33%. In the United States, however, an average of 10.5 million sheep were annually slaughtered and federally inspected from 1967 to 1971 without encountering any actinobacillosis. The eventual mortality is high, and the course varies from weeks to months.

At necropsy, facial tissues of emaciated carcasses contain abscess-like lesions 1 to 5 cm in diameter, and sinus tracts interconnect abscesses and surfaces. The green tenacious pus discharges to the skin surface, where it forms scabs. Grass awns may be identified in tissue. Parotid and submaxillary lymph nodes may be secondarily infected. Similar lesions may exist in nasal mucosa, epididymis, udder, and lungs. Histopathologically, purulent exudate containing rosettes is surrounded by epithelioid cells, giant cells, and fibrous connective tissue.

DIAGNOSIS. Veterinarians diagnose actinobacillosis from the characteristic facial lesions and from finding rosettes in the exudate. The differential diagnosis must consider contagious ecthyma and caseous lymphadenitis.

PREVENTION AND TREATMENT. Producers prevent some cases of actinobacillosis by avoiding use of feed contaminated with excessive amounts of penetrating grass awns and cactus thorns. Effective treatment consists of surgical drainage and of weekly intravenous administrations of 80 mg/kg of a 10% solution of sodium iodide, or daily administration of dihydrostreptomycin at the rate of 20 mg/kg of body weight for 7 to 10 days.

Animal Health Yearbook. FAO-WHO-OIE (Italy), 1970.

Davis, C.L. and Stiles, G.W.: Actinobacillosis in rams. JAVMA, 95:754, 1939.

Federal Meat Inspection. Statistical summaries, USDA, 1967-1971.

Frost, B.A.: Thesis. Cornell University Library, 1940.

Fubini, S. and Campbell, S.: External lumps on sheep and goats. Vet. Clin. N. Am., 5:457-476, 1983.

Hayston, J.T.: Actinobacillosis in sheep. Aust. Vet. J., 24:64-66, 1948.

Johnson, K.G.: Nasal actinobacillosis in sheep. Aust. Vet. J., 30:105-106, 1954.

Kirk-Head, C. and Mullowney, P.: Nonparasitic skin diseases of sheep. Current Veterinary Therapy. Food Animal Practice. Edited by J. Howard. Philadelphia, W.B. Saunders Co., 1986.

Laws, L. and Elder, J.E.: Ovine epididymoorchitis caused by Actinobacillosis lignieresii. Aust. Vet. J., 45:384, 1969a.

Laws, L. and Elder, J.E.: Mastitis in sheep caused by Actinobacillus lignieresii. Aust. Vet. J., 45:401-403, 1969b.

Marsh, H. and Wilkins, H.W.: Actinobacillosis in sheep. JAVMA, 94:363-364, 1939.

Phillips, J.E.: The antigenic structure and serological typing of Actinobacillosis lignieresii. J. Pathol. Bacteriol., 93:463-475, 1967.

Wilson, G.: Actinomyces, Nocardia and Actinobacillus. In Topley and Wilson's Principles of Bacteriology, Virology and Immunity. 7th Edition. Baltimore, Williams & Wilkins, 1983-1984.

Bluetongue

(BT; catarrhal fever; sore muzzle)

Bluetongue, an acute noncontagious disease, is characterized by fever, leukopenia, stomatitis, panpoditis, and myositis, and is caused by a fly-transmitted virus. Although unmeasured, the biologic and financial waste from BT is extensive. Economic losses result from prolonged incapacitation of affected sheep, deaths, fetal deformities, damaged wool, possible spread to cattle, and the cost of preventive programs. Of equal economic significance is the loss of sales of breeding stock from endemic areas and the international sales of semen from bulls due to the presence of BT in the United States. The disease name derives from a clinical sign observed in some sheep.

OCCURRENCE. Bluetongue occurs in most species of ruminants, both domestic and wild. Among sheep, all breeds, sexes, and ages are susceptible, but breeds native to endemic areas probably are more resistant than breeds from BT-free regions. Native African and Asiatic breeds, such as Karakul and Black Head Persian, are more resistant than European breeds. Although most ruminants can be attacked, sheep appear to be the most susceptible, and the disease has major economic importance with this species. The susceptibilities of goats and cattle are approximately equal. Among wild ruminants, deer appear to be highly susceptible and may die from the disease. Antelope, bighorn, sheep, and moose are also susceptible, but the degree is unknown.

The seasonal variance of BT relates to availability of the vector. In America and other parts of the temperate zone the disease occurs during late summer and early fall. During summers of high rainfall, the disease appears early in the season. In the neotropics most animals become infected in late summer and fall.

During the first half-century of BT history, the disease was limited to Africa. Since 1949, however, it has been identified by virus isolation in Cyprus, Palestine, Syria, Turkey, United States, Portugal, Spain, and West Pakistan. The most recent extensions have been in Australia, the South American countries of Brazil, Guyana, Suriname, and the Caribbean countries of Jamaica, St. Kitts/Nevis, Antigua, St. Lucia, Barbados, Grenada, Trinidad, Tobago and the Bahamas.

ETIOLOGY AND PATHOGENESIS. The Bluetongue virus (BTV) is a member of the orbi virus genus, family Reoviridae with a buoyant density of 1.36 g/cm^3 in cesium chloride, a sedimentation rate of 550 s, and a diameter of 69 nm. It consists of a double-layered capsid containing a core particle, with a clearly defined capsomere structure surrounded by a structureless, diffuse outer layer. BTV possesses a double-stranded RNA (ds RNA) genome consisting of 10 segments. The segments can be separated into individual species by polyacrylamide gel electrophoresis (PAGE). The BTV contains seven polypeptides. Four of these polypeptides are major components and three are minor components of the virus. These components are involved in genetic changes involving the incidence of point mutations in the viral genome and genetic shift involving RNA segment reassortment which occur among Bluetongue viruses in nature. The relationship between the serotypes is determined by oligonucleotide fingerprinting technique of the ds RNA segments and peptide mapping of the polypeptides. Although not completely understood, the relationships of these viral components hold the answers to infectivity, antigenicity, stimulation of the immune system and ultimately selection of the antigenic determinants necessary to synthesize a subunit vaccine for the control of all BTV serotypes. There are currently 23 BTV serotypes recognized throughout the world with serotypes 2, 10, 11, 13, and 17 being identified in the United States. Serotype BTV 2 was the most recently (1983) announced serotype being isolated from a sentinel cattle herd in Florida.

BT virus is remarkably stable. Virus infectivity is relatively stable to lipid solvents and sodium deoxycholate. The non-purified virus is reasonably thermostable. In citrated blood or properly prepared splenic tissue stored at 4°C, infectivity persists for years. Even at room temperature, virus in citrated blood has remained viable for more than 25 years. Minimal losses in titer result from lyophilization and storage at −70°C. A number of serotypes have shown an inactivation of BTV infectivity below pH 6.5. At 60°C, the virus is inactivated in 30 minutes.

Outside the ruminant host and the vector insect, the virus adapts to and grows in artificial systems. In chicken eggs embryonated 8 days, it grows and concentrates at 33.5°C; embryo death usually occurs 3 to 4 days after inoculation. Following intracerebral inoculation of suckling mice, the virus grows in the central nervous system. In culture systems, the virus grows in cells of sheep kidney, bovine kidney, bovine lymph node, lamb testicle, Chang liver, Hela clones, and human amnion.

Culicoides breed in many habitats, particularly damp, muddy areas, running streams and fecal matter. Because of nocturnal feeding habits, the *Culicoides* attack the host sheep on night pastures or open pens. The females take a blood meal every 3 to 4 days during their life

which can be up to 70 days. The virus replicates in the cells in the hemocoel and salivary glands of the *Culicoides* after blood engorgement. After 7 to 10 days the virus is excreted in the saliva at which time transmission is possible. Once in the host animal the virus penetrates into the cell by pinocytosis. The primary virus replication appears to occur in the local draining lymph nodes, is disseminated through the blood with a second phase of generalized virus replication which is responsible for the rapid increase in viremic levels reaching a peak in about 7 days, and continues for around 30 days postinfection. A maximum febrile response (42 to 43°C) occurs at about the same time as the peak viremia and lasts from 24 to 48 hours. The viremic level drops to a low level but may persist for several months. A marked leukopenia develops about day 3 and lasts for about 5 to 7 days.

In North America the *Culicoides* gnat (*Culicoides varipennis*) (Fig. 12-4) is the only known vector in the biologic transmission of BTV. In Africa and western Asia, *Culicoides imicola* is responsible for transmission. In southern Florida, the Caribbean and South America neither *Culicoides varipennis* nor *Culicoides imicola* exist. The vector is unknown but *Culicoides insignis* is a possibility. Transovarian passage

Fig. 12-4. *Culicoides.* × 29. (Courtesy of James Kretzmeir)

has not been determined but could potentially be a method in continued propagation and genetic variation of BTV. Other vectors and inapparent hosts are possible but presently unknown. The BTV has been identified in the salivary glands of the experimentally infected argasid tick, *Ornithodoros coriaceus* suggesting a potential biologic vector and reservoir for continued infection as the tick can live up to 5 years.

Cattle act as a principal virus reservoir as BTV can be isolated from clinically normal animals. There is a close association of BTV with erythrocytes in the presence of virus-specific antibodies. The virus can circulate in the blood for as long as 4 months and possibly up to 5 years. Thus, it is possible for a continuous biologic cycle of BTV throughout the year. The host-vector relationships in perpetuation of BTV are not completely understood. If transovarian passage is possible, in some strains, an obligate replication cycle in a vertebrate host would not be necessary. There is evidence to suggest that persistence of BTV is due to the competence of *Culicoides* vectors to develop oral infection and subsequently transmit BTV. A competent vector is not required in perpetuation of BTV within a population as horizontal transmission via semen and dam to fetus can occur. The existence of other viral reservoirs, besides cattle and sheep, is suspected but not identified or adequately investigated.

Because of an affinity for epithelium, the virus attacks cells of the malpighian and spinose layers of the tongue, mouth, esophagus, rumen, and probably skin. The epithelial cells undergo ballooning degeneration and eventually necrose. Detachment of the dead cells produces erosions and ulcers. In pregnant sheep, the virus traverses the placenta and, during the first trimester, may seriously interfere with organogenesis, especially of the brain.

CLINICAL SIGNS AND POSTMORTEM LESIONS. Following an incubation period of 3 to 8 days, the body temperature begins to rise, reaches a peak of 42 to 43°C in 2 to 3 days, and then declines but continues, with fluctuations, above normal for a febrile period of 6 to 8 days. During the early days of high fever, the following signs appear: (1) mucous membranes of the mouth and skin of the face and feet are hyperemic; (2) after approximately 48 hours of fever, the temperature declines, and erosions up to 3 mm in diameter form on the lips, dental pad, tongue, and on papillae of the buccal cavity; (3) hemorrhages may develop in oral and buccal tissues (Fig. 12-5); (4) the nose discharges serous secretion that, after a few days, changes to mucopurulent material that dehydrates and forms crusts around the nostrils; (5) respirations are rapid and, in some sheep, difficult. Leukopenia forms early. Throughout early stages, affected animals remain agile and seldom die.

During the period following high fever, different signs are evident. Body temperature, although fluctuating above normal, is not high. The face, including lips, ears, and eyelids, swells. Salivation, anorexia, and lameness de-

Fig. 12-5. Mouth of sheep with bluetongue. × 0.6.

velop. Coronitis, with dermal hyperemia dorsal to the hooves and especially of the hind limbs, is prominent; vertical linear hemorrhages may appear at the coronet and in hooves of sheep with nonpigmented skin. Because of hot tender feet, affected sheep recline and, when forced to move, may knee-walk. Exuviation of hooves and wool may occur, and torticollis may form. Physical weakness, stiffness, and depression become prominent and deaths are numerous. In infected flocks, both morbidity and mortality vary from 10 to 80%; lambs become severely incapacitated, and mortality from natural deaths and euthanasia consequently is high. The course usually varies from 10 to 15 days.

Of the lambs produced by ewes vaccinated with live virus or experiencing infection during weeks 4 to 8 of pregnancy, 20% may show developmental defects. Hydrocephalus, cerebellar hypoplasia, and supernumerary gyri and sulci are among the conditions encountered.

At necropsy, important lesions may exist in the mouth, rumen, heart, muscles, skin, and feet. The mouth contains erosions, deeply reddened areas, and edema on the tongue, dental pad, hard palate, buccal mucosa, and lips. In some sheep, the tongue is cyanotic. The rumen, especially along the anterior pillar and esophageal groove, often contains dark red areas where the surface epithelium is ballooned and necrotic and the corium congested, hemorrhagic, and edematous (Fig. 12-6).

The heart and other organs contain multiple petechial and ecchymotic hemorrhages in the subserosal tissues. Both myocardium and voluntary muscles show red areas of hemorrhage and pale areas of necrosis and leukocytosis.

The nonpigmented skin, discolored from hyperemia and hemorrhage, may show areas of eczema. Removal of hair and wool from the limbs reveals reddening of the skin between the hooves and tarsus or carpus; the change, most intense near the hoof, gradually diminishes towards the tarsus and carpus. The coronet may contain punctiform or linear redness, extending in some feet into the hooves, from hyperemia and hemorrhage (Fig. 12-7).

Fig. 12-6. Hemorrhage and necrosis on ruminal pillar of sheep with bluetongue. × 0.6.

HOST IMMUNE RESPONSE. Recovery from infection with BTV is accompanied by type-specific neutralizing antibodies, group-specific precipitating and complement fixing antibodies. These appear in about 7 to 21 days after infection and persist in excess of 1 year. The mechanism of the protective immune response to BTV is unknown. Although neutralizing antibodies are basically serotype-specific and thought to play a major role in protection, the virus can persist in the body of the host animal in the presence of high levels of neutralizing antibodies. Conversely the host animal may be protected from viral attack without measurable neutralizing antibody titers. Cell-mediated immune (CMI) responses have been found to occur following exposure to BT virus antigens and may work independently, or at certain stages together with neutralizing anti-

Fig. 12-7. Congestion of distal part of a limb from sheep with bluetongue. × 0.8.

bodies and complement in protective immunity. The relative importance of the humoral and CMI response to BTV or the location of antigenic determinants for CMI response, or if other antigens are required for regulation of the immune response is not known. Different BTV types induce different levels of cross-reactive cytotoxic T lymphocytes and also display variations in susceptibility to their effect. Inoculation with a specific serotype gives rise to homologous antibodies to only that specific serotype. Serial inoculation of two different BTV types give rise to a heterotypic antibody response and protection from challenge with a third BTV type. Studies on sequentially administered monovalent vaccines may make huge multivalent combinations unnecessary. Passive antibody transfer with immune serum given to adults is capable of preventing infec-

tion and is type specific. Colostral immunity in lambs is variable and many times capable of preventing infection. This lack of colostral protection is not understood but possibly due to the immaturity of the reticuloendothelial system. The outcome of infection and the severity of the disease is probably due to the nature of the virus strain and the susceptibility of the host.

DIAGNOSIS. Veterinarians diagnose BT on evidence of typical signs and lesions. The prevalence of vectoring insects and the manifestation of fever, leukopenia, swelling and erosions of the mouth and lips, lameness, stiffness, and pododermatitis are highly indicative changes that, in endemic areas, justify a clinical diagnosis. Laboratory confirmation depends on technical serologic procedures. The virus can be isolated from sheep blood during the stage of high fever and identified as to antigenic type. Some strains of BTV can be isolated in cell culture; others require inoculation of sheep or IV inoculation of chicken embryos prior to adaptation to cell culture. Serologic tests are divided into those detecting antibody of group antigen and those used to identify antibody to the specific types. The enzyme-linked immunosorbent assay is a sensitive group-specific serologic assay available for diagnostic assistance. Serum neutralization and the agar gel immunodiffusion test are used identifying antigenic types.

The differential diagnosis requires consideration of foot-and-mouth disease, contagious ecthyma, and photosensitization. For technical assistance from a diagnostic laboratory, practitioners should submit samples of clotted and unclotted blood and affected tongue, oral and buccal mucosa, feet, and muscle.

PREVENTION. Due to the varied habitat and potential wind drift from distant localities control of the *Culicoides* is extremely difficult and in most cases economically unfeasible. As the *Culicoides* is nocturnal in nature, its habitat is usually low lying wet areas and it is reluctant to enter enclosures; housing the animals at night and grazing areas of high infestation during the day time may reduce the exposure. At present in the United States the only commercially available vaccine is an attenuated virus of type 10 which protects only the homologous type and surveys indicate it is the serotype in all regions of the U.S. Attenuated and inactivated multivalent vaccines are available in other parts of the world and being investigated, with the current serotypes, in the United States. The current vaccines and immunizing regimens have many disadvantages. With the advances in genetic engineering, work should be directed towards developing a subunit BTV vaccine designed to incorporate only those antigens responsible for protective immunity.

Treatment is primarily directed towards supportive therapy and nursing care with the use of antibiotics to prevent secondary bacterial infection. Separation of affected from healthy animals is essential to provide access to feed and water without competition. Also, the affected animals can be closely monitored and provided with supportive nutrition, electrolyte therapy, and correction of dehydration.

Alstad, A.D., et al.: Localization of BT virus in erythrocytes of infected sheep. Am. Assoc. Lab. Diagnost., 20: 273-290, 1977.

Anderson, C.K. and Jensen R.: Pathologic changes in placentas of ewes inoculated with bluetongue virus. AJVR, 30:987-999, 1969.

Aral, N., quoted from Gambles, R.M.: Bluetongue of sheep in Cyprus. J. Comp. Pathol. Ther., 59:176, 1949.

Bekker, J.F., DeKock, G.W., and Quinlan, J.B.: The occurrence and identification of bluetongue in cattle—the so-called pseudo foot and mouth disease in South Africa. Onderstepoort J. Vet. Sci. Anim. Husb., 2:393-507, 1934.

Bowne, J.G.: Bluetongue disease. Adv. Vet. Sci., 15: 1-40, 1971.

Bowne, J.G. and Jochim, M.M.: Cytopathologic changes and development of inclusion bodies in cultured cells infected with bluetongue virus. AJVR, 28:1091-1105, 1967.

Bowne, J.G. and Jones, R.H.: Observations of bluetongue virus in salivary glands of an insect vector, Culicoides variipennis. Virology, 30:127-133, 1966.

Bowne, J.G., Luedke, A.J., Foster, B.S., and Jochim, M.M.: Current aspects of bluetongue in cattle. JAVMA, 148:1177-1178, 1966.

Bowne, J.G. and Ritchie, A.E.: Some morphological features of bluetongue virus. Virology, 40:903-911, 1970.

Campbell, C. and Grubman, M.: Current knowledge on the biochemistry and immunology of bluetongue. Prog. Vet. Microbiol. Immun., 1:58-79, 1985.

Carlson, J.: Differential serotyping of bluetongue virus-positive serums obtained in a national survey. Double-Stranded RNA Viruses. Edited by R. Compans and D. Bishop. Amsterdam, Elsevier Science Publishers B.V., 1983, pp. 361-366.

DuToit, R.M.: The transmission of bluetongue and horsesickness by Culicoides. Onderstepoort J. Vet. Sci., 19:7-16, 1944.

Els, H.J. and Verwoerd, D.W.: Morphology of bluetongue virus. Virology, 38:213-219, 1969.

Foster, N.M., Jones, R.H., and McCrory, B.R.: Preliminary investigations on insect transmission of bluetongue virus in sheep. AJVR, 24:1195, 1963.

Gambles, R.M.: Bluetongue of sheep in Cyprus. J. Comp. Pathol. Ther., 59:176, 1949.

Ghalib, H., Cherrington, J., and Osburn, B.: Virological, clinical and serological responses of sheep infected with tissue culture adapted bluetongue virus serotypes 10, 11, 13 and 17. Vet. Microbiol., 10:179-188, 1984-1985.

Gibbs, E.: Bluetongue—A review for clinicians. Florida Vet. J., 12:33-36, 1983.

Gibbs, E.: Bluetongue. An analysis of current problems with particular reference to importation of ruminants to the United States. JAVMA, 182:1190-1199, 1983.

Griner, L.A., McCrory, B.R., Foster, N.M., and Meyer, H.: Bluetongue associated with abnormalities in newborn lambs. JAVMA, 145:1013-1019, 1964.

Hardy, W.T. and Price, D.A.: Soremuzzle of sheep. JAVMA, 120:23-25, 1952.

Howell, P.G.: The antigenic classification and distribution of naturally occurring strains of bluetongue virus. J. S. Afr. Vet. Med. Assoc., 41:215-223, 1970.

Howell, P.G.: A preliminary antigenical classification of strains of bluetongue virus. Onderstepoort J. Vet. Res., 28:357-363, 1960.

Howell, P.G., Verwoerd, D.W., and Oellermann, R.A.: Plaque formation by bluetongue virus. Onderstepoort J. Vet. Res., 34:317-332, 1967.

Hutcheon, D., quoted from Henning, M.W.: Animal Diseases in South Africa. 3rd Edition. South Africa, Central News Agency, 1956, p. 809.

Jeggo, M., Wardley, R., and Taylor, W.: Role of neutralizing antibody in passive immunity to bluetongue infection. Res. Vet. Sci., 36:81-85, 1984.

Jeggo, M., Gumm, I., and Taylor, W.: Clinical and serological response of sheep to serial challenge with different bluetongue virus types. Res. Vet. Sci., 34: 205-211, 1983.

Jeggo, M., Wardley, R., and Taylor, W.: Host response to bluetongue virus. Double-Stranded RNA Viruses. Edited by R. Compans and D. Bishop. Amsterdam, Elsevier Science Publishers B.V., 1983, pp. 353-359.

Jeggo, M., Wardley, R., and Taylor, W.: Clinical and serological outcome following the simultaneous inoculation of three bluetongue virus types into sheep. Res. Vet. Sci., 37:368-370, 1984.

Jochim, M.M. and Jones, R.H.: Multiplication of bluetongue virus in Culicoides variipennis following artificial infection. Am. J. Epidemiol., 84:241-246, 1966.

Kamarov, A. and Goldsmidt, L.: A disease similar to bluetongue in cattle and sheep in Israel. Refuah Vet., 8:96, 1951.

Letchworth, G., III and Appleton, J.: Passive protection of mice and sheep against bluetongue virus by a neutralizing monoclonal antibody. Inf. Imm., *39*:208-212, 1983.

Luedke, A.J., Jones, R.H., and Jochim, M.M.: Transmission of bluetongue between sheep and cattle by *Culicoides variipennis*. AJVR, *28*:457-460, 1967.

McConnell, S. and Livingston, C.: Progress in multivalent modified live virus bluetongue vaccines: Comments on safety and efficacy. Proc. Eighty-Sixth Ann. Mtg. U.S. An. Health Assn., 103-112, 1982.

McKercher, D.G., McGowan, B., Howarth, J.A., and Saito, J.K.: Preliminary report on the isolation and identification of bluetongue virus from sheep in California. JAVMA, *122*:300, 1953.

Neitz, W.O.: Immunological studies on bluetongue in sheep. Onderstepoort J. Vet. Sci. Anim. Ind., *23*:93-136, 1948.

Omori, T.: Bluetongue-like disease in Japan. Bull. Off. Int. Epizoot., *55*:1109-1117, 1961.

Owen, N.C. and Munz, E.K.: Observations on a strain of bluetongue virus by electron microscopy. Onderstepoort J. Vet. Res., *33*:9-14, 1966.

Price, D.A. and Hardy, W.T.: Isolation of the bluetongue virus from Texas sheep—*Culicoides* shown to be a vector. JAVMA, *124*:255-258, 1954.

Rao, C. and Roy, P.: Genetic variation of bluetongue virus serotype II isolated from host (sheep) vector (*Culicoides variipennis*) at the same site. Am. J. Vet. Res., *44*:911-914, 1983.

Rao, C., Sugiyama, K. and Roy, P.: Antigenic drift in bluetongue viruses. *Double-Stranded RNA Viruses*. Edited by R. Compans and D. Bishop. Amsterdam, Elsevier Science Publishers B.V., 1983, pp. 313-320.

Ribeiro, J.M. and Noronha, F.M.O.: Fievra catarrhale du mouton au Portugal (bluetongue). Bull. Off. Int. Epizoot., *50*:46, 1958.

Shulz, G. and DeLay, P.D.: Losses in newborn lambs associated with bluetongue vaccination of pregnant ewes. JAVMA, *127*:224, 1955.

Spreull, J.: Malarial catarrhal fever in South Africa. J. Comp. Pathol., *18*:321-337, 1905.

Stott, J., et al.: Epizootiology of bluetongue virus in western United States. Proc. U.S. An. Health Assn., *85*:170-180, 1981.

Stott, J., Barber, T., and Osburn, B.: Immunologic response of sheep to inactivated and virulent bluetongue virus. Am. J. Vet. Res., *46*:1043-1049, 1985.

Stott, J., Osburn, B., and Alexander, L.: *Ornithorodoros Coriaceus* (pajaroello tick) as a vector of bluetongue virus. Am. J. Vet. Res., *46*:1197-1199, 1985.

Studdert, M.J., Pangborn, J., and Addison, R.B.: Bluetongue virus structure. Virology, *29*:509-511, 1966.

Svehag, S.E., Leendertsen, L., and Gorham, J.R.: Sensitivity of bluetongue virus to lipid solvents, trypsin and pH changes and its serological relationship to arboviruses. J. Hyg. (Cambridge), *64*:339-346, 1966.

Theiler, A.: Bluetongue in sheep in Transvaal. Dir. Agric. Ann. Rep., 1904-1905, pp. 110-121, quoted from Henning, M.W.: *Animal Diseases in South Africa*. 3rd Edition. South Africa, Central News Agency, 1956, p. 809.

Verwoerd, D.W.: Purification and characterization of bluetongue virus. Virology, *38*:203-212, 1969.

Young S. and Cordy, D.R.: An ovine fetal encephalopathy caused by bluetongue vaccine virus. J. Neuropath. Exp. Neurol., *23*:635-659, 1964.

Foot-and-Mouth Disease

(FMD; maul und klauenseuche; fiebre aftosa; fievre aphtheuse)

Foot-and-mouth disease, an extremely contagious and ravaging disease, is characterized by vesicles in the mouth and on the feet and is caused by the foot-and-mouth disease virus. Although more devastating to cattle and swine, FMD seriously affects sheep in both panzootic and sporadic outbreaks.

Economic losses result from reduced capacity of affected animals to produce meat, milk, and wool, from dietary deficiencies among sheep-dependent people, from quarantine constraints on commerce, by forming potential reservoirs of infection to cattle and swine, from the high cost of necessary research programs, and from the excessive expense of preventive and eradicative programs. The Mexican eradication program of 1946-1953 cost the United States alone $130 million, and the British outbreak of 1967-1968 cost England approximately $240 million and required the slaughter of at least 28,000 sheep, including some valuable genetic lines.

OCCURRENCE. Under natural conditions, foot-and-mouth disease occurs in all breeds, sexes, and ages of sheep. Native breeds of North Africa, Middle East, and Asia have, for many centuries, coexisted with the disease and probably are more resistant than are sheep imported from North America, Australia, and New Zealand. Cattle and swine are more susceptible than sheep. Goats, deer, buffalo, and possibly other species of wild ruminants and swine are attacked. Because the virus has low pathogenicity in people, the disease has little importance to them.

Geographically, FMD occurs on all continents except Australia, Central and North America. New Zealand, Iceland, Greenland, Japan, the Irish Republic, Great Britian, Norway, and Sweden are also free of the disease. Most disease-free countries have had outbreaks that were eradicated.

ETIOLOGY AND PATHOGENESIS. A virus of the RNA family Picornaviridae causes foot-and-mouth disease. The spherical virion measures approximately 22 nm in diameter, has no envelope, and consequently is not sensitive to ether or chloroform. Single-stranded RNA forms the core and constitutes 31% of the virion. The virus is composed of a message-sense RNA and a viral capsid containing 4 proteins. One of these polypeptides (VPl) stimulates the protective immune response and is serotype specific. After replicating in the cytoplasm of infected cells, the virus locates in the blood, vesicular fluid, and saliva.

In composition, the virus contains 7 antigenic types and 53 subtypes; these are: type A with 23 subtypes, type O with 10, type C with 4, type SAT 1 with 7, SAT 2 with 3, SAT 3 with 4, and ASIA 1 with 2. Typing may be accomplished with the complement-fixation test or the Enzyme-Linked Immunosorbent Assay (ELISA). In the laboratory, the virus grows in embryonating chicken eggs, day-old chicks, unweaned mice, and cell-culture systems of calf and swine kidneys. At 4°C it is stable at pH 7.0 to 7.5, but is rapidly inactivated at pH values above 10.0 and below 6.5.

FMD transmits through direct and indirect contact. During febrile stages, the blood, tissues, secretions, and excretions contain virus; saliva, urine, feces, and milk commonly convey virus to the external environment. Virus in exhaled aerosol from infected animals may be inhaled and deposited on the muzzle, nostrils, and mouth of susceptible animals. Dissemination of virus also occurs through mechanical transfer of infected animals and contaminated feed, equipment, hides, meat, and bones. Virus particles on dust and other airborne material may be blown long distances, and carrion-eating birds may transport virus over natural barriers. After clinical recovery from the disease, some sheep and cattle carry the virus for as long as 9 months in the esophagus, pharynx, and tonsils and excrete infectious material to the external environment.

Scientists have researched the FMD virus more than any other animal virus. Although some aspects of the disease remain conjectural, much information on both the virus and the disease has been obtained. Susceptible sheep become infected by contacting the FMD virus either from other infected animals or from contaminated feed, bedding, or equipment. Under natural conditions, the virus usually penetrates tissues of the mouth or feet where the integument is continuously contused and abraded—the· mouth from prehending and masticating feed and the feet from walking.

At the point of inoculation, the virions penetrate epithelial cells, replicate in the cytoplasm, and cause a primary vesicle. After leaving the injured cells, the viral particles enter the blood, which transports them to all tissues. Usually within 24 to 48 hours after penetration, generalized vesicles develop in the mouth and on the feet. During viremia, affected sheep develop a biphasic fever that lasts 3 to 4 days. Neutralizing antibodies first appear approximately 7 to 8 days after inoculation, reach a peak level in 10 additional days, and continue for 150 days. Complement-fixing antibodies are detectable 10 days after inoculation, reach a peak level and continue for 105 days, and then decline

Healing usually occurs in 2 to 3 weeks. In some sheep, the virus localizes in the mucous membrane of the esophagus, pharynx, and tonsils, and the host animals remain carriers for 1 to 9 months or longer. Recovered animals are immune to the homologous virus for several years. In young lambs, the virus attacks myocardial cells and causes foci of necrosis. Lesions in the right ventricle may cause generalized passive congestion and edema, and in the left ventricle, passive congestion of the lungs and pulmonary edema.

CLINICAL SIGNS AND POSTMORTEM LESIONS. In sheep, FMD is generally milder than it is in cattle or swine; in sheep, however, the disease varies from asymptomatic to severe and incapacitating forms. Following an incubation period of 3 to 8 or more days, body temperature rises to 42 to 43°C and persists 3 to 4 days when affected sheep show lassitude and inappetence.

Soon after the beginning of fever, flat, white, fluidless vesicles form in the mouth and on the feet. Mouth vesicles, 1 to 15 mm in diameter, form commonly on the dental pad and less commonly on the dorsum of the tongue caudal to the dorsal eminence. In addition, the lips may contain less conspicuous lesions. After rupture, the vesicated tissue is hyperemic, swollen, raw, and tender. Mild oral lesions do not affect eating, but modest to severe stomatitis causes limited salivation and oral smacking.

Foot vesicles form along the coronary band and in the interdigital skin. In severely affected feet, the sensitive laminae necrose and the hoof may slough. Lameness, often a severe and dominant sign, may cause knee-walking and prostration. Young lambs affected with malignant FMD show lassitude, physical weakness, rapid breathing, prostration, and death. Vesicles may be scarce or absent.

The morbidity among adult sheep varies up to 80% or more, but the mortality is low. Morbidity among lambs may reach 90% and mortality 40%. The disease course varies with complications and severity, but usually is 2 to 3 weeks.

At necropsy of adult sheep, vesicles may be found in the mucous membrane of the rumen as well as in the mouth and on the feet. Lambs that die from FMD show multiple gray or yellow foci of necrosis several millimeters in diameter in the myocardium.

DIAGNOSIS. Veterinarians diagnose FMD on the basis of clinical and laboratory evidence. Following the identification or suspicion of vesicles on the feet and in the mouth, veterinarians and sheep producers should immediately notify the state veterinarian, who quarantines the premises and collects appropriate tissue for laboratory studies. Special federal laboratories are equipped and staffed for accurate and rapid isolation and identification of the virus. Either the ELISA or CF test, or the combination of the two, can be used for typing. The ELISA has the advantage of being more sensitive and specific.

If the disease occurs in sheep, and/or cattle, and/or swine, the differential diagnosis requires consideration of vesicular stomatitis and vesicular exanthema. Besides laboratory studies, selected animal inoculations on the premises may be made as follows:

	FMD	VS	VE
Horse, intralingual	−	+	±
Cow, intralingual	+	+	−
Cow, intramuscular	+	−	−
Guinea pig, intrafootpad	+	+	−

PREVENTION. Methods for preventing FMD vary. In the United States, Australia, Britain, and other FMD-free countries, the importation of susceptible and infected animals, meat, meat products, and garbage from countries where FMD is endemic is prohibited. In case of an outbreak, the contaminated premises are rigidly quarantined, and all infected and exposed animals are destroyed, covered with hydrated lime, and buried. Buildings of low value, such as thatched sheds, are burned, and all remaining surfaces are cleaned and disinfected with 2% lye or 4% sodium carbonate solution. After 30 days of rest, test animals enter the premises. If disease does not develop, restocking takes place 90 days after the cleaning and disinfecting process.

In endemic countries, FMD is controlled by quarantine and vaccination against homologous strains. Using the conventional whole virus, inactivated vaccines require 3 inoculations during the year to induce and maintain effective immunity. In endemic areas vaccination strategies vary considerably. Two strategies frequently employed are the barrier vaccination and the ring vaccination. In the barrier vaccination strategy, all susceptible animals in a buffer zone are immunized with the strain/strains prevalent to that area. This strategy is used mainly on a regional or national basis. In the ring vaccination strategy, all susceptible animals are immunized around an outbreak. Early diagnosis and typing is essential for success of this strategy. Quarantine and slaughter may also be incorporated into the control procedures.

A biosynthetic polypeptide FMD vaccine has been developed that produces an effective immune response for 7 to 11 months following 2 inoculations. This type of vaccine production is more economical to produce, requires no refrigeration, and there is no chance of spreading the virus as has been a problem with inactivated vaccines. Further investigations are needed in the development and efficacy of fusion protein vaccines.

Animal Health Yearbook. FAO-WHO-OIE (Italy), 1970.

Bachrach, H.L.: Foot-and-mouth disease. Ann. Rev. Microbiol., 22:201-244, 1968.

Bachrach, H.L. and Breese, S.S.: Purification and electron microscopy of foot-and-mouth disease virus. Proc. Soc. Exp. Biol. Med., 97:659-665, 1958.

Bachrach, H.L., Trautman, R., and Breese, S.S.: Chemical and physical properties of virtually pure foot-and-mouth disease virus. AJVR, 25:333-342, 1964.

Breese, S.S.: Observations on complete and empty capsids of foot-and-mouth disease virus. J. Gen. Virol., 2:465-468, 1968.

Breese, S.S., Trautman, R., and Bachrach, H.L.: Rotational symmetry in foot-and-mouth disease virus and models. Science, 150:1303-1305, 1965.

Burrows, R.: The persistence of foot-and-mouth disease virus in sheep. J. Hyg. (Cambridge), 66:633-640, 1968.

Burrows, R.: Studies on the carrier state of cattle exposed to foot-and-mouth disease virus. J. Hyg. (Cambridge), 64:81-90, 1966.

Cardassis, J., et al.: Test of infectivity and dose of foot-and-mouth disease vaccine in sheep. Bull. Off. Int. Epizool., 65:427-438, 1966.

Cottral, G.E., Cox, B.F., and Baldwin, D.E.: The survival of foot-and-mouth disease virus in cured and uncured meat. AJVR, 21:288-297, 1960.

Cox, B.F., Cottral, G.E., and Baldwin, D.E.: Further studies on survival of foot-and-mouth disease virus in meat. AJVR, 22:224-226, 1961.

Dellers, R.W. and Hyde, J.L.: Response of sheep to experimental infection with FMDV. AJVR, 25:469-473, 1964.

Eaton, G.: Differential diagnosis of disease conditions and abnormalities of the mouth and feet of cattle, sheep and swine with particular reference to FMD. Vet. Rec., 13:848-849, 1933.

Frenkel, H.S.: Research on foot-and-mouth disease. III. The cultivation of the virus on a practical scale in explantations of bovine tongue epithelium. AJVR, 12:187-190, 1951.

Geering, W.A.: Foot-and-mouth disease in sheep. Aust. Vet. J., 43:485-489, 1967.

Gillespie, J.H.: The propagation and effects of type A foot-and-mouth virus in the day-old chick. Cornell Vet., 44:425-433, 1954.

Goldsmit, L.: Experiments with an attenuated type SAT 1 foot-and-mouth disease virus strain. Bull. Off. Int. Epizool., 61:1177-1182, 1964.

Hamblin, C., Armstrong, R., and Hedger, R.: A rapid Enzyme-Linked Immunosorbent Assay for the detection of foot and mouth disease virus in epithelial tissue. Vet. Microbiol., 9:435-443, 1984.

Jivoin, P. and Surdan, C.: Susceptibility of newborn lambs to FMD virus. Arch. Vet., 2:21-29, 1967.

Kleid, D., et al.: Cloned viral protein for foot and mouth disease. Developments in Industrial Microbiol., 25:317-325, 1984.

Loeffler, F. and Frosch, P.: Berichte der kommission zur erforschung der maul-und-klauenseuche bei dem institute fur infectionskrankheiten in Berlin. Zentralbl. Bakteriol., 23:371, 1898.

Loeffler, F. and Frosch, P.: Summarischer bericht uber die ergebnisse der unter suchunger der kommission zur erforschung der maul-und-klauenseuche bei der institute fur infectionskrankheiten in Berlin. Zentralbl. Bakteriol., 22:257, 1897.

Martin, W.B., Davies, E.B., and Smith, I.M.: The immunization of cattle with a mouse-adapted strain of type SAT 2 of virus of FMD. Res. Vet. Sci., 3:357-367, 1962.

McCullough, K. and Crowther, J.: The protective immune response against foot and mouth disease virus: relationship to viron topography. Foot and Mouth Disease Bulletin, 23:81-102, 1985.

McKercher, D.G. and Giordano, A.R.: Immune response of steers to chemically treated FMD virus. Arch. Gesamte Virusforsch., 20:190-197, 1967.

McKercher, P.: Dose-response evaluation of a genetically engineered foot and mouth disease virus polypeptide immunogen in cattle. Am. J. Vet. Res., 46:587-590, 1985.

McVicar, J.W. and Sutmoller, P.: Sheep and goats as foot-and-mouth disease carriers. Proc. U.S. Livestock Sanit. Assoc., 72:400-406, 1968.

National Academy of Sciences-National Research Council. Studies on foot-and-mouth disease. Publication 1343. Washington, D.C., 1966.

News report: American veterinarians assist England in FMD fight. JAVMA, 152:213-217, 1968.

Rivenson, S., Segura, M., and Zakin, M.M.: Antibodies in sheep experimentally infected with or vaccinated against FMD. Rev. Fac. Cienc. Vet. LaPlata, 8:53-58, 1966.

Skinner, H.H., Henderson, W.M., and Brooksby, J.B.: Use of unweaned white mice in foot-and-mouth disease research. Nature, 169:794-795, 1952.

Skinner, H.H.: Infection of chickens and chick embryos with the virus of FMD and of vesicular stomatitis. Nature, 174:1052-1053, 1954.

Sutmoller, P. and Cottral, G.E.: Improved techniques for the detection of FMD virus in carrier cattle. Arch. Gesamte Virusforsch., 21:170-177, 1967.

Sutmoller, P., McVicar, J.W., and Cottral, G.E.: The epizootiological importance of FMD carriers. Arch. Gesamte Virusforsch., 23:227-235, 1968.

Rinderpest

(Cattle plague; pestis bovina)

Ovine rinderpest, an acute contagious disease, is characterized by fever, leukopenia and, in some outbreaks, by rhinitis, erosive pharyngitis, and enterocolitis and is caused by the rinderpest virus. Although a minor disease among world sheep, rinderpest may cause animal and financial waste to individual sheep enterprises in some countries of Africa, Middle East, and Asia, where it remains enzootic. Economic losses result from reduced productivity of affected sheep, deaths, quarantine and destruction of exposed flocks, possible spread to cattle, protein deficiencies among sheep-dependent people, and the cost of preventive and eradicative programs.

Despite its low significance to sheep, rinderpest as a continental scourge probably has attacked and killed more cattle than any other single disease. Throughout human history, rinderpest, coming from the east, has repeatedly invaded Europe and Africa. During periods of peace, politicians, veterinarians, and agriculturists researched, fought, and subdued the disease, but during times of wars, the malady reoccupied lost territory. Statisticians estimated that from 1750 to 1800, rinderpest killed 200 million European cattle.

OCCURRENCE. Although all sexes and breeds are susceptible, breeds vary in attack rates. Indigenous breeds of endemic areas possess some resistance, but breeds from rinderpest-free countries, such as the United States, Australia, Britain, and New Zealand, are fully susceptible. Adult sheep suffer a higher incidence than do lambs. In addition to cattle, sheep, goats, and swine, rinderpest may occur, especially in the inapparent form, in wild ruminants, such as buffalo, reedbuck, blue wildebeest, waterbuck, bushbuck, eland, bushpig, giant forest pig, and warthog.

Geographically, the disease is endemic in Sudan, Chad, Niger, Upper Volta, Mali, Senegal, Nigeria, Tanzania, Uganda, Iran, Afghanistan, Nepal, India, Laos, and Vietnam. Eradicated outbreaks occurred in Brazil in 1921 and Australia in 1923.

ETIOLOGY AND PATHOGENESIS. The rinderpest virus, a member of the RNA family *Paramyxoviridae,* is related to measles and canine distemper viruses. Containing lipoprotein in the envelope and single-stranded RNA in the core, the pleomorphic virion measures 120 nm and the nucleocapsid, 18 nm in diameter. Multiplication occurs in the cytoplasm of host cells. In an external environment, the delicate virus inactivates in 1 to 2 days on dried material, but at pH 7 and 0°C, it persists for 1 to 3 months; lyophilization further enhances duration.

In culture systems, the virus grows in embryonating chicken eggs and in cultures of cells from kidneys of cow, sheep, goat, man, dog, rabbit, and hamster. Although strains vary in virulence, they form a uniform antigenic structure. In infected sheep, the virus occurs in blood from 3 to 10 days after inoculation, in lymphoid tissue and occasionally in nasal secretions for unknown periods.

Rinderpest is transmitted by both direct and indirect contact; indirect contact is effective for short times only because of early inactivation of the virus. Virus excreted by any infected ruminant may contaminate feed and water and, in these media, may be ingested by susceptible animals. Some animals may inhale viral particles in infective aerosols.

The pathogenesis of ovine rinderpest has not been adequately investigated. A conjectured pathogenesis from information derived from cattle, however, can be projected. Following ingestion or inhalation of infectious material, the virus probably penetrates the mucous membrane of the pharynx and tonsils and rapidly enters the pharyngeal and submaxillary lymph nodes, where it multiplies. After leaving the primary lymphoid tissue, the virus enters the blood and distributes to all organs, especially other lymphoid tissue, such as Peyer's patches, mesenteric nodes, and spleen. In germinal centers, lymphocytes necrose. Depletion of lymphocytes results in leukopenia.

After inoculation, viremia forms by day 3, reaches a peak titer by days 5 to 6, and persists through day 10. Virus may be excreted to the external environment in nasal and other secretions. Healing often occurs without overt symptoms, and complement-fixing antibodies form by day 13 and increase by day 21.

In sheep affected with clinical rinderpest, the mucous membranes of the intestines are attacked and damaged, and these changes result in persistent diarrhea. The fluid feces contain water, Na^+, K^+, Cl^- and HCO_3^-. During a few days, affected animals may lose 12% of body water. The loss of water results in tissue dehydration and the loss of HCO_3^- in acidosis; these changes contribute to the cause of death.

CLINICAL SIGNS AND POSTMORTEM LESIONS. Following an incubation period of 2 to 8 days, either the inapparent or clinical form develops. Inapparent rinderpest usually follows experimental inoculation of virus into sheep. Body temperature elevates from day 2 to 9, and lymphocytopenia forms from day 2 to 13. Some sheep lose appetite and show nasal discharge.

Clinical rinderpest usually occurs as natural outbreaks. During the first 2 days, body temperature elevates, and pained sheep stand with arched backs. Serous nasal exudate and fluid feces containing flecks of mucus and blood discharge to the surface. Later, animals become physically weak and depressed. Coughing is common. Nasal discharge is mucopurulent, and the fluid feces are brown. The temperature descends to subnormal levels; the animals recline, pass into coma, and die.

Among sheep, rinderpest is rare. The morbidity in infected flocks is high, and the mortality varies from 30 to 40%. The course ranges from 5 to 10 days.

At necropsy, most changes are in the gastrointestinal and respiratory systems. During early stages, mucous membranes of the nasal cavity, pharynx, abomasum, and intestines are congested. The soft palate contains erosions, and the crests of longitudinal mucosal folds of the colon, cecum, and rectum show bright red parallel stripes of hemorrhages. In advanced stages, the hemorrhagic stripes are brown, and over the hemorrhages the mucosa is eroded. Peyer's patches may show ulcers. Many organs contain petechial hemorrhages, and the lungs contain areas of pneumonia.

DIAGNOSIS. Veterinarians in endemic areas diagnose clinical rinderpest on evidence of typical signs and lesions in both sheep and cohabiting cattle. Rapid spread among sheep and cattle, leukopenia, fever, diarrhea, soft palatal erosions, and striped hemorrhages in the colon, cecum, and rectum are indicative changes. In rinderpest-free regions, clinically suspected animals should be referred to a state veterinarian, who may quarantine the herd and collect blood and lymphoid tissue for virus isolation and identification. Convalescent sheep have ascending titers of complement-fixing and virus-neutralizing antibodies.

A rapid diagnosis can be made from nasal and ocular secretions using the indirect immunofluorescence antibody test. Special laboratories, staffed with specially trained personnel, make the confirming diagnosis.

The differential diagnosis requires consideration of Nairobi sheep disease, which also produces striped hemorrhages in the colon, but does not spread by contact to either sheep or cattle.

PREVENTION. In endemic areas, veterinarians and producers prevent rinderpest by applying sanitary and management principles that protect animals against exposure to virus and by vaccination. Effective vaccines, containing virus attenuated by adaptation to chick embryos, by rabbit passages, or by cell-culture modification, are available and should be applied annually before breeding. In rinderpest-free regions, disease outbreaks are eradicated by quarantine, slaughter of diseased and exposed ruminants, disinfecting and resting contaminated premises, and cautious restocking.

Animal Health Yearbook. FAO-WHO-OIE (Italy), 1970.

Barber, T.L. and DeBoer, C.J.: Response of calves, sheep, and pigs to a cell-culture-modified rinderpest virus. Cornell Vet., 55:590-598, 1965.

Barber, T.L. and Heuschele, W.P.: Experimental rinderpest in sheep. 67th Proc. U.S. Livestock Sanit. Assoc., 1963, pp. 155-162.

Breese, S.S. and DeBoer, C.J.: Electron microscopy of rinderpest virus in bovine kidney tissue culture cells. Virology, 19:340-348, 1963.

Bussell, R.H. and Karzon, D.T.: Measles-canine distemper-rinderpest group. In Basic Medical Virology. Edited by J.E. Prior. Baltimore, Williams & Wilkins, 1966, pp. 313-336.

DeLay, P.D., et al.: Clinical and immune response of alien hosts to inoculation with measles, rinderpest, and canine distemper. AJVR, 26:1359-1373, 1965.

Dhanda, M.R. and Manjrekar, S.L.: Observations on rinderpest amongst sheep and goats in the State of Bombay. Indian Vet. J., 28:306-319, 1952.

Heuschele, W.P. and Barber, T.L.: Changes in certain blood components of rinderpest-infected cattle. AJVR, 27:1001-1006, 1966.

Johnson, R.H.: An outbreak of rinderpest involving cattle and sheep. Vet. Rec., 70:457-461, 1958.

Lall, H.K.: Some observations on the immunization of sheep and goats against rinderpest. Indian J. Vet. Sci., 17:11-12, 1947.

Lewis, C.D.: The Georgics of Virgil. Book III. London, Jonathan Cape, 1940, pp. 464-466.

Mushi, E., Wafula, J., and Erei, R.: Detection of rinderpest virus antigens in ocular and nasal secretions by immunofluorescence. Trop. Vet., 2:11-14, 1984.

Nicolle, M. and Adil-Bey: Etudes sur la peste bovine. Ann. Inst. Pasteur, *16*:56, 1902.

Plowright, W.: Observations on the behavior of rinderpest in indigenous African sheep. Br. Vet. J., *108*:450-457, 1952.

Plowright, W., Cruickshank, J.G., and Waterson, A.P.: The morphology of rinderpest virus. Virology, *17*: 118-122, 1962.

Polding, J.B. and Simpson, R.M.: A possible immunological relationship between canine distemper and rinderpest. Vet. Rec., *69*:582, 1957.

Srikantaiah, G.N.: Rinderpest in sheep, with special reference to artificial infection. Indian Vet. J., *11*: 104-108, 1934.

Taylor, W.P. and Plowright, W.: Studies on the pathogenesis of rinderpest in experimental cattle. III. Proliferation of an attenuated strain in various tissues following subcutaneous inoculation. J. Hyg. (Cambridge), *63*:263-275, 1965.

Taylor, W.P., et al.: Studies on the pathogenesis of rinderpest in experimental cattle. IV. Proliferation of the virus following contact infection. J. Hyg. (Cambridge), *63*:497-506, 1965.

Zwart, D. and Macadam, I.: I. Transmission of rinderpest by contact from cattle to sheep and goats. II. Observations on rinderpest in sheep and goats and transmission to cattle. Res. Vet. Sci., *8*:37-44, 1967.

Esophageal Obstruction

(*Esophageal occlusion; choke*)

Esophageal obstruction is the accidental lodgment of ingesta in the lumen of that organ. Occlusion may be partial or complete; if partial, limited amounts of fluid and gas may bypass the static mass, but if complete, gases cannot traverse the esophagus, and they consequently accumulate within the forestomachs. Since the disease occurs sporadically, it is of little economic importance to the sheep industry, but under certain conditions, the disease may cause serious losses to individual enterprises.

OCCURRENCE. Esophageal obstructions occur in all breeds and sexes, but feedlot lambs 4 to 6 months of age commonly are affected. During late summer and early autumn, weaned lambs grazing harvested fields commonly develop obstruction.

ETIOLOGY AND PATHOGENESIS. Esophageal obstruction results from eating globular feeds whose particle diameters are too large to pass freely through the esophagus. Common offending feeds include fragments of sugar-beet crowns, sugar beets, table beets, ear corn, fruits, turnips, potatoes, and carrots. These feeds may be grazed from fields or fed from crop surpluses.

The prehended food particles may be too large for free passage through the esophagus or too large, tough, hard, or smooth for easy mastication. When attempts at mastication are unsuccessful, the large unwieldy particle is forced into the pharynx and swallowed. Because the peristaltic pressures are inadequate to push the rigidly shaped food through the lumen, the food mass lodges at some part of the esophagus. In sheep, obstructing food usually lodges near the cranial entrance or at some point along the cervical part of the esophagus, but in some cases, the obstruction locates in the thorax near the cardia.

Lodgment stimulates forceful peristaltic contractions, which may eventually move the food along, but if the obstruction is firm and immovable, local pressure at the points where tissue contacts the obstructing body causes necrosis of the esophageal wall. Saliva accumulates cranial to the obstruction and, by overfilling or by reversed peristalsis, is forced through the mouth and nose to the exterior. Some food particles, saliva, and water may enter the larynx, trachea, bronchi, and lungs. Unless the obstruction is relieved, death from pneumonia or bloat ensues.

CLINICAL SIGNS AND POSTMORTEM LESIONS. Since the onset of esophageal obstruction is sudden, the affected animal becomes distressed and alarmed. Prehension of feed usually ceases immediately. The head is extended, and mastication and swallowing movements are strong and repetitive. Saliva and feed particles drip from the mouth and nose. With the obstruction near the larynx, breathing may be difficult, oral, and gasping. Coughing is frequent. The animal strains and often changes the position of the head and neck. Bloat develops rapidly and aggravates the animal's distress. Careful palpation along the cervical part of the esophagus may reveal the obstruction.

In fatal cases, lesions are found in the alimentary and respiratory systems. The obstructing mass is present in the esophagus, and although usually located in the cervical part, a mass is occasionally in the thoracic portion. In prolonged obstructions, the esophageal mucosa, and even the musculature, may be necrotic and infected. The trachea may show aspirated feed and the lungs pneumonia.

DIAGNOSIS. A positive clinical diagnosis requires typical signs, mechanical probing, and a history of available obstructing feed particles. Important indicative signs are drooling of saliva and feed particles, repeated chewing and swallowing movements, bloating, straining, and coughing. Confirmation can be obtained by dextrous palpation of cervical obstructions and by instrumental probing of the thoracic part of the esophagus.

The differential diagnosis should include a consideration of primary bloat, diphtheria, and pneumonia.

TREATMENT. Treatment includes both relief of acute bloat and removal of the obstructing mass. If bloat is severe and threatens fatality, the rumen should be pierced with a trocar or large gauge needle. In animals with moderate or less bloating, attention should be directed towards removal of the obstruction. The anatomic location of the obstruction may be determined by cervical palpation and/or esophageal probing. Obstructions within the cervical part of the esophagus may be manually pushed forward to the pharynx or to a position accessible to grasping instruments. In some cases, a loop of doubled wire may be passed in the esophagus beyond the obstruction, then repeatedly pulled forward to engage the obstruction and draw it forward into the pharynx and mouth.

Obstructions located in the thoracic part of the esophagus may be pushed with a stomach tube or a firmer hose along the esophagus into the rumen. If probing indicates that the object is immovable, lubricating mineral oil or water and detergents should be pumped against the mass.

Braxy

(Bradsot)

Braxy, an acute infectious but noncontagious toxemia, is characterized by sudden deaths and acute focal infection in the abomasum and is caused by anaerobic bacteria. Although braxy may cause severe monetary damages to individual producers, it is of minor importance to the sheep industry because an effective vaccine is available for control and because of its declining incidence within endemic areas and its limited geographic distribution. Economic losses, however, accrue from deaths of affected sheep, depreciation in market value of affected property, and from the cost of control programs.

OCCURRENCE. As a disease of limited economic importance to sheep producers, braxy occurs in Britain, Scandinavia, Iceland, and Tasmania. Isolated cases develop rarely in other countries, such as the United States. Although all sexes and breeds are susceptible, the disease usually develops in prime-conditioned sheep 6 to 18 months of age. Young lambs and animals over 3 years of age are seldom attacked. Most cases occur during autumn and early winter, and outbreaks cease when ambient temperatures reach freezing degrees, although chilling of the abomasum by ingestion of frosted forages has been suggested as a predisposing factor.

ETIOLOGY AND PATHOGENESIS. *Clostridium septicum,* a producer of specific exotoxin, causes braxy. Occasionally *C. novyi* and *C. perfringens* also inhabit the characteristic abomasal lesion. *C. septicum,* a motile, sporing anaerobe, lives in soil, manure, and alimentary tracts and on animal skin surfaces. The vegetative form measures 0.6 to 0.8 × 3 to 8 μm. The oval spore has a subterminal position in the cell. Organisms in tissues and in young cultures are gram-positive, but in old cultures, many cells become gram-negative. The bacteria tend to form short chains, but single cells are also observed. On peritoneal surfaces of infected guinea pigs, short chains predominate.

The exotoxin in tissues and cultures contains two antigenic components: alpha, which is necrotizing and lethal, and beta, a hemolytic deoxyribonuclease. Vegetative forms are susceptible to drying, high temperatures, and chemical disinfectants; spores are resistant and withstand 120°C for 10 minutes and endure in soil and dried tissues for many years. Spores are readily killed by a 3% solution of formaldehyde.

The pathogenesis of braxy has not been completely determined, but information on the cause and pathology makes a reasonable conjecture possible. The causative organism, *C. septicum,* resides usually as spores in soil and manure, and if these materials contaminate feed and water, the spores are ingested along with forage. In the fundus, and less commonly the pylorus of the abomasum, fibrous ingesta penetrate the mucous membrane and mechanically transport either spores or vegetative cells of *C. septicum* into the lamina propria and the submucosa. Damage to the mucosal lining of the abomasum from chemicals and high levels of volatile fatty acids have produced braxy in experimental sheep.

Within the tissues and under favorable conditions, the spores vegetate, and the irritating bacteria grow, proliferate, and produce exotoxin. The alpha component of toxin necroses mucosal tissue and provokes a strong inflammatory reaction. Inflammatory exudates along with some organisms pass from the lesion into the peritoneal cavity. Exotoxin formed by the bacteria is absorbed into the circulatory system and carried to all organs. Toxin, acting on the central nervous system, and acute shock cause profound illness and usually death. If the animal survives, antitoxin and other types of antibodies develop, and the abomasum heals. The bacteria are discharged back into the soil with feces from live animals and with decomposing tissues of dead animals.

CLINICAL SIGNS AND POSTMORTEM LESIONS. After a brief but unmeasured incubation period, braxy runs a short and usually fatal course. Commonly, the husbandman finds the dead animal without any awareness of the sheep's previous sickness. Astute husbandmen, by objective observations of the animals, may identify some sheep during periods of sickness. Such animals separate from the flock and, at frequent intervals, alternate standing and reclining positions. Muscular movements, as in forced walking, are weak and uncoordinated.

The tense abdomen may distend with feed and gas, and manipulation of the sheep may cause discomfort and pain. Body temperature ranges from normal to 42°C. In advanced stages, the recumbent sheep becomes severely depressed, passes into coma, and dies. The clinical course varies up to 1 hour. Over a prolonged period, the morbidity varies from 10 to 20% and may reach 50%. Most affected sheep die.

At necropsy of killed or recently deceased sheep, characteristic pathologic changes can usually be found. The fundus of the abomasum contains one or more darkened areas visible through the thin wall of the unopened stomach. After opening the abomasum with a longitudinal incision along the lesser curvature and cleaning the mucosa with water, gastric lesions are easily discernible. Each one measures up to 50 mm in diameter and is circular or irregular in outline. The reddened tissue, necrotic on the surface, is slightly depressed below the level of surrounding healthy mucosa. The necrotic surface has a rough, firm texture. The abomasal wall over the lesions commonly is edematous with widespread emphysema, especially in the submucosa. The abdominal cavity, thoracic cavity, and/or pericardial sac may contain an increased amount of fluid, which tends to coagulate when exposed to air. The subendocardium, especially of the left ventricle, and the subepicardium often contain multiple petechial hemorrhages. Subserosal hemorrhages may also be found in other organs, such as intestines and lungs. Histopathologic examination of the abomasal lesions reveals the presence of masses of chained and *C. septicum,* as well as individual cells of the organism. Microscopic changes in the mucosa consist of foci of coagulation necrosis with distended vessels, extravasated erythrocytes, and bacterial colonies.

DIAGNOSIS. The clinical diagnosis of braxy is based on observing typical signs in the living sheep and on finding characteristic lesions at necropsy. In the laboratory, *C. septicum* can be identified by immunofluorescence, or isolated from the abomasal lesion and peritoneal fluid and occasionally from the blood.

The differential diagnosis requires consideration of black disease, enterotoxemia, anthrax, plant poisoning, and mineral poisoning.

PREVENTION AND TREATMENT. The need for preventive programs, of course, is limited to endemic areas where the disease is expected to occur. Under these circumstances, susceptible sheep should be immunized. Reputable vaccines are commercially available for this specific purpose. The vaccine should be administered several weeks in advance of the expected disease outbreak. An additional precaution is the protection of the environment against further contamination with *C. septicum* by incineration or deep burial in quicklime of all dead animals.

Dumaresq, J.A.: Braxy in Tasmania. Aust. Vet. J., *15*: 252-255, 1939.

Dungal, N.: Recherches bacteriologiques sur le bradsot du muton islandais. Pathologenie et vaccination. Ann. Inst. Pasteur, *48*:604-616, 1932.

Ellis, T., Rowe, J., and Lloyd, J.: Acute abomasitis due to *Clostridium septicum* infection in experimental sheep. Aust. Vet. J. *60*:308-309, 1983.

Eustis, S. and Bergland, M.: Suppurative abomasitis associated with *Clostridium septicum* infection. JAVMA, *178*:732-734, 1981.

Gaiger, S.H.: Investigations in braxy. J. Comp. Pathol. Ther., 35:191-223; 236-256, 1922.

Garcia, M.M. and McKay, K.A.: On the growth and survival of *Clostridium septicum* in soil. J. Appl. Bacteriol., *32*:362-370, 1969.

Jensen, C.O.: Ueber bradsot und deren oetiology. Dtsch. Z. Tiermed. Vergl. Pathol., 22:249-274, 1896.

Jungherr, E. and Welch, H.A.: A report on lamb diseases. JAVMA, 72:317-326, 1927.

Kerimov, C.: Survival of *Clostridium septicum* and *Clostridium novyi*, the agents of sheep braxy, in external environment. Development of a method for disinfecting sheep pens. Tr. Vses. Inst. Vet. Sanit., *28*:126-136, 1967.

Nielsen, I.: Bradsot hos faaret (gastromycosis). T. Vet., 1888.

Struck

An acute infectious but noncontagious toxemia of adult sheep, struck is characterized by sudden and unexpected deaths, peritonitis, and ulcerative enteritis and is caused by anaerobic bacteria that commonly reside in soil. Since struck has a low incidence and a limited geographic distribution, it is of minor economic importance even to endemic regions. Some individual sheep enterprises, however, may experience considerable economic waste from the disease. Financial loss results from deaths of adult sheep, property depreciation, and the cost of preventive programs. The term "struck" presumably refers to the suddenness of deaths of affected sheep.

OCCURRENCE. Struck occurs in all breeds and sexes of adult sheep. Even though all classes of adults develop the malady, sheep 0.5 to 2 years old develop a higher incidence than do other age groups. Most cases of the disease form during winter and spring. The geographic distribution includes England, Wales, and Sardinia—where the incidence of the disease is of economic importance. In Germany, New Zealand, and Mongolia, the number of cases is low. In the United States, cases develop in feedlot lambs that are moved from fattening pens, held for 1 to 2 days for shearing with little or no feed, and then returned to the fattening pens and full ration.

ETIOLOGY AND PATHOGENESIS. *Clostridium perfringens* type C, the cause of struck, lives in soil, manure, and the alimentary tracts of some sheep and cattle. This anaerobic bacterium is a gram-positive, nonmotile, encapsulated, spore-bearing bacillus that measures 4 to 8 × 0.8 to 1.5 μm. Except for mannitol, the bacterium ferments most sugars and produces acid and gas. On the basis of toxin-antitoxin neutralization tests, the species is divided into 6 types: A, B, C, D, E, and F. The species produces 12 exotoxins, which are named with Greek letters. Each type produces one major toxin and one or more minor toxins. The major toxin of type C is beta toxin, which is necrotizing. Table 6-1 presents types, toxins, and diseases.

Although little information is available on the pathogenesis of struck, on the basis of what is known about struck and related diseases, a pathogenesis can be suggested. In areas where struck is endemic, spores of the causative organism reside in soil and enter the alimentary tract with contaminated feed or water. In the small intestine, especially the duodenum and jejunum, the bacteria multiply and produce beta toxin. After causing acute enteritis, both bacteria and toxin pass into the intestinal wall and enter the blood. Injury to capillaries of the abdominal and thoracic viscera increases the permeability to plasma proteins and results in the accumulation of transudate and exudate in the body cavities. The bacteria enter the transudate, spleen, and other organs and accumulate in skeletal muscles.

Death results from toxic injury to vital neurons and shock. During the 8 hours following death, the bacteria multiply in the muscles and produce changes that closely resemble the muscle lesions of blackleg. The bacteria pass to the exterior in feces and decomposing tissues, form spores, and re-enter the soil. Sublethal doses of toxin stimulate the formation of specific antibodies.

CLINICAL SIGNS AND POSTMORTEM LESIONS. Struck in most affected sheep has a short disease course and consequently, shepherds commonly find dead animals without observing previous signs of illness. When observed, however, affected sheep separate from the flock, recline, and display uneasiness, depression, and convulsions. Death follows promptly.

At necropsy, gross changes are evident in the digestive and circulatory systems. Parts of the duodenum and jejunum may show congestion, cyanosis, and erosions of the mucous membrane. In some areas, the intestinal changes may have progressed into ulcers of varying size. The peritoneal and thoracic cavities as well as the pericardial sac usually contain excessive amounts of clear fluid that, on exposure to air, forms strands of fibrin. Small hemorrhages discolor many serosal surfaces.

Immediately after death, the skeletal muscles appear normal, but within 8 hours, the intermuscular septa contains sanguineous fluid, and the muscle is hemorrhagic and gaseous in foci; these changes closely resemble lesions of blackleg. *C. perfringens* type C can be found in smears of transudate and infected organs and isolated from the same places.

DIAGNOSIS. Veterinarians diagnose struck on the basis of characteristic signs and lesions among adult sheep. Cyanotic, erosive and ulcerative enteritis, peritonitis, and fluid in the body cavities and pericardial sac suggest struck. In the laboratory, scientists can estab-

lish or confirm the diagnosis by isolating and identifying the bacterium from body-cavity fluids and spleen and by finding beta toxin in the contents of the small intestine.

The differential diagnosis requires consideration of other diseases that cause sudden deaths, such as anthrax, black disease, and acute poisoning.

PREVENTION.   If losses from struck are anticipated, the animals should be immunized with commercial vaccine containing antigens of beta toxin. The vaccine should be administered several weeks before expected exposure to the disease.

Buddle, M.B.: "Degraded" strains of *Clostridium welchii* type C isolated from sheep in New Zealand. J. Comp. Pathol. Ther., *64*:217-224, 1954.

Dedie, K., Schreibner, G., and Preuss, H.: Enterotoxemia of sheep in Germany caused by *Clostridium welchii* type C. Arch. Exp. Vet. Med., *11*:921-929, 1957.

Ipatenko, N.G.: Infectious enterotoxemia of camels in Mongolia, caused by *C. perfringens* type C. Veterinariia (Moscow), No. 11, *43*:32-35, 1966.

McEwen, A.D.: *B. paludis*: a new species of pathogenic anaerobic bacterium. J. Comp. Pathol. Ther., *43*:1-21, 1929.

McEwen, A.D. and Roberts, R.S.: "Struck": enteritis and peritonitis of sheep caused by a bacterial toxin derived from the alimentary tract. J. Comp. Pathol. Ther., *44*:26-49, 1931.

Montgomerie, R.F. and Rowlands, W.T.: *Clostridium welchii* type C Wilsdon (*B. paludis* McEwen) isolated from sheep in North Wales. Vet. Rec., *48*:829-832, 1936.

Quesada, A.: Gastro-entero-tossiemie degli ovini (studie recherche). Clin. Vet. Milano, *76*:324-344, 1953.

Wilsdon, A.J.: Observations on the classification of *Bacillus welchii*. Second Rep. Univ. Cambridge Inst. Anim. Pathol., 1931.

Nairobi Sheep Disease

(*NSD*)

Nairobi sheep disease, an acute infectious but noncontagious malady, is characterized by fever, diarrhea, and hemorrhagic gastroenteritis, and is caused by a virus. Even though NSD occurs only in the central part of Africa, it causes serious waste to the sheep enterprises of the endemic areas. Economic losses come from deaths of infected animals, the cost of preventive programs, the threat of spread to new geographic areas, and dietary deficiencies among sheep-dependent people.

OCCURRENCE.   Although NSD develops in all breeds and sexes of sheep, the virus more commonly attacks adult animals than lambs. In addition to sheep, the disease occurs in adult goats and possibly some wild ruminants, especially the duiker. The rodent *Arvicanthis abyssinicus* is susceptible to artificial exposure. Antibody titers in human sera indicate that NSD may result in a nosocomial subclinical infection in people working with infected animals.

Vectoring ticks transmit NSD, and because environmental moisture favors their survival, the malady develops highest incidence during seasons of high rainfall. Extensive grazing also exposes susceptible sheep to the vectors.

Geographically, NSD occurs in Kenya, especially between Nairobi and Mount Kenya, and Naivasha area in the Rift Valley, in Uganda, Sudan, and probably in the Congo and northern Tanzania.

ETIOLOGY.   Nairobi sheep disease is caused by a virus of the genus Nairovirus within the family Bunyaviridae. The spherical virion contains a core of single-stranded RNA, measures approximately 40 to 60 nm in diameter, and replicates in the cytoplasm of host cells. The virus persists for considerable time on contaminated fomites and, when lyophilized and stored at low temperatures, retains viability for many months. Although strains may vary in virulence, they form a uniform antigenic structure. The virus is more stable in a slightly alkaline environment and has its optimal stability at pH 7.4 to 8.0.

In the laboratory, the virus grows in infant and adult mice and also in cultured cells from lamb testes and kidneys, hamster kidneys, and goat testes and kidneys. During febrile stages of the disease, the virus is concentrated in affected sheep spleen, blood, liver, mesenteric lymph nodes, and kidney, and in vectoring larvae, nymphs, and adults of the brown tick, *Rhipicephalus appendiculatus.*

TRANSMISSION.   The three-host brown tick, *R. appendiculatus,* is the common vector of NSD virus, and is the only tick in which transovarial transmission is known to occur. The larvae, nymphs, and adults become infec-

tive by feeding on viremic sheep, carry the virus into the next life stage and, in that stage, transmit the NSD virus by feeding on susceptible sheep. Under field conditions, unfed adult ticks may retain and transmit virulent virus for up to 18 months. Infected ticks are cleansed of infection if they feed on immune sheep or nonsusceptible hosts. Other species of vectoring tick include *Amblyomma variegatum*; this arthropod inefficiently transmits the virus and presumably has little importance in the disease economy.

No wild host reservoir for the virus has been identified. A rodent, *Arvicanthis abyssinicus,* when artificially inoculated, becomes viremic, and epizootiologists have suspected that the animal forms a natural reservoir.

PATHOGENESIS.   Many aspects of NSD have not been studied; consequently, some factors in the pathogenesis are conjectural. As the infective vector feeds on a susceptible sheep, the NSD virus, along with vector saliva, enters the host blood and distributes to all organs. Although target organs and cells for virus attack are incompletely known, they probably include epithelial cells of the mucosa of the ileum, cecum, and large intestine.

From the blood, the virus penetrates the cytoplasm, where it replicates. The release of newly formed virions maintains viremia during febrile stages. Injury to and necrosis of epithelial cells cause congestion and rupture of capillaries of the mucosa, especially along longitudinal ridges of the intestinal mucosa. The initial effect of virus on bone marrow is leukocytosis followed by severe suppression and leukopenia.

Injury and irritation to the intestine accelerate peristaltic movements and initiate diarrhea. The fluid feces contain microorganisms, water, Na^+, Cl^-, K^+ and HCO_3^-. After a few days, the infected sheep probably lose as much as 12% of their body water, and approximately 50% of the lost water probably comes from the plasma. The loss of water results in tissue dehydration, and the loss of HCO_3^- in acidosis.

Following clinical recovery, affected sheep are immune for several months and possibly for life. In fatal cases, death results from the combined effect of cell damage, tissue dehydration, acidosis, and shock.

CLINICAL SIGNS AND POSTMORTEM LESIONS. After an incubation period of 1 to 6 days, temperature rises and reaches a peak of approximately 42°C within 36 to 48 hours, remains elevated for 4 to 9 days, and then abruptly declines to subnormal levels when death occurs. In some animals, fever abates for 3 to 7 days and then rises to levels higher than preceding episodes. With the beginning of fever, affected sheep isolate from the flock, appear depressed and listless, and decline food. Diarrhea begins on day 2 or 3 of sickness; the feces become fluid and green but, during advanced stages, contain variable amounts of blood and mucus. Respiration becomes difficult, and mucopurulent exudate discharges from the nose.

During advanced stages, the external genitalia swell, and pregnant ewes may abort. The total leukocyte count changes from normal 4500 up to 5300, then decreases to 1000 per cmm. The usual clinical course of 3 to 4 days may extend to 9 days. Mortality varies from 30 to 70% in adult sheep.

At necropsy, the affected sheep may contain numerous brown ticks and show nasal discharge, diarrhea, and swollen genitalia. Salient internal changes are in the alimentary and respiratory systems. The abomasum, small intestine, and colon, but especially the ileocecal valve, contain petechial to ecchymotic hemorrhages in the lamina propria and submucosa. In the cecum and colon, hemorrhages form along longitudinal folds in the mucosa, thus giving the colon a striped appearance. Some blood may be mixed with feces. Mesenteric lymph nodes are swollen, and the spleen may be enlarged. The nasal mucosa is congested and swollen, and lungs may contain fluid.

DIAGNOSIS. Veterinarians clinically diagnose NSD from evidence of typical signs and lesions. In endemic areas, brown-tick parasitism, high fever, green or bloody fluid feces, and leukopenia are indicative signs; hemorrhagic ileocecocolitis is additional evidence. Laboratory isolation and identification of the NSD virus or the demonstration of a rising titer in recovering sheep confirm the diagnosis. The indirect haemagglutination (IHA), the enzyme-linked immunosorbent assay (ELISA), and the indirect immunofluorescence-antibody test (IFAT) can be used to detect antibodies in sera. The IHA and ELISA are suitable tests for large scale seroepidemiologic surveys because they are quick and simple. The IFAT is used to check doubtful reactions.

The differential diagnosis requires consideration of acute coccidiosis and intestinal helminthosis.

PREVENTION. Veterinarians and producers prevent NSD by controlling the brown tick and by annually vaccinating adult sheep, if vaccine is available. Recovery from NSD leads to a strong immunity which is probably permanent. Application of tickcides to sheep at weekly intervals reduces the number of ticks and lowers the exposure rate. Vaccines, prepared from attenuated mouse-adapted virus, should be annually administered prior to the anticipated tick season.

TREATMENT. There is no specific treatment for NSD although replacement of fluids, electrolytes, and correcting the acid base balance is helpful. Oral administration electrolyte products, such as those products used in the treatment of calf scours, can be used as a fluid and energy replacement. Antibiotics are advised to suppress secondary bacterial infections.

Ansell, R.H.: Attenuation of Nairobi sheep disease virus in the mouse brain. Vet. Rec., 69:410-412, 1957.
Bugyaki, L.: La "maladie de Kisenyi" du mouton, due à un virus filtrable et transmise par des tiques. Bull. Agric. Congo Belge, 46:1455-1562, 1955.
Coackley, W. and Pini, A.: The effect of Nairobi sheep disease virus on tissue culture systems. J. Pathol. Bacteriol., 90:672-675, 1965.
Daubney, R. and Hudson, J.R.: Nairobi sheep disease. Parasitology, 23:507-524, 1931.
Haddow, A.J.: East African High Commission. Rep. East Afr. Virus Res. Inst., 1957-1958, Nairobi (Abst. Vet. Bull., 29:435, 1959).
Howarth, J.A. and Terpstra, C.: The propagation of Nairobi sheep disease virus in tissue culture. J. Comp. Pathol., 75:437-441, 1965.
Konnerup, N.: Nairobi sheep disease U.S. livestock sanitary ASSN. Foreign Animal Diseases, 1964, pp. 183-187.
Lewis, E.A.: Nairobi sheep disease. The survival of the virus in the tick Rhipicephalus appendiculatus. Parasitology, 37:55-59, 1945.

Montgomery, R.E.: Tick-borne gastroenteritis of sheep and goats in East Africa. J. Comp. Pathol. Ther., *30*:28, 1917.

Munz, E., Reiman, M., Fritz, Th., and Meier, K.: An enzyme-linked immunosorbent assay (ELISA) for the detection of antibodies to Nairobi sheep disease virus in comparison with an indirect immunofluorescent and haemagglutination test. Zbl. Vet. Med. B., *31*: 537-549, 1984.

Neitz, W.O.: Viral disease. Rep. FAO/OIE Int. Conf. on Sheep Diseases. Rome, 1966, pp. 43-54.

Terpstra, C.: Physical and biological properties of Nairobi sheep disease virus. Vet. Microbiol., *8*:531-541, 1983.

Weinbren, M.P., Gourlay, R.N., Lumsden, W.H.R. and Weinbren, B.M.: An epizootic of Nairobi sheep disease in Uganda. J. Comp. Pathol. Ther., *68*:174-187, 1955.

Paratuberculosis

(PTB; Johne's disease)

Paratuberculosis, a chronic contagious infection of adult sheep and cattle, is characterized by intermittent febrile diarrhea and emaciation and is caused by acid-fast bacteria. The condition is thought to have minor importance, but reliable estimates of the economic significance cannot be made due to undetermined prevalence and the effects of subclinical infection. Individual enterprises, especially newly infected flocks in previously clean regions, may experience high financial waste. Losses result from prolonged unthriftiness of affected sheep, eventual deaths, testing and disposal of infected animals, and legal constraints against domestic and international sheep commerce. The occurrence of PTB as a major disease in cattle and also in deer, goats, and camels adds economic importance to the malady.

OCCURRENCE. PTB occurs in all breeds and sexes of sheep 1 year of age and older. The age incidence results from the prolonged incubation period. Sheep of regions where the disease has been absent for long periods are especially susceptible and, on exposure, develop high incidence and experience high mortality. Although PTB occurs in all climatic seasons, ewes may show recrudescence of clinical signs during the spring because of the stresses and devitalization from parturition and lactation. Animals confined to pens, small pastures, and farms, because of exposure to infected feces, develop more cases than do flocks that graze continuously on large pastures and open ranges.

Geographically, PTB occurs at least sporadically in some localities among flocks of New Zealand, United States, Canada, Iceland, Britain, The Netherlands, Germany, Italy, Turkey, Israel, Yugoslavia, USSR, Pakistan, India, and Japan.

ETIOLOGY AND PATHOGENESIS. *Mycobacterium paratuberculosis,* the specific bacterial cause of both ovine and bovine PTB, is a gram-positive, acid-fast, nonsporing rod measuring 1 to 2 $\times$ 0.5 μm. This fastidious organism does not grow on many standard laboratory media, but it metabolizes and proliferates slowly and with difficulty on egg-yolk agar containing mycobacterin, a growth factor derived from extract of mycobacteria or dead tubercle bacilli. After incubation at 37°C for 4 weeks, small white colonies become visible. In infected sheep, the organism locates in the intestinal mucosa, mesenteric lymph nodes, and feces. Other *Mycobacterium spp* are slow growing and mycobactin-dependent requiring growth on Herrold's egg yolk medium (HEYM) with mycobactin and subsequent analysis by gas-liquid chromatography to identify *M. paratuberculosis* and distinguish it from other *Mycobacterium spp.*

In the external environment, the bacteria possess moderate resistance to inimical factors. They survive in water and manure for 270 and 246 days, respectively, but die from exposure for 15 minutes to cresylic compounds diluted 1:64, phenol diluted 1:40, sodium orthophenylphenate diluted 1:200, 70% ethyl alcohol and 0.1% mercuric chloride.

Even though the organism's antigenic structure is incompletely known, in lambs it produces delayed hypersensitivity, complement-fixing antibodies, hemagglutinins, and precipitins against *M. paratuberculosis.* The delayed sensitivity cross-reacts, to some extent, with antigens of *M. avium.*

PTB is probably transmitted by direct or indirect contact between diseased and susceptible young animals. Infected animal feces, heavily contaminated with *M. paratuberculosis,* often contaminate, either continuously or intermittently, flock feed and water, and all members of the flock, including susceptible sheep, ingest the pathogens along with the feed. In addition, some sheep may inhale contaminated manure dust, which enables the bacteria to penetrate the respiratory system or, after cough expulsion from the lungs, to enter the alimentary tract. Development of the disease is probably an interaction of age, genetic variability, stress factors, nutritional management, and continuous exposure to high numbers of infective organisms.

Disease development begins, usually in young animals, with ingestion of the causative organisms. In the intestines, especially ileum, cecum, and colon, the viable bacteria penetrate the epithelial membrane and enter the lamina propria. The presence of organisms in this mesenchymal tissue provokes a series of changes. Initially, neutrophils accumulate around and among the bacteria; later, macrophages and lymphocytes assemble in the area, and finally, fibrocytes proliferate. The numerous macrophages phagocytize the slowly proliferating bacteria, and some eventually enter the afferent lymph vessels and go to the mesenteric lymph nodes, where they accumulate. These changes slowly thicken the infected mucosa and enlarge the lymph nodes.

Some affected animals may show progressive debility and emaciation with normal to a slightly softened feces, but the presence of the pathogens stimulates other general reactions. Following oral inoculation, lambs develop delayed sensitivity through weeks 4 to 40, titers of complement-fixing antibodies through weeks 18 to 56, titers of hemagglutinins through weeks 7 to 60, and strong titers of precipitins through weeks 8 to 66.

EPIDEMIOLOGY AND TRANSMISSION. The infectious organism escapes from the host animal via the feces. This shedding may be intermittent contaminating the environment. The organism enters the new host via contaminated feed or water. In the case of lambs, the organism is transmitted via feces contaminated teats. In utero infection can be acquired if ewes are in

advanced stages of the disease. The outcome is dependent on the infective dose of organism and the host response to elicit a cell-mediated immune response with delayed-type hypersensitivity. If the infective dose is not overwhelming and the host defense is adequate, disease does not develop. Depending on the outcome of the agent-host interaction, the development and manifestations of the disease are extremely variable. Exposure at an early age with establishment of infection usually results in clinical manifestations, whereas older sheep tend to be more resistant with less overt disease signs.

The organism may establish a low grade infection which the host responses are unable to eliminate, thus becoming an asymptomatic carrier capable of shedding the organism. If the infectious process develops, intestinal lesions slowly progress with the cellular changes in the intestine gradually interfering with its function followed by clinical manifestations of wasting. The clinical pathologic changes include a loss of plasma proteins into the lumen with concurrent malabsorption of amino acids and enhancement of protein metabolism in the liver, the substrates which are probably metabolized from the muscles resulting in wasting. The initial agent-host interaction determines the disease outcome and is not influenced by subsequent exposures.

CLINICAL SIGNS AND POSTMORTEM LESIONS. Following an incubation period of months to years, the prominent clinical sign is loss of body condition due to muscle deterioration with no specific clinical signs. Inconsistent with the disease in cattle, diarrhea is not a common clinical feature. In advanced cases the feces may become soft and lack form. The disease becomes chronic with extreme variations in the time period between the appearance of the initial ill-thrift, emaciation, weakness, and epilation prostration. Appetite persists. Body temperatures vary and have episodes of elevation. During terminal stages, other diseases such as pneumonia supervene and accelerate the course. Hematologic studies may reveal anemia, hypoproteinemia and depression of blood levels of calcium and magnesium below normal values of 10.7 and 2.6 mg/dl.

Among infected flocks, the morbidity ranges from 1 to 10%, and most but not all affected animals eventually die. The course varies from 1 month to many, with periods of improvement and exacerbation.

At necropsy, emaciation is prominent and anemia evident. Internal lesions are limited to the alimentary system. The mucous membrane of the ileum, cecum, and colon may show general or focal thickening with or without transverse or longitudinal ridging. As viewed from the serosal surface, lymph vessels are prominent, pale, and firm, and the mesenteric lymph nodes are pale, firm, and enlarged.

Histopathologically, the changes vary quantitatively. The lamina propria of affected parts of the intestine contain variable numbers of mononuclear macrophages, lymphocytes, multinucleated giant cells, eosinophils, and proliferated fibrocytes. The macrophages, varying from small numbers to nodular masses to diffuse infiltrations, frequently contain one or more phagocytized acid-fast bacteria. Some organisms may be free among the cells. In advanced stages, the cell infiltrations extend into the submucosa. Affected lymph nodes contain, especially in the cortices, variable numbers of macrophages with phagocytized bacteria.

DIAGNOSIS. Veterinarians clinically suspect PTB in adult sheep that show characteristic signs and lesions. Gradual loss of live weight associated with intermittent or continuous diarrhea is a suggestive sign, and thickened mucosa of the ileum, cecum, or colon and enlarged mesenteric lymph nodes are indicative lesions. Confirmation of the diagnosis within a flock requires demonstration of *M. paratuberculosis*; this may be achieved in smears or sections of suspected mucosa stained for acid-fast bacilli and by culturing the bacteria from tissues or feces. Biopsy of the ileocecal lymph node may provide positive diagnosis even in early stages of infection.

Cultural isolation requires several months, and for that reason, the method has limited diagnostic value. In live animals, the johnin intradermal test, with tissue swelling at the injected site indicating reaction, and the intravenous johnin test, with rise in body temperature indicating reaction, may be used, but give unpredictable results. Serologic tests for antibodies to *M. paratuberculosis* include the complement-fixation, hemagglutination, and agar-gel immunodiffusion. These tests become more positive as the disease progresses but may give false-positive reactions due to *Corynebacterium sp* and *Nocardia sp*. As research progresses in identifying and purifying the antigenic portions of the *M. paratuberculosis* organism the enzyme-linked immunosorbent assay test will become a practical test for screening and early detection of the disease.

The differential diagnosis requires consideration of chronic gastrointestinal parasitism, internal abscesses, and chronic hepatic disease.

PREVENTION. Veterinarians and producers prevent PTB by eradicating the disease from an area. This purification is achieved by eliminating infected animals, cleaning and disinfecting premises, and avoiding new exposures. All infected flocks should be quarantined. Producers with flocks with extensive infection, as revealed by clinical signs or laboratory tests, should institute the following eradicative measures:

1. Slaughter or destroy the entire flock and all other associated animals, such as cattle.

2. Clean and disinfect the premises with cresylic compounds diluted 1:64 or with sodium orthophenylphenate diluted 1:200. Organic iodine disinfectants at manufacturers recommended levels are effective. Detergents improve the effectiveness.

3. Rest the premises for approximately 12 months.

4. Restock with healthy sheep.

5. Maintain active vigilance for clinical signs and positive reactions to johnin tests; remove and slaughter all new cases and reactors.

6. Introduce only known clean animals into the flock.

Producers with infected flocks containing valuable genetic lines should:

1. Remove for slaughter or destruction all clinical cases, johnin reactors, or feces-infected animals.

2. Transfer the remaining flock members to clean pens or pastures, and clean and disinfect the contaminated premises.

3. Continue testing until no new cases develop.

4. Vaccinate lambs, only once at 3 months of age, intended for flock replacements. Treatment is ineffective.

Animal Health Yearbook. FAO-WHO-OIE (Italy), 1970.
Chandler, R.L.: Development of vaccines for Johne's disease in sheep. N.Z. Vet. J., 5:39-43, 1957.
Chiodini, R. and VanKruiningen, H.: Characterization of *Mycobacterium paratuberculosis* of bovine, caprine and ovine origin by gas-liquid chromatographic analysis of fatty acids in whole-cell extracts. Am. J. Vet. Res., 46:1980-1989, 1985.
Gilmour, N. and Angus, K.: Johne's disease. In *Diseases of Sheep*. Edited by W.B. Martin. Oxford, Blackwell Scientific, 1983.
Howarth, J.A.: Paratuberculosis enteritis in sheep caused by an acid-fast organism. JAVMA, 81:383-387, 1932.
Hutchinson, L.: Johne's disease. Animal Health and Nutrition, 41:24-28, 1986.
Kluge, J.P., et al.: Experimental paratuberculosis in sheep after oral, intratracheal, or intravenous inoculation: lesions and demonstrations of etiologic agent. AJVR, 29:953-962, 1968.
Larsen, A.B.: Recent developments in paratuberculosis (Johne's disease) research. 68th Proc. U.S. Livestock Sanit. Assoc., 1964, pp. 342-347.
Larsen, A.B., Hawkins, W.W., and Merkal, R.S.: Experimental vaccination of sheep against Johne's disease. AJVR, 25:974-976, 1964.
Lovell, R., Levi, M., and Francis, J.: Studies on the survival of Johne's bacilli. J. Comp. Pathol., 54:120-129, 1944.
Marsh, H.: Johne's disease in an experimental flock of sheep. JAVMA, 120:20-22, 1952.
Merkal, R.S., et al.: Experimental paratuberculosis in sheep after oral, intratracheal, or intravenous inoculation: serologic and intradermal tests. AJVR, 29:963-969, 1968.
Merkal, R. and Whipple, D.: Effectiveness of disinfectants on *Mycobacterium paratuberculosis*. Proc. Eighty-Sixth Annual Mtg. U.S. Animal Health Assn., 1982, pp. 514-518.
Nakamatsu, M., Fujimoto, Y., and Satoh, H.: The pathological study of paratuberculosis in goats, centered around the formation of remote lesions. Jpn. J. Vet. Res., 16:103-120, 1968.
Seaman, J. and Thompson, D.: Johne's disease in sheep. Aust. Vet. J., 61:227-229, 1984.
Sigurdsson, B.: A killed vaccine against paratuberculosis (Johne's disease) in sheep. AJVR, 21:54-67, 1960.
Stamp, J.T. and Watt, J.A.: Johne's disease in sheep. J. Comp. Pathol., 64:26-40, 1954.
Stewart, J., McCallum, J.W., and Taylor, A.W.: Observations on the blood picture of Johne's disease in sheep and cattle with special reference to magnesium content of the blood. J. Comp. Pathol., 55:45-48, 1945.
Stockman, S.: Johne's disease in sheep. J. Comp. Pathol., 24:66-69, 1911.
Sweeney, R., Divers, T., and Shaw, D.: Paratuberculosis in a ram. JAVMA, 185:444-445, 1984.

Sneezeweed Poisoning

(*SWP; spewing sickness*)

Sneezeweed poisoning is an acute or sub-acute intoxication of range sheep, and occasionally goats and cattle that eat plants of the genus *Helenium*. The disease is characterized by weakness, incoordination, abdominal pain, and profuse vomiting that often leads to inhalation pneumonia. Various species of sneezeweed are widely distributed throughout North America and have caused considerable economic losses as a result of general unthriftiness, poor weight gains, and mortality of affected sheep. Incalculable losses also occur as a result of sneezeweed establishing itself in disturbed soils and overgrazed range land with the exclusion of useful forage plants.

OCCURRENCE. SWP occurs in all breeds, sexes, and ages of adult sheep grazing sneezeweed-infested ranges. The incidence is high on overgrazed ranges where nutritious feed is scarce and sneezeweed is abundant. Most cases develop during middle and late summer when flocks normally graze at high altitudes. Poisoning may occur, however, during spring and autumn when sneezeweed is the only green forage available.

Geographically, sneezeweed grows at altitudes between 1500 to 4000 m on ranges of western U.S., especially Colorado and Utah. Other *Helenium* species occur in the eastern states, in Texas, and in South Africa.

ETIOLOGY AND PATHOGENESIS. There are 25 known sneezeweeds (bitterweeds) belonging to the genera *Helenium* and *Dugaldia,* family Compositae. Of these at least 3 are major sources of livestock poisoning in North America: *Helenium microcephalum,* small head sneezeweed of the southwestern U.S., *H. autumnale,* eastern bitterweed (sneezeweed) of the eastern U.S., and *Dugaldia hoopesii* (H. hoopesii), orange sneezeweed of the western U.S. Orange sneezeweed is a perennial with one to four erect, terminally branched stems, which bear orange-yellow flowers and attain heights of 30 to 60 cm. The alternating leaves are pubescent and glabrous in young and mature plants, respectively (Fig. 12-8). The plant grows in association with sagebrush and aspen trees on drained, loamy soil, and may attain densities of one or more plants per m² especially in overgrazed areas. It is not generally palatable to sheep. In South Africa, *Geigeria passerinoides* causes vomeersiekte.

Sneezeweeds contain sesqinterpene lactones, several of which are known to be toxic to livestock. Helanalin is the most important of these compounds and is highly irritating to mucous membranes of the mouth and gastrointestinal tract. Similar lactones are found in *Hymenoxys* species (rubberweed) and *Baileya multiradiata,* common plants in the rangelands of the western and southwestern U.S. The ovine lethal dose of helanalin ranges between 85 to 150 mg/kg, and the toxic single oral dose of green orange sneezeweed is about 5% of body weight. The plants retain their toxicity when dried in hay.

After daily consumption of subtoxic doses of orange sneezeweed for 2 to 3 weeks, physical weakness and vomiting begin and exacerbate to the point of death if consumption continues. Removing sneezeweed from the diets of early, mild, and moderate cases rapidly abates the disease, but dietary correction for severe cases usually does not relieve the signs, and the poisoning progresses to fatal inanition, often with inhalation pneumonia.

CLINICAL SIGNS AND POSTMORTEM LESIONS. Signs begin after daily consumption of small but significant amounts of sneezeweed for 2 to 3 weeks. The first signs of sneezeweed poisoning observed by herders include coughing, vomiting, and the presence of rumen contents around the lips and nares. Depression, muscular weakness, and weight loss usually precede

Fig. 12-8. Orange sneezeweed *Dugaldia hoopesii.* × 0.4.

the onset of vomiting, the latter being the origin of the term "spewing sickness." Vomiting animals, except during the act, elevate their heads, salivate, and drip vomitus from their mouths. Coughing from inhaled ingesta is frequent and conspicuous. The pulse is weak, rapid, and irregular, and breathing is shallow, rapid, and difficult. Weak and incoordinated movements result in stumbling and falling gaits. The morbidity commonly reaches 10% but may go higher, and the eventual mortality of affected sheep is about 50%.

At necropsy, no primary changes are discernible, but secondary pneumonia from inhaled vomitus may exist.

DIAGNOSIS. Veterinarians and producers diagnose SWP on the basis of typical signs and history of continuous access to sneezeweed.

PREVENTION AND TREATMENT. Producers and herders prevent SWP by weed avoidance and herd management. Heavily infested ranges should not be grazed by sheep, but may be used for less susceptible cattle. Where avoidance is not feasible, management should include: (1) preventing overgrazing of marginal range lands by keeping stock density low, (2) providing free access to mineralized salt, and (3) ensuring sheep are not hungry by frequently moving the flock to new range as nutritious forages are depleted.

Control or eradication of sneezeweed is difficult owing to the vast range areas affected. The indiscriminate use of herbicides and soil sterilants should be avoided because of the detrimental effects of these compounds on useful vegetation.

Treatment consists of moving affected flocks from heavily infested ranges to areas less infested or preferably free of the weed. Alternating at 10-day intervals between weed-infested and weed-free range reduces the incidence of poisoning. Severely poisoned sheep should be identified for early culling and replacement.

Dollahite, J.W., Hardy, W.T., and Hensen, J.B.: Toxicity of *Helenium microcephalum*. JAVMA, 145:694-696, 1964.

Grosskopf, J.F.W.: Present knowledge of "vomeersiekte." Dep. Agric. Pretoria. Bull. No. 21, 1964 (VB, 35:312, 1965).

Heiz, W.: Sesquiterpene lactones from livestock poisons. In *Effects of Poisonous Plants on Livestock.* Edited by R.F. Keeler, K.R. VanKampen, and L.F. James. New York, Academic Press, 1978, pp. 487-497.

Marsh, C.D., Clawson, A.B., Couch, J.F., and Marsh, H.: Western sneezeweed: a poisonous plant. USDA Bull. 947, 1921, pp. 1-46.

Merrill, L.B. and Schuster, J.L.: Grazing management practices affect livestock losses from poisonous plants. J. Range Manage., 31(5):351-354, 1978.

Nielson, D.B.: The economic impact of poisonous plants on the range livestock industry in the 17 western states. J. Range Manage., 31(5):325-328, 1978.

Witzel, D.A., Ivie, G.W., and Dollahite, J.W.: Mammalian toxicity of helenalin, toxic principle of *Helenium microcephalum* (smallhead sneezehead). AJVR, 37:859-861, 1976.

Lupine Poisoning

Lupines grow in many parts of the world both as natural range plants and as a crop plant for the high protein content (30 to 40%) of the lupine seeds. Lupines have been developed especially in Australia as an important supplement for livestock, whereas in North America they are rarely grown as a crop plant. Livestock poisoning from the consumption of lupines is of extreme economic importance due to their toxic effects causing deaths, weight

Fig. 12-9. *Lupinus argenteus.* Portion of plant. × 0.5.

TABLE 12-1. *Lupines Associated Alkaloidal Lupinosis*

Names		Distribution
Scientific	Common	
L. leucophyllus	wooly lupine	U.S.: drylands of Washington and Montana to Utah and California
L. sericeus	silky lupine	U.S.: hills and valleys of Utah and Wyoming to Montana and Canada
L. argenteus	silvery lupine	U.S.: slopes and plains in Montana to California and New Mexico
L. leucopsis	big bend lupine	U.S.: hills and valleys of Oregon and Washington

loss, abortion, and deformed fetuses. Lupine poisoning occurs most commonly in sheep and cattle and results from the toxic effects of quinolizidine alkaloids in the plants, or the formation of mycotoxins from the fungus *Phomopsis leptostromiformis* growing in the plant.

Alkaloidal Lupinosis

Alkaloidal lupinosis is an acute plant intoxication, is characterized by nervous excitement, muscular weakness, and respiratory disturbance. It is caused by quinolizidine alkaloids from several species of lupines, plants prevalent in the western U.S. and other countries. The disease occasionally results in mass mortalities of sheep on the range. Economic losses result from deaths and incomplete use of lupine-infected ranges and pastures. Although the alkaloid anagyrine present in some lupines is teratogenic in cows which consume the plants between the 40th to 70th days of gestation, this potential effect has not been proven in sheep.

OCCURRENCE. Alkaloidal lupinosis occurs in all breeds, sexes, and ages of grazing sheep. Most episodes develop during late summer and early autumn when transported or driven sheep suddenly gain access to and voraciously consume large amounts of growing leaves and stems or of mature pods and seeds. Geographically, the disease develops on ranges of the western U.S. and on cultivated pastures of some other countries.

ETIOLOGY. The botanical genus *Lupinus* contains at least 100 species, some of which are toxic (Table 12-1). Lupines are perennial or annual herbs ranging in height from 15 to 180 cm. The linear leaflets, palmately arranged, number 3 to 17, and terminal racemes form varicolored flowers and flattened seed pods (Fig. 12-9). The various species grow on plains, valleys, hills, and forests in association with other plants of these habitats. Growing leaves and stems as well as mature seeds are toxic, and the toxicity persists in lupine hay.

Four of the alkaloids that are present in greatest quantity in the seeds are: 5,6-dehydrolupanine, lupanine, 13-epimethoxylupanine, and sparteine. Anagyrine, an alkaloid not toxic to sheep, when eaten by pregnant cows at the rate of 6 to 12 mg/kg, is teratogenic to bovine embryos during gestation days 40 to 75.

The development of alkaloidal intoxication is enigmatically variable. Western ranges, many with concentrated and dispersed growths of lupine, annually support sheep that are rarely seriously poisoned by the plant. Frequently, hungry flocks consume the plant with impunity, yet serious outbreaks of poisoning occasionally occur. Most losses develop when hungry sheep—after prolonged marches, following corral confinements, and after vehicular transport—consume large amounts of lupine. Under these circumstances, 50% or more of the members of large flocks may become intoxicated, and many may die. The toxic dose of lupine for sheep is approximately 0.25 to 0.5% of body weight for seeds, and 1.5% of body weight for pods and seeds. The severity of poisoning is enhanced when the seeds are consumed over a short period. The specific alkaloids responsible for lupinosis in range sheep are not well defined, nor are their effects on the animal well understood.

CLINICAL SIGNS AND POSTMORTEM LESIONS. In alkaloidal lupinosis, signs suddenly develop after a latent period of 1 to 24 hours. Affected sheep become excited, run, leap, butt, tremble, and convulse. They head-push, stagger, and fall. As the disease progresses, the animals grind their teeth, froth at the mouth, and breathe with difficulty. Morbidity ranges up to 60% and the mortality up to 80%. The course varies from 2 to 24 hours. Some animals show rapid and complete recovery. At necropsy, no specific lesions exist, but identifiable fragments of lupine leaves and pods may be discernible in the rumen.

DIAGNOSIS. Diagnosis of alkaloidal lupinosis can be difficult, and must rely on the clinical signs and evidence of sheep having grazing access to mature lupine with seed pods. Grazing access of hungry sheep to large amounts of lupine, especially containing pods and seeds, and typical manifestations suggest the disease. Identifying parts of lupine in the rumens of dead animals confirms the diagnosis. The differential diagnosis requires consideration of acute poisoning from death camas, milkweed, and other sources.

PREVENTION. Producers avoid the disease by denying hungry sheep access to large amounts of lupine. Supplementary feed should be provided to sheep during long marches over lupine-infested trails and to sheep unloaded from transporting vehicles onto lupine-infected range or pasture. Correction of hunger reduces risk.

Cheeke, P.R.: Quinolizidine alkaloids. In *Natural Toxicants in Feeds and Poisonous Plants.* Connecticut, AVI Publishing Company, Inc., 1985, pp. 127-131.
James, L.F., Binns, W., and Shupe, T.L.: Blood changes in cattle and sheep fed lupine. AJVR, *29*:557-560, 1968.
Keeler, R.F.: Lupine alkaloids from teratogenic and nonteratogenic lupines. III. Identification of anagyrine. J. Toxicol. Environ. Health, *1*:887-898, 1976.
Keeler, R.F. and Cronin, E.H.: Lupine alkaloids from teratogenic and nonteratogenic lupines. IV. Concentration of total alkaloids and anagyrine as a function of plant parts and growth stage. J. Toxicol. Environ. Health, *1*:899-908, 1976.
Kingsbury, J.M.: *Poisonous Plants of the U.S. and Canada.* Englewood Cliffs, N.J., Prentice-Hall, 1964.
Marsh, C.D., Clawson, A.B., and Marsh, H.: Lupines as poisonous plants. USDA Bull. 405, 1916.
Shupe, J.L., Binns, W., James, L.F., and Keeler, R.F.: Lupine, a cause of crooked calf disease. JAVMA, *151*:198-203, 1967.

Mycotic Lupinosis

Mycotic lupinosis is a worldwide disease of sheep and cattle that consume lupines containing a hepatic mycotoxin produced by the fungus *Phomopsis leptostromiformis.* The disease is characterized by weight loss, depression, and icterus that develop secondarily to hepatic necrosis. Lupinosis has attained economic significance in many countries, especially Australia, where lupines are grown as crop plants for their high protein content. The disease concerns the sheep industry because it is widespread and causes mass mortalities. Development of the disease in cattle also adds economic significance to the malady.

OCCURRENCE. Mycotic lupinosis occurs sporadically in all breeds, sexes, and ages of grazing sheep, but susceptibility among animals is not uniform. It usually develops in late summer or early autumn after heavy precipitation when humidity and temperature favor fungal growth. Geographically, mycotic lupinosis affects sheep of Europe, South Africa, and Australia where farmers cultivate lupines as an agronomic crop. Mycotic lupinosis is rarely encountered under American range conditions.

ETIOLOGY. The fungus *Phomopsis leptostromiformis* growing initially in the green and later the dry lupine plant produces toxic metabolites, the most important of which are Phomopsin A and B. Wet, humid conditions and high sheep stocking rates seem to enhance the growth of the fungus. Heavily infected lupine stubble or seed pods may have a gray-brown discoloration. All lupine stubble should be considered potentially toxic and managed accordingly. Phomopsins are potent toxins, requiring as little as 10 μg/kg body weight to kill a sheep. The primary effect of the phomopsins is to inhibit mitosis in liver cells with resulting hepatic degeneration.

The lupine stalks or the stubble remaining after harvesting contain the highest concentrations of fungus. Not all species of lupine are susceptible to the fungus, a factor that has enabled the selection of fungal resistant varieties of lupine.

CLINICAL SIGNS AND LESIONS.   Within a few days of consuming lupine containing phomopsins, sheep become anorexic, depressed, and may die in 1 to 2 days after the onset of signs. Subacute cases may survive for months but are emaciated, weak, depressed, and tend to stand by themselves or wander aimlessly (hepatic encephalopathy). Icterus is a predominant clinical feature of the disease. Plasma bilirubin levels are significantly elevated. Liver enzymes in the acute stages of the disease are markedly elevated reflecting hepatic necrosis. Serum and liver copper levels are frequently elevated due to liver necrosis and signs of chronic copper poisoning may prevail. Photosensitization is rarely a feature of the disease in sheep. Liver selenium levels are often increased and zinc levels decreased in mycotic lupinosis. A lupinosis-associated myopathy occurs in sheep that resembles that seen with a vitamin E-selenium deficiency. However, the myopathy is not preventable or treatable with vitamin E or selenium. The morbidity in sheep with mycotic lupinosis may exceed 50%, and the mortality may reach 80%.

At necropsy, lost weight and icterus are obvious. Hepatic lipidosis is extreme in acute cases and moderate in subacute cases. Kidneys may be darkened. Histologically, hepatocytes of centrolobular zones show cytoplasmic fat, cell enlargement, nuclear enlargement, and karyorrhexis. Enlarged reticuloendothelial cells contain phagocytized yellow-brown granules. Fibrosis occurs around central veins, and proliferated capillaries occur around triads.

Myopathy involving skeletal and myocardial muscle is also reported in sheep with mycotic lupinosis. Spongioform encephalopathy occurs in natural and experimentally induced lupinosis in sheep.

DIAGNOSIS.   Mycotic lupinosis can be diagnosed in sheep from the history of grazing lupine, the clinical signs, and the presence of hepatic necrosis. The identification of fungi of the genus *Phomopsis* and the isolation of Phomopsin from lupine, on which the animals have been grazing, would confirm the diagnosis.

The differential diagnosis requires consideration of pyrrolizidine alkaloid poisoning and chronic copper poisoning.

PREVENTION.   Lupinosis can be prevented by limiting access to fungus infected lupine stubble. If sheep or cattle are fed lupine, careful monitoring of the lupine for evidence of fungal infection should be performed regularly. Experimentally at least, supplementing zinc in the ration helps reduce the severity of liver damage. Selection of fungus resistant varieties of lupine may be the solution to overcoming the lupinosis problem.

Allen, J.G.: The emergence of a lupinosis-associated myopathy in sheep in western Australia. Aust. Vet. J., 54:548-549, 1978.

Allen, J.G.: An evaluation of lupinosis cattle in western Australia. Aust. Vet. J., 57:212-215, 1981.

Allen, J.G. and Masters, H.G.: Prevention of ovine lupinosis by the oral administration of zinc sulfate and the effect of such therapy on liver and pancreas zinc and liver copper. Aust. Vet. J., 56:168-171, 1980.

Allen, J.G., Masters, H.G., and Wallace, S.R.: The effect of lupinosis on liver copper, selenium and zinc concentrations in Merino sheep. Vet. Rec., 105:434-436, 1979.

Allen, J.G., Moir, R.J., and McIntosh, J.B.: Ovine lupinosis resulting from the ingestion of lupin seed naturally infected with *Phomopsis leptostromiformis*. Aust. Vet. J., 60:206-208, 1983.

Bennetts, H.W.: Lupine poisoning in sheep of western Australia. Aust. Vet. J., 33:277-283, 1957.

Culvenor, C.C.J., Smith, L.W., Frahn, J.C., and Cockram, P.A.: Lupinosis: Chemical properties of Phomopsin A, the main toxic metabolite of *Phomopsis leptostromiformis*. In *Effects of Poisonous Plants on Livestock*. Edited by R.F. Keeler, K.R. VanKampen, and L.F. James. New York, Academic Press, 1978, pp. 565-573.

Gardiner, M.R.: Fungus-induced toxicity in lupinosis. Br. Vet. J., 122:508-516, 1966.

Gardiner, M.R. and Parr, W.H.: Acute lupinosis of sheep. J. Comp. Pathol., 77:51-52, 1967.

Jago, M.V., Peterson, J.E., Payne, A.L., and Campbell, D.G.: Response of sheep to different doses of Phompsin. Aust. J. Exp. Biol. Sci., 60:239-251, 1982.

Van Warmelo, K.T., Marasas, W.F.O., Adelaar, T.F., and Kellerman, T.S.: Evidence that sheep lupinosis is caused by fungus. J. S. Afr. Vet. Med. Assoc., 41:235-247, 1970.

TABLE 12-2. *Species of Zigadenus*

Name Scientific (common)	Latent Period (Hours)	Clinical Course (Hours)	MTD (% body Weight)	MLD (% body Weight)	Distribution
Z. gramineus (grassy)	2	12	0.4	0.6	U.S.: high plains, west Canada: west
Z. nuttallii (Nuttall's)	8	48	0.2	0.5	Tennessee to Texas Oklahoma
Z. venenosus (meadow)	3	29	0.4	2.0	U.S.: west Canada: west
Z. paniculatus (foothill)	3	36	1.0	2.5	U.S.: west

(Compiled from Kingsbury, 1964.)

Death Camas Poisoning

(*Zigadenus poisoning*)

Death camas poisoning, an acute plant intoxication of sheep, is characterized by digestive and locomotor disturbances and is caused by alkaloids from several species of *Zigadenus,* a common lily of western North America. Its wide distribution in pastures and ranges grazed by sheep and its retained toxicity when dried in hay makes death camas a significant problem to sheep producers. Some enterprises encounter high incidence and financial waste. Economic losses result from deaths of affected sheep and from the costs of prevention. Occurrence of the disease in cattle and horses and (rarely) in people also adds both economic importance and public health significance to the malady.

OCCURRENCE. Death camas poisoning occurs in all breeds, sexes, and ages of grazing sheep. Most cases develop during early spring because the emergence of camas precedes the growth of most other range plants and becomes available to sheep hungry after marching, transporting, or shearing. Geographically, the disease occurs on most range habitats of the high plains and western states and provinces of the United States and Canada.

ETIOLOGY. There are at least 15 species of *Zigadenus*, at least 4 of which have proven toxicity (Table 12-2). This perennial herb, growing from an onion-like bulb produces grasslike, glabrous, basal linear leaves, and greenish white to yellow flowers on a terminal raceme (Fig. 12-10).

Zigadenus species often grow in the same habitat as wild onion, a plant that may be confused with death camas by people with often fatal results. The surest way to differentiate death camas from wild onion is to crush the leaves or bulbs and detect the smell of onion that is absent in death camas.

Fig. 12-10. *Zigadenus gramineus.* × 0.3.

Various species, either separately or in combinations, occupy habitats commonly grazed by sheep. After its early spring emergence, the plant forms sparse to abundant growths on plains, hills, and meadows at altitudes of up to 2500 m.

The poisonous substance includes complex ester alkaloids, glycoalkaloids, and steroid alkaloids, such as zigacine. The compounds are distributed in all parts of the plant, including the bulb, but the amounts in leaves and flowers, the consumed plant parts, usually cause poisoning.

Sheep generally find zigadenus unpalatable and selectively exclude it from their diets when alternative forage is available. Circumstances of sheep hunger and plant availability usually induce consumption: laborious spring marching along camas-containing trails, prolonged transportation and unloading on infested areas, confinement for shearing and release to camas-infested range, and winter feeding of camas-contaminated hay. Following the consumption of death camas in amounts ranging from 0.2 to 1.0% of body weight, sheep sicken; they recover or die depending on the amount of toxin and the rate of consumption.

CLINICAL SIGNS. Following ingestion of the minimal toxic dose of green camas, ranging from 0.2 to 1.0% of sheep weight, the affected animals become ill within 2 to 8 hours. Early signs are salivation, nausea, and vomiting; these are followed by mental depression and physical weakness. Body temperature ranges from normal to subnormal values. In terminal stages, the pulse becomes weak and irregular. Pregnant ewes may abort or bear stillborn lambs.

The morbidity varies up to 25% of a flock, and the mortality among affected sheep commonly reaches 20%. The short course ranges from 12 to 48 hours.

DIAGNOSIS. Veterinarians diagnose death camas poisoning on evidence of typical signs and the presence of species of Zigadenus in the diet of fresh or preserved forage. Fragments of the causative plant may be identified in the rumen contents. The differential diagnosis requires consideration of other quick-acting poisons, such as cyanogenic plants and greasewood, and metabolic tetanies.

TREATMENT. There is no effective treatment for sheep with acute death camas poisoning, although in the early stages of poisoning 2 mg atropine sulfate and 8 mg picrotoxin per 100 lbs body weight may be helpful.

PREVENTION. Producers prevent death camas poisoning by avoiding simultaneous sheep hunger and zigadenus availability. Marching, transported, and corralled sheep should receive supplementary feed before gaining access to camas. Fed animals usually reject the plant. Concentrated pasture growths in early prebloom stage can be effectively sprayed with herbicide such as 2,4-D ester.

Beath, O.A., Eppson, H.F., Draize, J.H., and Justice, R.S.: Species of *Zygadenus*. Wyoming Agric. Exp. Stat. Bull. 194, 1933.

Jeger, O. and Prelog, V.: Steroid alkaloids. In *Alkaloids.* Vol. VII. New York, Academic Press, 1960.

Kingsbury, J.M.: *Poisonous Plants in the United States and Canada.* Englewood Cliffs, N.J., Prentice-Hall, 1964, pp. 461-466.

Kupchan, S.M. and Diliwala, C.V.: *Zygadenus* alkaloids. J. Am. Chem. Soc., 75:1025, 1953.

Marsh, C.D. and Clawson, A.B.: Meadow death camas (*Z. venenosus*) as a poisonous plant. USDA Bull. 1240, 1924.

Marsh, C.D., Clawson, A.B., and Marsh, H.: *Zygadenus* or death *camas.* USDA Bull. 125, 1915.

Marsh, C.D., Clawson, A.B., and Roe, G.C.: Nuttall's death camas as a poisonous plant. USDA Bull. 1376, 1926.

Oxalate Poisoning

(Halogeton poisoning; greasewood poisoning)

Oxalate poisoning in sheep is generally an acute intoxication caused by the ingestion of plants high in sodium and potassium oxalates. In North America oxalate toxicity is most frequently associated with the ingestion of Halogeton and greasewood, whereas in Australia soursob (*Oxalis spp*) is most commonly incriminated. Halogeton is of prime economic importance because it has infested at least 10 million acres of semiarid western rangeland that are chiefly used for livestock production. In addition to being toxic to sheep and cattle that consume them, halogeton and greasewood displace useful forage from the rangelands.

OCCURRENCE. Oxalate poisoning occurs in all breeds and sexes of sheep 1 year of age and older. The disease usually develops under circumstances of sheep hunger and oxalate availability. Poisoning from halogeton usually occurs in autumn following prolonged transportation and during winter when snow covers wholesome forage. Poisoning from consuming greasewood occurs during spring among hungry sheep unaccustomed to the plant.

Geographically, oxalate poisoning is encountered among sheep grazing open ranges of the western United States. It may also occur in the USSR, Tibet, and Kashmir where sheep and halogeton coexist, and in Australia where *Oxalis cernua* contaminates forage.

Fig. 12-11. *Halogeton glomeratus* showing characteristic terminal fiber on rounded fleshy leaves.

ETIOLOGY AND PATHOGENESIS. In North America the two most important oxalate forming plants are *Halogeton glomeratus* and *Sarcobatus vermiculatus* (greasewood). In Australia *Oxalis pes-caprae* (soursob) is a prime source of oxalate poisoning. Other plant species capable of accumulating smaller quantities of oxalates include *Amaranthus retroflexus* (red rooted pigweed), *Kochia scoparia* (kochia weed), *Rumex crispus* (dock, sorrel), *Chenopodium album* (lamb's quarter), *Salsola rali* (Russian thistle), and *Beta vulgaris* (beet). Certain grasses have also been shown to form oxalates in sufficient quantity to impair normal dietary mineral utilization e.g. *Cenchrus ciliaris Setaria sphacelata, pennisetum clandestinum* (kikuyn grass). The minimum lethal doses of soluble oxalates for fed and fasted adult sheep are 44 and 28 g, respectively.

H. glomeratus grows 100 to 500 mm high and typically develops four upturned branches arranged in cruciform pattern. During vegetative growth, the stems are pink to purple and the leaves blue-green, but on maturation, the entire plant becomes pale yellow. The round fleshy leaves measure 6 to 18 mm in length, form repeating clusters along stems, and possess a terminal fiber (Fig. 12-11). The two types of seeds—brown and black—are abundant and measure about 1 mm in diameter. The species grows in arid and semiarid climates on saline soil in disturbed areas, such as roadsides, trails, watering sites, and corrals. Wind, vehicles, and sheep disperse the prolific seeds, some of which maintain viability for 10 years. Leaf concentrations of oxalates range from 8% of dry matter in spring to 30% in autumn.

S. vermiculatus, an erect woody perennial shrub, has spiny branches and alternating, green, fleshy, deciduous leaves 7 to 32 mm long. The sexes are separate in bushes 1 to 2 m in height (Fig. 12-12). The leaf concentrations of sodium and potassium oxalates range from 10 to 22% of dry weight. The plant grows on thousands of square kilometers of saline alkaline soil of arid and semiarid ranges of the western United States, often in association with Halogeton.

Fig. 12-12. Greasewood *Sarcobatus vermiculatus.*
× 0.1.

The toxicity of oxalates varies with size of animal, other components of the diet, nutritional state, and adaptation to oxalates. In general, feed consisting of a mixture of oxalate-containing and oxalate-free plants has low toxicity for fully fed sheep, whereas feed consisting mainly of oxalate-containing plants has high toxicity for hungry animals. Sheep that are slowly adapted to diets high in oxalate are able to tolerate much higher levels of oxalate than nonadapted sheep. High oxalate rations enhance the development of rumen microorganisms capable of degrading oxalate to formate and carbon dioxide in the process of using it in their growth requirements. It requires about 4 days for rumen microorganisms to reach effective oxalate-degrading capacity. The minimum lethal dose of soluble oxalates for fed and fasted adult sheep is 44 g and 28 g respectively.

Range circumstances that lead to hunger and thus to oxalate vulnerability include: (1) prolonged marches in which nutritious feed is scarce and oxalate-bearing plants are abundant, (2) prolonged shipment by truck or rail and unloading where oxalate-bearing plants abound, (3) autumn or winter grazing where snow covers most forage except oxalate-bearing plants, and (4) watering thirsty and consequently hungry sheep where halogeton is available. Under any of these conditions, hungry sheep indiscriminantly consume available forage, including oxalate-bearing plants, and may suffer fatal intoxication.

The pathogenesis of poisoning begins with ingestion of a minimum toxic dose of sodium and potassium oxalates. In the rumen, the compounds undergo three dispositional actions: (1) one portion, acted on by ruminal microflora, degrades to carbonates and bicarbonates, (2) an amount precipitates as insoluble calcium oxalate and remains with the feces, and (3) a moiety absorbs into the blood and other tissues, where it precipitates as calcium oxalate crystals in vessel walls and nephron tubules. These tissue changes may reduce the plasma calcium by nearly 50%, elevate blood urea, and possibly derange carbohydrate metabolism. Mortality in oxalate poisoning is not simply due to the effects of hypocalcemia since treatment with calcium gluconate does not alter the fatal course of the acute disease in sheep.

An exception to the pathogenesis exists, in some areas at least, among sheep grazing greasewood. Hungry flocks, unaccustomed to greasewood, consume spring stands of the plants and suffer mass mortalities. But flocks gradually adapted over 4 to 7 days to greasewood can continuously graze it as a major dietary component with impunity and, in the process, support lambs and gain weight. This adaptation to dietary oxalates probably results from qualitative and quantitative changes in ruminal microflora whereby the bacteria rapidly degrade large amounts of the compounds.

CLINICAL SIGNS AND POSTMORTEM LESIONS. Signs of oxalate poisoning develop within 2 to 12 hours after sheep consume toxic amounts of the source plants. Initial signs are depression, weakness, and inability to march with the flock. Within a few hours, the pulse accelerates, and respiration becomes rapid, shallow, and difficult. Foam may form in the mouth. Affected animals prostrate, pass into coma, and die from cardiac failure. When large flocks consume the causative plants, many hundreds of animals may succumb to a single disease episode. The mortality of affected sheep is high; the course ranges from 1 to 6 hours.

At necropsy, the rumen contains identifiable fragments of the toxic plants and may show edema, hemorrhage, and necrosis from corrosive action of the oxalates. Histopathologic changes include deposition of oxalate crystals in the walls of some ruminal vessels and in tubules of the kidneys.

DIAGNOSIS. Veterinarians diagnose oxalate poisoning on evidence of history, signs, and laboratory findings. Sudden deaths among hungry sheep with access to halogeton or greasewood suggest the disease. Finding hypocalcemia in terminal stages or crystals in the kidneys confirms the diagnosis.

PREVENTION AND TREATMENT. Producers prevent oxalate poisoning by prudent management:

1. Avoid grazing sheep on range heavily infested with halogeton and greasewood.

2. Avoid grazing hungry sheep on range moderately infested with halogeton; provide feed supplement to sheep grazing such ranges.

3. Avoid grazing sheep where only halogeton projects above snow cover.

4. Avoid watering thirsty and therefore hungry sheep where halogeton predominates as available feed; provide supplementary feed under these circumstances.

5. Provide water and supplementary feed, fortified with 25% dicalcium phosphate, to sheep marching along roads and trails where halogeton grows abundantly.

6. Provide water and supplementary feed, fortified with 25% dicalcium phosphate, to sheep before loading onto and after unloading from vehicles for transport into range containing halogeton.

7. Avoid grazing spring stands of greasewood with sheep unaccustomed to the plant.

8. If sheep must be ranged where halogeton is abundant, provide supplemental feed for the first 4 days to allow time for the sheep's rumen microflora to adapt to the oxalates in the diet.

Treatment, usually unfeasible and unsuccessful, is unsatisfactory to both producers and practitioners. Sheep should be removed from areas with dense stands of halogeton, and fed hay supplemented with a balanced mineral with dicalcium phosphate.

Allison, M.J., Littledike, E.T., and James, L.F.: Changes in ruminal oxalate degradation rates associated with adaptation to oxalate ingestion. J. Anim. Sci., 45:1173-1178, 1977.

Allison, M.J., Cook, H.M., and Dawson, K.A.: Selection of oxalate degrading rumen bacteria in continuous cultures. J. Anim. Sci., 53:810-816, 1981.

ARS Bulletin 327. 22 plants poisonous to livestock, 1968.

Blaney, G.J., Gartner, B.J.W., and Head, T.A.: The effects of oxalate in tropical grasses on calcium, phosphorus and magnesium availability to cattle. J. Agric. Sci., 99:533-546, 1982.

Cook, W.C. and Stoddard, L.A.: Halogeton problem in Utah. Utah Agric. Exp. Stat. Bull., 346, 1953.

Couch, J.F.: Toxic constituent of greasewood. Am. J. Pharm., 94:631, 1922.

Cronin, E.H.: Ecological and physical factors influencing *Halogeton glomeratus*. USDA Tech. Bull., 1325: 1-65, 1965.

Dodson, M.E.: Oxalate ingestion in sheep. Aust. Vet. J., 35:225, 1959.

James, L.F.: Oxalate metabolism in sheep. J. Anim. Sci., 27:718-723, 1968a.

James, L.F.: Serum electrolyte acid-base balance in halogeton poisoning. Can. J. Comp. Med., 32:539-543, 1968b.

James, L.F.: Oxalate toxicosis. Clin. Toxicol., 5:231-243, 1972.

James, L.F., Butcher, J.E., and Van Kampen, K.R.: Relationship between halogeton consumption and water intake. J. Range Manag., 23:123-127, 1970.

James, L.F. and Johnson, A.E.: Prevention of fatal halogeton poisoning in sheep. JAVMA, 157:437-442, 1970.

James, L.F. and Cronin, E.H.: Management practices to minimize death losses in sheep grazing halogeton infested range. J. Range Management, 27:424-426, 1974.

James, L.F.: Oxalate poisoning in livestock. In *Effects of Poisonous Plants on Livestock*. Edited by R.F. Keeler, K.R. VanKampen, and L.R. James. New York, Academic Press, 1978, pp. 139-145.

Kingsbury, J.M.: *Poisonous Plants of the United States and Canada*. Englewood Cliffs, N.J., Prentice-Hall, 1964, p. 240.

Littledike, E.T., James, L.F., and Cook, H.: Oxalate (halogeton) poisoning of sheep; certain physiopathologic changes. Am. J. Vet. Res., 37:661-666, 1976.

McIntosh, G.H.: Chronic oxalate poisoning in sheep. Aust. Vet. J., 48:535, 1972.

Osguthorp, D.A.: Preventing oxalate poisoning in sheep. Personal communications, 1972.

Shupe, J.L. and James, L.F.: Physiologic changes in halogeton poisoning in sheep. Cornell Vet., 59:41-55, 1969.

VanKampen, K.R. and James, L.F.: Acute halogeton poisoning in sheep: lesions. AJVR, 30:1779-1783, 1969.

Watts, P.S.: Oxalic acid ingestion in sheep. J. Agric. Sci., 52:244-249; 250-255, 1959.

Williams, M.C. and Cronin, E.H.: Poisonous range weeds. J. Range Manag., 19:274-279, 1966.

Zappettini, G.: Taxonomy of *Halogeton glomeratus*. Am. Mid. Nat., 50:238-247, 1953.

Rubberweed Poisoning

(*RWP*)

Rubberweed poisoning occurring primarily in sheep is caused by the consumption of toxic amounts of rubberweed or pingue (*Hymenoxys spp*). Annual loss of sheep attributed to rubberweed toxicity in Texas have been estimated to be several million dollars. Goats and less frequently cattle may also be affected by rubberweed.

OCCURRENCE. RWP can occur in all sexes, breeds, and ages of weaned grazing sheep. It develops during plant-growing periods from early spring through summer and autumn. It is more common, however, during early and late seasons when salubrious forage plants are scarce, or when rubberweeds predominate over all other types of forage. Geographically, the disease exists where plants grow: bitter-weed from Kansas south to Mexico and from Central Texas west to California, and pingue from Montana south to Mexico.

ETIOLOGY AND PATHOGENESIS. Two species of rubberweed—*Hymenoxys odorata*, commonly called bitterweed, and *H. richardsoni*, also known as pingue or Colorado rubberweed, both of the family Compositae—cause the disease in the U.S. These related annual or perennial herbs have one or more erect, usually pubescent, sometimes branched, leafy stems up to 60 cm in height, and usually with alternate and very narrow leaves. The yellow flower heads have three-lobed ray flowers. Involucral bracts of flower heads are in two series; those of the outer one are partially united at the base (Fig. 12-13). These highly unpalatable plants are rejected by sheep except under critical conditions of hunger and weed availability.

Bitterweeds contain sesquiterpene lactones, the most toxic of which is hymenoxon, a highly irritating compound that inhibits cellular functions by alkylating sulfhydril groups of cellular enzymes. Feeding of cysteine and methionine helps to reduce the toxicity of hymenoxon. The oral LD50 of dried bitterweed in sheep is 2.9 to 8.5 g/kg body weight. Sheep will develop severe poisoning if they eat 0.5 to 1.3% of the body weight in green plant or 1 g/kg/

Fig. 12-13. Pingue (*H. richardsoni*).

day for 15 days. The minimum lethal dose of hymenoxon is approximately 100 mg/kg body weight. Similar sesquiterpene lactones occur in other common range land plants of the genera *Helenium, Dugaldia* and *Baileya.*

CLINICAL SIGNS AND POSTMORTEM LESIONS. Following the ingestion of toxic amounts of rubberweed, acutely sick sheep show anorexia, cessation of rumination, oral frothing, mucoid nasal discharge, vomiting, arched back, and disinclination to move. Mental depression progresses to recumbency, semicoma, opisthotonos, convulsions, tachycardia, dyspnea, and death. During the disease course, serum total protein, albumin, and glucose decrease, while serum urea nitrogen, creatinine, total bilirubin, aspartate transferase, lactic acid, and creatine kinase levels increase. Arterial blood pH decreases, and urine acidity increases. The fatal course ranges up to 7 days. Animals in early stages commonly recover when moved to nutritious feed free of the weed. Losses are greater during seasons of drought than during times of rainfall.

At necropsy, mucous membranes of the rumen and abomasum show some edema and petechial hemorrhages. Kidneys may have glomerulonephrosis.

DIAGNOSIS. Rubberweed poisoning should be diagnosed on the basis of clinical signs and evidence of rubberweed consumption. Hungry sheep on overgrazed pastures are likely to consume rubberweed if it is the predominant plant available.

PREVENTION AND TREATMENT. RWP can be prevented by appropriate management procedures. Grazing sheep, especially when hungry and fatigued, should not be exposed to forage consisting mainly of rubberweed, and if unavoidably exposed, they should be given supplementary feed, preferably in advance.

Heavy stands of rubberweed on pasture or range can be controlled by spraying the plants, in the budding stage, with an ester of 2,4-D at the rate of 11 kg/hectare. Indiscriminant use of herbicides and soil sterilants should be avoided to safeguard other useful range plants. Overgrazing range land should be prevented to discourage the overgrowth of rubberweeds.

Treatment consists of transferring affected sheep during early stages of poisoning from rubberweed-infested to weed-free range.

Aanes, W.A.: Pingue (*Hymenoxys richardsoni*) poisoning in sheep. AJVR, *22*:47-51, 1961.

Calhoun, M.C., Meckert, D.N., Livingston, C.W., and Baldwin, B.C.: Effects of bitterweed (*Hymenoxys odorata*) on voluntary feed intake and serum constituents of sheep. Am. J. Vet. Res., *42*:1713-1716, 1981.

Cheeke, P.R.: *Natural Toxicants in Feeds and Poisonous Plants.* Westport, Connecticut, AVI Publishing Company, Inc., 1985, pp. 359-363.

Herz, W.: Sesquiterpene lactones from livestock poisons. In *Effects of Poisonous Plants on Livestock.* Edited by R.F. Keeler, K.R. VanKampen, L.F. James. New York, Academic Press, 1978, pp. 487-497.

Ivie, G.W., et al.: Hymenoxon, major toxic constituent of western bitterweed (*H. odorata*). J. Agric. Food Chem., *23*:841-845, 1975.

Kim, H.L., Rowe, L.D., and Camp, B.G.: Hymenovin, a poisonous sesquiterpene lactone, from *H. odorata.* Res. Commun. Chem. Pathol. Pharmacol., *11*:647-650, 1975.

Rowe, L.D., Kim, H.L., and Camp, B.J.: The antagonistic effect of L-Cysteine in experimental *Hymenoxon* intoxication in sheep. Am. J. Vet. Res., *41*:484-486, 1980.

Witzel, D.A., Jones, L.P., and Ivie, G.W.: Pathology of subacute bitterweed (*H. odorata*) poisoning in sheep. Vet. Pathol., *14*:73-78, 1977.

Witzel, D.A., Rowe, L.D., and Clark, D.E.: Physiopathologic studies on acute *H. odorata* (bitterweed) poisoning in sheep. AJVR, *35*:931-934, 1974.

Urea Poisoning

(*UP; Ammonia-urea toxicosis*)

Urea poisoning, an acute ammoniac intoxication, is characterized by tetany, circulatory failure, and a short course and is caused by excessive hydrolysis of dietary urea, ammonia or ammonia salts. Because the disease is uncommon and generally avoidable, it causes little concern to the sheep industry. Accidental poisonings, however, may cause financial waste to individual enterprises from deaths and the cost of treatments. The disease also occurs in goats and cattle, especially farm flocks and herds and feedlot animals.

OCCURRENCE. UP occurs in all breeds, sexes, and ages except in unweaned lambs, but only among animals consuming rations containing urea or those accidentally feeding on extradietary sources of the compound. Usually the condition develops during the fall when sheep change from a ration of roughage to one that is supplemented with urea. In feed-lot lambs, the poisoning occurs when animals are first adapting to new rations and during periods of resumed feeding after anorexia and declined adaptation. Other sources of toxicity may occur from accidental consumption of urea, ammonia, or ammonium salts used as farm fertilizers. Geographically, it occurs in all industrialized countries where sheep are maintained or fattened on rations with urea constituents.

ETIOLOGY AND PATHOGENESIS. Urea is hydrolyzed in the rumen with the aid of urease to ammonia (NH_3) and carbon dioxide (CO_2) within about 1 hour of ingestion. The ammonia (NH_3) is utilized by rumen microorganisms along with carbohydrates to synthesize amino acids and protein. Excess amounts of urea or NH_3 are absorbed by the portal circulation and detoxified by the liver or cleared by the kidney. Toxicity results from rapid ingestion of urea or ammonia salts in excess of the metabolic requirements and the capacity of the liver and kidney to synthesize or clear these products from the system. Factors enhancing animal susceptibility to the condition include fasting, nonadaptation to the compound, incomplete mixing of the urea with other ration ingredients, and inadequate amounts of carbohydrate or protein in the diet.

Normal amounts of rumen NH_3 up to 50 μmol/L of fluid are used by bacteria to synthesize their cellular amino acids and proteins, and as such bacteria die, their proteins are digested and absorbed by the host ruminant. In an acidic medium, however, the NH_3 converts to ammonium ion, which is absorbed slowly, but toxic amounts of NH_3 (60 μmol/L) form a strong concentration gradient that transports the NH_3 across the epithelium into portal blood. Normal levels of portal blood NH_3 (0.3 to 0.5 μmol/L) enter the liver and are converted to urea, but larger amounts exceed the detoxifying capacity of the liver and leak past the liver into peripheral blood. Ammonia inhibits the energy yielding processes including the Krebs cycle and oxidative-phosphorylation, whereas high concentrations of urea adversely affect urogenesis, lipogenesis, water and mineral metabolism, and respiration. The toxicity of NH_3, whether from ammonia salts and urea or protein feeds is related to ammonia levels and rumen pH values. Only nonionized or free NH_3 diffuses from the rumen into the portal blood. High rumen pH (8.4) favors NH_3 and toxicity, although toxicity may occur at lower levels (pH 6.0) depending on the diet and variety of environmental influences. Normal $NH_3 - N$ levels in the blood range from 0.1 to 0.2 mg/dl. Toxic levels range from 3.0 to 6.0 mg/dl with clinical signs appearing at 1.0 mg/dl. Toxic levels of peripheral blood NH_3 (3 to 6 μmol/L) act directly on the cardiovascular system, increasing the permeability of capillaries to plasma proteins and damaging the heart. Fluids pass out of the vessels, and the blood undergoes concentration. Death is probably due to hyperkalemic cardiac shock and cessation of respiration.

The following rates of intake are safe for adapted sheep: 33% of the dietary protein, 2 to 3% of dietary concentrate, or 1% of the total dry ration. Fatal doses are 0.4 to 0.5 g/kg of body weight in fasted or starved sheep and 0.7 to 0.8 g/kg in well-nourished animals. In practice there is a narrow margin between toxic symptoms and a lethal dose (0.05 g/kg body weight).

CLINICAL SIGNS AND POSTMORTEM LESIONS. Affected animals show illness within 20 to 60 minutes after ingesting toxic amounts of urea. Signs begin with depression and dullness, followed by uneasiness and hyperesthesia. Later, ruminations cease and bloating begins. Muscles twitch and tremble, and movements become incoordinated. Tetany supervenes, and the animal may fall with extended limbs, labored breathing, accelerated pulse, and salivation. There is a significant increase in packed cell volume (10 to 15%) with elevations in blood glucose, potassium, phosphorus, SGOT, SGPT, and BUN. The disease course lasts for 1.5 to 2.5 hours. Morbidity ranges up to 50%, and the case mortality reaches 80%.

At necropsy, the opened rumen emits a faint to strong ammoniac odor and contains ammonia at 60 to 120 μmol/L of contents. The heart has subepicardial and subendocardial hemorrhages.

DIAGNOSIS. Veterinarians clinically suspect UP on evidence of typical signs in animals whose rations contain a significant amount of urea, and they confirm the diagnosis in a laboratory by finding toxic levels of ammonia in the blood or rumen. The differential diagnosis requires consideration of strychnine, hydrocyanic acid, lead and organophosphorus poisoning, vitamin A deficiency, polioencephalomalacia, nitrate and cyanide poisoning and grain overload. For technical assistance from a diagnostic laboratory, fresh blood should be collected, the serum separated and frozen until analyzed. A composite sample of fluid taken from different locations in the rumen should be frozen or preserved with 1% mercuric chloride. Autolyzed blood or rumenal contents are diagnostically worthless. At least two of the suspected feed samples should be analyzed.

PREVENTION AND TREATMENT. Sheep owners and herdsmen avoid UP by (1) accurately formulating rations with safe amounts of urea, (2) thoroughly mixing all ration ingredients, (3) including correct amounts of carbohydrate and protein, (4) gradually adapting sheep to urea in new rations, and in old rations after a period of anorexia and diminished tolerance.

Veterinarians treat the ammonia-urea toxicosis by orally acidifying the rumen with strong vinegar or 5% acetic acid (5 ml/kg body weight) followed by drenching with cold water. Retreatment in 6 to 8 hours may be necessary. In expensive breeding stocks a rumenotomy to remove the source may be effective.

Clark, R., Oyaert, W., and Quin, J.I.: Toxicity of urea to sheep under different conditions. Onderstepoort J. Vet. Res., 25:73, 1951.

Emmanuel, B., et al.: Interrelationships between urea, ammonia, glucose, insulin and adrenaline during ammonia-urea toxicosis in sheep (ovis aries). Comp. Biochem. Physiol., 72A:697-702, 1982.

Hogan, J.P.: Absorption of ammonia through the rumen of sheep. Aust. J. Biol. Sci., 14:448-460, 1961.

Jones, G.A., MacLeod, R.A., and Blackwood, A.C.: Ureolytic rumen bacteria from urea-fed sheep. Can. J. Microbiol., 10:371-378, 1964.

Kennedy, P., Christopherson, R., and Milligan, L.: Effect of cold exposure on feed protein degradation, microbial protein synthesis and transfer of plasma urea to the rumen of sheep. Br. J. Nutr., 47:521-535, 1982.

Kirkpatrick, W.C., Roller, M.H., and Swanson, R.N.: Hemogram of sheep acutely intoxicated with ammonia. AJVR, 34:587-589, 1973.

Lewis, D.: Ammonia toxicity in the ruminant. J. Agric. Sci., 55:111-117, 1960.

Lewis, D., Hill, J.K., and Annison, E.F.: Absorption of ammonia from the rumen of sheep. Biochem. J., 66:587-592, 1957.

Lloyd, W.: Urea and other non-protein nitrogen sources. Current Veterinary Therapy. 2. Food Animal Practice. Edited by J. Howard. Philadelphia, W.B. Saunders Co., 1986.

McBarron, E.J. and McInnes, P.: Urea toxicity in sheep. Aust. Vet. J., 44:90-96, 1968.

McDonald, I.W.: Ammonia in ruminal digestion of protein. Biochem. J., 51:86-90, 1952.

Nawaz, M., Shah, B.: Renal clearance of endogenous creatinine and urea in sheep during summer and winter. Res. Vet. Sci., 36:220-224, 1984.

Rattenbury, J., et al.: Effect of propionic acid on urea synthesis by sheep liver. Res. Vet. Sci., 35:61-63, 1983.

Wilson, R.P., et al.: Toxicologic effects of ammonium carbamate and related compounds. AJVR, 29:897-906, 1968.

Word, J.D., et al.: Urea toxicity in cattle. J. Anim. Sci., 29:786-791, 1969.

Yelverton, C.C., Roller, M.H., and Swanson, R.N.: Ammonium nitrogen in fetuses of urea-treated sheep. AJVR, 36:191-192, 1975.

Lead Poisoning

Lead poisoning, an acute or subacute systemic intoxication, is characterized by digestive and nervous disturbances and is usually caused by ingested compounds and metals of lead. Throughout much of agricultural history, lead poisoning has affected livestock, especially sheep and cattle, but during recent decades, the incidence has increased because of greater use of the element and its compounds in industrial products and hence greater exposure of animals to concentrations in consumer goods and to residues in the environment.

Because most poisonings are preventable by sanitary management, the sheep industry has little concern for the condition. Economic losses, however, accrue to some livestock enterprises from deaths, unthriftiness, costs of prevention and treatment, and incomplete utilization of lead-contaminated feeds. Occurrence of the condition in most other species of domestic animals as well as in people adds economic importance and public health significance to the malady.

OCCURRENCE. Lead poisoning occurs in all breeds, sexes, and ages, but sheep up to 2 years old are more susceptible than are those of other age groups. Feedlot lambs are fully susceptible. Cattle and other domestic animals are also affected. Because of shortage of feeds and availability of lead, the disease develops more commonly during winter and spring than during summer and fall. Geographically, it occurs in all countries where sheep production has been commercialized.

ETIOLOGY AND PATHOGENESIS. Metallic lead and compounds of lead cause lead poisoning. Metallic lead is usually in the form of fragments from fixtures, weights, pipes, sheets, toys, projectiles and batteries, but lead compounds— red lead (triplumbic tetroxide, Pb_3O_4), white lead (lead carbonate, $2\ PbCO_3 \bullet Pb\ [OH]_2$), and lead chromate ($PbCrO_4$)—are usually components of industrial and natural products: red lead of paint and plumbing articles; white lead of paint, linoleum, asphalt, and medicines; lead carbonate and lead chromate of paints; lead oxides and sulfides of motor and smelter emissions, of crank case oil, and of mine tailings. Most of these substances cause poisoning by ingestion, but occasionally by inhalation.

Ingestive poisonings result from willful or accidental consumption of various forms of lead. Animals with depraved appetites willfully bite, masticate, and swallow metallic fragments of batteries, pipes, and plates; paint lead from surfaces of buckets, fences, troughs, and vehicles; lubricant lead from machinery and cans; and fuel lead from crankcase oil. Animals with normal appetites accidentally consume feeds contaminated with metallic lead comminuted in a grain grinder, compound lead deposited on forage, and compound lead from vehicles and containers.

The fatal single-day dose of lead oxide or basic carbonate is 40 to 80 and 120 to 150 mg/kg of body weight, respectively, for lambs and adults, whereas the fatal cumulative dose is about 1 to 2 mg/kg daily.

Following ingestion, lead interacts with proteins and anions to form complex groups and compounds. Some of these dissolve in digestive secretions, and about 1 to 2% of the ingested amounts are absorbed. The portal blood carries them to the liver, where a large portion is held. Some, however, escapes into the systemic blood, which distributes them to all organs. As a result, the blood level rises to a peak concentration and then descends to an intermediate plateau that persists for many weeks or months. Organ analyses for lead show a body distribution of about 60% in bones, 25% in liver, and 4% in kidneys. The amount in kidneys, however, is concentrated. Lead is excreted largely by the liver through the bile into the intestinal contents, but small amounts are excreted by the intestinal wall into feces and by the kidneys into the urine.

Lead probably affects all organs by interrupting their metabolic processes. One such process is the synthesis of heme, the iron protoporphyrin of hemoglobin. Heme is formed from succinyl CoA and glycine. An intermediate step in the process produces delta-aminolevulinic acid (ALA), two molecules of which, in the presence of dehydrase, form one molecule of porphobilinogen. Lead, by blocking the enzyme, causes an excess of ALA, which is variably excreted through the urine, and a deficit of hemoglobin, which variably stipples the erythrocytes.

CLINICAL SIGNS AND POSTMORTEM LESIONS. Clinical signs usually begin 2 to 3 days after exposure to a heavy dose of lead and several weeks after light daily doses. Signs are elevated but later normal body temperatures, twitching of face and neck muscles, violent blinking of eyelids, walking in circles or into fences because of blindness, salivation, excitement, maniacal bleating and climbing, convulsions, head pressing, incoordination, and depression. Cerebral edema is considered to be the primary cause of the neurologic signs. Depression, ruminal stasis, anorexia, constipation, dehydration, chewing movements, dental stridor, some nervous manifestations, moderate anemia, and basophilic stippling of some erythrocytes develop in some prolonged cases. The course ranges from a few hours to several days. Morbidity is usually 10 to 15% and the case mortality 50 to 80%.

Necropsy may reveal few lesions. The source of the ingested lead—oil, paint, asphalt, linoleum, metal—may be discernible in the stomachs. The abomasum and intestines may show inflammation, the liver, centrilobular necrosis, and the brain, edema. About 70% of affected animals contain acid-fast intranuclear inclusion bodies in the liver and kidneys.

DIAGNOSIS. Veterinarians diagnose lead poisoning on evidence of typical signs and laboratory findings. Chemical analyses for lead show concentrations as listed in Table 12-3. Although these ranges are the usual values, deviations above and below also occur. Live animals may be analyzed for ALA in the urine, for dehydrase, lead, and stippling in the blood, and for lead in ingesta and feces. The differential diagnosis requires consideration of rabies, listeriosis, polioencephalomalacia, poisoning from urea, hydrocyanic acid, or organophosphorus insecticides, and vitamin A deficiency.

For technical assistance from a diagnostic laboratory, practitioners should submit heparin-treated blood; fresh liver; kidney and ruminal contents; and formalin-fixed liver, kidney, and brain.

PREVENTION AND TREATMENT. Producers prevent lead poisoning by not allowing sheep access to lead paint, discarded refuse, lubricants on machinery, crankcase oil, fragments of batteries, chopped lead in ground feed, and feed grown near busy highways and lead smelters.

Veterinarians treat poisoned animals by emptying the alimentary tract and precipitating lead with magnesium sulfate purge. In addition, they administer intraperitoneally, subcutaneously, or intravenously a 1 to 2% solution of Ca EDTA in 5% glucose solution at the rate of 110 to 220 mg/kg on each of 2 successive days and repeat the dose after a 2-day interval. The division of the total daily dose is more effective as is slow intravenous drip but often impractical. Treatment with thiamine HCl (5 to 10 mg/kg intravenously or intramuscularly) BID is recommended and may be repeated daily along with EDTA. Dexamethasone (0.1 to 0.2 mg/kg given intravenously or intramuscularly) aids in reducing cerebral edema. Although the prognosis of animals showing severe nervous signs is grave, the nervous condition may be controlled with intravenous pentobarbital given to effect. Supportive therapy of oral nutrients, water and electrolytes is essential for blind or incapacitated animals. Animals with blood levels below and above one mg/L have favorable and unfavorable prognoses, respectively.

Allcroft, R.: Distribution of lead in tissues of cattle after ingesting lead. J. Comp. Pathol., *60*:190-208, 1950.

Bratton, G., et al.: An ultrastructural comparison of two potential treatments for lead poisoning in calves. J. World Assn. Vet. Anatomists, *14*:80, 1985.

Bratton, G., et al.: Thiamine as treatment of lead poisoning in ruminants. Modern Veterinary Practice, *62*:441-446, 1981.

Davis, L.: Clinical management of lead poisoning. JAVMA, *184*:858-860, 1984.

Fassbender, C.P.: Enzyme diagnosis of subclinical lead poisoning in sheep. Inaugural dissertation. Tieraerztl. Hochschule, Hanover, 1973, p. 90.

Hammond, P.B. and Arnson, A.L.: Mobilization and excretion of lead in cattle with chelating agents. N.Y. Acad. Sci., *88*:498-511, 1960.

Hammond, P.B. and Arnson, A.L.: Lead poisoning in cattle and horses in vicinity of a smelter. N.Y. Acad. Sci., *111*:595-611, 1964.

Hapke, H.J. and Priggs, E.: Lead poisoning in ruminants. Berl. Muench. Tieraerztl. Wochenschr., *86*:410-413, 1973.

McSherry, B.J., Willoughby, R.A., and Thomson, R.G.: Urinary delta-aminolevulenic acid in cattle. Can. J. Comp. Med., *35*:136-140, 1971.

Osweiler, G.D., Buck, W.B., and Lloyd, W.E.: Epidemiology of lead poisoning in cattle. Clin. Toxicol., *6*:367-376, 1973.

Rolton, C.E., Horton, B.J., and Pass, D.A.: Evaluation of tests for the diagnosis of lead exposure in sheep. Aust. Vet. J., *54*:393-397, 1978.

Sexton, J. and Buck, W.: Lead. In *Current Veterinary Therapy. 2. Food Animal Practice.* Edited by J. Howard. Philadelphia, W.B. Saunders Co., 1986.

Smith, J.: Toxic encephalopathies in cattle. *Current Veterinary Therapy. 2. Food Animal Practice.* Edited by J. Howard. Philadelphia, W.B. Saunders Co., 1986.

TABLE 12-3. *Normal and Pathologic Lead Concentrations*

Location	Lead Concentration (mg/kg)	
	Normal	Pathologic
Blood	0.10–1.13	0.4–4.0
Liver	0.3–1.5	10–40
Renal cortex	0.3–1.25	15–300
Ruminal contents	0–10	50–2000

Black Disease

(Infectious necrotic hepatitis)

An acute infectious toxemia of sheep, black disease is characterized by liver necrosis and sudden death and is caused by interaction of bacteria and flukes. Economic losses result from deaths and depreciation of infected property and from the costs of preventive programs and sanitary disposal of dead sheep affected with the disease. Although not precisely measured, financial losses to the industry are high because vaccinations are not universally practiced; in the United States, however, the monetary loss is low because of limited geographic distribution and the sporadic nature of the disease. The term "black disease" derives from the cyanotic venous blood in the subcutaneous tissues and the apparent darkening of the removed hide.

OCCURRENCE. Black disease develops in sheep 1 year of age and older, but it is most common in animals 2 to 4 years of age. The disease does not attack young lambs. Prevalence is highest in animals in excellent physical condition. Although black disease primarily affects sheep, it also occurs in cattle and rarely in pigs. Most cases develop during late summer and autumn. Freezing temperatures probably destroy metacercariae and interrupt the development of new cases during the winter months.

Geographically, black disease occurs in areas containing both *Fasciola hepatica* infestations and *C. novyi* infections. Snails, the intermediate hosts of the fluke, occupy moist habitats around streams, swamps, lakes, springs, and frequently irrigated land. Black disease exists in Australia, New Zealand, Britain, Rumania, Yugoslavia, and probably Germany. In the United States, it occurs in Montana and Oregon and probably in some other states known to contain areas of infestation with *Fasciola hepatica*; incidence of the disease in the United States, however, is low.

ETIOLOGY AND PATHOGENESIS. The cause of black disease is an interaction of bacteria, *C. novyi*, especially type B, and immature flukes, *Fasciola hepatica*.

C. novyi, widely distributed and prevalent bacteria, are gram-positive, sporing, strictly anaerobic bacilli measuring 0.8 to 1.5 × 5 to 10 μ m. With rounded ends and parallel sides, they occur singly, in pairs, and in filaments. Oval subterminal spores form in media. These slightly motile organisms grow well on media and ferment glucose and maltose but not lactose, sucrose, or salicin, and liquefy gelatin but not serum. Their resistance to germicidal factors simulates other species of *Clostridium.*

Microbiologists have classified *C. novyi* into types A, B, C, and D; all produce exotoxins. Type A produces alpha, gamma, delta, and epsilon exotoxins, and type B generates alpha, beta, and zeta exotoxins. Type D shares beta, eta, and theta toxins with type B but is considered a separate species. *C. novyi* inhabits soil, manure, alimentary tracts of ruminants, and, in some areas, normal livers of sheep. They may be participating pathogens in blackleg and malignant edema lesions of sheep and cattle, and in wound infections of people.

The common liver fluke, *Fasciola hepatica,* develops through a complex life cycle involving two major phases: the asexual phase that parasitizes snails, and the sexual phase that parasitizes the livers of sheep and cattle. The sexual forms consist of immature flukes and adult flukes. The immature flukes originate in the small intestine from excystation of ingested metacercariae. The newly formed immature flukes penetrate the intestinal wall and move through the peritoneal cavity to the liver, which they penetrate. Containing two suckers and a spiny cuticle, each oval-shaped immature fluke measures 3 to 6 mm in length. Collectively, the immature flukes are one factor in the cause of black disease. For a discussion of the entire life cycle, see the section on liver fluke disease in Chapter 4.

In the pathogenesis of black disease, both *C. novyi* and the immature flukes contribute to the malady. The soil spores of *C. novyi* contaminate forage and are ingested by sheep. Some penetrate the gastrointestinal wall, enter the portal blood system or lymphatic system, and are transported into the liver. In the normal liver, because the oxidation-reduction potential is too high for germination, the viable spores may remain latent and innocuous for several weeks.

Following fluke penetration and migration, and the production of massive necrosis in the spore-bearing liver, the oxidation-reduction potential lowers sufficiently to allow the spores of *C. novyi* to germinate. Other conditions, such as liver biopsy or invasion by other parasites (*Cysticercus tenuicollis*) causing local liver damage may precipitate the proliferation of *C. novyi*. The vegetative forms then metabolize and multiply in the dead tissue. Exotoxin forms and enters the general circulatory system. Toxemia damages neurons and other vital cells.

In rare cases of survival from the disease, antitoxin forms against the specific exotoxins and probably protects the animal against subsequent attacks, but nearly all affected sheep die from action of the exotoxin and acute shock. Some of the bacteria sporulate in the decomposing tissues and return to the soil.

In black disease, the sheep, the immature flukes, and the bacteria establish an apparently disastrous relationship that results in high mortality. The sheep, the flukes, and some of the bacteria die. This fatal catastrophe suggests that the tripartite association is recent in evolutionary time and that tolerable adjustments among the three participants have not yet developed.

CLINICAL SIGNS AND POSTMORTEM LESIONS. Because of its acute nature and short course, black disease usually escapes detection in the clinical phase. Early in the morning and without previous clues of sickness, husbandmen simply find the dead sheep. Careful and persistent scrutiny of the flock may, however, identify incipient cases. Affected sheep, always in excellent physical condition, lag behind an exercised flock, separate from other animals, and usually manifest depression, incoordinated movements, weakness, elevation of body temperature to 41 to 42°C, and shallow and rapid breathing. After a course of 10 to 60 minutes, the reclining animal becomes comatose and quietly dies. The morbidity usually varies from 15 to 30% but may go higher. Nearly 100% of affected sheep die. Usually, a sequence of deaths occur over a period of weeks.

At necropsy, the pathologist finds grossly observable changes in the liver, body cavities, and circulatory system. The swollen, congested liver constantly contains one or more foci of coagulative necrosis. Each focus measures up to 3 to 4 cm in diameter, feels firm, and appears pale. The globular but irregularly shaped mass of dead tissue extends deeply into the organ, but is visible or palpable from the surface. On dissection of the liver, careful examiners may also find bore tracts, immature flukes in the tracts, and dead tissue.

The pericardial sac usually contains approximately 60 ml of clear fluid and the peritoneal and thoracic cavities 100 ml each. The fluid coagulates on exposure to air. Petechial and ecchymotic hemorrhages discolor the subendocardium of the left ventricle. The congestion of subcutaneous tissues with cyanotic venous blood darkens the hide.

Significant histopathologic changes are seen in the liver. Coagulative necrosis extends through many contiguous lobules. Leukocytes, especially neutrophils and eosinophils, infiltrate the dead tissue and the surrounding viable tissue. A dense zone of neutrophils and mononuclear cells forms near the junction of dead and living tissue. Numerous bacteria, *C. novyi,* accumulate immediately inside the leukocytic zone. The bore tracts contain a cavity filled with necrotic liver cells, blood, leukocytes and, in some sections, the immature flukes.

DIAGNOSIS. Veterinarians diagnose black disease on the basis of typical signs and lesions in sheep residing in regions endemic for liver fluke. For laboratory assistance one should present refrigerated and formalin fixed samples of the liver lesions for bacterial isolation and histology. The specimens must be taken prior to autolysis otherwise the anaerobic conditions may allow multiplication of *C. novyi* giving false positive results. Fluorescent antibody or culture can be used to identify the organisms.

The differential diagnosis requires the consideration of acute fascioliasis, enterotoxemia, anthrax, hydrocyanic acid poisoning, and metallic poisoning.

PREVENTION AND TREATMENT. Since invasion of the sheep liver by immature flukes is an essential factor in the cause of black disease, controlling the flukes prevents black disease. In addition, an efficient toxoid against infection from *C. novyi* is commercially available. For maximum immune response sheep should receive the initial immunizing dose 6 weeks prior to exposure followed in 2 weeks with a booster. Although *C. novyi* toxoids give a solid immune response, annual boosters may be necessary. All dead sheep should be burned or buried in quicklime to avoid pollution with *C. novyi*.

Treatment for black disease has not been developed and, if available, probably would not be feasible for use because the disease develops suddenly and runs a short fatal course.

Albiston, H.E.: Infectious necrotic hepatitis of sheep in Victoria. J. Exp. Biol. Med. Sci., 4:113-123, 1927.

Dodd, S.: The etiology of black disease. J. Comp. Pathol. Ther., 34:1-26, 1921.

Dodd, S.: Studies in black disease—a braxy-like disease of sheep. J. Comp. Pathol. Ther., 31:1-35, 1918.

Duncan, I.: Liver biopsy and black disease in a sheep. Aust. Vet. J., 61:272-273, 1984.

Edgar, G.: On the occurrence of black disease bacilli in the livers of normal sheep. Aust. Vet. J., 4:133-141, 1928.

Gilruth, J.A.: A disease of sheep in Tasmania. Vet. J., 66:254-265, 1911.

Hopkirk, C.S.M.: Braxy-like disease of sheep in Hawke's Bay. N.Z. J. Agric., 35:141-150, 1927.

Jamieson, S.: The identification of *Clostridium oedematiens* and an experimental investigation of its role in the pathogenesis of infectious necrotic hepatitis (black disease) of sheep. J. Pathol. Bacteriol., 61:389-402, 1949.

Jamieson, S., Thompson, J.J., and Brotherston, J.G.: Studies in black disease. I. The occurrence of the disease in the North Scotland. Vet. Rec., 60:11-14, 1948.

Katitch, R.V., et al.: Attempts to reproduce necrotic hepatitis experimentally. Bull. Acad. Vet. Fr., 42:33-39, 1969.

Nakamura, S., Kimura, I., Yamakawa, K., and Nishida, S.: Taxonomic relationships among *Clostridium novyi* Types A and B, *Clostridium haemolyticum* and *Clostridium botulinum* Type C. J. Gen. Microbiol., 129:1473-1479, 1983.

Oakley, C.L., Warrack, G.H., and Clarke, P.H.: The toxins of *Clostridium oedematiens* (*C. novyi*). J. Gen. Bacteriol., 1:91-106, 1947.

Shaw, J.N., Muth, O.H., and Seghetti, L.: Black disease. Oregon Agric. Exp. Stat. Bull. 360, 1939.

Taylor, E.L.: Fascioliasis and the liver fluke. FAO (Rome), 1964.

Tunnicliff, E.A.: Persistence of immunity against infectious necrotic hepatitis in sheep vaccinated with an alum-precipitated toxoid. JAVMA, 103:368-370, 1943.

Tunnicliff, E.A.: Black disease immunization. JAVMA, 90:105-106, 1940.

Tunnicliff, E.A. and Marsh, H.: An alum-precipitated toxoid as an immunizing agent against infectious necrotic hepatitis (black disease) in sheep. JAVMA, 94:98-110, 1939.

Turner, A.W.: Black disease (infectious necrotic hepatitis) of sheep in Australia. Aust. CSIRO. Bull. 46, 1930.

Turner, A.W. and Davesne, J.: Role du *B. oedematiens* dans l'etiologie de l'hepatite infectieuse du muton Austraien. Ann. Inst. Pasteur, 41:1078, 1927.

Echinococcosis

(Hydatidosis; hydatid cyst; hydatid disease)

Echinococcosis, a chronic two-host zoonosis of sheep and other herbivorous and omnivorous mammals, is characterized by the formation of variably sized cysts in the liver and lungs and is caused by the larvae of *Echinococcus granulosus,* a tapeworm of dogs, wolves, and coyotes. Because the disease has worldwide distribution and generally high incidence, it causes significant financial waste to the sheep industry except in the United States, Iceland, and Scandinavia. Economic losses result from condemnation of infected food carcasses, from the costs of preventive and eradicative programs, and from incapacitation of infected people.

Occurrence of the disease in cattle, horses, swine, and people greatly enhances the economic importance and public health significance of the malady.

OCCURRENCE. Echinococcosis occurs in all breeds, sexes, and ages of sheep, but animals 5 years of age and older have higher infection rates and greater numbers of cysts per animal than do younger age groups. Sheep acquire the infection during grazing seasons but continue the cysts throughout all seasons.

Geographically, echinococcosis occurs in nearly all sheep-producing countries, but it is widespread and concentrated in eastern Australia, Peru, Chile, Argentina, Uruguay, Mediterranean Basin, Balkans, Middle East, and southern USSR; it is naturally uncommon in North America and Scandinavia and significantly suppressed in Iceland, New Zealand, and Tasmania.

ETIOLOGY AND PATHOGENESIS. A tapeworm causes echinococcosis. The adult worm, *Echinococcus granulosus,* inhabits the small intestines of dogs, wolves, and coyotes, and the larvae, hydatid cysts, reside in the liver, lungs, and other organs of sheep, cattle, swine, horses, camels, wild ruminants, and people. The mature tapeworm, measuring 4 to 6 mm in length, contains a scolex and 2 to 4 segments, and the scolex possesses a rostellum with 2 rows of 28 to 46 hooks (Fig. 12-14).

The hydatid cyst, a spherical monolocular vesicle, consists of a wall and cavity filled with fluid, and commonly measures 5 to 10 cm in diameter. The cyst wall has an outer circle of laminated connective tissue and an inner layer of germinal epithelium. Secondary epithelial vesicles project into the main cavity, and protoscolices may form from the germinal epithelium. Each secondary vesicle contains 30 to

Fig. 12-14. Adult tapeworm *Echinococcus granulosis.* × 30.

40 protoscolices and constitutes a brood capsule which, when detached, becomes hydatid sand. A single liver may contain many cysts, each with several million protoscolices, but about 8% of ovine cysts are sterile and, consequently, contain no protoscolices.

The life cycle begins with expulsion of embryonated ova and gravid segments to the exterior. When eaten by sheep or other intermediate hosts, the eggs hatch, and the oncospheres penetrate the small intestine, enter blood vessels, and transport to the liver, lungs, and, uncommonly, other organs. In the liver, a vesicle grows to 4 to 5 mm in diameter in 3 months and to 10 mm in 5 months. Cyst ruptures and outbuddings form new cysts. The protoscolices remain viable throughout the life of the host. Following ingestion by a dog, the protoscolices enter the small intestine, evaginate, attach to the mucosa, and mature through a prepatent period of about 45 days. A single dog may harbor 40,000 worms, which live up to 2 years, and each adult worm sheds a gravid segment, containing 200 to 400 eggs, every 14 days.

CLINICAL SIGNS AND POSTMORTEM LESIONS. Most cases of ovine echinococcosis are asymptomatic. Large cysts and excessive numbers of cysts, however, may cause hepatic insufficiency and pulmonary atelectasis, with signs of weakness, anorexia, dyspnea, loss of live weight, and finally death.

At necropsy, single or multiple cysts are found in the liver and/or lungs and occasionally other organs (Fig. 12-15). Opened fertile cysts show brood capsules, up to 1 mm in diameter, attached to the germinal surface (Fig. 12-16).

DIAGNOSIS. Veterinarians seldom diagnose echinococcosis in live sheep. Finding the hydatid cysts at necropsy of dead sheep or at inspection of slaughtered animals establishes a diagnosis. The differential diagnosis requires consideration of *E. multilocularis*, cystic bile ducts, and cystic neoplasms. Gross and histopathologic features help differentiate those conditions.

Veterinarians diagnose intestinal tapeworm infections in dogs by administering a purge of arecoline and identifying the expelled worms.

Fig. 12-15. Echinococcal cysts in liver. × 0.3.

PREVENTION.   Producers, veterinarians, and public health officials prevent and in some cases eradicate echinococcosis by developing and persistently pursuing regional programs as follows:

1. Control the movements of all working dogs and eliminate stray animals to avoid contaminating pastures and other feeds with tapeworm ova.

2. Apply an arecoline hydrobromide purge to each dog and examine the feces for *E. granulosus* tapeworms. Animals who show positive results with the test should be treated twice at 2-day intervals with bunamidine hydrochloride at a rate of 50 mg/kg body weight. In eradication programs, the procedure should be repeated at 6-week intervals.

3. Eliminate all raw viscera from the diets of dogs, and deactivate all viscera from sheep, cattle, and swine by heating or burying.

4. Obtain active public support for control programs by educating the local people

Fig. 12-16. Opened echinococcal cyst in lung. Note brood capsules. × 1.0.

to understand the disease, to appreciate the public benefits from control, and to believe in the possibility of achieving control.

Animal Health Yearbook. FAO-WHO-OIE (Italy), 1970.
Genis, D.E.: Epizootiology of echinococcosis in Kazakhstan. Med. Parazitol., 39:302-306, 1970.
Hercus, C.E., Williams, R.J., Gemmell, M.A., and Parnell, I.W.: Formalin is not hydatid ovicide. Vet. Rec., 74:1515, 1962.
McCristell, T.: Rep. New Zealand Hydatid Council. Wellington, 1968, p. 24.
Meymarian, E. and Schwabe, C.W.: Resistance of ova of *Echinococcus granulosus* to germicides. Am. J. Trop. Med. Hyg., 11:360-364, 1962.
Mozgovi, A.A., Rizhikov, K.M., and Sudarikov, V.E.: Tr. Gelm. Lab. Akad. Nauk. USSR. In Helm. Abst., 25:543d, 1956.
Nenow, S.: Wystepowanie bablowcow (Echinococcus) W. Bulgarii. Helm. Abst., 30:850, 1961.
Peisley, H.R.: Survey of echinococcosis in sheep. Aust. Vet. J., 32:61-62, 1956.
Pellegrini, D. and Cilli, V.: Hydatidosis in Italy. Helm. Abst., 24:65, 1955.

Popov, A.: Echinococcosis in Bulgarie. Bull. Off. Int. Epizoot., *62*:1023-1029, 1964.

Schantz, P.M. and Schwabe, C.W.: Status of hydatid disease control. JAVMA, *155*:2104-2120, 1969.

Simitch, T.: Frequency of echinococcosis. Bull. Off. Int. Epizoot., *62*:1031-1061, 1964.

Smyth, J.D.: *In vitro* studies of echinococcosis. Bull. WHO, *39*:5-12, 1968.

Smyth, J.D., Howkins, A.B., and Barton, M.: Factors controlling differentiation of hydatid organisms. Nature, *211*:1374-1377, 1966.

Thomson, G.A.: Hydatids eradication in Iceland. New Zealand Nat. Hydatids Coun. Bull. 15, 1965.

Von Siebold, 1852, quoted from Craig, C.F. and Faust, E.C.: *Clinical Pathology.* 5th Edition. Philadelphia, Lea & Febiger, 1951, p. 589.

Paramphistomosis

(*Rumen fluke infection*)

Paramphistomosis, a parasitic disease of domestic ruminants, is characterized in the early stage by hemorrhagic duodenitis and in late stages by innocuous rumen flukes. It is caused by numerous species of cone flukes, uncommon trematodes in the U.S. The duodenal form adversely affects some sheep and causes major losses from illness, death, loss of live weight, incomplete use of infested pastures and ranges, and the costs of preventive and treatment procedures. Development of paramphistomosis also in cattle and goats adds economic importance and general interest to the disease.

OCCURRENCE.   Both duodenal and ruminal paramphistomosis occurs in sheep. They affect all breeds and sexes, but animals aged 4 to 24 months have higher infection rates than do other age groups. Most cases develop during summer and autumn, but once established, infections persist throughout many consecutive seasons. Geographically, the disease exists in Australia, New Zealand, East and South Africa, Mediterranean basin, Middle East, USSR, Asia, and America; in the United States, it exists at low incidence in the southern states.

ETIOLOGY AND PATHOGENESIS. Numerous species of cone flukes, including *Calicophoron calicophorum, Paramphistomum ichikauai, P. microbothrium,* and *P. cervi,* cause paramphistomosis in livestock. The two latter species predominate in the U.S. Massive doses of metacercariae are necessary to cause the

disease. The adults, light pink in color, are cone-shaped, rounded in cross section, and measure 5 to 12 mm in length. With large subterminal posterior suckers, they are slightly convex dorsally and concave ventrally.

The life cycle begins with the extrusion of eggs mixed with feces to the exterior. Under favorable moisture and temperature, they hatch in approximately 1 month. The miracidia utilize, as intermediate hosts, species of snails of the genera *Bulinas, Glyptanisus, Indoplanorbis, Lymnaea, Planorbis, Pseudosuccinea,* and *Pygmanisus*; important species are *Bulinas tropicus* and *B. truncatus.* The development of cercariae within the snail requires approximately 1 month. Emerging cercariae encyst on grass or other edible vegetation, and the resulting metacercariae may endure for several months. When eaten by sheep or cattle, the metacercariae pass along the alimentary system into the duodenum, where excystation occurs. The resulting young flukes attach to and penetrate the mucosa and finally migrate craniad in the tissues. Ultimately, they move through the lumen of the abomasum into the rumen and reticulum where, among papillae, they attach to the mucosa, their definitive positions. The entire life cycle requires about 100 days; the prepatency period is 56 to 70 days.

Pathogenicity varies directly with the number of parasites. A minimum burden of 2000 to 23,000 causes disease and even death. By severely injuring the duodenal mucosa, the young flukes interfere with digestion, provoke diarrhea, and cause leakage of plasma albumin. Those pathologic changes may result in unthriftiness, edema, emaciation, and even death of the host. Within the rumen, the flukes inflict little or no injury. As a result of penetration of the duodenum by flukes, their antigens probably stimulate the synthesis of IgG and IgA immunoglobulins and thereby induce immunity that endures for several years.

CLINICAL SIGNS AND POSTMORTEM LESIONS. Feedlot sheep harboring flukes in their rumens, except for the presence of eggs in their feces, manifest no signs. In grazing sheep with duodenitis, however, signs commence 16 to

28 days after infection and consist of anorexia, bloody diarrhea, straining, dehydration, weakness, and loss of live weight. Feces may contain young flukes, and plasma may have only 50% normal levels of albumin. Morbidity varies up to 100%, and the case mortality may reach 25%. Sheep with nonfatal infection may have reduced capacity to gain weight.

At necropsy and inspection of slaughtered sheep, the adult pink flukes are attached to the mucosa among papillae near the anterior and posterior pillars and in the reticulum (Fig. 12-17). They may be inconspicuous and, to be detected, require close inspection of the cleaned rumen. In fatal duodenitis, primary lesions are concentrated in the cranial 2 m of the small intestine. The mucosa is thickened, swollen, rugous, and ulcerated. Young flukes 1 to 2 mm in diameter usually are attached to the surface. The large intestine may contain

Fig. 12-17. *Paramphistomum cervi* among ruminal papillae (a). × 1.2.

bloody fluid, and the abomasum may be edematous.

DIAGNOSIS. Veterinarians diagnose paramphistomosis at necropsy of dead sheep and at inspection of slaughtered sheep by finding the adult flukes in the rumen and/or reticulum, or in live animals by finding specific eggs in the feces. They diagnose the duodenal form in grazing sheep on evidence of characteristic signs and lesions and of young flukes in feces.

The differential diagnosis requires consideration of coccidiosis, salmonellosis, fascioliasis, and helminthosis. For technical assistance from a diagnostic laboratory, practitioners should submit adult flukes from the rumen, feces from the rectum, and segments of suspect duodenum.

PREVENTION AND TREATMENT. Producers prevent paramphistomosis by avoiding grazing sheep on metacercaria-infested pastures, by destroying molluscian intermediate hosts through treatment and drainage of infested land (as for fascioliasis), and by treating carrier livestock to prevent reseeding of clean grazing lands with new eggs.

Infected sheep should be treated with one of the following anthelmintic agents: (1) albendazole in an oral dose of 10 to 15 mg/kg of body weight, (2) niclosamide, 90 mg/kg, (3) menichlopholan (Niclofolan), 6 mg/kg or (4) resorantel, 65 mg/kg. Only albendazole is approved for use in the U.S.

Boray, J.C.: Antihelmintic efficiency of niclosamide and menichlopholan as treatment for paramphistomosis. Aust. Vet. J., *45*:133-134, 1969.

Cvetkovic, I.: Acute intestinal paramphistomiasis in sheep. Vet. Glasn., *22*:41-49, 1968. (Abst. Vet. Bull., *38*: 609, 1968).

Horak, I.G.: Pathogenesis of paramphistomosis in sheep. J. S. Afr. Vet. Med. Assoc., 37:428-430, 1966.

Horak, I.G.: Host parasite relationships *Paramphistomum microbothrium* and sheep. Onderstepoort J. Vet. Res., *34*:451-540, 1967.

Horak, I.G. and Clark, R.: Pathologic physiology of acute paramphistomosis in sheep. Onderstepoort J. Vet. Sci., *30*:145-159, 1963.

Roach, R.W. and Lopes, V.: Mortality of adult ewes resulting from intestinal infestation with immature paramphistomes. Bull. Epizoot. Dis. Afr., *14*:317-323, 1966.

Sharma Deorani, V.P. and Katiyar, R.D.: Pathogenicity of immature amphistomes among sheep and goats. Indian Vet. J., *44*:199-205, 1967.

Whitten, L.K.: Paramphistomiasis in sheep. N.Z. Vet. J., *3*:144, 1955.

Carcinoma of the Small Intestine

(SIA; small intestine adenocarcinoma)

Carcinoma of the small intestine, a malignant neoplasm, is characterized by intestinal obstruction, ascites, prostration, and death. In some countries, the disease commonly causes death of ewes, but because affected sheep are old, the economic loss is low. The extraordinarily high incidence in sheep, however, enhances veterinary and biologic interest in the entity. Similar neoplasms occur at lower incidences in other species of domestic animals.

OCCURRENCE.   The disease develops often in British and Merino breeds. Ewes 5 years of age and older are attacked. Old rams may be equally susceptible, but the population of such sheep may be too small for the disease to develop enough to attract attention. Seasons are not an influential factor. Geographically, the disease occurs commonly in New Zealand, Australia, and Iceland, and less commonly in Scotland, South Africa, and in the U.S. in Colorado.

ETIOLOGY AND PATHOGENESIS.   Although the exact cause or interactive agents of small intestine adenocarcinoma are unknown, there is a highly significant increase in tumor rate when sheep are exposed to pastures sprayed with phenoxy, picolinic acid herbicides, or both. The tumor rate is indirectly proportional to the time lapse between spraying and grazing. The sooner grazing is allowed, the higher the tumor rate. These herbicides or other carcinogens act on the intestinal epithelial cells over a prolonged period and eventually induce a change at one or more locations from normal to neoplastic cells. Once the transformation has occurred, it does not reverse. The neoplastic cells proliferate, form a mass in the lumen, invade the entire wall, enter blood and lymph vessels, metastasize to other organs, and ultimately cause death by constricting the intestine and occluding the lumen. The prevalence of small intestine adenocarcinoma in sheep and carcinoma of the colon in man are higher in regions of New Zealand than anywhere in the world leading to the speculation of some common factors of the two conditions.

CLINICAL SIGNS AND POSTMORTEM LESIONS. Affected sheep develop anorexia and gradually lose weight. The abdomen may fill with fluid. Physical weakness and prolonged recumbency precede death. Some animals are found dead without the shepherd's knowledge of the illness. In endemic areas, the morbidity ranges from 0.2 to 0.9%, and the mortality is 100%. The course usually extends over many weeks.

At necropsy, the primary problem is centered at one or more points in the jejunum or ileum. At the point of origin, a neoplastic mass, often ulcerous and necrotic, projects into and partially or completely fills the lumen. White, scirrhous plaques of tumor form on serous surfaces along the sides of the intestine and extend cephalad. Afferent lymphatics are dilated and may be nodular. Metastases through lymphatics may form white, firm masses in regional lymph nodes and through veins in the liver. Transplant metastases to serous surfaces may be widely distributed throughout the peritoneal cavity. Cranial to the neoplasm, the intestinal muscularis is hypertrophied, and the lumen is distended with ingesta.

Microscopically, the neoplastic epithelial cells may contain cytoplasmic mucus and form small aggregates, sheets, and trabeculae within the stroma. All layers of the wall and many vessels may be invaded. The ratio of fibrous stroma to epithelial cells is high.

DIAGNOSIS.   Veterinarians seldom if ever clinically diagnose carcinoma of the small intestine. At necropsy of dead sheep and inspection of slaughtered animals, they suspect the disease from gross lesions and confirm it through histopathologic studies. For technical assistance from a diagnostic laboratory, practitioners should submit tissues from primary intestinal lesions, involved mesenteric nodes, affected liver, and peritoneal transplants.

TREATMENT.   Because of the low economic value of old ewes, surgical excision and other antitumor procedures are not applied.

Anderson, B.: Adenocarcinoma of the small intestine of a yearling ewe. JAVMA, *183*:1467-1468, 1983.

Bastianello, S.: A survey on neoplasia in domestic species over a 40-year period from 1935 to 1974 in the Republic of South Africa. II. Tumors occurring in sheep. Onderstepoort J. Vet. Res., *49*:205-209, 1982.

Dodd, D.C.: Adenocarcinoma of small intestine of sheep. N.Z. Vet. J., *8*:109-112, 1960.

Georgsson, G. and Vigfusson, H.: Carcinoma of the small intestine of sheep in Iceland. A pathologic and epizootiologic study. Acta Vet. Scand., *14*:392-409, 1973.

McDonald, J.W. and Leaver, D.D.: Adenocarcinoma of the small intestine of Merino sheep. Aust. Vet. J., *41*:269-271, 1965.

Moulton, J.E.: *Tumors of Domestic Animals.* 2nd Edition. Berkeley, University of California Press, 1978, pp. 263-266.

Newell, K., Ross, A., and Renner, R.: Phenoxy and picolinic acid herbicides and small intestinal adenocarcinoma in sheep. The Lancet, *2*:1301-1304, 1984.

Simpson, B.H. and Jolly, R.D.: Carcinoma of the small intestine in sheep. J. Pathol., *112*:83-92, 1974.

Ruminal Papillomatosis

Ruminal papillomatosis is a recently reported condition of sheep in areas of Scotland and Northern England characterized by fibropapillomas along a pillar of muscle between the dorsal and ventral rumen. Cutaneous papillomas are common to man and other animals but rare in sheep. The causative agent is a papilloma virus of the family *Papovaviridae.* The papilloma virus is a double-stranded, covalently closed circular DNA molecule. Classification is based on polynucleotide sequence, tissue tropism, and the histology of the lesion. The sheep papilloma virus belong to a group which includes bovine type 1 and 2 and European elk papilloma virus which induces not only a cutaneous papilloma, but, in addition, an underlying fibroma of connective tissue (fibropapilloma). Although insignificant to the overall sheep industry, the prevalence of ruminal papillomatosis is high in certain areas of Scotland (12.5% of adult ewes slaughtered at Edinburgh) and could possibly be a problem in other parts of the world where similar ecologic and environmental conditions exist. The high prevalence is associated with grazing of braken fern (*Pteridium aquilinum*). Studies on sheep grazing the North East Yorkshire area of Scotland showed a tumor prevalence of 14% of 219 casualties and the leading cause of death on certain farms grazing braken. In cattle there is frequent conversion of multiple alimentary papillomas to carcinomas if braken fern is present in the diet. Similar conversion has been seen in sheep but not fully investigated. Rumen papillomas occurring in conjunction with adenocarcinoma of the small intestine have been reported. The high prevalence of ruminal papillomas and tumors in specific geographic areas suggests a multifactorial process involving a papilloma virus, genetic background, and environmental factors.

The papillomas may occur singly or in multiple numbers. Histologically, they are a fibropapilloma with a branching ventral core of coarse collagenous connective tissue. Electron microscopy shows enlarging, actively growing epithelial cells in the germinal and spinous layers with increase in tonofibrils and desmosomes. The degenerating cells in the spinous layer show a loss of tonofibrils, detachment of desmosomes, focal necrosis, vacuoles in the cytoplasm, and condense marginated chromatin. Diagnosis is accomplished at slaughter and the full significance of the problem awaits investigation into the possibility that the papilloma virus acts as a precursor to carcinogenesis.

Lancaster, W. and Olson, C.: Animal papilloma viruses. Microbiologic Review, *46*:191-207, 1982.

McCrea, C. and Head, K.: Sheep tumors in North East Yorkshire. I. Prevalence on seven moorland farms. Br. Vet. J., *134*:454-461, 1978.

Norval, M., Michie, J., and Apps, M.: Rumen papillomas in sheep. Vet. Microbiol., *10*:219-229, 1984/85.

13

DISEASES OF THE RESPIRATORY SYSTEM

Nasal Myiosis

(Nasal bot; head bot; head grub)

Nasal myiosis, a chronic rhinitis and sinusitis of sheep, is characterized by persistent annoyance and mucopurulent discharge and is caused by invading maggots. Even though the disease prevails in most sheep-producing areas and maintains high incidence within flocks, it causes little measurable damage and for that reason attracts insignificant concern from the general sheep industry. Limited material waste accrues, however, to some enterprises from interference by the adult flies with peaceful sheep grazing, from complications of nasal infestations, and from aberrant locations of the larvae. Occurrence of the disease among goats, deer, elk, dogs, and people adds some scientific interest and public health significance to the condition.

OCCURRENCE. Nasal myiosis occurs in all breeds, sexes, and ages of sheep. In warm geographic zones of the world, both adult and larval phases of the disease persist throughout all seasons, but in temperate zones, adult flies emerge, mate, and oviposit only during summer, and the myiosis continues throughout the cold seasons. Geographically, the disease prevails among sheep of all continents and probably all countries. The incidence is high in Australia, United States, Argentina, Brazil, Africa, Europe, and USSR.

ETIOLOGY AND PATHOGENESIS. *Oestrus ovis,* a prevalent fly, causes nasal myiosis. Both the adult insects and their larvae attack sheep. The gray adult females, measuring 10 to 12 mm in length, possess black thoracic spots, yellow body hairs, and rudimentary mouth parts. They live for 2 to 28 days in protected areas such as property fences and building walls. During that time, each female mates and produces up to 500 larvae which, on warm middays, she deposits on the nostrils of sheep. The first instar larva is translucent white and measures 2 mm in length, but the mature third instar is opaque gray and possesses two black oral hooks, two black posterior spiracles, ventral spines, and dorsal transverse bands of pigment, and measures 30 x 8 mm.

The life cycle begins with deposition of the larvae on sheep nostrils. The first instars enter the nasal cavity and feed on mucus and desquamated cells. The second instars pass into the frontal or maxillary sinuses, where they grow into third instars. After 2 to 10 months, the mature larvae return to the nostrils and are sneezed to the exterior. They enter the soil and pupate through a period of 27 to 36 days. The adult females deposit larvae throughout the summer in temperate zones and throughout most seasons in hot zones.

Even though they are minor sheep pests, both adults and larvae of *Oestrus ovis* attack and torment sheep. The swarming, buzzing flies agitate and harass the animals and send them in urgent search for cover. These frenzied episodes interrupt feeding and resting and may cause loss of live weight. The movements

265

of numerous maggots in the nasal cavities and paranasal sinuses also annoy the hosts. In the sinuses, dead larvae apparently result in allergic and inflammatory reactions; these changes cause discomfort and interrupt the animal's feeding. Some larvae wander along the trachea into the lungs and there produce fatal reactions. Recovered sheep, except for frenetic behavior, do not resist reinfestation.

CLINICAL SIGNS AND POSTMORTEM LESIONS. Sheep attacked by ovipositing flies stamp their feet, shake their heads, sneeze, blow, and ram their noses against the ground or other sheep. In some cases, these acts traumatize and infect the nostrils. The animals also seek cool areas, such as damp shade, where the flies do not frequent. During the time the larvae occupy the nose and sinuses, affected sheep may hold their heads towards the ground and persistently discharge mucopurulent exudate from the nostrils. Breathing may be difficult because of swollen nasal membranes and plugged nostrils. The morbidity may reach 80% of a flock, but mortality is nil. The course of adult fly attack periodically extends through the summer, and the rhinitis and sinusitis continue up to 10 months.

At necropsy of dead sheep or at inspection of slaughtered animals, up to 20 larvae of different instars and sizes are found in the frontal and maxillary sinuses (Fig. 13-1). Living larvae rapidly retreat from opened sinuses through the nasosinus aperture into the nasal cavity. Sinuses with live larvae usually appear near normal, but sinuses containing one or more dead larvae show edema-thickened membranes and exudate-filled cavities.

DIAGNOSIS. Veterinarians diagnose adult fly attacks from restlessness and frenzied behavior of sheep during hot middays and from observing the furtive flies. They suspect myiosis in sheep with chronic nasal discharge and confirm the diagnosis by finding larvae in the sinuses.

TREATMENT. Sheep should be treated for nasal myiosis during the autumn when most larvae are small. Killing mature larvae in the sinuses may result in severe reactions in the sinus membranes. Either of the following compounds and dosage rates are highly effective:

1. Rafoxanide administered orally at the dose rate of 7.5 mg/kg of body weight (not approved for use in the U.S.).

2. Ivermectin, at the rate of 50 μg/kg.

Fig. 13-1. *Oestrus ovis* in dissected frontal sinuses. × 1.0.

Animal Health Yearbook. FAO-WHO-OIE (Italy), 1970.

Cobbett, N.G. and Mitchell, W.C.: Further observations in the life cycle of *Oe. ovis.* AJVR, *2*:258-266, 1941.

Horak, I.G., Louw, J.P., and Raymond, S.M.: Trials with rafoxanide against larvae of sheep nasal bots. S. Afr. Vet. Med. Assoc., *42*:337-339, 1971.

Lloyd, J.E. and Pfadt, R.E.: University of Wyoming records, 1980.

Roncalli, R.: Efficacy of ivermectin against *Oestrus ovis* in sheep. Vet. Med., *79*:1095-1097, 1984.

Roncalli, R.A., Barbosa, A., and Fernandez, J.F.: Efficacy of rafoxanide against larval *Oestrus ovis* in sheep. Vet. Rec., *88*:289-290, 1971.

Semenov, P.V.: Drugs for preventing and treating sheep nasal bots. Izd. Kolos, 1964, pp. 262-268.

Tuberculosis

(*TB*)

Tuberculosis, a chronic contagious disease of sheep, is characterized by primary caseous nodules in the lungs and pulmonary lymph nodes and by disseminated caseous nodules in many other organs and is caused by acid-fast bacteria. Generally, tuberculosis in sheep is rare. Prior to 1957, the United States annually slaughtered and inspected about 14 million sheep and found tuberculosis in only a few animals; since that time, the nation slaughtered 10 to 12 million sheep and found no cases of tuberculosis. Because of insignificant incidence, the sheep industry has little concern for the disease.

Occurrence of the condition in other species of domestic animals and man gives major economic importance and public health significance to the general malady.

OCCURRENCE. Tuberculosis occurs in all breeds and sexes of sheep 2 years of age and older. Most cases, however, develop among farm flocks in close, crowded, and unsanitary confinement. Probably, most cases begin during winter when animals are housed, but the characteristically long course extends into other seasons. Geographically, the disease probably occurs at low incidence in all sheep-producing countries. It does not develop, however, among feedlot lambs because of the short fattening period and young-age slaughter; neither does it develop among range flocks of the western United States because such animals

continuously move to clean, new, open habitats. Prevalence rates are dependent upon management practices, ecologic habitat, and exposure as sheep are highly susceptible to *Mycobacterium bovis.*

ETIOLOGY. *Mycobacterium avium* and *M. bovis* usually, and *M. tuberculosis* rarely, cause tuberculosis in sheep. These pleomorphic, aerobic, nonmotile, nonsporing bacteria measure 1.5 to 4 x 0.2 to 0.6 μm. In staining affinity they are acid-fast and gram-positive. Organisms in old cultures often contain granules. Bacteriologists type the three species on the basis of their pathogenicity for experimental animals as indicated in Table 13-1.

Outside the host animal tissues, these organisms vary in resistance to bactericidal agents. When exposed to direct concentrated sunlight, they die in 2 hours. In milk heated to 70°C, they survive less than 5 minutes. In dry media, such as dust, exudates, and discharges, not exposed to direct sunlight, they endure for several months.

TRANSMISSION. Susceptible sheep acquire infection from their immediate environment. Infected animals, including sheep, cattle, and poultry, excrete the tubercle bacilli in cough-expelled sputum, salivary secretions, nasal discharges, and other excretions. Susceptible sheep usually acquire the disease by inhalation of infective aerosols or by ingestion of feed or water contaminated with infective sputum, saliva, milk, urine, or feces. In addition, animals may acquire infection by contact with tuberculous people or by exposure to human tuberculous excretions or human infective sewage.

TABLE 13-1. *Pathogenicity of Mycobacteria*

Bacterial Species	Pathogenicity for		
	Guinea Pig	Rabbit	Chicken
M. bovis	+	+	0
M. tuberculosis	+	±	0
M. avium	±	+	+

Fetuses may occasionally acquire the disease through the umbilical vein as a result of uterine infections. Rarely, infected genitalia mechanically transmit the pathogens during coitus.

PATHOGENESIS. Pathologists have investigated only small numbers of sheep with tuberculosis. Consequently, little factual information on the pathogenesis is available. Because ovine tuberculosis and bovine tuberculosis appear similar, information on cattle is herein extrapolated to sheep.

In adult sheep, tuberculosis develops in animals maintained in a tuberculous environment. Housing sheep in a building that is unhygienic because of crowding, poor ventilation, and inadequate lighting favors disease transmission. When a focus of infection develops, spread occurs. The route of transmission may be through the respiratory system. In some cases, however, infection may be acquired through the digestive system. A primary complex is the combination of an original organic tubercle and the near contemporaneous lesion in the regional lymph node. The anatomic location of a primary complex is evidence of the primary route of infection. Since this complex commonly occurs in the thorax, it is assumed in the following account that the route of infection is through the respiratory system.

Tuberculous animals expel bacilli into the air. Susceptible sheep inhale infected droplets as an aerosol. The virulent organisms may enter the alveoli or be arrested on the mucous membrane of the bronchial tree. In the alveoli, the first tissue reaction is the accumulation of neutrophils around the bacilli. After a short period, the neutrophils undergo necrosis, and epithelioid cells accumulate to form a multilayered zone around the bacteria and dead cells. Some epithelioid cells fuse to form Langhans' giant cells. Some bacilli are phagocytized, and some of these are destroyed. A zone of lymphocytes and fibrous connective tissue forms around the zone of epithelioid cells.

Vascularity is low. Towards the center of the lesion, many epithelioid cells and normal tissue cells undergo caseation necrosis. Calcium salts may precipitate in foci in the necrotic tissue. Some foci of infection coalesce and thus form a macroscopic tubercle. Healing of the primary lesion may occur. Some bacilli escape from the lesion, enter lymphatics, and are moved to the bronchial or mediastinal lymph nodes, where a new focus of infection develops.

In some cases, the initial lesion erodes into a bronchus or bronchiole. In this event, virulent bacilli enter the lumen of the bronchus. From here they may descend into many alveoli and produce tuberculous bronchopneumonia. The organisms may also be coughed out of the infected bronchus into the atmosphere or into saliva of the mouth or secretions of the nose. Infected sputum may be swallowed into the alimentary tract, where secondary foci of infection form.

In either the primary or secondary lesions, blood vessels, especially veins, may be eroded and penetrated by organisms. This entrance creates a bacteremia and causes hematogenous dissemination of the bacilli. By this means, new foci of infection may establish in any and many organs.

Metabolism of the infectious tubercle bacilli synthesizes specific protein foreign to the host. The host response to the tubercle bacilli is primarily cell mediated stimulating a delayed hypersensitivity, although exposure to certain mycobacterium often stimulates a humoral response. There is a variable relationship between the cell mediated immune response and the number of bacilli occurring in the lesions of different animals and animal species infected with *M. bovis*. Early in the disease and continuing through most of the course, the host tissues become sensitized to the protein. In some advanced stages, the tissues are exposed to large amounts of the protein and become desensitized, thus, there is an inverse relationship between the number of bacilli occurring in the lesion and the degree of allergy (measured by the intradermal delayed hypersensitivity test) and the amount of caseation in the lesion. The sensitization is the basis for the tuberculin reaction used in diagnosis.

CLINICAL SIGNS AND POSTMORTEM LESIONS. Since tuberculosis usually is an insidious disease, clinical signs commonly are inconspicuous. Infected animals, however, slowly lose body weight despite availability of adequate feed. Deep cough and nasal discharge persist. In some cases, pneumonia develops. The morbidity is extremely low, but the mortality of affected sheep is high. The course is often prolonged for many months and sometimes years. Hematogenous dissemination shortens the fatal course.

At necropsy, lesions are usually in the respiratory system (Figs. 13-2 and 13-3). Primary tubercles, frequently located in the dorsal part of the lungs, are single or few in number and measure 1 to 2 cm in diameter. They are firm and encapsulated and, on the cut surface,

Fig. 13-3. Caseous tubercle in the mediastinal lymph node of a cow with tuberculosis. × 0.8.

show gray to yellow caseous necrosis. Mineralization may be discernible as grittiness. The enlarged bronchial or mediastinal lymph nodes also contain gross tubercles. The two first tubercles—lung component and lymph node component—constitute the primary complex. In addition, caseous acinar bronchopneumonia and caseous lobular bronchopneumonia may exist.

In case of hematogenous dissemination from the primary complex, multiple tubercles, often miliary, are distributed to many organs, but especially the spleen, liver, kidneys, alimentary tract, mesenteric and hepatic lymph nodes, and lungs. This distribution of lesions constitutes generalization of the disease.

DIAGNOSIS. Veterinarians diagnose ovine tuberculosis in living animals on evidence of clinical signs, positive tuberculin reactions, or isolation of tubercle bacilli from secretions or excretions. In the United States, the intradermal tuberculin test in the caudal fold is universally used. Most serologic tests have not been widely accepted. The development of the Enzyme-Linked Immunosorbent Assay (ELISA) with evaluation of the biologically active components of *M. bovis* and antigen fractions obtained from other mycobacterium holds promise for a rapid screening test with a high degree of sensitivity and specificity. In dead animals, the diagnosis is based on the demonstration of tubercle bacilli in typical lesions. Usually, laboratory animals are inoculated with lesion tissue, and media isolations are made from them.

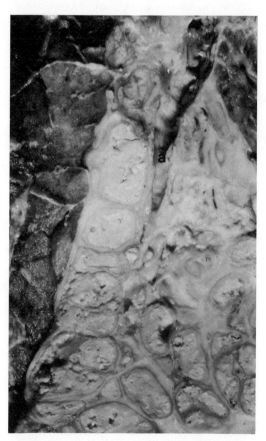

Fig. 13-2. Caseous lobular bronchopneumonia in the lung of a cow with tuberculosis; bronchus (*a*). × 0.8.

The differential diagnosis requires consideration of spreading caseous lymphadenitis, metastasizing neoplasms, and other chronic infections.

PREVENTION.   In the United States and some other countries, such as Denmark, Finland, and the Netherlands, the bovine type of tuberculosis in both sheep and cattle is now prevented by successfully eradicating the disease from populations of those species. In the United States, eradication is achieved in individual states by applying the intradermal tuberculin test and removing and slaughtering all reactor animals. After removing reactors, the premises are cleaned and disinfected. In some cases, premises are vacated for variable periods. Since sheep are highly susceptible to avian tuberculosis, tuberculous chickens should not associate with sheep.

Providing sanitary environment also reduces spread of the disease. Producers should eliminate excessive crowding and adequately ventilate and illuminate the quarters.

Clean herds and flocks should be protected against the introduction of disease. Additions to the flock should be free of tuberculosis. This state should be established by isolating and performing a tuberculin test on any suspected animals prior to cohabitation with the flock. Clean animals should not enter public shows or graze public range or pasture unless all animals in the public assemblage are proven free of tuberculosis by proper application of the tuberculin test.

Although sheep are highly susceptible to *M. bovis*, the prevalence in cattle is extremely low with some states designated as tuberculosis free. Therefore, the exposure potential in the United States is virtually nonexistent.

Carmichael, J.: Tuberculosis of sheep in Uganda. Vet. Rec., 50:1138-1147, 1938.
Cordes, D., Bullians, J., Lake, D., and Carter, M.: Observations on tuberculosis caused by mycobacterium bovis in sheep. N.Z. Vet. J., 29:60-62, 1981.
Creech, G.T.: Bovine type tuberculosis in sheep. AJVR, 1:23-25, 1940.
Davidson, R., Alley, M., and Beaston, N.: Tuberculosis in a flock of sheep. N.Z. Vet. J., 29:1-2, 1981.
Francis, J.: *Tuberculosis in Man and Animals*. London, Cassells & Co., 1958.
Harshfield, J.S. and Roderick, L.M.: Avian tuberculosis in sheep. JAVMA, 85:597-610, 1934.
Jowett, W.: Two cases of tuberculosis in sheep. J. Comp. Pathol., 41:255-258, 1928.
M'Fadyean, J.: Tuberculosis of sheep. J. Comp. Pathol., 13:59-60, 1900.
Mantovani, A.: A case of human tuberculosis in a sheep. Rev. Med. Vet., Parma, 6:65-68, 1954.
Prieto, C.: Two cases of natural tuberculosis in sheep. Rev. Fac. Agric. Vet., Buenos Aires, 9:219-232, 1942.
Robinson, E.M.: Tuberculosis in sheep and goats. J. S. Afr. Vet. Med. Assoc., 26:95-104, 1955.
Shishkina, E.Y.: Tuberculosis and tuberculin testing in sheep. Veterinariia (Moscow), No. 6, 32:43-44, 1955.
Stubbs, E.L. and Live, I.: A case of sheep tuberculosis due to bovine type. JAVMA, 95:173-176, 1939.
Swartz, K., et al.: Comparison of ELISA reactions and tuberculin skin responses in elk (Cervus Elaphus) in a herd in which Mycobacterium bovis was previously diagnosed. Proceedings U.S. Animal Health Assn., 87:552-558, 603-610, 1983.
Thoen, C., Hall, M., Petersburg, T., and Harrington, R.: Detection of mycobacterial antibodies in sera of cattle experimentally exposed to Mycobacterium bovis by use of a modified enzyme-linked immunosorbent assay. An. Assn. Vet. Lab. Diagnosticians, 28th Annual Proceedings, 25-38, 1983.
Thorns, C., Morris, J., and Little, T.: A spectrum of immune responses and pathological conditions between certain animal species to experimental Mycobacterium bovis infection. Br. J. Exp. Path., 62:562-572, 1982.

Pulmonary Adenomatosis

(SPA; jaagsiekte; pulmonary carcinoma of sheep)

Pulmonary adenomatosis, a contagious neoplastic disease of adult sheep, is characterized by insidious but continuous development, physical weakness, dyspnea, nasal discharge, and fatal termination. It is caused by a virus. Pulmonary adenomatosis and ovine progressive pneumonia may simultaneously affect the same flock and the same animal; both produce similar signs and lesions.

Because of wide geographic distribution and high mortality, SPA, a major disease of the sheep industry, causes extensive financial waste. Economic losses result from unthriftiness of affected sheep, inevitable deaths, interference with sheep commerce; protein deficiencies among sheep-dependent people, the costs of eradicative and preventive programs, and disposal procedures.

OCCURRENCE. SPA probably occurs in all breeds and sexes. Susceptibility among breeds varies, however, and Merino sheep are highly susceptible. Sheep of SPA-free regions are especially susceptible and develop a high disease incidence following exposure to the virus. Rams, wethers, and ewes develop SPA, but, because of prevailing numbers of each group, cases among ewes attract attention. Although all ages of sheep are susceptible to the virus, the clinical disease, because of long incubation period, appears primarily among adult sheep, especially animals 3 to 5 years of age. In addition to sheep, SPA may occur in goats.

Exacerbations and deaths among affected sheep may be numerically increased during winter. Inclement weather predisposes all sheep to bacterial pneumonia, and this intercurrent infection may shorten the clinical course of SPA.

Geographically, the disease is widely distributed and occurs among sheep of South Africa, Kenya, Israel, Turkey, India, Bulgaria, Greece, Czechoslovakia, USSR, Germany, France, Italy, Spain, Great Britain, Iceland, Chile, Peru, Ireland, Netherlands, and the U.S.A. Some other countries bordering areas of known infection may also contain the disease.

ETIOLOGY AND PATHOGENESIS. SPA is caused by a relatively new retrovirus of the family retroviridae, i.e. a 60 to 70S single-stranded RNA virus, and unrelated to any of the other members of this group. This group of retroviruses are generally divided into 6 main classes, designated A, B, C, D, E and F types. Early work indicated A and C type viral particles were involved, although recent biophysical and immunologic findings suggest a relationship with type B and D retroviruses. SPA tumor and lung fluids all contain a particle-associated reverse transcriptase. In the lung exudate some of the virions are present in the form of immune complexes, primarily IgA. Gel filtration experiments suggest the majority of virions present in lung fluid is complexed with IgA, which may explain the low infectivity of the virus in nature and cell culture. This may also explain the lack of metastasis and that the immune response of the host is mainly an IgA-mediated local response. Further evidence indicates that herpes-virus does not produce SPA.

SPA is transmitted horizontally by means of the transplantation of whole cells or by infection with SPA retrovirus. Affected sheep, by coughing and blowing, discharge virus-infected cells into the atmosphere. Nearby susceptible sheep inhale the cells and contract the disease. Crowding sheep into pens, especially closed buildings, facilitates spread of infection from diseased to healthy animals.

The target cells are the type II alveolar epithelial cells and less frequently the nonciliated bronchiolar epithelial cells. In early lesions the transformed cells proliferate forming a single layer lining the alveolar lumen and develop into a papilliform mass. These masses proliferate further to fill the alveolar space and spread from one alveolus to the other. The tumor cells on the periphery of the lesions contain secretory granules resembling those found in normal sheep granular pneumocytes. However, tumor granules contain more osmiophilic substance. The content of the secretory granules may be related to the rate of surfactant production. The great increase in the number of cells producing surfactant in the diseased sheep explains the large amount of lung exudate. The tumor cells undergo rapid protein synthesis and cell division with virus replication during the process.

Eventually, small foci of neoplasia, by expansion or coalescence, form large nodules that may finally incapacitate parts of the affected lungs. After a course of many months or even years, metastases may form and grow in regional lymph nodes but rarely in extrathoracic organs. The growth of extensive neoplastic tissue within the lungs may increase the resistance to pulmonary circulation and result in hypertrophy of the right ventricle and, in some animals, eventual failure.

During the long course, complement-fixing and serum-neutralizing antibodies form, but these substances do not influence progress of the disease. The most prevalent cell of the immune system found in the SPA lung is the alveolar macrophage. The role of the alveolar macrophage in SPA is uncertain except in the clearance of surfactant material and possibly some effects on limiting metastasis. Plasma cells found in the interstitial space probably play a role in the production of local immunoglobulins against SPA. A hypergammaglobulinemia develops with persistent hyper-7S-immunoglobulinemia.

Death results from failure of the right ventricle and hypoxia; many affected sheep develop acute bacterial pneumonia and die prematurely. The virus particles return to the external environment in expelled cells and there may infect susceptible sheep.

CLINICAL SIGNS AND POSTMORTEM LESIONS. The symptoms of PA relate to incapacitation of lung tissue. The incubation period varies from 2 months to 2 years and is followed by insidious development of dyspnea. During early stages, although the affected animal has good physical condition, breathing accelerates excessively during forced exercise or work performance, such as upgrade drives. Later, respirations remain continuously fast and shallow, and the affected animal may, in the struggle for oxygen, extend its head and dilate its nostrils.

Coughing is frequent, and when the head is lowered and the animal upended, fluid pours from the nostrils. Auscultation and percussion of the thorax reveal rales and areas of lung consolidation, especially in the ventral planes. In terminal stages, physical weakness and emaciation supervene, but the animal maintains the standing position because recumbency exacerbates dyspnea.

The annual morbidity among infected flocks averages 2%, and the mortality of affected animals is 100%. The clinical course varies from a few weeks to several months.

At necropsy or at organ inspection following slaughter, most changes are limited to the lungs and heart and vary with disease development. During early stages, the lungs show a diffuse distribution of gray-blue nodules measuring 1 to 20 mm in diameter. In advanced stages, the heavy lungs contain both small nodules and large masses of neoplastic tissue (Fig. 13-4). Regional lymph nodes may be

Fig. 13-4. Part of left lung from a sheep with pulmonary adenomatosis. × 0.8.

enlarged from metastases; extrathoracic metastases rarely occur. The right ventricle may be hypertrophied and also dilated, and small amounts of transudate may have accumulated in the body cavities.

Histopathologically, the neoplasm consists of proliferating alveolar and/or bronchiolar epithelium (Fig. 13-5). The granular pneumocyte is the major site of transformation. The adenoma is composed of fetal type II alveolar epithelial cells. Papillary masses of cuboidal epithelial cells form in and eventually replace alveoli. Affected bronchioles show both hyperplastic and neoplastic epithelia, which also form papillary masses entering the adjacent alveoli. In some nodules, fibrous stoma quantitatively dominates the tumor. Metastatic foci usually resemble the primary tumor.

DIAGNOSIS. Veterinarians diagnose SPA on evidence of typical signs and lesions. In en-

Fig. 13-5. Lung of a sheep with pulmonary adenomatosis. HE stain. × 120.

demic areas, the gradually and continuously increasing dyspnea and the nasal discharge of fluid from upended sheep are suggestive changes. At necropsy of dead or sacrificed animals, the presence of gray-blue nodules throughout the lungs gives further support to clinical diagnosis. Laboratory confirmation depends on finding histopathologic features of the pulmonary tumor.

The differential diagnosis requires consideration of chronic progressive pneumonia, pasteurellosis, verminous pneumonia, and other lung infections. None of these diseases causes the nasal discharge of fluid; each has characteristic histopathologic features.

PREVENTION. Veterinarians and producers prevent SPA by establishing and maintaining

disease-free flocks. In the absence of a simple diagnostic test, preventive and eradication programs depend on the slaughter of infected and contact animals. Following depopulation the premises should be cleaned and disinfected prior to replacing with sheep from clean flocks. All clean flocks must be operated on a closed basis. Replacement ewes and rams should be raised by the flock or purchased only from other clean flocks.

Alibasoglu, M.: Studies on ovine pulmonary adenomatosis. Vet. Fac. Derg. Ankara Univ., 16:337-351, 1969.

Aliev, D.I.: Dynamics of the pathological changes in pulmonary adenomatosis of sheep. Veterinariia (Moscow), No. 7, 55-56, 1967.

Blackmore, F. and Bosworth, T.J.: The occurrence of jaagsiekte in England. Vet. Rec., 53:35-37, 1941.

Cortizie, S., Els, H.J., and Verwoerd, D.W.: Transmission of jaagsiekte (ovine pulmonary adenomatosis) by means of a permanent epithelial cell line established from affected lungs. Onderstepoort J. Vet. Res., 43:133-141, 1976.

Cowdry, E.V.: Studies on the etiology of jaagsiekte. II. The origin of the epithelial proliferations and the subsequent changes. J. Exp. Med., 42:335-346, 1925.

Cowdry, E.V. and Marsh, H.: Comparative pathology of South African jaagsiekte and Montana progressive pneumonia of sheep. J. Exp. Med., 45:571-585, 1927.

Cuba-Caparo, A.: Adenomatosis pulmonar de los ovinos en el Peru. Bull. Off. Int. Epizoot., 56:840-849, 1961.

Cuba-Caparo, A., de la Vega, E., and Copaira, M.: Pulmonary adenomatosis of sheep-metastasizing bronchial tumors. AJVR, 20:673-682, 1961.

Cuba-Caparo, A., de la Vega, E., and Durand, W.: Experimental transmission of ovine pulmonary adenomatosis. Rev. Fac. Med. Vet. Univ. Nac., Lima, 18:97-124, 1967.

Cutlip, R. and Young, S.: Sheep pulmonary adenomatosis (jaagsiekte) in the United States. Am. J. Vet. Res., 43:2108-2113, 1982.

Cvjetanovic, V., Forsek, Z., and Nevjestic, A.: Ovine pulmonary adenomatosis in Crna Gora, Yugoslavia. I. Epidemiological and pathological studies. Veterinaria (Saraj), 19:315-319, 1970.

Cvjetanovic, V. and Martincic, M.: Pulmonary adenomatosis in sheep of Yugoslavia. Vet. Arch., 32:77-82, 1962.

Damodaran, S.: Ovine pulmonary adenomatosis (jaagsiekte). Indian Vet. J., 37:127-138, 1960.

Deiana, S. and Ceretto, F.: Histoimmunological findings in ovine pulmonary adenomatosis in Sardinia. Atti Soc. Ital. Sci. Vet., 21:612-615, 1968.

DeKock, G.: Are the lesions of jaagsiekte in sheep in the nature of a neoplasm? 15th Ann. Rept. Dir. Vet. Serv., S. Afr., 1929, pp. 611-641.

Dungal, N.: Epizootic adenomatosis of the lungs of sheep: its relation to verminous pneumonia and jaagsiekte. Proc. R. Soc. Med., 31:497-505, 1938.

Enchev, S.: Reproduction of pulmonary adenomatosis (jaagsiekte) in sheep. II. Vet. Med. Nauki (Sofia), 5:13-24, 1968.

Enchev, S.: Experimentally induced pulmonary adenomatosis in sheep. Vet. Med. Nauki (Sofia), 3:947-954, 1966.

Enchev, S.: Pulmonary adenomatosis of sheep in Bulgaria. I. Epidemiology, symptoms and pathology. II. Metastases in pulmonary lymph nodes. Izv. Vet. Inst. Zaraz. Parszit. Bolesti, Sofia, 1:345-356, 1961; 2:177-186, 1961.

Herring, A., Sharp, J., Scott, F., and Angus, K.: Further evidence for a retrovirus as the etiologic agent of sheep pulmonary adenomatosis (jaagsiekte). Vet. Microbiol., 8:237-249, 1983.

Hod, I., Herz, A., and Zimber, A.: Pulmonary carcinoma (jaagsiekte) of sheep: Ultrastructure study of early and advanced tumor lesions. Am. J. Pathol., 86:545-558, 1977.

Hod, I., Zimber, A., and Kloffer, U.: Long term serum protein values in sheep with pulmonary adenomatosis or other chronic pulmonary disease. Br. Vet. J., 133:56-61, 1977.

Hunter, A. and Munro, R.: The diagnosis, occurrence and distribution of sheep pulmonary adenomatosis in Scotland 1975 to 1981. Br. Vet. J., 139:153-164, 1983.

Jakob, W. and Krause, H.: Pulmonary adenomatosis in sheep. Mh. Vet. Med., 6:217-223, 1965.

Kostenko, Y.G.: Adenomatosis in sheep. Veterinariia (Moscow), No. 11, 41:34-36, 1964.

Malmquist, W.A., Krauss, H.H., Moulton, J.E., and Wandera, J.G.: Morphologic study of virus-infected lung cell cultures from sheep pulmonary adenomatosis. Lab. Invest., 26:528-533, 1972.

Markson, L.M. and Terlecki, S.: The experimental transmission of ovine pulmonary adenomatosis. Pathol. Vet. 1:269, 1964.

Martin, W.B., Angus, K.W., Robinson, G.W., and Scott, F.M.M.: The herpes virus of sheep pulmonary adenomatosis. Comp. Immunol. Microbiol. Infect. Dis., 2:313-325, 1979.

Mitrofano, V.M.: Metastasizing pulmonary adenomatosis in sheep. Arch. Pathol., 26:68-74, 1964.

Nesbit, D.I., Mackay, J.M.K., Smith, W., and Gray, E.W.: Ultrastructure of sheep pulmonary adenomatosis (jaagsiekte). J. Pathol., 103:157-162, 1971.

Nevjestic, A., Rukavina, L., Forsek, Z., and Cvjetanovic, V.: Ovine pulmonary adenomatosis in Crna Gora, Yugo. II. Detection of diseased sheep by the complement fixation test. Veterinaria (Saraj), 19:429-434, 1970.

Nobel, T.A.: Pulmonary adenomatosis (jaagsiekte) in sheep with special reference to its occurrence in Israel. Refuah Vet., 15:98-101, 1958.

Nobel, T.A., Neumann, F., and Klopfer, V.: Histological patterns of the metastases in pulmonary adenomatosis of sheep (jaagsiekte). J. Comp. Pathol., 79:537-540, 1969.

Nobel, T.A., Neumann, F., and Klopfer, V.: Metastases in pulmonary adenomatosis of sheep. Refuah Vet., 25:5-6, 1968.

Payne, A. and Verwoerd, D.: A scanning and transmission electron microscopy study of jaagsiekte lesions. Onderstepoort J. Vet. Res., 51:1-13, 1984.

Perk, K.: Slow virus infections of ovine lungs. Advances in Vet. Sci. and Comp. Med., 26:267-287, 1982.

Perk, K. and Hod, I.: Demonstration of virus particles in ovine pulmonary adenomata. Experimentia, 27:437-438, 1971.

Perk, K., Hod, I., and Nobel, T.A.: Pulmonary adenomatosis of sheep (jaagsiekte). I. Ultrastructure of the tumor. J. Natl. Cancer Inst., 46:525-537, 1971.

Perk, K., Michalides, R., Spiegelman, S., and Schlorn, J.: Biochemical and morphologic evidence for the presence of an RNA tumor virus in pulmonary carcinoma of sheep (jaagsiekte). J. Natl. Cancer Inst., 53:131-135, 1974.

Perk, K. and Yaniv, A.: Lack of maedi viral related RNA in pulmonary carcinoma of sheep (jaagsiekte). Res. Vet. Sci., 24:46-48, 1978.

Romboli, B.: Pneumonopatie displastiche (progressive jaagsiekte) nelle pecore macellate in Toscana. Ann. Fac. Med. Vet., Pisa, 12:50-96, 1959.

Schulz, L.C., Somoza, A., and Weiland, F.: Neoplastic character of pulmonary adenomatosis of sheep. Comparative studies in Chile and Federal Germany. DTW, 72:458-461, 1965.

Scott, F., Sharp, J., Angus, K., and Gray, E.: Infection of specific-pathogen free lambs with a herpesvirus isolated from pulmonary adenomatosis. Arch. Vir., 80:147-162, 1984.

Shirlaw, J.F.: Studies on jaagsiekte in Kenya. Bull. Epizoot. Dis. Afr., 7:287-302, 1959.

Sigurdsson, B.: Adenomatosis of sheep's lungs. Experimental transmission. Arch. Gesamte Virusforsch., 8:51-58, 1958.

Snyder, S., DeMartini, J., Ameghino, E., and Caletti, E.: Coexistence of pulmonary adenomatosis and progressive pneumonia in sheep in the central Sierra of Peru. Am. J. Vet. Res., 44:1334-1338, 1983.

Tustin, R.C.: Ovine jaagsiekte, J. S. Afr. Vet. Med. Assoc., 40:3-23, 1969.

Tustin, R.C. and Geyer, S.M.: Transmission of ovine jaagsiekte using neoplastic cells grown in tissue culture. J. S. Afr. Vet. Med. Assoc., 42:181-182, 1971.

Verwoerd, D., Payne, A., York, D., and Myer, M.: Isolation and preliminary characterization of the jaagsiekte retrovirus (JSRV). Onderstepoort J. Vet. Res., 50:309-316, 1983.

Wandera, J.G.: Clinical pulmonary adenomatosis of sheep produced experimentally. Br. Vet. J., 126:185-193, 1970.

Wandera, J.G.: Experimental transmission of sheep pulmonary adenomatosis (jaagsiekte). Vet. Rec., 83:478-482, 1968.

Ovine Progressive Pneumonia

(OPP; maedi; visna-maedi; lunger disease; la bouita; zwoegerziekte; Graaf-Reint disease; laikipia disease; visna)

Although the above-named diseases may not be clinically and pathologically identical, they have the same etiologic characteristics and therefore are considered together. Visna-Maedi (visna meaning wasting, maedi meaning shortness of breath) was originally described in Iceland as two clinical syndromes involving the lung and brain with a high morbidity and annual losses exceeding 50% in infected flocks of Icelandic sheep. Morphogenesis, molecular hydridization, serology, and animal experiments have shown these to be caused by the same virus. Visna-Maedi is similar in clinical and etiologic characteristics to Montana progressive pneumonia and ovine progressive pneumonia of North America, Zwoegerziekte in Holland, Great Renet in South Africa, and LaBouhite in France.

Ovine progressive pneumonia, a slow virus disease of adult sheep, is characterized by a lymphoproliferative pneumonia, meningeal arteritis with encephalitis, nonsuppurative arthritis and lymphocytic mastitis. An insidious but continuously advancing and eventually fatal pneumonitis, physical weakness, dyspnea, and emaciation are the predominant clinical features. Because of distribution to most major sheep-producing countries and a high morbidity, OPP is a major disease of the sheep industry and annually results in financial waste. Losses come from deaths, unthriftiness during the long course of the disease, the cost of expensive research and control programs, and protein deficiencies among sheep-dependent people.

OCCURRENCE. Seroprevalence of OPP in cull ewes in western and midwestern United States ranges from 1 to 70% depending on the geographic location with greater than 50% of the flocks having some infection. All breeds of sheep are susceptible. It is undetermined if a variation in breed susceptibility, management practices, or variations in the genetic make up of the virus account for difference in prevalence rates of various geographic locations. The age-specific prevalence shows that the proportion of infected sheep increases with age. Serologic responses may occur months to years in advance of the clinical signs. Although the number of animals with clinical signs and serologic responses increase with age, these responses can occur within the first year of life

depending on the exposure dose and host-virus interaction. Geographically the disease has been observed and reported from most Eastern and Western European countries, the Mediterranean countries, Africa, South America, North America, Russia, the Baltic countries, and the near East. Especially high prevalence rates are observed in the western range flocks of the United States.

ETIOLOGY AND PATHOGENESIS.   OPP is caused by a nononcogenic retrovirus of the subfamily Lentivirinae (lenti is Latin for slow). The lentiviruses, caprine arthritis-encephalitis virus (CAEV), visna virus (VV) and ovine progressive pneumonia virus (OPPV) cause complex multisystemic disease processes in sheep and goats. Although related, comparative studies using virus morphogenesis, nucleic acid hybridization, and radioimmunoassay have determined major differences in the viral genomes and the virion-associated proteins and glycoproteins of CAEV, VV, and OPPV. On the basis of protein and nucleic acid content, analysis of naturally present OPPV, a highly lytic (type I) and a persistent (type II), genetically distinct viruses have been identified. The highly lytic type I being closely related to the Icelandic prototype strains of visna virus and the persistent type II more related to CAEV. The virus is remarkably similar to the RNA tumor viruses with the existence of a 60 to 70 S RNA genome, RNA-dependent DNA polymerase activity, and similar morphologic properties. Two types of virus are visible under the electron microscope: a large particle (120 to 140 nm) with an electron-lucent center and a dense laminated outer rim, and a small particle (80 to 110 nm) with an electron-dense core surrounded by a single membrane. It replicates slowly in the cytoplasm of host cells and matures by budding from the cell membrane. The target cells for OPPV are lung tissue with extrathoracic replication occurring in the brain, choroid plexus, spleen, lymph nodes, buffy coat, kidney, liver, the synovial membrane of joints, mammary tissue, and possibly other locations. Macrophages have proven to be an invariable source of virus and provide a major site of viral replication within the infected host. Although infection stimulates production of complement-fixing and serum-neutralizing antibodies, these are extremely variable. Early transient cell-mediated immune responses to OPPV have been demonstrated and humoral antibodies may be delayed for months or the possibility exists that OPPV infection can occur without antibody production. The exact mechanisms which allow an agent-host compatibility evolving into a disease of such chronicity is unknown. Hybridization techniques have shown that relatively few cells in visna-infected sheep contain proviral DNA or viral RNA indicating a low level of replication. Thus, chronic low level antigen presentation, perhaps controlled by a block at the level of proviral DNA transcription, may account for continued stimulation and the resultant slowly developing lymphoid hyperplasia. It is inactivated in 10 minutes by a temperature of 56°C, by 0.04% formaldehyde, and by a pH of 4.2.

The virus is transmitted in aerosols and inhaled, by the feces and ingested or by viral infected lymphocytes in the colostrum or milk and ingested by the newborn. One case of vertical transmission, from infected dam to fetal lamb, has been reported. Prolonged and heavy exposure dose to the virus will accelerate seroconversion and appearance of lesions in lambs which can become seropositive within a year of age. The number of infected sheep, stage of infection, amounts of virus being shed, and intensive management practices will influence the proportion of seropositive animals in a flock. These can easily reach 80%.

Although not fully investigated, some aspects of the pathogenesis of OPP are known; others are conjectural. Following the entrance of virus by inhalation into the respiratory system, the target cells are invaded and, in some animals, the virus spreads into the bronchial and mediastinal lymph nodes, blood, spleen, and kidneys. The invaded pulmonary cells, probably reticular cells and B-lymphocytes, are not seriously damaged but are stimulated to proliferate. Consequently, the interalveolar septa thicken from the presence of numerous new histiocytes and some new fibrocytes and

collagenous fibers. As the septa enlarge, the squamous epithelial cells lining the alveoli morphologically transform into cuboidal cells.

In addition, the peribronchiolar and perivascular lymphoreticular tissues may undergo hyperplasia and form active germinal centers. The combined septal, bronchiolar, and vascular changes reduce and obliterate alveoli, lower the efficiency of gaseous exchange, and produce gradually increasing and eventually fatal hypoxia. The apparent reduction in patency of septal capillaries probably causes pulmonary arterial hypertension and possibly right ventricular hypertrophy. Death may occur early in the long disease course from intercurrent acute bacterial pneumonia.

Furthermore, some extrapulmonary effects may develop; lymphocytic meningitis, pleocytosis, choroiditis, leukoencephalitis, meningeal arteritis, and demyelination of subependymal white matter have been reported. In some experimental sheep, the pleocytosis eventually abates without clinical signs developing; in others, the lesions of the central nervous system progress relentlessly and eventually kill. Chronic nonsuppurative arthritis may develop, concurrently with interstitial pneumonitis, in the carpal and tarsal joints of sheep naturally infected with OPPV. The initial articular lesions are edema, hyperemia, and hyperplasia of the joint and bursal linings followed by necrosis of these tissues. Lymphoid hyperplasia occurs in the mammary gland parenchyma, with massive periductular lymphoid proliferation, including follicle formation, intralobular infiltration of lymphocytes and occasional plasma cells. During the prolonged incubation period and clinical course, serum-neutralizing antibodies form in some infected sheep, but probably do not substantially influence the disease.

CLINICAL SIGNS AND POSTMORTEM LESIONS. Following a prolonged incubation period of 1 to 2 years, sheep with OPP develop advanced pulmonary lesions and then evince gradually increasing respiratory distress. During early stages, the animals, under physical stress of a drive especially on uphill grades, are unable to work and thus lag behind the flock. Respirations accelerate and physical condition declines. As the disease worsens, breathing increases to 80 to 120 respirations per minute during exertion and remains fast during rest. With nostrils dilated and head held high, the animal struggles, sometimes with oral breathing, for adequate amounts of oxygen.

Despite a persisting appetite, the loss of live weight continues, and the sheep becomes generally emaciated and physically weak. Animals usually remain standing because recumbency forces the diaphragm forward, which further belabors respiration. Auscultation and percussion of the thorax reveal aeration in dorsal parts of the lungs and consolidation in the ventral parts. Body temperature is usually normal.

Concurrent with or separate from the clinical respiratory distress animals may show lameness due to involvement of the carpal and tarsal joints. The joints are firm and swollen without increased fluid or exudate. A clinical mastitis characterized by edema and homogeneous firmness of the udder is also a frequent clinical finding.

Laboratory findings include mild hypochromic anemia, hypogammaglobulinemia, persisting leukocytosis, pleocytosis in those with central nervous system (CNS) disease, and a positive result from an agar gel immunodiffusion test. Death results from hypoxia and may occur prematurely from intercurrent acute bacterial pneumonia.

CNS lesions form 1 to 2 months after exposure of sheep to virus; pleocytosis, the earliest sign, forms and continues for a few weeks to several months. After several months, other clinical signs insidiously develop. Extensor muscles of the hind feet weaken, and consequently, the fetlocks and pastern joints involuntarily flex during locomotion; this feature can be induced or exaggerated by forced and excessive locomotion. Later, inconspicuous tremors form in the lips, and the head may be deflected to one side. Paresis slowly exacerbates and progresses to paralysis, prostration, and death. The respiratory form is seen most commonly in sheep in the western U.S., although sheep may develop respiratory and CNS lesions simultaneously.

At necropsy, overt changes are seen in the lungs (Fig. 13-6), pulmonary lymph nodes, carpal and tarsal joints, mammary gland, and CNS. On opening the thorax, the lungs do not

Fig. 13-6. Left lung from a sheep with progressive pneumonia.

collapse.. Adhesions unite one lobe with another and connect the lung to the thoracic wall. Both pleural and cut lung surfaces show firm gray-brown pneumonic tissue in the anteroventral part and functional aerating tissue in the dorsal part. Lung weights are increased from the normal range of 300 to 500 g to an average of 1200 g. Bronchial lymph nodes also show marked lymphoid proliferation with enlargement from a normal weight range of 10 to 15 g to an average of 40 g. In the CNS, there is a moderate meningitis, with edema over the convexity of the hemispheres and piriform lobes. The choroid plexuses of the lateral ventricles show diffuse and nodular thickening. The spinal ganglia may contain lymphoid nodules. There are foci of leukoencephalomalacia up to 10 mm in diameter (Fig. 13-7). Carpal and tarsal joint lesions include necrosis of synovial tissue, necrosis and erosion of articular cartilage, necrosis of subchondral bone, and fibrous amylosis of the joint. Histologically, extensive perivascular lymphocytic and plasma cell infiltration occur in the synovium. In the subsynovial and periarticular tissues, areas of necrosis and mineralization, fibrosis, and perivascular mononuclear infiltration occur.

Histopathologic changes consist of thickening of interalveolar septa and lymphoid tissue hyperplasia. The septa are thickened from the existence of numerous new histiocytes, some new fibrocytes, and collagenous and reticular fibers, and in some lung areas, from cuboidal epithelialization of alveoli. In pneumonic areas, most alveoli are either obliterated or reduced

Fig. 13-8. Lung from a sheep with progressive pneumonia. Note lymphoid tissue around bronchioles. HE stain. × 120.

Fig. 13-7. Gross slice of brain with lesions of leukoencephalomalacia (a) from a sheep with progressive pneumonia.

in size. In addition, hyperplasia of lymphoid tissue surrounding or adjacent to bronchioles and vessels is prominent and may show active germinal centers (Fig. 13-8). Bronchiolar bundles of smooth muscle cells are hypertrophied.

CNS lesions consist of chronic meningitis, with fibroplasia and lymphocytic infiltration uniformly extending over the spinal cord and basal part of the brain. In the nerve tissue, early stages show foci of astrocytosis around blood vessels, and in more advanced stages, the foci coalesce to form sheets, which may be dense at the margins and microcavitated towards the center. Secondary changes include glial fibrosis, mild demyelination, and perivascular lymphoplasmacytosis. The changes may show extensive spread from the initial subependymal location into brain and spinal cord parenchyma. Sites of predilection for lesions include periependymal gray matter of the spinal cord, anterior horns, anterior columns, walls of the aqueduct, floors and walls of the ventricles, corpus callosum, and hippocampal and hypothalamic region.

DIAGNOSIS. Veterinarians diagnose OPP clinically on evidence of characteristic signs and lesions. Laboratory confirmation by positive results from complement-fixation tests, agar gel immunodiffusion tests, enzyme-linked immunosorbent assay, virus isolation, and histopathologic findings can be obtained.

The differential diagnosis requires consideration of pulmonary adenomatosis, verminous pneumonia, pulmonary abscesses, other lung diseases, and scrapie. The identification or elimination of these diseases depends on necropsy and laboratory findings.

PREVENTION, TREATMENT AND ERADICATION. Prevention is accomplished by avoiding exposure of healthy sheep to diseased animals. Additions to the flock should be considered only when the status of the originating flock is known to be free of OPP. With the serologic tests (C.F. AGID and ELISA) available, flock and individual status can be assessed. It is important to recognize that the development of antibodies following infection can take several months. Therefore, testing of lambs that have been infected from colostrum or milk, or adults recently exposed may give erroneous results. Also, some infected animals never show a serologic response. OPP free lambs can be obtained by removing them from their dam at birth prior to receiving colostrum from the infected dam and rearing in a clean atmosphere away from infected sheep. Iceland eradicated visna-maedi by a strict slaughter program of all infected and contact animals. These approaches are extremely expensive and may not be cost effective. Fortunately, there are alternative solutions made possible by serologic tests that can be tailored to meet the needs and economic constraints of the producer. Some of the options are alterations for control or eradication programs: (1) Containment: animals from infected flocks

cannot be sold live, taken to common pastures or to shows, thus restricting spread. (2) Selective culling: the economic losses caused by OPP may not be sufficient to justify removal of all infected sheep. (3) Testing for antibodies every 6 months and culling all reactors, maintaining a closed herd and selecting replacements from seronegative ewes. This procedure is effective in eradication of OPP and maintaining an OPP free flock. Testing may be reduced to once a year, as a surveillance, following 2 negative tests. Neither an effective vaccine against OPP nor rational treatment of disease has been developed.

Barban, V., et al.: Lentiviruses are naturally resident in a latent form in long-term ovine fibroblast cultures. J. Virol., *52*:680-682, 1984.

Chauhan, H.V.S. and Singh, C.M.: The clinical pathology of maedi of sheep in India. Br. Vet. J., *126*:364-367, 1970.

Crowdry, E.V. and Marsh, H.: Comparative pathology of South African jaagsiekte and Montana progressive pneumonia of sheep. J. Exp. Med., *45*:571-585, 1927.

Cross, R.F., Smith, C.K., and Moorhead, P.D.: Vertical transmission of progressive pneumonia of sheep. AJVR, *36*:465-468, 1975.

Cutlip, R.C. and Laird, G.A.: Isolation and characterization of a virus associated with progressive pneumonia (maedi) of sheep. AJVR, *37*:1377-1382, 1976.

Cutlip, R., Lehmkuhl, H., Brogden, K., and McClurkin, A.: Vasculitis associated with ovine progressive pneumonia virus infection in sheep. Am. J. Vet. Res., *46*:61-63, 1985.

Cutlip, R., Lehmkuhl, H., Wood, R., and Brogden, K.: Arthritis associated with ovine progressive pneumonia. Am. J. Vet. Res., *46*:65-68, 1985.

Cutlip, R.C., Jackson, T.A., and Lehmkuhl, H.D.: Lesions of ovine progressive pneumonia. Interstitial pneumonitis and encephalitis. AJVR, *40*:1370-1374, 1979.

Cutlip, R.C., Jackson, T.A., and Lehmkuhl, H.D.: Diagnostic features of ovine progressive pneumonia. JAVMA, *173*:1578-1579, 1978.

Cutlip, R.C., Jackson, T.A., and Laird, G.A.: Immunodiffusion test for ovine progressive pneumonia. AJVR, *38*:1081-1084, 1977.

DeKock, G.: Are the lesions of jaagsiekte in sheep in the nature of a neoplasm? 15th Ann. Rep. Dir. Vet. Ser., S. Afr., 1929, pp. 611-641.

Eklund, C.M. and Hadlow, W.J.: Pathogenesis of slow viral diseases. JAVMA, *155*:2094-2099, 1969.

Ellis, J. and DeMartini, J.: Evidence of decreased concanavalin an induced suppressor cell activity in the peripheral blood and pulmonary lymph nodes of sheep with ovine progressive pneumonia. Vet. Immunology Immunopath., *8*:93-106, 1985.

Ellis, J. and DeMartini, J.: Immunomorphologic and morphometric changes in pulmonary lymph nodes of sheep with progressive pneumonia. Vet. Pathol., *22*:32-41, 1985.

Georgsson, G. and Palsson, P.A.: The histopathology of maedi. Vet. Pathol., *8*:63-80, 1971.

Gogolewski, R., et al.: Antigenic cross-reactivity between caprine arthritis-encephalitis, visna and progressive pneumonia viruses. Involves all virion-associated protein and glycoproteins. J. Gen. Virol., *66*:1233-1240, 1985.

Gudnadottir, M. and Palsson, P.A.: Transmission of maedi by inoculation of a virus grown in tissue culture from maedi-affected lungs. J. Infect. Dis., *117*:1-6, 1967.

Gudnadottir, M. and Palsson, P.A.: Successful transmission of visna by intrapulmonary inoculation. J. Infect. Dis. *115*:217-225, 1965.

Harter, D.II., Hsu, K.C., and Rose, H.M.: Immunofluorescence and cytochemical studies of visna virus in cell cultures. J. Virol., *1*:1265-1270, 1967.

Harter, D.H., Rosenkranz, H.S., and Rose, H.M.: Nucleic acid content of visna virus. Proc. Soc. Exp. Biol. Med., *131*:927-933, 1969.

Harter, D.H., Scholm, J., and Spiegelman, H.: Characterization of visna virus nucleic acid. Biochem. Biophys., *240*:435-441, 1971.

Huffman, E., Kirk, J., Winward, L., and Gorhman, J.: Serological prevalence of ovine progressive pneumonia in a western range flock of sheep. JAVMA, *178*:708-710, 1981.

Kimberling, R.: Problems of long incubation viral diseases and their eradication. In *Sheep Production*. Proceedings 35th Easter School in Agricultural Science. In *Sheep Production*. Edited by W. Haresign. London, Butterworths, 1983, pp. 299-316.

Malmquist, W.A., Krauss, H.H., Moulton, J.E., and Wandera, J.G.: Morphologic study of virus-infected lung cell cultures from sheep pulmonary adenomatosis. Lab. Invest., *26*:528-533, 1972.

Marsh, H.: Progressive pneumonia in sheep. JAVMA, *62*:458-473, 1932.

Oliver, R., Gorham, J., Perryman, L., and Spencer, G.: Ovine progressive pneumonia: Experimental intrathoracic, intracerebral, and intraarticular infections. Am. J. Vet. Res., *42*:1560-1564, 1981.

Oliver, R., et al.: Ovine progressive pneumonia: Pathologic and virologic studies on the natural occurring disease. Am. J. Vet. Res., *42*:1554-1559, 1981.

Pautrat, G., Tamalet, J., Chippaux-Hyppolite, C., and Brahic, M.: Electron microscopic study of the structure of visna virus. C.R. Hebdo. Acad. Sci., *273D*:653-655, 1971.

Perk, K.: Slow virus infections of ovine lung. Advances in Vet. Sci. Comp. Med., *26*:267-287, 1982.

Perk, K., Irving, S., Yaniv, A., and Gazit, A.: Appearance of ovine progressive pneumonia virus outside the United States. Am. J. Vet. Res., *46*:2133-2135, 1985.

Querat, G., et al.: Highly lytic and persistent lentiviruses naturally present in sheep with progressive pneumonia are genetically distinct. J. Virology, *52*:672-679, 1984.

Ressang, A.A., Stam, F.C., and DeBoer, G.F.: A mengoleucoencephalomyelitis resembling visna in Dutch Zuoeger sheep. Pathol. Vet., *3*:401-411, 1966.

Schipper, I., Light, M., and Ludeman, L.: Control of ovine progressive pneumonia. North Dakota Farm Research, *43*:30-31, 1984.

Schipper, I., et al.: Ovine progressive pneumonia infection via the oral route. VM/SAC, 415-417, 1983.

Sigurdsson, B., Palsson, P.A., and Grimsson, H.: Visna, a demyelinating transmissible disease of sheep. J. Neuropath. Exp. Neurol., *16*:389-403, 1957.

Sigurdsson, B., Palsson, P.A., and Van Bogaert, L.: Pathology of visna. Acta Neuropath., *1*:343-362, 1962.

Sigurdsson, B., Thomar, H., and Palsson, P.A.: Cultivation of visna virus in tissue culture. Arch. Gesamte Virusforsch., *10*:368-381, 1961.

Sihvonen, K.: Late immune responses in experimental maedi. Vet. Microbiol., *9*:205-213, 1984.

Stevenson, R. and Boufford, A.: Chronic viral respiratory diseases of sheep. Can. Vet. J., *25*:34-37, 1984.

Stone, L.B., Takemoto, K.K., and Martin, M.A.: Physical and biochemical properties of progressive pneumonia virus, J. Virol., *8*:575-578, 1971.

Straub, O.C.: Isolation of maedi/visna virus (MVV) from a flock of sheep in Germany. Berl. Muench. Tieraerztl. Wochenschr., *83*:357-360, 1970.

Takemoto, K.K., et al.: Antigenic and morphological similarities of progressive pneumonia virus, a recently isolated "slow virus" of sheep, to visna and maedi virus. J. Virol., *7*:301-308, 1971.

Thormar, H.: A comparison of visna and maedi viruses. I. Physical, chemical and biological properties. Res. Vet. Sci., *6*:117-129, 1965a.

Thormar, H.: Stability of visna virus in infectious tissue culture fluid. Arch. Gesamte Virusforsch., *10*:501-509, 1961.

Thormar, H. and Cruickshank, J.G.: The structure of visna virus studied by the negative staining technique. Virology, *25*:145-148, 1965.

Thormar, H. and Helgadottir, H.: A comparison of visna and maedi viruses. II. Serological relationship. Res. Vet. Sci., *6*:456-465, 1965.

Wandera, J.G.: Progressive interstitial pneumonia (maedi) of sheep in Kenya. Vet. Rec., *86*:434-438, 1970.

Weiland, F. and Behrens, H.: Progressive interstitial pneumonia (maedi) in sheep in northern Germany. DTW, *77*:373-376, 1970.

Hydrocyanic Acid Poisoning

(*Prussic acid poisoning; cyanide poisoning*)

Hydrocyanic acid poisoning, an acute cellular asphyxiation, is characterized by sudden deaths and is caused by hydrogen cyanide (HCN) released from certain species of ingested plants. Even though the disease has wide geographic distribution, its sporadic occurrence and low incidence give it little significance in the economy of the sheep industry. Individual enterprises, however, may encounter high incidence and financial waste. Economic losses result from deaths and incomplete use of affected pastures and ranges. Development of the disease in cattle also adds economic importance to the malady.

OCCURRENCE. Cyanide poisoning occurs in all breeds, sexes, and ages of grazing sheep. Animals on natural range encounter more cyanogenic plants and therefore develop higher incidence of poisoning than do sheep on cultivated pasture. The disease develops during droughty summers and frosty autumns because these climatic adversities alter plant metabolism towards the production of cyanogenic glycosides. It also occurs in transported sheep because the associated fasting enhances susceptibility to feeds, such as linseed meal, that contain small and usually harmless amounts of cyanogenic glycosides.

Geographically, cyanide poisoning occurs among sheep of most countries where animal agriculture has developed, as Table 13-2 indicates.

ETIOLOGY AND PATHOGENESIS. Over 1000 plant species contain cyanogenic glycosides. Table 13-2 presents eight culpable species (Figs. 13-9, 13-10, 13-11). The content of cyanogenic glycosides in plants is especially high under conditions of plant wilting, retarded growth, drought damage, and frost injury. The quick intake by fed sheep of the equivalent of 2 to 4 mg HCN/kg of body weight is usually lethal. The lethal dose, however, for fasted sheep may be lower.

Following ingestion of innocuous cyanogenic glycoside, ruminal microorganisms, by enzymatic action, hydrolyze the glycoside and thereby release deadly HCN, which is absorbed into the blood and transported to vital cells. The cyanide ion produces cellular anoxia by inactivating the cytochrome oxidase enzyme that is essential to cell respiration. A lethal dose of HCN rapidly incapacitates and kills vital neurons of the central nervous system, and these changes cause respiratory failure and death. Cyanide is usually rapidly detoxified in the liver and kidney by the enzyme rhodanase that catalyzes the conversion of cyanide to thiocyanate. Thiocyanate is relatively innocuous and is excreted in the urine. Cyanide poisoning will only occur therefore when the quantity of cyanide absorbed exceeds the detoxifying capabilities of the liver and kidneys. Because of rapid detoxifica-

Fig. 13-9. Arrowgrass, *Triglochin maritima.* × 0.2.

tion, the slow consumption and absorption of doses in excess of 4 mg/kg of body weight may not kill the consuming animal. Further-

TABLE 13-2. *Cyanogenic Plants*

Names		Potential HCN (mg/100 g Plant)	Geographic Locations
Scientific	Common		
Bahia oppositifolia	bahia	30	U.S.: high plains
Linum usitatissimum	flax (linseed meal)	60	universal
Prunus virginiana	chokecherry	200	U.S.
Prunus serotina	wild black cherry	200	U.S.: east Canada: east
Suckleya suckleyana	suckleya	240	U.S.: high plains
Sorghum vulgare	sorghum	340	universal
Sorghum halpense	Johnson grass	340	universal
Triglochin maritima	arrowgrass	600	U.S.; Canada

more, HCN in the blood readily combines with methemoglobin to form stable and harmless cyanmethemoglobin.

CLINICAL SIGNS AND POSTMORTEM LESIONS. Cyanides and HCN act rapidly on cells, and lethal doses may cause death within 1 to 60 minutes. Sheep affected with large doses have convulsions, pass into coma, and quickly die, but animals receiving the minimal lethal dose salivate, become excited, and often bloat. Muscle groups, including those of the eyes and limbs, twitch and spastically contract and cause the animal to stagger and fall in opisthotonos. Terminally, animals exhibit open-mouthed, gasping respirations, and die from anoxia. The blood of cyanide victims remains bright red in color despite severe respiratory distress.

At necropsy, the blood retains a bright red color, and the ruminal ingesta emits a characteristic almond odor. Petechial hemorrhages on epicardium and other serosal membranes

Fig. 13-10. Western chokecherry, *Prunus virginiana.*

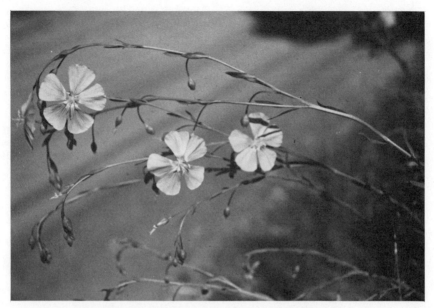

Fig. 13-11.   Blue flax, *Linum usitatissimum*

may be discernible. Fragments of cyanogenic plants are identifiable in the rumen.

DIAGNOSIS. Veterinarians diagnose cyanide poisoning on evidence of typical signs and positive results from chemical tests. Sudden deaths among sheep with access to known cyanogenic plants are highly suggestive. Finding 1.4 and 10 μg of hydrocyanic acid/g of liver and ruminal contents, respectively, confirms the diagnosis; lesser amounts may occur in sheep killed by other causes. If testing is delayed a day or longer, the materials for tests should be stored in 1% aqueous solution of mercuric chloride to avoid dissipation of the HCN.

The picrate paper test for identifying HCN is useful under field conditions. In practice, strips of filter paper are dipped in an aqueous solution containing 5% sodium carbonate and 0.5% picric acid. The paper is suspended over shredded leaves, ruminal content, or minced liver containing a few drops of chloroform or dilute acetic acid and incubated for 30 to 60 minutes at 30 to 35°C. The formation of a maroon color on the paper constitutes a positive reaction, and the amount of coloring quantitatively correlates with the amount of HCN present. The differential diagnosis re-

quires consideration of other causes of quick death, such as arsenic poisoning, lightning strike, oxalate poisoning, bloat, and clostridium perfringens enterotoxemia.

PREVENTION AND TREATMENT. Producers prevent cyanide poisoning by grazing sheep on ranges and pastures free of heavy infestations with cyanogenic plants. If the use of infested range is unavoidable, supplementary feed should be provided. After fasting during prolonged periods of shipment, sheep should not receive feed, such as linseed meal, known to contain small and usually safe amounts of HCN.

Treatment consists of converting the cyanide ion in the blood to an insoluble and excretable salt. This can be achieved by intravenously administering 22 mg/kg sodium nitrite and 660 mg/kg sodium thiosulfate. The nitrite converts hemoglobin to methemoglobin. Methemoglobin, having a greater affinity for cyanide than cytochrome oxidase, splits off and binds the cyanide in the form of an active cyanomethemoglobin. Sodium thiosulfate then binds with the cyanide to form excretable thiocyanate. The administration of cobaltous chloride and vitamin B_{12} may also be beneficial in early cases of cyanide intoxication.

Briese, R.R. and Couch, J.F.: Hydrocyanide in sorghum silage. Vet. Med., *35*:86-88, 1940.

Bunyea, H.: Treatments for HCN poisoning in sheep and cattle. JAVMA, *86*:656-661, 1935.

Burrows, G.E. and Way, J.L.: Cyanide intoxication: Enhancement of efficacy of sodium nitrite, sodium thiosulfate and cobaltous chloride. AJVR, *40*:613-617, 1979.

Cheeke, P.R.: Cyanogens. In *Natural Toxicants in Feeds and Poisonous Plants.* Edited by P.R. Cheeke. Connecticut, AVI Publishing Company, Inc., 1985, pp. 173-186.

Franklin, M.C. and MacGregory, C.H.: Cause of death among Merino rams after long journey by rail. Aust. Vet. J., *20*:328-331, 1944.

Franklin, M.C. and Reid, R.L.: Cyanogenic linseed nuts. I. Feeding trials with sheep. Aust. Vet. J., *20*:332-337, 1944.

Moran, E.A.: Cyanogenic compounds in plants and their significance. AJVR, *15*:171, 1954.

Muenscher, W.C.: *Poisonous Plants of the United States.* New York, The Macmillan Co., 1949, p. 109.

Thorp, F. and Deem, A.W.: *Suckleya suckleyana,* a poisonous plant. JAVMA, *94*:192-197, 1939.

Van der Walt, S.J.: Toxicology of hydrocyanic acid in ruminants. Onderstepoort J. Vet. Sci., *19*:79-153, 1944.

14

DISEASES OF THE SKIN

Sheep Pox

(*Variola ovina; clavelee; pockenseuche*)

Sheep pox, an acute, contagious, and often fatal disease, is characterized by generalized papules on the skin and plaques on mucous membranes and is caused by a virus. Because of its wide though not universal distribution and high incidence, sheep pox causes extensive commercial damage to the sheep industry. Economic losses result from high mortality, reduced yields of meat, milk, and wool, commercial inhibitions from quarantine, and the cost of repetitive disease-prevention programs. Additional losses come to sheep-dependent people from protein-deficient diets and, consequently, increased human suffering and reduced human productivity, and from the common practice in some countries of eating infected and sometimes moribund animals.

OCCURRENCE. Sheep pox occurs in all breeds, sexes, and ages of sheep, but the fine-wooled breeds, such as Merinos, are more susceptible than the coarse-wooled breeds, especially those that are native to endemic areas. Lambs suffer a higher disease incidence and often more severe lesions than do mature animals. Under natural conditions, no other species of animals, including goats, develop sheep pox.

A biseasonal disease, sheep pox commonly prevails in certain periods of both winter and summer. During December, January, and February, the severe form of the disease occurs, often with considerable mortality. Inclement wet weather exacerbates the disease. The mild form, with lower incidence, occurs during late spring and summer.

Geographically, sheep pox is widespread in Morocco, Algeria, Libya, Ethiopia, Turkey, Syria, Lebanon, Iraq, Iran, India, and Afghanistan, and less common but still troublesome in Tunisia, Sudan, Kenya, Tanzania, Portugal, USSR, Israel, Jordan, Saudi Arabia, and West Pakistan.

ETIOLOGY AND PATHOGENESIS. The sheep pox virus, a member of the DNA family Poxviridae, produces disease in sheep only. The brick-shaped virion measures approximately $300 \times 200 \times 100$ nm and contains an outer membrane of tube-shaped lipoprotein that encloses a core. The core contains double-stranded DNA and protein. Replicating in the cytoplasm, the virus produces cytoplasmic inclusion bodies.

The virion contains several antigens. Some are shared by other members of the same subgroup and one by the poxvirus group. Sheep pox, goat pox and contagious pustular dermatitis viruses share proteins having common charges and considerable antigenic cross-reactivity. The virus has been adapted to growth in the chorioallantoic membrane of embryonating chicken eggs and cell cultures from embryonic sheep lungs, sheep thyroid, sheep testes, and lamb kidneys. In sheep affected with pox, the virus is located in the blood during early stages of the disease, in lymph and cells of infected skin, and in lymph nodes, spleen, kidneys, and lungs. The virus retains viability in wool for 2 months, in open sheep pens for 6 months, and in protected areas for longer periods. ·

Experimentally, sheep inoculated intradermally with goat pox virus do not show any reaction, but are immune to sheep pox virus when challenged after 21 days. Similarly, goats inoculated with sheep pox virus are immune to goat pox virus, although goats show local and thermal reactions to inoculation.

Transmission probably occurs through inhalation but also takes place, in some cases, through skin abrasions. Infected droplets are sprayed into the air by coughing of infected sheep. Inhalation of virus-contaminated droplets and dust by susceptible sheep inoculates the respiratory system, and the deposit of airborne virus, contaminated saliva, or nasal secretion on susceptible skin may result in the penetration of tissues. In some instances, inoculation through the oral mucosa may occur, but not throughout the entire alimentary system.

Veterinarians have studied some aspects of sheep pox by inoculating the causative virus into the skin of susceptible sheep and then following the progress of the disease. After inoculation, the virus probably enters the regional lymph nodes and, in the reticuloendothelial cells, replicates and discharges through efferent lymphatics into the blood. Viremia develops within 3 to 4 days after inoculation and persists through the eighth day; the maximal concentration occurs on the fifth day.

Infected blood transports virus to all tissues and organs, and by the eighth day, the virus settles in lymph nodes, spleen, kidneys, lungs, and skin. Papules develop in skin, especially of the face, eyelids, nostrils, perineum, prepuce, and other nonwooled surfaces, and plaques form in mucosal surfaces of nose, trachea, mouth, pharynx, larynx, esophagus, forestomachs, and abomasum. After intradermal inoculation, and in some animals after a short eclipse phase, the concentration of virus logarithmically increases to a peak titer of 10^7

TCD_{50} per gram of tissue during days 7 to 12 and then decreases to approximately 10^5 TCD_{50} per gram of tissue by day 20.

A febrile reaction persists through the fifth to eighth days and is followed by the development of complement-fixing and neutralizing antibodies. Approximately one third of inoculated sheep develop lung lesions, which become visible on day 5 and begin to regress on day 16. Deaths result from severe generalized dermatitis and mucositis. Virus discharges to the external environment through nasal secretions, dermal lesion excretions, milk, and possibly urine.

CLINICAL SIGNS AND POSTMORTEM LESIONS. After an incubation period of 6 to 8 days, body temperature rises to 41 to 42°C and dermal eruption occurs. Physical depression and weakness develop and appetite wanes. Because of swelling of nostrils and nasal mucosa, breathing may become difficult and noisy. After 1 to 2 days of fever, circular hyperemic maculae form on swollen eyelids, nostrils, lips, cheeks, perineum, prepuce, and udder, and on some animals, over the neck, thorax, and abdomen. Each round macula measures from 1 to 3 cm in diameter, and closely placed lesions become confluent. Within 1 day, the maculae progress into papules, which are firm, flat, circular masses elevated 2 to 3 mm above the normal skin.

Small amounts of serum exude from the tissue and, after several days, a delicate layer of tissue readily detaches from the surface. After an additional few days, the flat surface umbilicates and undergoes necrosis. Eventually a firm, dry scab forms and detaches, leaving a glistening, denuded scar. Papules in the eye may lead to keratitis and those in the coronary band to lameness. In severe reactions, hemorrhage may occur in the tissue and impart a dark color to the papule. Typical cases of sheep pox do not develop vesicles. The oral mucosa may form elevated plaques, resembling papules, on the tongue, hard palate, and buccal surface. Pregnant ewes may abort.

The average course of sheep pox is 3 to 4 weeks, but the flock may retain infection 6 to 8 weeks or longer. Morbidity may reach 70%, and mortality of infected sheep may be 5 to 50%.

At necropsy, most lesions are in the skin and mucous membranes of the alimentary system. Numerically concentrated in skin of the face, perineum, prepuce, and scrotum, papules in fatal cases may also extend over skin of the neck, thorax, abdomen, and feet. During early stages of development, a small amount of lymph exudes from the papules; the moistness results in matting of wool or hair. Internally, the mucous membranes of the nasal cavity, larynx, trachea, mouth, forestomachs, and abomasum may contain plaques that are circular or oval in outline and elevated 1 to 2 mm from the surrounding surface; surface ulceration may have occurred.

Histopathologic changes occur in both the derma and epidermis of papules. Early dermal changes are edema and accumulation of neutrophils and histiocytes. In lesions a few days old, the histiocytes contain enlarged vacuolated nuclei and cytoplasm with inclusion bodies. In papules 7 to 10 days old, the capillaries are thrombosed. Simultaneous epidermal changes are hyperplasia and limited hydropic degeneration in the spinose layer of the epithelium.

As a result of thrombosis of capillaries, the overlying epidermis is necrosed and often invaded by saprophytic bacteria. Plaques in mucous membranes contain edema, lymphocytes, and mononuclear macrophages. Nodules of the lungs consist of increased numbers of mesenchymal cells of interalveolar septa and of alveolar epithelium transformed from squamous to cuboidal type.

DIAGNOSIS. Veterinarians diagnose sheep pox on the evidence of typical lesions and systemic reactions. In endemic areas, the presence of papules on skin of the face, perineum and, in some animals, neck, thorax, and abdomen suggests sheep pox. In the laboratory, the clinical diagnosis can be confirmed by: (1) isolating sheep pox virus from blood or from lymph of papules, (2) finding characteristic histiopathologic changes in papules, and (3) demonstrating in serially collected blood samples an ascending titer of complement-fixing or virus-neutralizing antibodies.

The differential diagnosis requires consideration of contagious ecthyma and ulcerative dermatosis.

PREVENTION AND TREATMENT. Veterinarians and producers prevent sheep pox by methods appropriate to the circumstance of the disease outbreak. In endemic areas, sheep are protected by annual vaccination. Either of the three following products, when applied as recommended, gives effective immunity for approximately 1 year: (1) virus adsorbed on aluminum gel and inactivated with 0.01% formaldehyde or thimerosol (Merthiolate), (2) a mixture of attenuated anthrax spores and avianized sheep pox virus, or (3) vaccine attenuated in tissue culture.

In addition, all dead sheep and contaminated feed and manure should be incinerated, and after cleaning, the premises and equipment should be disinfected with 2% lye solution. In outbreaks of sheep pox in areas otherwise free of the disease, the infection may be eradicated by quarantining the area, destroying diseased and exposed sheep, cleaning and disinfecting premises, and resting the premises until test sheep placed in the quarantined area do not contract the disease.

Treatment consists of both vaccination and medication. During early stages of an outbreak, vaccination benefits the flock by immunizing and thus protecting uninfected sheep. Ointments containing antibiotics provide some comfort to infected animals by softening dried papules and skin and by controlling bacterial infection of papules.

Abdussalam, M.: Elementary bodies of sheep pox. AJVR, *18*:614-617, 1957.
Animal Health Yearbook. FAO-WHO-OIE (Italy), 1970.
Borisovich, Y.F.: Immunological properties of dried chick embryo virus vaccine against sheep pox. Tr. Nauchkontrol Inst. Vet. Prepar., *10*:105-109, 1962.
Borisovich, Y.F., Koval, G.L., Bagmet, L.G., and Palgov, A.A.: Chick-embryo sheep pox vaccine. Tr. Nauchkontrol Inst. Vet. Prepar., *13*:29-33, 1966.
Heintl, 1822, quoted from Hutyra, F., Marek, J., and Manninger, R.: *Special Pathology and Therapeutics of Diseases of Domestic Animals.* Vol. I. Chicago, Alexander Eger, 1938, p. 353.

288 DISEASES OF ADULT SHEEP

388 DISEASES OF ADULT SHEEP

Likhachev, N.V., Kolesov, S.G., Borisovich, Y.F., and Presnov, I.N.: Combined vaccine against anthrax and sheep pox. Tr. Gosudarst Nauch-kontrol Inst. Vet. Prepar., *14*:35-45, 1967.

Likhachev, N.V., Sakalinskii, E.I., Formenko, A.S., and Pimburgskaya, N.A.: Some studies on pathogenesis of sheep pox. Tr. Nauch-kontrol Inst. Vet. Prepar., *12*:9-12, 1964.

Murray, M., Martin, W.B., and Korylu, A.: Experimental sheep pox: A histological and ultrastructural study. Res. Vet. Sci., *15*:201-208, 1973.

Nitzschke, E., Buckley, L.S., and Ergin, H.: Isolation and titration of sheep and goat pox viruses in sheep thyroid cell cultures. Vet. Rec., *18*:216-217, 1967.

Pandey, A.K., Malik, B.S., and Bansal, M.P.: Studies on sheep pox virus. I. Adaptation and propagation of the virus in cell cultures. Indian Vet. J., *46*:925-929, 1969.

Penkova, V.M., Jassium, F.A., Thompson, J.R., and Al-Doori, T.M.: The propagation of an attenuated sheep pox virus and its use as a vaccine. Bull. Off. Int. Epizoot., *81*:329-339, 1974.

Plowright, W. and Ferris, R.D.: Growth and cytopathogenicity of sheep pox virus in tissue culture. Br. J. Exp. Path., *39*:424-435, 1958.

Plowright, W., MacLeod, W.G., and Ferris, R.D.: The pathogenesis of sheep pox in the skin of sheep. J. Comp. Pathol., *69*:400-412, 1959.

Rafyi, A. and Chamsy, M.: Seven years control of sheep pox in Iran with an adsorbed tissue vaccine on aluminum gel. Br. Vet. J., *112*:541-547, 1956.

Ramachandran, S.: Observations on the histopathology of lung lesions in experimental pox infection in sheep and goats. Ceylon Vet J., *15*:78-82, 1967.

Ramyar, H. and Baharsefat, M.: A new approach to active immunization of sheep by a combination of sheep pox and anthrax vaccine. Zentralbl. Veterinaermed., *16B*:585-592, 1969.

Sabban, M.S.: Sheep pox and its control in Egypt using a dessicated live virus vaccine. AJVR, *16*:209-213, 1955.

Salmuth, 1804, quoted from Hutyra, F., Marek, J., and Manninger, R.: Special Pathology and Therapeutics of Diseases of Domestic Animals. Vol. I. Chicago, Alexander Eger, 1938, p. 353.

Sharma, S.N. and Dhanda, M.R.: Studies on the interrelationship between sheep and goat pox viruses. Indian J. Anim. Sci., *41*:267-272, 1971.

Subba, M., Malik, B., and Sharma, S.: Antigenic relationships among sheep pox, goat pox and contagious pustular dermatitis viruses. Acta. Virol., *28*:380-387, 1984.

Trotsenko, N.I.: Multiplication of sheep pox virus in cultured tissues. Tr. Nauch-kontrol Inst. Vet. Prepar., *9*:17-23, 1961.

Vegad, J.L. and Sharman, G.L.: Cutaneous and pulmonary lesions of sheep-pox. Indian J. Anim. Sci., *43*:1061-1067, 1973.

Papillomatosis

(*Warts; fibropapillomatosis*)

Papillomatosis, a benign surface proliferation, is characterized by multiple digitations, especially on the skin of face and legs, and is caused by a virus. Because of low incidence, the disease is of little concern to the sheep industry. It may result, however, in economic losses to some enterprises by partially incapacitating affected animals and by disqualifying them for public exhibitions and sales.

This uncommon disease attacks sheep of all sexes, all breeds, all ages between 1 and 5 years, and probably of all countries, including the United States and Britain. In comparison to other sheep producing countries, Australia reports a higher prevalence of ovine squamous cell carcinomas, especially on the unwooled areas of the muzzle and ears. These squamous cell carcinomas arise from sites of papillomas and histologically it appears that the papillomatous changes precede carcinogenesis. Similar maladies affect goats, cattle, horses, and people, but transfer between animal species probably does not occur.

A virus of the DNA family Papovaviridae causes papillomatosis. The papilloma virus genome is a double-stranded, covalently closed circular DNA molecule. Virion protein and polypeptides allow identification into types. The ovine papilloma virus has not been subtyped. Although the viral etiology of papillomatosis is established, the transformation of papillomas to carcinoma appears to involve not only virus, but other extensive factors, such as genetic background or environmental factors. The multifactorial carcinogenesis is suspected in areas of Australia where facial and aural lesions are more prevalent. It is possible that ovine facial and aural carcinomas have a complex etiology involving unpigmented skin, exposure to sunlight, and infection with papilloma virus. It probably is transmitted by direct or indirect contact, and cutaneous abrasions and lacerations may facilitate virus inoculation and growth. Secondary bacterial infections following trauma exacerbate the host effects. Individual papillomas, when first observed, measure 1 to 4 cm in diameter and 0.5 to 2 cm in height. Each has multiple spines that project from the surface. They are located on the hairy skin of limbs, ears, and face, but the papillomas usually are hairless (Fig. 14-1).

When located at critical anatomic areas and especially if traumatized and secondarily infected, the lesions adversely affect the animal: those over joints cause lameness, those on lips inhibit prehension, those near nostrils obstruct airways, and those on eyelids block vision. The incidence is low, and the course may be up to several months. The papilloma virus of sheep induces not only a cutaneous papilloma, but, in addition, an underlying fibroma of connective tissue (fibropapilloma). Papilloma virus infection of epithelial cells results in hyperplasia of cells in the spinous layer (acanthosis). The affected cells show an increase in size

Fig. 14-1. Limb of a yearling sheep with three papillomas (a). These lesions caused lameness. The same animal had facial papillomas.

and number of desmosomes and tonofibrils, whereas other epithelial cells show degenerative changes with loss of tonofibrils, detachment of desmosomes, focal nuclear atypia, and cytoplasmic vacuolization. The granular layer is characterized by evidence of nuclear degeneration with margination and condensation of chromatin. The virions appear in crystalline array in nuclei of degenerated cells in the keratinizing layer. Clinical diagnosis is achieved by identifying the papillomas at their predilection sites. Histologic examination, if necessary, can be conducted on excised tumors fixed in 10% formalin or Bouin's fixative. The differential diagnosis requires consideration of contagious ecthyma, ulcerative dermatosis, sheep pox, and strawberry foot rot.

TREATMENT.   Commercial vaccines are not available for sheep and the low incidence or economic feasibility usually does not warrant preparation of autogenous vaccines. Wart maceration and cryosurgical wart destruction have been utilized in cattle to hasten wart resolution, although documentation of success is lacking. Surgical excision may be followed by cure or, in some cases, by recurrence. Application of topical antibiotic ointments will aid in preventing secondary bacterial infections.

Gibbs, E.P.J., Smale, C.J., and Lawman, M.J.P.: Warts in sheep. J. Comp. Pathol., *85*:327, 1975.
Hunt, E.: Bovine neoplastic skin diseases. In *Current Veterinary Therapy*. Edited by J. Howard. Philadelphia, W.B. Saunders Co., 1986, 936-937.
Lancaster, W. and Olson, C.: Animal papilloma viruses. Microbiol Rev., *46*:191-207, 1982.
Vanselow, B. and Spradbrow, P.: Papilloma viruses, papillomas and squamous cell carcinomas in sheep. Vet. Rec., *110*:561-562, 1982.
Vanselow, B. and Spradbrow, P.: Squamous cell carcinoma of the vulva, hyperkeratosis and papilloma virus in a ewe. Aust. Vet. J., *60*:194-195, 1983.

Swelled Head

(*Big head*)

An acute infectious but noncontagious toxemia of young rams, swelled head is characterized by inflammatory edema of the head and neck, rapid development, and short course and is caused by anaerobic bacteria that commonly live on skin and in soil. Because swelled head has low incidence and limited geographic distribution, the disease is of little economic importance to the general sheep industry, but in some individual enterprises it may cause serious financial waste. Economic loss may result from deaths among high-quality and expensive rams and from the cost of disposal of dead animals and preventive programs. The industry, however, has not precisely measured the losses.

OCCURRENCE. Swelled head occurs exclusively in rams 1 to 2 years of age. Although all breeds are susceptible, the disease more commonly develops in the belligerent horned breeds. Animals exposed to high concentrations of spores, such as may occur in habitually used corrals and small pastures, may also suffer a high incidence. Even though swelled head can develop during any season, most cases occur during summer and early autumn when fighting is common. The geographic distribution includes Australia, South Africa, and Montana of the United States. Since fighting among rams is universal and the bacteria are widely distributed, the disease probably has a broader geographic range than scientific reports indicate.

ETIOLOGY AND PATHOGENESIS. *Clostridium novyi,* the usual cause of swelled head, lives in soil, on skin surfaces, and in alimentary tracts of sheep and cattle. This anaerobic, gram-positive, spore-bearing and motile bacterium measures 0.8 to 1.5 × 5 to 10 μm. With rounded ends and parallel sides, the bacilli occur singly, in pairs, and in filaments. They readily grow in media, form subterminal spores, and ferment glucose and maltose, but not lactose, sucrose, or salicin, and liquefy gelatin but not serum. Their resistance to germicidal factors simulates that of other species of *Clostridia*. On the basis of toxin-antitoxin neutralization tests, *C. novyi* is divided into four types: A, B, C, and D. The species produces six exotoxins.

Only a modicum of research has been conducted on swelled head; consequently, the hypothesis for pathogenesis is conjectural. Spores of the causative bacterium, *C. novyi,* commonly reside in soil of sheep corrals, pas-

tures, and ranges, and from the soil they are easily and mechanically transferred to the skin surfaces of the rams' heads where, under normal conditions, the organisms are innocuous.

As the breeding season approaches, young aggressive rams fight and, in the process, lacerate and contuse the skin and other soft tissues around the horns. The bacterial spores may be forced into the lacerations. Crusts develop over the injuries and exclude atmospheric oxygen. Under anaerobic conditions, the spores germinate, and the resulting vegetative cells multiply and produce toxin, but the bacteria tend to remain localized in and around the inoculation area.

Diffusing into soft tissues over the face and neck, the toxin increases the permeability of blood capillaries. Protein molecules pass through the capillary walls into the tissue, where the osmolarity is elevated sufficiently to force water from the plasma into the tissues. The resulting edematous fluid, clear or pale yellow, swells the skin and other soft tissues. Diffusion and gravity move the fluid and the toxin ventrally along the throat and neck. Swelling of the eyelids obstructs vision, and swelling of the nasal membranes and skin interferes with breathing.

Toxemia and shock are the probable causes of death. Although pure infections with *C. novyi* produce a clear edematous fluid, mixed infections may cause hemorrhage and hemolysis with discoloration of the fluid. Through decomposing tissues, the pathogenic *C. novyi* return to the exterior, sporulate, and re-enter the soil.

CLINICAL SIGNS AND POSTMORTEM LESIONS. In rams with swelled head, the body temperature rises to a range from 41 to 43°C. Affected animals separate from the flock and prefer the reclining position. Edema of the subcutaneous and muscular tissues of the head, throat, and neck rapidly develops, and drops of fluid may exude from the swollen skin. Swollen eyelids may be forcibly closed. Partial closure of the external nares and nasal meatuses may result in noisy, difficult, and rapid breathing. Because of physical weakness and discomfort, affected rams decline feed. Death comes after a disease course of 48 to 72 hours. The incidence usually involves 2 to 4% of the ram flock, but may go as high as 15%. Most affected animals die.

At necropsy, the prominent changes are seen in soft tissue of the head and neck. Lacerations in skin around the horns may be discernible. The skin of the ears and the mucous membranes of the mouth usually remain normal, but the subcutis and intermuscular septa of the face, throat, and neck usually contain a large amount of clear, edematous fluid.

Mixed infection may add hemoglobin and opaque exudate to the fluid. Fluid may also accumulate in the thoracic cavity and pericardial sac and in the lungs. Petechial hemorrhages in the subendocardial and subepicardial tissues are common. Histopathologically, the effect of fluid is evident. Around the lacerated and inoculated tissue, bacteria and leukocytes can be found.

DIAGNOSIS. Veterinarians diagnose swelled head on the basis of typical signs and lesions. Rapidly developing edema of the face, throat, and neck among rams strongly indicates this disease, and finding clear edematous fluid in the swollen tissue and the skin lacerations further substantiates the diagnosis. In the laboratory, *C. novyi* and related organisms, such as *C. sordelli* and *C. perfringens,* may be isolated from tissues near the lacerations.

The differential diagnosis requires consideration of photosensitization, blackleg, malignant edema, and bites from venomous animals. Photosensitization results in edematous swelling of the head, but the disease occurs in all sexes and individuals having nonpigmented skin. Blackleg occurs in both sexes and usually follows wounds from shearing, vaccinating, docking, castrating, and parturition. Characteristic muscle lesions are present, and the fluid usually is colored with hemoglobin. *C. chauvoei* can be isolated. Malignant edema, an acute focal infection around a wound, contains gas, blood-stained fluid, and necrotic tissue. *C. chauvoei* and *C. septicum* may be isolated. Venomous bites usually involve a single sheep and may be in either sex. The ac-

cumulated fluid contains hemoglobin or extravasated blood.

PREVENTION AND TREATMENT. Veterinarians and owners can protect rams against swelled head by immunization and management. The use of vaccine containing antigens of *C. novyi* significantly reduces the incidence of the disease. For the most effective results, the vaccine should be administered at least 6 weeks before the fighting season begins. During the time of anticipated disease outbreaks, the young rams should be excluded from corrals and other facilities known or suspected to be heavily seeded with *C. novyi.*

Infected rams should receive treatment during early stages of the disease. To provide comfort and promote recovery, affected animals should receive daily intramuscular injections of tetracycline antibiotic at the rate of 11 mg/kg and should quietly rest in a dark stall where cool water and appetizing feed are available.

Bull, L.B.: "Swell head" or "big head" in rams due to localized infection by *Clostridium oedematiens*. Serous, non-gaseous malignant edema of the head of rams. J. Comp. Pathol. Ther., *48*:21-35, 1935.
DeKock, G.: Swelled head, big-head or dikkopsiekte in rams. J. S. Afr. Vet. Med. Assoc., *1*:39, 1928.
Marsh, H., Welch, H., and Jungherr, E.: Blackleg in sheep. JAVMA, *27*:63-88, 1928.
Smith, L.D.S., Safford, J.W., and Hawkins, W.W.: *Clostridium sordellii,* infection in sheep. Cornell Vet., *52*:62-68, 1962.

Dermatophilosis

Dermatophilosis, a chronic exudative skin infection, is characterized by focal or general crusting and is caused by a species of filamentous bacteria. In sheep, the disease has two clinical forms: (1) lumpy wool and (2) strawberry foot rot. It has minor importance to the sheep industry in North America because of infrequent occurrence, but greater importance in Africa, Europe, and Australia because of common occurrence. A major economic impact to the Australian sheep industry is not only from reduced fleece and pelt values, but the major economic cost is that the lesions attract blow fly *Lucilia cuprina* to oviposit with subsequent cutaneous myiasis. A large increment from homologous caprine and bovine diseases enhances the economic importance of the general malady.

ETIOLOGY AND PATHOGENESIS. *D. congolensis* is a gram-positive, non-acid-fast, facultative anaerobic actinomycete in the genus *Dermatophilus,* family *Dermatophileaceae,* and order *Actinomycetales*. The natural habitat of *D. congolensis* is unknown, it possibly has a saprophytic existence in soil but isolations have only been made from the integument of various animals and man. *D. congolensis* has the capability of existing in quiescent form until climatic and microenvironmental factors are favorable for its infectivity. The reservoir of infection probably is chronically infected inapparent carrier animals as a free living state of *D. congolensis* is not known.

D. congolensis has two distinct morphologic forms, filamentous hyphae and motile zoospores. The filamentous hyphae develop through the germination of zoospores with branching filaments which fragment by transverse and longitudinal division into clusters of coccoid cells. The coccoid cells dissociate into multi-flagellated motile zoospores. *D. congolensis* completes its life cycle in the living layers of the epidermis. Its reproduction and spread is influenced by carbon dioxide tension of the tissues and lesions.

Natural resistance to *D. congolensis* infection is provided by the outer layers of the stratum corneum. The sebaceous lipids add a physical protective covering, while phagocytosis of the infective zoospores by neutrophils completes the host defense mechanisms. The dry wool coat itself provides a form of protection. Infection is established by damage or disruption of this protective barrier by injury such as shearing, external parasites, and prolonged wetness. The fine wool breeds, especially young Merino sheep, are highly susceptible. Once the defense barrier is disrupted the zoospores penetrate the stratum corneum, germinate to produce hyphae, which penetrate into the living epidermis inducing an acute inflammatory response with the accumulation of neutrophils, accelerated keratinization, and proliferation of the epidermis. The

hyphae continue to spread in all directions from the initial focus of infection. The invaded epidermis cornifies and separates from the dermal matrix by infiltration of granulocytes. The epithelium is cast off in the form of a scab. Hyphae continue to invade new hair follicles and epidermis resulting in additional build up of scab or crust. The entire process occurs in about 10 to 12 days. A delayed hypersensitivity and granulocytic infiltration are thought to be the factors limiting the invasion of zoospores or hyphae which results in accelerated healing of the lesion. Healing takes place without scar formation. The factors underlying the severity or chronicity of dermatophilosis in certain regions is not understood. Transmission is dependent upon the zoospores being present when the natural protective barriers of the skin are disrupted by prolonged wetting, or trauma from mechanical or biologic injuries, such as shearing or insect bites. *D. congolensis* can be transmitted directly from sheep to sheep or indirectly by vectors such as insects.

CLINICAL SIGNS AND LESIONS. 1. Lumpy wool. This disease develops during months of high rainfall and humidity. Early infections over the back and sides in adults consist of foci of erythema up to 4 cm in diameter. This stage persists for about 2 weeks. Later, pyramidal crusts and wool mats form. Still later, when healing has progressed, the crust is separated from the epidermis but may be held in position by attached wool fibers. Forcibly detached crusts leave a bleeding, inflamed surface. Lambs often develop confluent facial lesions and, if highly susceptible, generalized infection as well. The incidence in adults varies up to 15% and in lambs to nearly 100%.

Histopathologically, lesions show crusts of serum, leukocytes, necrotic epithelium, and wool. Superficial layers of epidermis are necrotic, but parts of the stratum germinativum remain viable. Swollen wool follicles contain necrotic cells, exudate, and parts of wool fibers. The derma is hyperemic, edematous, and infiltrated with leukocytes, especially lymphocytes. Hyphae of *D. congolensis* form tangled masses in follicles and lesser concentrations in crust and derma.

Dermatophilosis is usually considered a lesion confined to the living epidermis although an atypical granulomatous inflammatory lesion in the subcutaneous tissues has been reported. These differ histologically from the superficial lesions by the presence of monocytes, macrophages, epithelioid cells and giant cells rather than neutrophils.

2. Strawberry foot rot. This infection develops in animals in Britain and Australia during humid summers. All ages, especially lambs and yearlings, are susceptible. The incidence varies up to 100%. The disease develops when sheep are exposed to infected pasture, and the first signs appear after 0.5 to 3 months. Lesions consist of dry crusts 1 to 3 cm in diameter on skin between coronary bands and carpi and/or tarsi. Confluent crusts may form limb encasements. Forceful removal of the crusts exposes strawberry-like tissue. Lesions on interdigital skin and on more proximal flexion surfaces cause lameness. Recovered animals are not immune. The histopathologic features are similar to those of mycotic dermatitis.

DIAGNOSIS. Veterinarians suspect dermatophilosis because of the presence of characteristic skin lesions, and they confirm the diagnosis in a laboratory by isolating *D. congolensis* from the dermal lesions.

PREVENTION AND TREATMENT. Some cases of dermatophilosis, particularly strawberry foot rot, can be prevented by avoiding exposure of healthy sheep to infected animals and to premises recently occupied by infected sheep or goats, or by cattle affected with streptothricosis. As dermatophilosis occurs under such a wide array of management and ecologic systems, a simple preventive solution is not possible. Management and husbandry practices should be based upon preventing spread by isolation, sanitation, disinfection, and control of external parasites. Treatment consists of high doses of parenteral penicillin (5000 IU/kg) and Streptomycin (5 mg/kg) daily for a minimum of 5 days or a single intramuscular dose of long acting oxytetracycline (20 mg/kg). Experimental vaccines show some effectiveness and may be the control procedure in the future.

Austwick, P.K.C.: Cutaneous streptothricosis, mycotic dermatitis and strawberry footrot and the genus *Dermatophilus*. Vet. Rev. Annot., *4*:44-48, 1958.

Bisset, K.A. and Thompson, R.E.M.: Note on the morphology of organism isolated from strawberry footrot. J. Pathol. Bacteriol., *72*:322, 1956.

Bull, L.B.: Dermatomycosis of sheep due to *Actinomyces dermatonomus*. Aust. J. Exp. Biol. Med. Sci., *6*:301-314, 1929.

Gherardi, S., Lewer, R., Sutherland, S., and Howe, R.: Development of an artificial infection technique for examining the susceptibility of sheep to *Dermatophilus congolensis*. Aust. Vet. J., *61*:304, 1984.

Gheradi, S., Sutherland, S., and Monzu, N.: "Dermo" fleece rot and body strike on sheep. J. of Agri. Western Aust., *26*(2):57-59, 1985.

Harriss, S.T.: Proliferative dermatitis of the legs in sheep. J. Comp. Pathol. Ther., *58*:314-328, 1948.

Lloyd, D.: Immunology of dermatophilosis: Recent developments and prospects for control. Preventive Vet. Med., *2*:93-102, 1984.

Momotani, E., Inui, S., Ishikawa, Y., and Azuma, R.: Granulomatous sub-dermal lesions in sheep inoculated with *Dermatophilus congolensis*. J. Comp. Path., *94*:33-34, 1984.

Oyejide, A., Makinde, A., and Ezeh, A.: Prevalence of antibodies to *Dermatophilus congolensis* in sheep and goats in Nigeria. Vet. Quart., *6*:44-45, 1984.

Scanlan, C., Garrett, P., and Geiger, D.: *Dermatophilus congolensis* infections of cattle and sheep. Compendium on continuing education for the practicing veterinarian. *6*:54-59, 1984.

Thompson, R.E.M.: *Rhizobium* isolated from strawberry footrot in sheep. J. Pathol. Bacteriol., *68*:445-452, 1954.

Van Saceghem, R.: Dermatose contagieuse. Bull. Soc. Pathol. Exot., *8*:354-359, 1915.

Photosensitization

(*Big head; swelled head*)

Photosensitization, an acute dermatitis in nonpigmented sheep, is characterized by irritation, edema, and necrosis of the ears, eyelids, lips, face, vulva, and coronets and is caused by interaction of plant-formed pigments and sunlight. Because the disease occurs throughout all sheep-producing countries often at high incidence, it causes significant financial waste and concerns the entire sheep industry. In South Africa, geeldikkop, a specific photosensitivity, annually kills thousands of sheep. In the United States, up to 1000 sheep may develop the condition in one disease episode. Losses result from deaths, prolonged illnesses, wool damage, incomplete utilization of affected range, and the cost of treatments. Sporadic occurrence of the con-

Fig. 14-2. Buckwheat *Fagopyrum esculentum*.

dition among cattle and other domestic mammals adds economic importance to the malady.

OCCURRENCE. Photosensitization occurs in all breeds, ages, and sexes of nonpigmented sheep. Toxicosis from consuming St. John's wort occurs during early summer when plant growth is rapid. American big head develops during early spring, especially April and May, from eating *Tetradymia glabrata* and *T. canescens* (Fig. 14-3), and South African geeldikkop follows summer rains. Table 14-1 presents the geographic distribution of the specific forms of photosensitization.

ETIOLOGY AND PATHOGENESIS. The interaction of a photodynamic pigment and sunlight in nonpigmented skin causes photosensitization. In primary photosensitization, the photodynamic pigment originates from uncommonly ingested plants and exogenous drugs such as phenothiazine, whereas in secondary photosensitization, phylloerythrin is the photodynamic pigment.

In normal ruminant digestion, chlorophyll from ingested plants, by microbial action in the rumen, degrades into phylloerythrin. This compound is absorbed in the portal blood and transported to the liver, where it is transferred into the bile for excretion; consequently, the peripheral blood of normal sheep contains no phylloerythrin.

Animals with injured livers or with bile duct occlusion as from dietary hepatotoxins, however, are unable to excrete phylloerythrin, which consequently accumulates and causes generalized phylloerythrinemia. Pathogenic blood levels of photodynamic pigments are as little as 0.005 mg/dl. Table 14-1 presents the photodynamic pigments and the hepatotoxic substances for the different photosensitive diseases.

Photodynamic pigments in nonpigmented skin absorb quanta of sunlight and thus become activated. By collision with other molecules, such as proteins and amino acids, the energy is transferred and, in the presence of molecular oxygen, these compounds oxidize forming toxic compounds that increase the permeability of capillaries to plasma proteins, force water into affected tissues, and necrose cells. Death may result from secondary infections, inability to feed, and liver dysfunction. Sheep possessing hemoglobin A or AB, exposed to conditions that normally produce geeldikkop (hepatogenous photosensitization) and enzootic icterus are able to form hemoglobin C and are resistant to these conditions, whereas sheep with hemoglobin B are susceptible and die.

Considerable losses have occurred in sheep grazing *Tetradymia canescens* (spineless horsebrush) (Fig 14-3) and *Tetradymia glabrata* (little leaf horsebrush, coal oil brush). However, before sheep will develop classical photosensitization (big head), they must have previously consumed black sagebrush (*Artemisia nova*) before eating horsebrush. The apparent synergistic effects of these plants results in liver disease and secondary photosensitization. Both plants contain hepatotoxins; horsebrush contains several furanosesquiterpenes (tetradymol) and sages contain sesquiterpene lactones.

Secondary photosensitization due to the effects of pyrrolizidine-alkaloid containing plants

TABLE 14-1. *Forms of Photosensitization in Sheep*

Name	Cause		Location
	Plants	Agents	
A. Primary photosensitivity			
1. St. John's wort	*Hypericum perforatum*	hypericin	Canada, northwest, southeast and northeast U.S. Australia, New Zealand, Africa
2. Buckwheat	*Fagopyrum esculentum* (Fig. 14-2.)	fagopyrin	Australia, Europe, New Zealand, U.S.
3. Bishops weed	*Ammi majus*	furocoumarins	Texas
4. Spring parsley	*Cymopterus watsonii*	furocoumarins	Western U.S.
5. Dutchmans britches	*Thamnosma spp*	furocoumarins	North America
B. Secondary or hepatogenous			
1. Facial eczema	*Pithomyces chartarum*	sporidesmin	New Zealand, Australia, South Africa
2. Swelled head	*Agave lecheguilla*	saponins	U.S.: Texas, New Mexico, Mexico
3. Big head	*Tetradymia glabrata* *T. canescens*	tetradymol	Western U.S.
4. Geeldikkop	*Tribulus terrestris*	mycotoxins	South Africa, Australia
5. Alveld	*Narthecium ossifragum*	saponins	Norway
—	*Asaemia axillaris* *Lasiospermum bipinnatum*	not known	South Africa
C. Congenital			
1. Southdown sensitivity	genetic	—	New Zealand

rarely occurs in sheep. However, severe losses in sheep from eating plants with pyrrolizidine alkaloids *Echium plantagineum* (Paterson's curse), and *Heliotropeum europaeum* occur as a result of the accumulation of toxic levels of copper within the damaged livers of affected sheep.

CLINICAL SIGNS AND POSTMORTEM LESIONS. The time from ingestion of photodynamic pigment or hepatotoxic substances to the appearance of photosensitive signs ranges from several hours to 10 days. The disease begins with photophobia, erythema, and irritation of the cornea, lips, eyelids, face, vulva, and coronets (Fig. 14-4). Diseased sheep rub and kick the affected parts. These changes rapidly progress into facial edema. At this stage, the heavy ears droop, swollen nostrils constrict, and thickened lips are immobilized; consequently, affected sheep show dyspnea and anorexia.

Icterus may occur in secondary photosensitization. Severely depressed sheep separate from the flock and recline. Convalescent animals may show dry gangrene and sloughing of

Fig. 14-3.   Spineless horsebrush, *Tetradymia canescens.* × 0.2.

the skin, especially the ears. The morbidity ranges up to 80% of a flock, and the mortality may reach 20% of affected animals. The course varies from a few hours to a week.

At necropsy, the facial, vulvar, and pedal skin commonly is edematous. Icterus may be generalized in cases of secondary photosensitization, such as facial eczema, big head, and geeldikkop. The liver may show gross reticulation, pigmentation, and biliary cirrhosis, and microscopic bile duct necrosis, obstruction, and obliteration.

DIAGNOSIS.   Veterinarians diagnose photosensitization from evidence of signs, access to photosensitizing plants, and lesions. Photophobia and edema of affected skin strongly suggest the disease. Finding typical liver lesions, grazed culpable plants, history of administered drugs, and limitation of the disease to sheep with nonpigmented skins corroborates other suggestive changes. Although the process is usually not feasible, the chemical identification of a photodynamic pigment such as phylloerythrin in affected tissue confirms the diagnosis. The differential diagnosis re-

quires distinguishing between primary and secondary photosensitization. Primary photosensitivity has a far better prognosis than does secondary or hepatogenous photosensitivity. In addition to the known plants and drugs that cause photosensitivity, consideration should be given to other causes of liver disease, e.g. aflatoxicosis, liver abscesses, cor pulmonale. In the southwestern U.S., skin lesions due to *Elaeophora schneideri* can be mistaken for photosensitization.

PREVENTION AND TREATMENT.   Producers prevent photosensitization by avoiding the grazing of sheep during dangerous periods on ranges and pastures known to contain photosensitizing plants and agents. Spraying pastures containing the fungus, *Pithomyces chartarum,* with inhibiting chemicals, such as thiabendazole, may prevent facial eczema. Treatment, although not satisfactory, consists of removal of photosensitizing plants from the diet and confining the affected animals in shade where cool water and palatable feed are easily available. Sheep with chronic liver disease rarely recover.

Fig. 14-4. Photosensitization in a ewe with dermal necrosis (*A*), depilation (*B*), and keratitis (*C*).

Caterhoff, D.R.: Haemoglobin types and the geeldikkopenzootic icterus disease complex in sheep. Anim. Blood Groups Biochem. Genet. *2*:181-184, 1971.

Clare, N.T.: Photosensitization in animals. In *Advances in Veterinary Science.* New York, Academic Press, 1955, pp. 182-211.

Coetzer, I.A.W., Kellerman, T.S., Sadler, W., and Bath, G.F.: Photosensitivity in South Africa. A comparative study of the pathology of the ovine hepatogenous photosensitivity diseases, facial eczema and geeldikkop (*Tribulosis ovis*) with special reference to their pathogenesis. Onderstepoort J. Vet. Res., *50*:59-71, 1983.

Dertli, E.H., et al.: Phototoxic effect of *Thamnosma texana* (Dutchman's breeches) in sheep. Am. J. Vet. Res., *44*:1126-1129, 1983.

Dollahite, J.W., Younger, R.L., and Hoffman, G.O.: Photosensitization in cattle and sheep caused by feeding *Ammi majus* (greater ammi; Bishop's weed). Am. J. Vet. Res., *39*:193-197, 1978.

Filmer, J.F.: Pathogenic photosensitization of animals in New Zealand. Conf. Agric. Aust., 1949.

Glastonbury, I.R.W., Doughty, F.R., Whitaker, S.J., and Sergeant, E.: A syndrome of hepatogenous photosensitization resembling geeldikkop in sheep grazing *Tribulus terrestris.* Aust Vet. J., *61*:314-316, 1984.

Hore, D.E.: Facial eczema. Aust. Vet. J., *36*:172-176, 1960.

Jennings, P.W., et al.: Toxic constituents and hepatotoxicity of the plant *Tetradymia glabrata* (Asteroceae). In *Effects of Poisonous Plants on Livestock.* Edited by R.F. Keeler, K.R. VanKampen, L.F. James. New York, Academic Press, 1978, pp. 217-228.

Kellerman, T.S., et al.: Photosensitivity in South Africa. I. A comparative study of *Asaemia axillaris* (Thunb.) Harv. Ex Jackson and *Lasiospermum bipinnatum* (Thunb.) Druce poisoning in sheep. Onderstepoort J. Vet. Res., *40*:115-126, 1973.

Laksisvela, B., et al.: "Alveld" (Photosensitization due to *Narthecium ossifragum*) in lambs, review and research results. Nord. Vet. *89*:199-209, 1977.

Mitchell, K.J., Thomas, R.G., and Clarke, R.T.J.: Factors influencing growth of *Pithomyces chartarum* in pasture. N.Z. J. Agric. Res., *4*:566, 1961.

Mortimer, P.H.: Intoxication of sheep with sporidesmin. Histology and histochemistry of orally dosed sheep. Res. Vet. Sci., *4*:166, 1963.

Mortimer, P.H. and Standridge, T.A.: Excretion of sporidesmin given to sheep by mouth. J. Comp. Pathol., *78*:505-512, 1968.

Naude, T.W.: Facial eczema in South Africa, Onderstepoort Vet. Res. Inst. Personal communication, 1973.

Percival, J.C.: Association of *Sporidesmium bakeri* with facial eczema. N.Z. J. Agric. Res., *12*:1041-1056, 1959.

Quin, J.I.: Photosensitization in animals. VI. Effect of ligation of the bile duct. Onderstepoort J. Vet. Sci. Anim. Ind., *1*:505-526, 1933.

Rimington, C. and Quin, J.I.: Photosensitization in animals. VII. Nature of sensitizing agent in geeldikkop. Onderstepoort J. Vet. Sci. Anim. Ind., *3*:137-157, 1934.

Seaman, J.T.: Hepatogenous chronic copper poisoning in sheep associated with grazing *Echium plantigineum.* Aust. Vet. J., *62*:247-248, 1985.

Sinclair, D.P.: Thiabendazole shows promise for facial eczema control. N.Z. J. Agric. Res., *114*:23, 1967.

Sinclair, D.P. and Howe, M.W.: Effect of thiabendazole on *Pithomyces chartarum*. N.Z. J. Agric. Res., *11*:59-62, 1968.

Synge, R.L.M. and White, E.P.: Sporidesmin: substance from *Sporidesmium bakeri* causing lesions of facial eczema. Chem. Ind., 1959, pp. 1546-1547.

Taber, R.A., Pettit, R.E., Taber, W.A., and Dollahite, J.W.: Isolation of *Pithomyces chartarum* in Texas. Mycologia, *60*:727-733, 1968.

Witzel, D.A., Dollahite, J.W., and Jones, L.P.: Photosensitization in sheep fed *Ammi majus* (Bishop's weed) seed. Am. J. Vet. Res., *39*:320-321, 1978.

Elaeophorosis

(*Sore head*)

Elaeophorosis, a chronic vascular disease of the head and limbs of sheep, is characterized by dermatitis, mucositis, and oculitis. It is caused by microfilariae of a nematode of the western United States. Because the disease has limited geographic distribution, low incidence, and low mortality, it has little importance for the sheep industry. Some enterprises, how-ever, incur financial waste from the condition. Economic losses result from unthriftiness and unsalability of affected sheep during the prolonged course. Occurrence of elaeophorosis in game species adds scientific interest to the disease.

OCCURRENCE. Elaeophorosis occurs in all breeds of ewes beyond 2 years of age. Skin lesions develop during winter following summer grazing in endemic areas. In addition to sheep, the disease occurs in deer, elk, and moose. Geographically, it occurs in the United States in New Mexico, Colorado, Utah, Arizona, California, and Oregon. Endemic areas are grazing ranges above 1830 m altitude.

ETIOLOGY AND PATHOGENESIS. *Elaeophora schneideri,* an intra-arterial nematode, causes elaeophorosis. The adults, measuring 60 to 110 × 0.27 mm, occupy the lumina of arteries, such as the carotid and digital arteries, while the microfilariae, measuring 230 to 260 × 10 to 13 μm, inhabit the capillaries, dermas, and laminae propriae of skins and membranes

Fig. 14-5. Unilateral facial dermatitis and keratitis from *Elaeophora schneideri* larvae.

with blood supply from the parasitized arteries. In sheep, the adult worms occasionally cause arterial damage and circulatory impairment, but the irritating microfilariae provoke prolonged and debilitating dermatitis, stomatitis, rhinitis, and oculitis.

The life cycle of the worm begins with discharge of microfilariae from mature females and their movement to a network of skin capillaries, where they locate. The horsefly, *Hybomitra laticornis,* is the main intermediate host. Female horseflies acquire infection by obtaining blood meals from head skin lesions of sheep or from head skin of larvae-carrying deer. Microfilariae enter the fly along with blood and within 2 weeks develop into infective larvae, which move into the head and mouth parts of the fly. During blood-feeding at this stage, larvae, along with saliva, pass into a susceptible sheep, migrate to a definitive arterial position, and mature. Migration and maturation of the third-stage larvae require 5 to 6 months. Mature worms live 3 to 4 years.

Ovine lesions originate from two factors: (1) inflammatory reaction against microfilariae and (2) ischemia from vessel occlusion. Skin and mucosal changes are inflammatory reactions, but some eye and brain changes come from ischemia and result from necrosis and atrophy. The inflammatory lesions endure for several years but eventually heal.

CLINICAL SIGNS AND POSTMORTEM LESIONS. Following transmission of elaeophorosis by the bite of larvae-infected horseflies, dermatitis develops insidiously on the heads and feet and mucositis in the mouths, noses, and eyes of adult sheep. Most head lesions are ipsilateral. All diagnosed sheep have cephalic dermatitis. Of these, 25 to 50% also have oral and rhinal mucositis, and 25% have hind-foot dermatitis. Diseased tissues show specific changes: infected skin loses wool and hair and accumulates a crust of dried serum and exudate, infected eyes show conjunctivitis and corneal opacity, infected mouths develop palatal ulcers, infected turbinates are thick and nodular, and infected coronets have hoof deformities. Because of their general discomfort, affected sheep become unthrifty and may show lame-

Fig. 14-6. Unilateral stomatitis from larvae of *Elaeophora schneideri.* × 0.6.

ness and difficult breathing. Brain lesions may cause locomotor disturbances.

The morbidity usually is less than 0.5%, and few cases die. Healing occurs after a course of 3 to 4 years.

At necropsy, grossly discernible lesions are found in skin and membranes, and adult worms inhabit arteries supplying blood to the lesions. Consequently, parasitized arteries and head lesions are ipsilateral; for example, a sheep with adult worms in the right carotid artery only may have right-face dermatitis, right-side stomatitis, right-side rhinitis, and right-eye infections (Figs. 14-5 and 14-6).

Histopathologically, lesions contain microfilariae and cuticular fragments, and masses of eosinophils, lymphocytes, plasma cells, macrophages, and foreign body giant cells accumulate around these irritants.

DIAGNOSIS. Veterinarians diagnose elaeophorosis on evidence of skin and mouth lesions in adult sheep of endemic areas. Finding adult nematodes in the arteries at necropsy or microfilariae in lesions at biopsy confirms the diagnosis. The differential diagnosis requires consideration of the type of photosensitization that causes extensive facial edema.

PREVENTION. Producers prevent or reduce elaeophorosis by avoiding grazing sheep during fly seasons on mountain ranges known to contain infected deer and vectoring horseflies.

Adcock, J.L. and Hibler, C.P.: Vascular and neuro-oph-thalmic pathology of elaeophorosis in elk. Pathol. Vet., 6:185-213, 1969.

Clark, G.C. and Hibler, C.P.: Horseflies and *Elaeophora schneideri*. J. Wildlife Dis., 9:21-25, 1973.

Davis, C.L. and Kemper, H.E.: Histologic diagnosis of filarial dermatosis in sheep. JAVMA, 118:103-106, 1951.

Douglas, J.R., Cordy, D.R., and Spurlock, G.M.: *Elaeophora schneideri* in California sheep. Cornell Vet., 44:252-258, 1954.

Herman, C.M.: Worm parasites of deer in California. Calif. Fish Game, 3:201-208, 1945.

Hibler, C.P., Adcock, J.L., Davis, R.W., and Abdelbaki, Y.Z.: Elaeophorosis in deer and elk. Bull. Wildlife Dis. Assoc., 5:27-30, 1969.

Hibler, C.P., Adcock, J.L., Gates, G.H., and White, R.: Experimental infection of sheep and deer with *Elaeophora schneideri*. J. Wildlife Dis., 6:110-111, 1970.

Jensen, R. and Seghetti, L.: Elaeophoriasis in sheep. JAVMA, 127:499-505, 1955.

Kemper, H.E.: Filarial dermatosis in sheep. North Am. Vet., 19:36-41, Sept., 1938.

Kemper, H.E. and Roberts, I.H.: Treatment of filarial dermatosis of sheep. AJVR, 7:350-354, 1946.

Tick Infestation

Tick infestation, an acute dermatitis of sheep and other animals, is characterized primarily by irritation and annoyance and secondarily by anemia and transmitted diseases. Sheep are infested by many species of Ixodidae, the family of hard ticks, and some species of Argasidae, the family of soft ticks.

Because tick infestation occurs universally and usually affects all classes of sheep and other species of domestic animals and hence causes extensive material waste, it seriously concerns the entire livestock industry. Economic losses result from sheep deaths, annoyances, diminished productivity, transmitted diseases, protein deficiencies among sheep-dependent people, and the costs of preventive, eradicative, and treatment programs. The occurrence of tick infestations and tick-transmitted diseases among cattle, horses, poultry, and people adds both economic importance and public health significance to the maladies.

In the United States, four species of hard ticks—*Dermacentor andersoni, Amblyomma americanum, A. cajennense,* and *Rhipicephalus sanguineus*—and one species of soft tick—*Otobius megnini*—attack sheep. Animals acquire the parasites from western and southwestern ranges and pastures and may carry them into feedlots and other enterprises. Table 14-2 presents the common ticks of sheep, their distribution, and transmitted diseases.

The injury to sheep from tick parasitism varies directly, in most cases, with numbers of parasites. Ticks feed exclusively on blood, and when several hundred parasitize the same host, the animal becomes exsanguinated and anemic. Affected sheep are, therefore, unthrifty and may lose body weight. During warm seasons, the skin injuries attract gravid blowflies and screwworm flies, which may oviposit on the wounds and cause fatal cutaneous myiosis. In addition to hematophagous feeding, some species, such as nymphs of the spinose ear tick, occupy the external auditory canal, where they cause excruciating annoyance and occasionally middle ear infection. Furthermore, some engorging females generate a salivary toxin.

Tick Paralysis

Tick paralysis, an acute neurointoxication of sheep, is characterized by ascending and progressive paralysis and is caused by salivary toxin from some, but not all, engorging female ticks. Even though the disease has wide geographic distribution, the incidence within affected flocks is invariably low, and for that reason it attracts little attention from the sheep industry. The disease occurs in all breeds, sexes, and ages, but young sheep have a higher incidence than do other age groups. In addition to sheep, the malady occurs in cattle

TABLE 14-2. *Some Ticks of Sheep*

Families	Names — Scientific	Names — Common	Distribution	Diseases Transmitted or Produced in Sheep
	Dermacentor andersoni	Rocky Mountain wood tick	U.S., west; Canada, west	Tularemia, paralysis
	Rhipicephalus sanguineus	Brown dog tick	U.S.; world	Tularemia, Nairoba sheep disease
	Rhipicephalus evertsi	Red-legged tick	Africa	Paralysis
	Rhipicephalus bursa	—	Southern Europe; Africa	Babesiosis, eperythrozoonosis, gonderiosis, Nairobi sheep disease
	Rhipicephalus apppendicularius	Brown ear tick	Africa	Nairobi sheep disease, louping-ill
Ixodidae (hard ticks)	*Amblyomma americanum*	Lone star tick	Texas north to Iowa, east to Atlantic; Mexico; Central America; South America	Tularemia, paralysis
	Amblyomma cajennense	Cayenne tick	Southern Texas; Mexico; Central America; South America	Brucellosis
	Amblyomma hebraeum	Bont tick	South, Central Africa	Heart water
	Hyalomma plumbeum	—	Southern Europe; USSR; Egypt	Eperythrozoonosis
	Ixodes ricinus	Castor bean tick	Europe; USSR	Louping-ill, tick-borne fever, paralysis
	Ixodes holocyclus	Paralysis tick	Australia	Paralysis
	Ixodes rubicundus	Paralysis tick	South Africa	Paralysis
Argasidae (soft ticks)	*Otobius megnini*	Spinose ear tick	U.S., west; Canada; west Africa	Paralysis

and horses. Most cases develop during early spring when ticks actively seek suitable host animals.

ETIOLOGY AND PATHOGENESIS. Causative tick species include *Dermacentor andersoni* and *Amblyomma americanum* in the United States and Canada, *A. variegatum* in Nigeria, *Ixodes holocyclus* in Australia, *I. ricinus* in the Balkans, and *I. rubicundus* and *Rhipicephalus evertsi* in South Africa.

The parasites usually attach to host skin around the head and neck. Four to 6 days of initial tick feeding are required to produce the disease, but when the toxin-producing ticks are experimentally transferred to a second host, only 1 day is necessary to produce signs. The toxin, injected at the time of tick feeding, interrupts impulse transmission at the myoneural junction and possibly along the spinal cord. Unless the parasites are removed, the paralysis progresses anteriorly into the medulla and induces fatal respiratory failure. Intensity of paralysis is related to the number of feeding ticks. Presumably, sheep rapidly excrete or detoxify the toxin, because they may recover within hours after removing the toxin-forming ticks.

Experiments using mice with tick paralysis produced by *Ixodes holocyclus* indicate that motor paralysis can be explained by interference at the neuromuscular junction. It is suggested that the toxin from *I. holocyclus* has a direct temperature-sensitive action on the excitation-sensitive coupling mechanism, which results in an inhibition of transmitter release at the neuromuscular junction.

CLINICAL SIGNS AND POSTMORTEM LESIONS. Following tick feeding for about 4 days, paralysis begins with weakness and incoordinated movements in the caudal limbs. Within a few hours, these impaired functions change to paralysis, which progresses forward to involve the forelimbs, neck, and head. Some sheep may be found paralyzed without the observation of prodromic weakness. The eyes bulge and appear alert. Anemia may exist from heavy parasitism. Unless other diseases such as tularemia coexist, the body temperature is normal. The incidence is usually low and seldom exceeds a half-dozen cases per flock. The course ranges from 2 to 4 days and, unless successfully treated, terminates in death. Cohabitating cattle and horses may also contract the disease.

At necropsy, no significant changes, except the presence of ticks or their attachment wounds and possibly anemia, are apparent. Although a large number of ticks may be attached to the head and neck, only a few toxin-producing females are necessary to cause the disease.

DIAGNOSIS. Veterinarians diagnose tick infestation from evidence of pathologic numbers of ticks parasitizing sheep and anemia. They diagnose tick paralysis on the basis of signs and response. The presence of some ticks parasitizing paralyzed sheep during early spring strongly suggests the disease. Prompt recovery of some animals following removal of ticks confirms the diagnosis. The differential diagnosis requires consideration of tularemia, which also develops from spring tick parasitism. Tularemia, however, causes fever and the development of an ascending titer of agglutinating antibodies specific to *Francisella tularensis*. This organism can be isolated from ticks and sheep lymph nodes, spleen, and liver.

PREVENTION AND TREATMENT. Tick infestation, and hence tick paralysis, can be prevented by management or medication. Producers should avoid grazing sheep on infested areas during spring when ticks are active. If this precaution is not feasible, animals should be treated with a pesticide. Ticks should be removed by hand from tick-paralyzed sheep; if the number of infested animals or ticks is large, sheep should be hand-sprayed or dipped (see Table 14-5).

Baldwin, A.F.: Tick paralysis in sheep. Vet. Med., *20*:507-509, 1925.

Bootes, B.W.: Fatal paralysis in foals from *Ixodes holocyclus* infestation. Aust. Vet. J., *38*:168-69, 1962.

Clark, R.: Lamb paralysis caused by *Rhipicephalus evertsi*. J. S. Afr. Vet. Med. Assoc., *9*:143-145, 1938.

Cooper, B.J. and Spruce, I.: Temperature dependent inhibition of evoked acetylcholine release in tick paralysis. Nature, *263*:693-695, 1976.

Diplolu, O.O.: Tick paralysis of sheep caused by nymphs of *Amblyomma variegatum*. A preliminary report. Z. Parasitenk., *49*:293-295, 1976.

Eddy, G.W. and Bushland, R.C.: Fleeceworms. In *Yearbook of Agriculture*. USDA, 1956.

Gregson, J.D.: Tick paralysis in groundhogs, guinea pigs and hamsters. Can. J. Comp. Med., 23:266-268, 1959.

Gregson, J.D.: Tick paralysis: an appraisal of natural and experimental data. Can. Dep. Agric., 1973, p. 109.

Hadwen, S.: Tick paralysis in sheep and man following bites of *Dermacentor andersoni*. Parasitology, 6:283, 1914.

Jellison, W.L. and Kohls, G.M.: Tick-host anemia induced by *Dermacentor andersoni*. J. Parasitol., 24:143-154, 1938.

Jellison, W.L., Stoenner, H.G., Kramis, N.J., and Beardmore, H.R.: Tick paralysis in western Montana. Vet Med., 46:163-166, 1951.

Kozinc, M.: Tick paralysis in sheep. Yugoslavia Vet. Glasn., 16:252-254, 1938.

Legg, J.: Infestation of sheep with ticks. Aust. Vet. J., 3:12-14, 1927.

Manual on Livestock Ticks. USDA/ARS, 1965.

Murnaghan, M.F.: Tick paralysis in a dog: a neurological study. Proc. 10th Int. Cong. Entomol., 3:841-848, 1956.

Nietz, W.O., Baughton, F., and Walter, H.S.: Laboratory investigations on the life cycle of the karoo paralysis tick (*Ixodes rubicundus*). Onderstepoort J. Vet. Res., 38:215-223, 1971.

Scabies

(*Mange; scab; itch; acariasis*)

Scabies, a chronic contagious dermatitis of sheep and other domestic animals, is characterized by encrustation, denudation, and itching of the skin and is caused by five species of pathogenic mites. Although most species of domestic animals are attacked by scabies, a high degree of host specificity prevents transfer of parasites between host species. This fact validates the separate control and eradicative programs for scabies of sheep and scabies of cattle.

Throughout their histories, the USDA and the state departments of agriculture have conscientiously fought and researched scabies of both species. Finally, in 1973, the United States, except for inconsequential demodectic mange, became free of sheep scabies. In many sheep-producing countries, however, some form of the disease persists, causes waste, and worries the sheep industry. Economic losses result from damaged wool, reduced production of meat and wool, interference to sheep commerce, and the costs of control programs.

TYPES OF SCABIES. Ovine scabies is classified according to the type of causative mite. Five genera are involved. Although each type in early stages possesses differential characteristics, the positive diagnosis requires isolation and identification of the specific mite. The types, their causative agents, and some specific characteristics are compared in Table 14-3.

1. Psoroptic scabies. The economic importance of common scabies exceeds any other type and possibly all other types combined. It occurs in all ages, but more often in adults than in lambs. The clinical disease is limited to late autumn, winter, and early spring. Geographically, it is prevalent in regions of temperate climatic zones including Iceland, Europe, Africa, Middle East, Balkans, Pakistan, India, and South and Central America. Australia, New Zealand, Canada, and the United States have eradicated the disease. In addition to sheep, the species infests cattle, horses, donkeys, mules, and probably bighorn sheep and water buffalo.

Psoroptes ovis, the causative mites, are oval-shaped, 0.5 to 0.6 mm in length, and have heads that are longer than they are wide. All legs project beyond the body edge, and the third pair has two long hairs. Leg pairs 1, 2, and 3 in males and 1, 2, and 4 in females bear a sucker on a jointed pedicle.

These obligate parasitic mites live entirely on the host skin surface. Their life cycle has five stages, of which the final two are sexually dimorphic: (1) egg, (2) larva, (3) protonymph, (4) deutonymph male and pubescent female, and (5) adult male and ovigerous female. Cycle time from egg to egg is 10 to 12 days. During autumn, when microclimatic fleece temperature decreases, light concentration diminishes, and humidity increases, the mite populations vastly increase and severely injure host skin. In spring, however, when microclimatic temperature increases, light concentration increases, and humidity decreases, the populations abate and become latent, and the skin heals and wool grows.

Throughout summer latency, surviving mites hide in infraorbital fossae, inguinal folds, perineum, scrotum, tail, interdigital fossae, and

TABLE 14-3. *Sheep Scabies*

		Mites			Lesions	
Mange type	Species	Life Cycle (days)	Eggs per Female	Length (mm)	Early Locations	Characteristics
1. Psoroptic (common scabies)	Psoroptes ovis	10–12	15–25	F 0.6 M 0.5	Rump, shoulders, sides	Central crust; denuded
2. Sarcoptic (head scabies)	Sarcoptes scabiei ovis	17	10–40	F 0.3–0.6 M 0.2–0.4	Head	Thick, crusty, wrinkled, denuded
3. Psorergatic (itch scabies)	Psorergates ovis	—	—	F 0.19 M 0.17	Side, flank, thigh	Dry, scurfy, broken wool
4. Chorioptic (foot scabies)	Chorioptes communis ovis	19–23	3–16	F 0.4 M 0.3	Hind feet, pasterns	Crusty, brown, thickened, fissured
5. Demodectic (follicular mange)	Demodex ovis	—	—	0.2–0.4	Eyelids, prepuce, vulva, neck, back	Normal to nodular, pustular

vulvar furrows, and from these shelters they emerge in the autumn.

Transmission is usually by direct contact, but it can occur by indirect contact. Live mites can survive off the ovine hosts for more than 30 days under ideal laboratory conditions, but cannot infest new hosts after 1 to 2 weeks in vacated sheep pens.

Active mites feed by piercing the host epidermis; hyperemia, swelling, vesication, and pustulation subsequently develop at each point. The mite then ingests the exuding lymph and tissue fluids. Excess fluids mix with keratinized cells, wool, soil, and manure and coagulate and thus form crusts that dehydrate and fissure. The dermal changes at the points eventually render feeding impossible. Consequently, as mites continually move further and further to the lesion peripheries to feed on normal tissue, the individual lesions expand and adjacent lesions coalesce.

Mite saliva injected during feeding and mite movements on sensitive skin surface provoke itching. Clinical signs of the disease relate to the itching. The tormented sheep bite, kick, and rub the infested skin of the wethers, rump, and back, and these actions break and extirpate the wool. During winter, the lesions consist of thickened, fissured, denuded crusts surrounded by zones of hyperemia. Later, in spring and summer, lesions gradually heal, and new wool covers the area (Fig. 14-7).

Veterinarians suspect the disease from evidence of typical signs and lesions, and they confirm the diagnosis by finding the specific mites in skin scrapings from the peripheral zones of lesions. Multiple samples may be necessary to find the mites in declining populations, and during summer latency, samples should be scraped from sites of predilection for hiding. A dissecting microscope gives adequate magnification for identification and efficiency for processing numerous samples. The differential diagnosis requires consideration of other itch-provoking diseases, such as other types of scabies, pediculosis, scrapie, and photosensitization.

2. Sarcoptic scabies. Head scabies occurs among sheep of Europe, Africa, Middle East,

Fig. 14-7. Sheep with common scabies in spring when lesions over withers and shoulders are healing and growing new wool. (Courtesy of Dr. Miguel Galina)

Balkans, India, South America, and Central America. The disease usually develops in undernourished sheep during late winter and persists for long periods. *Sarcoptes scabiei ovis,* the causative mites, selectively infect skin of the head, especially around the eyes and ears. The round-bodied and round-headed adults have short legs, with pairs 1 and 2 pro-

jecting beyond the body edge, and with suckers on long unjointed stalks of pairs 1, 2, and 4 in males and pairs 1 and 2 in females. The dorsal surface has transverse striations. They burrow in the epidermis, feed on tissue fluids, and thereby cause intense itching. Infected skin becomes thickened from crusts of exudate, epithelial keratinization, and dermal fi-

TABLE 14-4. *Characteristics of Sheep Lice*

Names	Female length (mm)	Color	Type of mouth parts	Predilection sites on hosts	Seasons of high activity	Egg incubation (days)	Life cycle (days)
Damalinia ovis (body louse)	1.2	white-yellow	biting	upper sides, withers	winter, spring	9–10	24–36
Linognathus ovillus (blue body louse; face louse)	2.5	blue-gray	sucking	face, body	winter	11–13	35
Linognathus pedalis (foot louse)	2.0	blue-gray	sucking	hairy legs, scrotum	winter, spring	17	43

TABLE 14-5. *Treatment of Lice, Ticks, Keds*

Pesticide	Application	Withdrawal Days
Coumaphos	Spray or dip—0.06–0.12%	15
Dioxathion	Spray or dip—0.15%	0
Dioxathion & DDVP	Spray or dip—0.15 & 0.005%	0
Diazinon	Spray high pressure—0.03%	14
	Spray low pressure —0.06%	14
Malathion	Spray or dip—0.05%	0
Chlorfenvinphos	Spray—0.05%	0
	Dip —0.01%	0
Crotoxyphos	Spray—0.25%	0
Crotoxyphos & DDVP	Spray	1
Methoxychlor	Spray or dip—0.5%	0

brosis. By persistently rubbing their lesions, infected sheep traumatize the skin and exacerbate the infection.

The disease spreads among sheep by direct contact and mite transfer. Veterinarians clinically diagnose sarcoptic scabies on evidence of signs and lesions, and they confirm the diagnosis by finding mites in deep skin scrapings from the peripheries of lesions.

3. Psorergatic scabies. Itch mange has occurred among Merino breeds in Australia, New Zealand, South Africa, Argentina, and the United States. *Psorergates ovis,* the causative mites, have round bodies, body indentations between legs, and long setae and an inward-curving spine on each femur. They selectively infect skin surfaces of sides, flanks, and thighs. They feed by piercing the epidermis and ingesting the exuding fluids. The infected skin is dry, scurfy, and hyperkeratotic; fibers easily break, but persisting wool agglomerates into ragged tufts. Intense itching causes infected sheep to bite, kick, and rub the parasitized areas. Even though the lesions spread slowly, they may become generalized after a course of several years. The disease spreads by direct contact and mite transfer. Veterinarians diagnose the disease from evidence of signs and lesions and confirm the diagnosis by finding the causative mites in skin scrapings from the lesions. The differential diagnosis requires consideration of lousiness.

4. Chorioptic scabies. Foot mange occurs in low incidence among sheep of Australia. *Chorioptes ovis,* the causative mites, have ovoid bodies and campanulate suckers attached to unsegmented pedicles on leg pairs 1, 2, 3, and 4 of adult males, and on pairs 1, 2, and 4 of females. They live on the skin surface and infect hind feet, especially the pastern and interdigital areas. The dermatitic lesions consist of yellow-brown crusts with hemorrhaging fissures. Intense itching causes foot stamping and biting. Veterinarians diagnose the disease from evidence of signs and lesions and finding the causative mites in lesion scrapings. The differential diagnosis requires consideration of trombidiosis and strawberry foot rot.

5. Demodectic mange. Follicular mange, an invasion of hair follicles and sebaceous glands, has two forms: (1) innocuous commensalism in the prepuce, vulva, and eyelids, and (2) parasitism of skin. The condition probably occurs in some animals in most sheep-producing countries, including France, Britain, Australia, Germany, and the United States.

Demodex ovis, the causative mites, possess short legs and elongated, striated abdomens. They selectively parasitize follicles and sebaceous glands of the feet, face, eyelids, ears, and back. Infected follicles become distended with mites, exoskeletons, eggs, and epithelial cells and thereby form nodules; pyogenic bacteria may convert the nodules into pustules.

Hughes, C.A. and Iwan, L.G.R.: *Psorergates ovis* of Merino sheep in Patagonia. Rev. Med. Vet., Buenos Aires, *41*:19-29, 1960.

Imes, M.: Sheep Scab. USDA Farmers Bull. 713, 1935.

Jensen, R., et al.: Psoroptic cattle scabies research. U.S. Nat. Res. Council., Natl. Acad. Sci. Washington, D.C., 1979.

Klein, W.: Scabies of sheep from *Demodex folliculorum*. DTW, *29*:105, 1921.

McKenna, C.T. and Pulsford, M.F.: *Chorioptes communis ovis* on sheep in Australia. Aust. Vet. J., *23*:146-147, 1947.

Murray, M.D.: Demodectic mange in sheep. Aust. Vet. J., *35*:93, 1959.

Palimpestov, N.A., et al.: Effect of physical and chemical factors on itch mites. Veterinariia (Moscow), *27*:38-40, 1950.

Roberts, I.H., Blachut, K., and Meleney, W.P.: Oversummering locations of *Psoroptes ovis* on sheep. Entomol. Soc. Amer. Annals, *64*:105-108, 1971.

Shilston, A.W.: Life history of *Ps communis ovis* in South Africa. 3rd and 4th Dep. Dir. Vet. Res., Union S. Afr. Dep. Agric., 1915, pp. 69-107.

Spence, T.: Latent phase of sheep scab. J. Comp. Pathol. Ther., *59*:305-318, 1949.

Sweatman, G.K.: Life cycle of *Chorioptes bovis*. J. Parasitol. *41*:Suppl. 34, 1955.

Sweatman, G.K.: Life history and validity of species of *Psoroptes*. Can. J. Zool., *36*:905-929, 1958.

Whitten, L.K. and Elliot, D.C.: *Psorergates ovis* on New Zealand sheep. N.Z. Vet. J., *4*:19, 1956.

Wilson, G.I., Blachut, K., and Roberts, I.H.: Infectivity of scabies mites, *Psoroptes ovis*, to sheep. Res. Vet. Sci., *22*:292-297, 1977.

TABLE 14-6. *Treatment of Mange Mites*

Pesticide	Method of Application
Coumaphos	Dip—3%
Toxophene	Dip—0.5%
Phosmet	Dip—0.15-0.25%
Lime sulfur	Dip—2.0%

Skin with advanced lesions is thickened, scaly, denuded, nodular, and pustular. Itching may stimulate kicking, biting, and rubbing of the lesions. In general, the disease has low incidence and little importance.

PREVENTION AND TREATMENT. Producers and veterinarians prevent scabies by avoiding exposure of susceptible sheep to infected animals. Before admitting animals into a clean flock, suspected sheep should be dipped or sprayed with a state-approved acaricide. Eradicating the disease, of course, provides long-term prevention.

In the United States, psoroptic, sarcoptic, psorergatic, and chorioptic scabies must be reported to state or USDA officials. In most states, infected flocks are quarantined until properly treated and declared free of the disease (Table 14-6).

Animal Health Yearbook. FAO-WHO-OIE (Italy), 1970.

Aynaud, M.: Kystes à *Demodex*, kystes sebaces et absces du mouton. Ann. Inst. Pasteur, *46*:306-319, 1931.

Baker, D.W. and Nutting, W.B.: Demodectic mange in New York State sheep. Cornell. Vet., *40*:140-142, 1950.

Bell, D.S., Pounden, W.D., Edgington, B.H., and Bentley, O.G.: *Psorergates ovis* in sheep. JAVMA, *120*:117-120, 1952.

Blake, B.H., et al.: Morphology of mouth parts of sheep scab mite. Ann. Entomol. Soc. Am., *72*:289-294, 1978.

Brownlee, A.A.: Demodex found in sheep in Britain. J. Comp. Pathol., *48*:68-73, 1935.

Carter, H.B.: Follicle mite (*Demodex*) in Australian sheep. Aust. Vet. J., *18*:120-124, 1942.

Carter, H.B.: Sheep skin disease due to *Psorergates ovis*. Aust. Vet. J., *17*:193-201, 1941.

Downing, W.: Life history of *Psoroptes communis ovis*. I. J. Comp. Pathol. Ther., *49*:163-180, 1936.

Fiedler, O.G.H. and DuToit, R.: Australian itch in South Africa. J. S. Afr. Vet. Med. Assoc., *25*:21-24, 1954.

Trombidiosis

(*Legitch; blacksoil itch*)

Trombidiosis, an acute dermatitis of the feet, is characterized by severe itching and is caused by the larvae of *Trombicula sarcina,* a soil mite. Because the disease is limited to Australia, has low incidence, and causes no deaths, it has little importance to the general sheep industry. Affected enterprises, however, may incur losses from unthriftiness and the cost of treatment of infected animals.

ETIOLOGY AND PATHOGENESIS. The causative larvae of *T. sarcina* parasitize animals, but nymphs and adults of the species are free-living; related mites include American chiggers and British harvest mites. Following summer rains the larvae move from infested soil onto the feet of sheep and adhere in clusters to the skin of the coronets, pasterns, metacarpi, and metatarsi. Each mite synthesizes a feeding tube, which the arachnid inserts into the derma. After feeding on tissue fluids for 3 to 5 days, the mites leave the tubes and the hosts and return to the soil. The irritating tubes, and possibly mite saliva, cause acute inflammation and provoke intense itching.

CLINICAL SIGNS AND LESIONS. During the early stages of trombidiosis, affected sheep violently stamp and bite their feet. Feed consumption diminishes, and the animals lose weight. The infected skin is swollen and contains clusters of larvae, 1 mm in diameter, attached to punctiform ulcers. Later, the traumatized skin shows denudation, ulcers, and crusts. The morbidity may reach 90%, and the course ranges from 6 to 8 weeks.

DIAGNOSIS. Veterinarians diagnose the disease in early stages by finding the larvae in scrapings from infected skin and in advanced stages, after mite departure, on evidence of signs and lesions.

TREATMENT. Although the efficacy of modern acaricides against the larvae has not been reported, their use is indicated.

Crogan, W.E.: Trombidiosis of sheep. Aust. Vet. J., 25:103-104, 1949.
Gill, D.A., Moule, G.R., and Riek, R.F.: Trombidiosis of sheep. Aust. Vet. J., 21:22-31, 1945.

Cutaneous Myiosis

(CM; blowfly myiasis; strike)

Cutaneous myiosis, an acute dermatitis of sheep, is characterized by denudation, thinning of the epidermis, and invasion of the subcutis and is caused by blowfly larvae. Presumably, the maggots do not attack and ingest live tissue, but they continuously irritate, injure, and kill surface cells, which they voraciously consume, and by this erosive process they gradually destroy and penetrate tissue.

Because the condition has high incidence throughout warm and temperate zones, where sheep and blowflies coexist, it causes major financial waste and seriously concerns the entire sheep industry. Economic losses result from deaths, disfigurements, wool damage, and the costs of preventive and therapeutic programs. In addition to sheep, CM occurs in most other species of domestic and wild mammals. The same species of maggots rapidly and beneficially invade and destroy all types of carrion.

OCCURRENCE. Although CM occurs in all breeds, sexes, and ages of sheep, adult Merinos have a higher incidence than do other classes of sheep: ewes develop breech myiosis, the most common type, and rams contract pole and preputial myiosis. The disease occurs only during warm seasons when adult flies are active. Geographically, it develops in all sheep-producing countries.

ETIOLOGY AND PATHOGENESIS. The larvae of blowflies cause CM. Although many types of flies are involved, predominating species include *Lucilia cuprina* and *Caliphora augur* in Australia, *Calliphora stygia* and *Lucilia sericata* in New Zealand, *Lucilia sericata* in Britain, *Lucilia cuprina* in South Africa, and *Phormia regina* in the United States. The adults of *Phormia regina*, commonly known as black blowflies, contain black to blue-green thoraces and abdomens and measure 6 to 11 mm in length. *Lucilia cuprina* and *L. sericata*, the greenbottle flies, have metallic green bodies and red-brown eyes and measure 8 to 10 mm in length. The mature larvae, measuring 10 to 14 mm in length, are gray, white, yellow, or pink and contain two oral hooks and two stigmal plates at the anterior and posterior ends, respectively. The cuticle is smooth. These genera are primary blowflies and hence are able to initiate ovine myiosis; some others, such as *Chrysomyia* and *Sarcophaga*, are secondary and unable to initiate lesions, but they can participate in the disease after a primary genus has started the condition.

The life cycles of all blowflies pass through four stages: egg, larva, pupa, and adult. Although the species have similar life cycles, the stages vary in period lengths. In general, each female fly lives about 1 month and lays 2000 to 3000 eggs, which hatch after an incubation period of 1 to 24 hours. Larvae rapidly grow to mature size in 3 to 6 days. Pupation occurs in the soil and endures 3 to 7 days. Under favorable conditions of food, temperature, and moisture, the entire life cycle is completed in 10 to 20 days.

Even though the fly larvae inflict the host damage, several factors contribute to their deposition and development; these include moisture, temperature, and skin topography. Moisture in the breech wool, especially from urine and fluid feces, attracts female flies and invites oviposition. Larval survival and development require abundant moisture and high humidity. Favorable temperature ranges from 15 to 26°C. Wrinkled skin with long fine wool retains moisture, maintains heat, and nourishes bacteria. These conditions attract blowflies and sustain their larvae.

The pathogenesis of CM begins with egg hatching and larval emergence. The maggots do not eat live tissue but consume dead cells, exudates, secretions, and debris. They irritate, injure, and kill successive layers of cells and provoke exudation. A large population of maggots rapidly consumes the dead cells and exudate and avidly competes for all exudative increments. After a short course, the maggots bore through the thinned epidermis into the subcutis, where they continue to feed on exudate and killed cells. The erosive process forms tissue cavities up to several centimeters in diameter. Unless the pathogenic process is arrested by appropriate treatment, the affected animals die from shock, intoxication, histolysis, and infection.

CLINICAL SIGNS AND POSTMORTEM LESIONS. Four anatomic locations for CM are breech, body, pole, and prepuce. Each area is predisposed to infestation under special circumstances: (1) breech—the most common form, in females with wool soiled by urine and fluid feces and in males with wool soiled by fluid feces (Fig. 14-8); (2) body—in both sexes along the neck, back, and sides, with prolonged moistening of the wool; (3) pole—in rams with tightly coiled horns and moist skin folds around the horns; and (4) prepuce—in males with urine-soiled and dew-moistened wool.

Affected sheep are restless, anxious, and preoccupied with their lesions. Animals with breech infestation shake their tails, flex their rump muscles, stamp their feet, and stand with lowered heads, and sheep infested in more

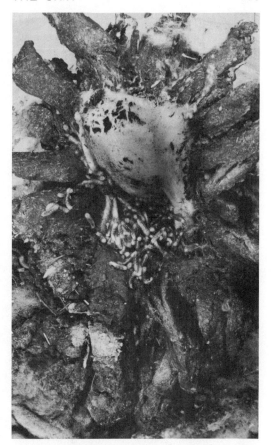

Fig. 14-8. Maggots of blowflies, *Phormia regina*, attacking the soiled perineum. × 0.8.

accessible areas kick, rub, and bite the affected skin.

Close examination of early lesions reveals moist skin, variable numbers of small maggots, and peculiar odor. The cleaned skin is red and tender. Advanced lesions show brown-stained wool and loosened fibers and contain up to several thousand eggs and maggots. The epidermis is thin and the skin inflamed, and some larvae occupy cavities in the subcutaneous tissue. At this stage, affected sheep are depressed, febrile, and usually prostrated.

At necropsy, the lesion is large and the tissue destruction extensive. Body cavities may be invaded and parts of muscles destroyed.

DIAGNOSIS. Veterinarians suspect CM in sheep showing typical signs, and they confirm the diagnosis by finding larval infestation. Early lesions need careful inspection for the immature maggots. The differential diagnosis requires consideration of screwworm infestation. Mature larvae of this species are about 15 mm long and contain pigmented tracheae and large posterior spiracles.

PREVENTION AND TREATMENT.   Producers and veterinarians prevent CM by combinations of the following procedures:

1. Dock animals, with tail incisions at a level 6 mm below the vulva.

2. Shear wool from the breech of ewes before parturition. Aeration avoids some soiling and skin moistness that attract ovipositing flies.

3. Spray the breech and other vulnerable areas with 0.04% solution of diazinon, an organophosphorus compound, under sufficient pressure to assure penetration of the wool to the skin. Proper spraying protects treated sheep for at least 12 to 14 weeks, but spraying the wool only does not give protection. Other organophosphorus compounds, such as coumaphos and ronnel, are also effective (Table 14-7).

4. Amputate skin from each side of the perineum using the Australian modified mules operation. This obliterates breech wrinkles and widens the bare surface of the perineum. A linear piece of skin, pointed at each end and 2 to 4 cm wide, is excised from each side of the bare perineum. The strip begins about 2 cm

TABLE 14-7.   *Treatment of Blowfly and Screwworm Larvae*

Pesticide	Method of Application
Lindane	Smear—3% Pressurized spray
Coumaphos	Spray foam—3% Dust—5%
Bonnel	Aerosol spray—2.5% Smear—5% Dust—5% Pressurized spray—5%

above and 2 cm lateral to the end of the docked tail, passes along the wooled skin adjacent to the bare perineum to a point 4 cm below the bare perineum, where it then deviates laterally onto the medial aspect of the thigh and terminates over the gastrocnemius tendon. The scar widens the bare perineum and, by contraction, obliterates skin wrinkles. The operation should be performed on ewe lambs 5 to 10 weeks of age.

Infested sheep should be treated by removing the wool from the affected skin and applying a topical dressing, such as one of the following larvicides, to deinfest the skin and to repel flies:

1. Ronnel in pressurized can as supplied by the manufacturer.

2. Diazinon in 0.04% concentration.

Eddy, G.W. and Bushland, R.C.: Fleeceworms. In *Yearbook of Agriculture.* USDA, 1956, pp. 175-177.
Hepburn, G.A.: Sheep blowfly research. Onderstepoort. J. Vet. Sci. Anim. Ind., *18*:13-17, 1943.
MacLeod, J.: Species of Diptera concerned in cutaneous myiasis in British sheep. Proc. R. Entomol. Soc. London (A), *12*:127-133, 1937.
Mackerras, I.M. and Mackerras, M.J.: Aust. CSIRO Bull. 181, 1944.
Miller, D.: New Zealand survey of the maggot problem. N.Z. J. Sci. Tech., *21*:240A-244A, 1939.
Sedden, H.R.: *Diseases of Domestic Animals in Australia. Arthropod Infestations.* Aust. Dept. Health., 1967.
Zumpt, F.: *Myiasis in Man and Animals in the Old World.* London, Butterworths, 1965.

Screwworm Myiosis

(SM)

Screwworm myiosis, an acute predation of livestock, is characterized by excruciating invasion and ingestion of injured but living tissues and is caused by the maggots of *Cochliomyia hominivorax,* a dipterous fly. The causative screwworm has been essentially eliminated from the United States. Prior to the eradication programs, however, screwworms annually attacked 1.5 million domestic animals and caused severe economic losses from deaths, disfigurements, and incapacitations, and from the costs of preventive and treatment programs.

OCCURRENCE. SM occurs in all breeds, sexes, and species of warm-blooded animals. The flies attack individuals in anatomic areas of tissue injury, such as accidental trauma, surgical incisions, and parturitional exposures. Favorable conditions for the insect flight and attack develop only during the warm months of late spring, summer, and early autumn.

Geographically, the screwworms of *C. hominivorax* occur only in South America, Central America, and Mexico. Prior to 1959, they also ranged through the southeastern states and the southwestern border states of the United States. From overwintering areas in Texas, New Mexico, Arizona, and Southern California, flies migrated northward during summer as far as Colorado and Nebraska. Related species of screwworms occur in Africa and parts of Asia.

ETIOLOGY AND PATHOGENESIS. Larvae of the fly, *Cochliomyia hominivorax,* cause SM. The blue-green adult flies, measuring 12 to 15 mm in length, contain an orange head and three longitudinal dark stripes on the thorax. Mature larvae taper from a large posterior to small anterior diameters and possess clusters of cuticular spines on each body segment (Fig. 14-9). The larva morphologically resembles a wood screw, from which it derives its common name.

The life cycle is typical of many dipterous flies. Female flies, attracted to animal injuries such as surgical incisions, accidental wounds, dog bites, bloody excretions, and severed umbilici, deposit clusters of about 250 overlapping eggs on or near the injuries. A single female may produce up to 4000 eggs. Hatching occurs after 10 to 12 hours. The larvae

Fig. 14-9. Screwworm larva, *Cochliomyia hominivorax.* × 4.

bore into the host and tear away and consume live tissue.

Growth is rapid, and after 3 to 6 days the larvae mature, drop from the host, enter the soil, and pupate. Pupation lasts 3 to 7 days in warm climates, but may extend to several weeks in cool climates. Following emergence, the adult flies mate and begin egg-laying within 5 to 6 days. The average length of the entire life cycle is 21 days. Adults and pupae overwinter in mild climates of the southern United States and Mexico. The strong flying adults may travel 21 km per week.

The newly hatched larvae crowd together, dig into, feed on, and rapidly devour live host tissue. Infested tissue attracts additional female flies, which oviposit new batches of eggs. Toxemia, continuous destruction of tissue, and shock cause agonizing death of the host.

CLINICAL SIGNS AND POSTMORTEM LESIONS. Sheep affected with SM manifest excruciating pain. Apprehensive and nervous, they separate from the flock and, in seclusion of shade, bite and scratch the infested wound. Body temperature may rise. The discharging wound exudate emits malodors and attracts many species of flies. Close examination of the cleaned wound reveals clusters of crowded screwworms and the cavities created by them. If untreated, the area of infestation continues to expand through the addition of new eggs. In terminal stages, the animal is depressed, disoriented, and usually prostrated. Death occurs after a course of about 10 days.

At necropsy of fatally infested animals, prominent changes are in the wounded tissue. Discharging exudates stain adjacent wool and skin. Removal of exudate and debris reveals crowded nests of larvae in various stages of growth. The tissue cavity may be several centimeters in diameter. Infestations in the abdominal wall may extend into the peritoneal cavity. Trauma from biting and scratching may exist.

DIAGNOSIS. Veterinarians diagnose SM by finding and identifying larvae of *C. hominivorax* in a wound. Suggestive signs attract attention: isolation from the flock and scratching, biting, and rubbing injured tissue. In-endemic areas, producers quickly learn to identify the disease and the infesting larvae.

The differential diagnosis requires consideration of infestation with the common blowfly that randomly deposits single eggs throughout the necrotic wound surface; its live larvae do not cluster together, but move independently about the wound surface.

TREATMENT AND PREVENTION. Animals in the early stages of infestation should be treated to remove all larvae and to protect against reinfestation. Wool from around the infestation should be clipped. The wound should be cleaned by removing larvae and debris, and dressed with one of the following preparations: (1) EQ 135 to kill and repel larvae and flies, or (2) coumaphos or ronnel spray.

Producers prevent SM by avoiding accidental injuries and by scheduling surgical procedures and parturition during fly-free seasons. When unavoidable injuries and operations do occur during fly season, the traumatized animals should receive topical applications of repellant preparations such as Smear 62, EQ 335, or sprays of coumaphos. Vulnerable animals should be observed frequently for possible screwworm attacks.

A more satisfactory method of prevention is regional or national eradication of screwworms. Although the initial costs are high, the subsequent economic savings to the livestock industry and the economy more than compensate for the investment. Successful eradication programs have been applied to Curaçao, southeastern United States, and southwestern United States. A successful eradicative program contains the following essential items: (1) systematic and strategic release of sterile male flies into the natural fly population, (2) inspection of all ingressing livestock for screwworm conveyors, (3) intraregional inspections for local outbreaks, and (4) dissemination of program information to the involved public.

Baumhover, A.H., et al.: Screwworm control through release of sterilized flies. J. Econ. Entomol., *48*:462-468, 1955.
Bushland, R.C. and Hopkins, D.E.: Experiments with screwworm flies sterilized by x-rays. J. Econ. Entomol., 44:725, 1951.
Facts about Screwworm Eradication. USDA ARS 91-22, 1963, pp. 1-13.
Knipling, E.F.: Possibilities of insect control through use of sexually sterile males. J. Econ. Entomol., *48*:459, 1955.
Knipling, E.F.: Sterile-male method of population control. Science, *130*:902-904, 1959.
Knipling, E.F.: The sterility principle. Agric. Sci., Rev., *1*:2-12, 1963.
Runner, G.S.: Effect of roentgen rays on tobacco or cigarette beetles. J. Agric. Res., 6:383-388, 1916.
Smith, C.L.: Mass production of screwworms for eradication programs. J. Econ. Entomol., 53:1110-1116, 1960.
Status of Screwworm in the United States. USDA ARS 22-79, June, 1962, pp. 1-13.

Ked Infestation

(*Sheep tick*)

Ked infestation, a chronic dermatitis of sheep, is characterized by itching annoyance and seasonal fluctuation and is caused by *Melophagus ovinus*, a wingless fly. Because this parasitic disease has universal distribution and high incidence, reduces productivity, and causes material waste, it concerns the entire sheep industry. Economic losses result from unthriftiness, reduced production of meat and wool, damage to wool, pelt damage, and the costs of control programs.

ETIOLOGY AND PATHOGENESIS. *Melophagus ovinus,* also known as keds and sheep ticks, causes the infestation. The adult fly, measuring 4 to 6 mm in length, has no wings but possesses three pairs of strong legs, each with a robust claw. The tough brown-gray pest has a broad head with stout piercing mouth parts.

The ked spends its entire life cycle as a parasite on the skin of sheep. Within 3 to 4 days after emergence from the pupa, the viviparous female mates and begins the production of a series of 10 to 15 larvae. The gestation period is 10 to 12 days. Following parturition, the female glues the larva, 3 to 4 mm in length, to a wool fiber, where it forms an external case and pupates for 19 and 24 days in summer and winter, respectively. Even though the female lives 4 to 5 months, a complete generation of the insect develops in 32 to 40 days.

Reproduction continues through all seasons, but climatic and other factors profoundly influence the seasonal population dynamics: following winter shearing, many keds immobilize or freeze and drop from the host; spring shearing removes large numbers of keds; summer solar energy generates intolerably high skin temperatures; and autumnal and winter environments create favorable skin temperatures. These factors cause regular summer population declines and winter population rises. The numbers per sheep in summer may be few and in winter, 300 to 400.

Adult keds feed by piercing the skin and ingesting sheep blood. The annoying process diverts the sheep's attention from peaceful feeding and thus reduces the production of both meat and wool. Large numbers of feeding keds gradually exsanguinate the host and cause variable degrees of anemia. In addition, excreta from the keds stain the wool and thereby increase the cost of processing. The bite of feeding keds causes an irritation and inflammation which causes a rash known as Cockle. This rash may not be detectable until the pelt is tanned causing a severe price discount. Ked transmission occurs by direct contact among crowding ewes and rams and between nursing ewes and their lambs. Although the entire life cycle of the sheep ked is completed on the sheep host and most transmission is from direct contact, it is possible for the sheep ked to drop from the host in a suitable environment, survive for 1 to 3 weeks and infest a new host.

CLINICAL SIGNS. Because of their size and color, both adult and pupal keds on lambs and shorn sheep are conspicuous to casual examination, but on wooled sheep they are concealed within the fleece, and their quantitation requires close inspection between parted fibers. Topographically, they concentrate on the skin of the neck, sides, rump, and abdomen.

Although small numbers of the parasite result in no disturbance, large numbers cause restlessness, reduced consumption of feed, and retarded growth rate. Affected sheep bite, kick, and rub their infested skins, and the mechanically damaged wool may be rough,

broken, and detached. In infested flocks, all individuals are continuously parasitized, but few if any sheep die from uncomplicated ked infestation.

DIAGNOSIS. Veterinarians diagnose ked infestation by finding pathogenic numbers of the parasites on the skin and in the fleece. Keds are readily distinguished from other arthropod parasites of the skin by size, color, and general morphologic characteristics having three pair of legs compared to eight for the true tick species.

TREATMENT. A successful voluntary ked eradication program is in progress in a number of the western states of the U.S.A. The program consists of treating of all sheep on a premises with an effective insecticide. This treatment is done on an annual basis following shearing and prior to lambing with monitoring to determine the effectiveness and need for further treatment. The success of the program is dependent upon treatment of all animals in the flock with quarantine and treatment of all introductions. Although the organophosphate pour-on insecticides are effective, Ectrin, a synthetic pyrethum with good residual activity and easily appliable, is an approved product for use on sheep. Dusts and dips listed in Table 14-5 are available and effective but each has disadvantages. Once treated and free of keds the sheep should not follow ked-infested sheep on a premise except after an interval of several weeks. Animals from unclean flocks should be quarantined and treated before joining flocks. Clean sheep should not follow ked-infested sheep on a premise except after an interval of several weeks.

Gecheva, G.: Pathogenic role of *M. ovinus* in sheep: Hematological aspects. Vet. Med. Nauki, (Sofia), 9:89-94, 1972.

Gecheva, G.: Seasonal dynamics of *Melophagus ovinus* in sheep. Vet. Med. Nauki (Sofia), 8:67-71, 1971.

Imes, M.: Sheep tick and its eradication. USDA Farmer's Bull. 798, 1944.

Nelson, W.A. and Qually, M.C.: Annual cycles in numbers of sheep ked. Can. J. Anim. Sci., 38:194-199, 1958.

Nelson, W.A. and Slen, S.B.: Weight gains and wool growth in sheep infested with *M. ovinus*. Exp. Parasitol., 22:223-226, 1968.

Strickman, Dr., Lloyd, J., and Kumar, R.: Relocation of hosts by the sheep ked (Diptera: Hippoboscidae). J. Econ. Entomol., 77:437-439, 1984.

Pediculosis

(*Lousiness*)

Lousiness, a chronic dermatitis of sheep, is characterized by constant annoyance, itching, and seasonal variation and is caused by pathogenic numbers of lice, which are ectoparasitic insects. Even though the condition has high incidence and probably occurs in most flocks of all sheep-producing countries, it attracts little attention from producers and insignificant research investment. Universally, it begets acceptance. Despite this neglect, the disease causes considerable, but unmeasured, material waste. Economic losses result from unthriftiness, retarded growth, damaged wool, and diminished production of meat and wool.

ETIOLOGY AND PATHOGENESIS. Three species of lice—*Damalinia ovis, Linognathus ovillus,* and *L. pedalis*—usually infest sheep. Table 14-4 presents some of their morphologic and biologic characteristics.

1. *Damalinia ovis.* The body louse is widely distributed throughout sheep-producing countries. The insect contains a broad head with chewing mouth parts that eat epithelial scales, fibers, and skin debris, and its movements irritate the skin and annoy the host. Although the entire life cycle is spent on the sheep, the numbers of lice and their topographic distribution are profoundly influenced by climatic factors. Because of summer solar radiation, the mean temperature of 3-cm length wool reaches 81°C at the tips and 42°C at the skin. But nymphs and adults are killed in 60 minutes at 48°C, in 30 minutes at 50°C, and in 5 minutes at 56°C, and females diminish oviposition after 4 hours at 55°C. Because of temperature gradients, females attach new eggs to wool fibers about 6 mm from the skin. Because of loss of insect numbers, partly from intolerably high fleece and skin temperatures, the population declines numerically during summer, increases during winter, and reaches a peak in early spring.

2. *Linognathus ovillus.* The blue body louse occurs in Australia, New Zealand, United States, Britain, and probably other sheep-producing countries. The thin, elongated lead contains piercing mouth parts that penetrate the host skin and ingest blood. This species inhabits the haired and wooled skin of the face and, as the population increases, the mobile individuals scatter over the wooled skin of the entire body. During spring shearing, large numbers of lice remain with the fleece and thus separate from the sheep. Furthermore, environmental temperatures of 28°C are accompanied by skin temperatures of 38°C, which inhibit egg development and hatching. These losses of insect numbers lead to summer population declines, but during subsequent months, a winter increase and an early spring peak occur in a regular pattern for seasonal population dynamics.

3. *L. pedalis.* The foot louse occurs in Australia, United States, Britain, South America, Africa, and possibly other sheep-producing countries. The thin head contains piercing mouth parts that penetrate host skin and ingest blood. This species inhabits the haired skin between the hooves and knees and hocks and usually forms stationary clusters.

Within a cluster, the density may reach several hundred insects per square centimeter, but between clusters the number may be nil. Under population pressure of rapidly increasing numbers, however, the colony may expand dorsally onto wooled skin of the scrotum and abdomen. Through adaptation to fluctuating climatic factors around sheep limbs, this species has acquired resistance to low environmental temperatures; consequently, when separated from the host, *L. pedalis* endures cold weather twice as long as some other species, such as *L. ovillus*.

Spring shearing decimates the population occupying the abdominal skin, but has essentially no reducing effect on the main population of the haired skin. Summer solar radiation, however, as with other species of lice, raises both environmental and skin temperatures to intolerable levels and thus reduces the population, but during autumn and winter, the population numerically increases and reaches a peak in early spring. This population pattern of summer decline and winter increase generally prevails, but the high and low levels vary with climatic factors.

CLINICAL SIGNS. The symptoms of lousiness vary with the degree of infestation. Small numbers occurring during summer cause no clinical manifestations, but the large numbers frequently prevailing during late winter cause skin irritation and itching. Sheep heavily infested with lice become restless, consume little feed, and may lose live weight. Animals with body infestation rub, bite, and kick the itching skin and thereby damage and detach parts of the wool. Dense accumulations of *L. ovillus* on the face discolor white wool and hair to a conspicuous gray. Heavy infestations with *L. pedalis* cause foot stamping and biting. Some sheep may develop a degree of anemia from prolonged support of sucking lice.

DIAGNOSIS. Veterinarians diagnose lousiness on evidence of skin irritation, itching, and dense accumulations of lice on the sites of predilection. The differential diagnosis requires consideration of trombidiosis, foot scabies, strawberry foot rot, and ked infestation. Each of these diseases produces prominent dermatitis, and the causative organisms can be identified in gross and microscopic examinations.

TREATMENT. All sheep of flocks infested with lice or ticks should be treated within 6 weeks of shearing with one of the procedures listed in Table 14-5. Animals from unclean flocks should be quarantined and treated before joining clean flocks. Clean sheep should not follow infested sheep on a property except after an interval of at least 21 days.

Hantsbarger, W.M.: Insect control handbook for Colorado. Coop. Ext. Serv. Exp. Stat, 1973.

MacFarlane, W.V., Morris, R.J.H., and Howard, B.: Heat and water in tropical Merino sheep. Aust. J. Agric. Res., 9:217-228, 1958.

Murray, M.D.: Biologies of *L. pedalis* and *L. ovillus*, Aust. J. Zool., 11:153-156, 1963a.

Murray, M.D.: Distribution of eggs of *Damalinia ovis* on sheep. Aust. J. Zool., 5173-182, 1957.

Murray, M.D.: Infestation of sheep with face louse. Aust. Vet. J., 31:22-26, 1955.

Murray, M.D.: Influence of shearing and solar energy on populations of *D. ovis*. Aust. J. Zool., 16:725-738, 1968.

Murray, M.D.: Influence of skin temperature on populations of *Linognathus pedalis*. Aust. J. Zool., 8:349-356, 1960a.

Murray, M.D.: Influence of temperature and humidity on development of eggs of *Damalinia ovis*. Aust. J. Zool., 8:357-362, 1960b.

Murray, M.D.: Populations of *L. ovillus*. Aust. J. Zool. 11:157-172, 1963b.

Murray, M.D. and Gordon, G.: Population dynamics of *D. ovis*. Aust. J. Zool., 17:179-186, 1969.

Peterson, H.O. and Bushland, R.C.: Lice of sheep. In *Yearbook of Agriculture*. USDA, 1956, pp. 411-414.

Scott, M.T.: Bionomics of *L. pedalis*. Aust. J. Agric. Res., 1:465-470, 1950.

Fleece Rot

Fleece rot is a lesion of the skin characterized by a superficial inflammatory condition and seropurulent exudation with a putrifactive odor which attracts blowfly (*Lucilia cuprina*) to oviposition. Fleece rot is an affliction causing severe financial loss through down grading of wool or subsequent body strike (cutaneous myosis) by blowfly. The condition is common to areas of Australia with prolonged rainy periods and possibly other regions with similar climatic and ecosystems. *P. aeruginosa* is a motile organism which is a normal inhabitant, along with numerous other bacteria, of the fleece and is activated to multiply on the skin surface when conditions of protein moisture and temperature become ideal. This generally occurs during periods of continued wetting of the fleece by rain which can also alter the protective resistance of normal skin. *P. aerugenosa* produces proteolytic enzymes which may contribute to the inflammatory process with resultant production of excessive protein on the skin surface. The protein on the skin surface is an ideal media for first-instar blowfly larvae. *P. aerugenosa* also produces a bacteriostatic inhibitor which prevents growth of other bacteria.

Histopathology *P. aerugenosa* produces a mild inflammation with an increase in thickness of the epidermis and dermis with hyperkeratinization especially noticeable in follicular openings, mild acanthosis, edema of the basal layers with focal spongiosis of the stratum spinosum, and stratum germination. There is a mild hyperemia, edema, and polymorphonuclear cell infiltration of the dermis with microabscesses in the stratum corneum. The dermis has an increase in numbers of mononuclear lymphocytes, mast cells, eosinophils, and basophils.

Clinically fleece rot is characterized by a greenish discoloration of the wool fibers with a crust covered seropurulent exudative lesion usually over the withers and down the sides and accompanied by a distinctive putrefactive odor. Diagnosis is based on a history of continuous wetting of the wool during prolonged rainy weather, the characteristics of the lesion, and, if needed, bacterial isolation of the causative agent. The lesions are treated by removing the wool, thorough cleansing with an iodine scrub, and applying a drying agent with antibiotics, such as one of the furacin topical sprays. Fleece rot caused by *P. aerugenosa* can be prevented by vaccination although the full implication of immunization needs further investigation.

Burrell, D.: Immunization of sheep against experimental *Pseudomonas aeruginosa* dermatitis and fleece rot associated body strike. Aust. Vet. J., *62*:55-57, 1985.

Burrell, D., Merritt, G., Watts, J., and Walker, K.: Experimental production of dermatitis in sheep with *Pseudomonas aeruginosa*. Aust. Vet. J., *59*:140-144, 1982.

Gtteradi, S., Sutherland, S., Monzu, N., and Johnson, K.: Field observations on body strike in sheep affected with dermatophilosis and fleece rot. Aust. Vet. J., *60*:27-28, 1983.

Merritt, G. and Watts, J.: An *in-vitro* technique for studying fleece rot and fly strike in sheep. Aust. Vet. J., *54*:513-516, 1978.

Merritt, G. and Watts, J.: The changes in protein concentration and bacteria of fleece and skin during the development of fleece rot and body strike in sheep. Aust. Vet. J., *54*:517-520, 1978.

Sutherland, S., Gheradi, S., and Monzu, N.: Body strike in sheep affected with dermatophilus with or without fleece rot. Aust. Vet. J., *60*:88-89, 1983.

15

DISEASES OF THE FEET

Contagious Foot Rot

*(CFR; foot rot; hoof rot;
pietin; pedero)*

Contagious foot rot, an acute or chronic contagious epidermitis of ovine feet, is characterized by lameness and bidigital separation of the hoof corneum from the basal epithelium and derma. It is caused by the interaction of two nonsporing anaerobic bacteria. Because the disease is universally distributed, affects all ages, and recurs, it is of major concern to the entire sheep industry.

Economic losses result from unthriftiness and loss of live weight, damage to wool quality, occasional deaths, legal restraints against national and international sheep commerce, and the cost in labor and materials for treatment, continuous vigilance for outbreaks, technical research, and eradicative programs. Even though research has established the principles and education has inculcated the skills for eradicating CFR, it persists in all sheep-producing countries and prevails at great cost against the industry. Foot rot of sheep and foot rot of cattle probably are not intertransferable.

OCCURRENCE. CFR occurs in all breeds, sexes, and ages of sheep, but Merinos are more susceptible than other breeds, and adults contract a higher incidence than do lambs. The disease develops in range, pasture, farm, and feedlot sheep and, following clinical recovery, may recur in the same flocks and indi-

viduals. Most outbreaks of CFR occur during the warm months of spring, summer, and autumn following prolonged periods of rainfall or continuous exposure to surface water in pasture. Besides sheep, the disease also affects goats.

Geographically, CFR develops in all sheep-producing countries, but the incidence is especially high in Australia, New Zealand, United States, Britain, and India.

ETIOLOGY AND PATHOGENESIS. *Bacterioides nodosus* and *Fusobacterium necrophorum,* pathogenic synergists, cause CFR. Other organisms, such as *Spirocheata penortha,* motile fusiforms, and *Corynebacterium pyogenes,* often enter the lesions and play an unknown role in the pathogenesis. *B. nodosus* is a nonsporing, nonmotile, noncapsulating, granular, gram-negative, anaerobic bacillus, measuring 0.6 to 1.2×2 to $10 \, \mu$m. Slightly curving sides and bulbous ends, distinguishing features of the rods, help identify the organisms in stained smears and tissue sections from infected feet.

The organism grows in media enriched with horse serum and cysteine at 37°C in an atmosphere of 5 to 10% CO_2. Flourishing surface colonies, usually small but often reaching diameters of 1 mm in 2 to 3 days, characteristically etch into the enriched medium surface. The bacteria settle in epidermal lesions of sheep hooves, where they persist for prolonged periods. In contaminated soil and manure, they survive for less than 2 weeks.

317

B. nodosus has at least 20 serotypes each with varying amounts of pili and production of protease. These two components constitute the variability in pathogenicity and to a degree the immunogenic response of the host. Although breed susceptibility and macro and microenvironment play a role in the severity of the lesions, the strains of *B. nodosus* vary in the amount of pili and protease production which are the dominant factors governing virulence; diffuse polar material and perhaps the additional layer may also be associated with virulence and immunoprotection. The invasive properties of various strains produce a spectrum of clinical entities ranging from benign (a mild dermatitis and inflammation of the skin in the interdigital space) to severe. The benign strains do not cause undermining lesions and heal spontaneously with dry conditions, do not recur or become chronic. Other strains with intermediate invasiveness cause lesions of the interdigital space with undermining of the sole, but have a tendency for self cure and do not become chronic. Strains with abundant pili and protease production have the ability to cause severe lesions with undermining of the sole, axial, and abaxial walls resulting in hoof deformities and a high incidence of chronic cases. The immunogenic properties of *B. nodosus* depend upon the pilus antigen for the major homologous protective immunogen. There are at least two other immunogens possibly located in the cell envelope which contribute to heterologous protection.

F. necrophorum is a nonsporing, nonmotile, noncapsulating, gram-negative, anaerobic bacterium. This pleomorphic organism, in young cultures and infected tissues, forms nonbranching filaments up to 100 μm in length and, in old cultures, coccobacillary rods 0.5 to 1.5 μm in length. Although difficult to culture, it grows in Rosenow's brainbroth and on blood agar, where small opaque colonies form.

The organism produces acid and gas from glucose, maltose, and glycerol, but not from xylose, rhamnose, mannose, raffinose, inulin, dulcitol, salicin, sorbitol, or inositol. It liquefies solid serum but not gelatin or albumin. In both liquid media and infected tissue, it produces an exotoxin, leukocidin, which kills leukocytes protecting itself and other bacteria from phagocytosis resulting in dermonecrosis. Various strains contain heterogeneous antigens. The two principal virulence determinants are leukotoxin and lipopolysaccharides. There are undetermined cellular and cytoplasmic antigens which may play a role in immunoprotection. Although animals that recover from necrophorus infection are not usually immune to subsequent attacks, advances are being made in developing a vaccine that will provide protective immunity. Animals that recover from necrophorus infections are not immune to subsequent attacks.

F. necrophorum universally exists in manure, in the alimentary tracts, and on skins and feet of all animals, and consequently is part of sheep environment. Its pathogenicity is low for healthy surface membranes but high for non-covering tissue.

CFR is transmitted by direct and indirect contact with *B. nodosus*. Following clinical recovery from CFR, some feet carry the viable organisms in cavities, crevices, cracks, and other deformities of hooves. Under conditions of warm temperatures and abundant moisture, the bacteria multiply and contaminate moist soil and manure, where they contact susceptible feet. Macerated feet and feet affected with scald, a moist superficial interdigital dermatitis, are highly susceptible to the pathogens. Sources of infection for flock outbreaks include introduced sheep, relapsed sheep, and infected premises.

The pathogenesis of CFR begins with transmission of *B. nodosus* from the environment to macerated or scald-affected interdigital skin. At the skin-horn junction near the axial bulbar notches, *F. necrophorum,* as the first step in the disease process, colonizes the moist epidermal surface; only then does *B. nodosus,* as the second step, adhere to the host tissue, colonize the sites on the feet that probably have lowered oxygen tension, penetrate the surface tissue and due to the pili action involve the epidermis of the hoof. By action of its powerful protease, *B. nodosus* liquefies the cells of the stratum granulosum and stratum spinosum and thus cleaves the cells and separates the hoof corneum from the basal epithelium and derma. *B. nodosus* stimulates no host reaction, but *F. necrophorum,* following *B. nodosus* into the tissue, provokes a strong and damaging inflammation. The failure of natural infection to stimulate agglutinin titers accounts for the lack of durable immunity. Protective antibodies are formed relative to the amount of pili present on the invading strain of *B. nodosus*. After clinical recovery, some feet carry *B. nodosus* in abnormal cavities, cracks, and deformities of the hoof.

CLINICAL SIGNS AND LESIONS. Within 10 to 20 days after susceptible sheep enter an infected area, lameness in one or more feet develops. Lameness varies in degree and may cause carriage of one foot, knee-walking, or recumbency. Although a complete spectrum of disease entities occur, the strain of *B. nodosus* and the amount of pili and protease production affect the severity of the lesion. Some strains with few pili and low protease production cause a benign foot rot or scald characterized by a mild inflammation of the interdigital skin and slight undermining of the hoof sole causing only slight lameness. These usually heal spontaneously and cause very little effect on production. Severely affected animals, because of discomfort and inability to graze, lose body weight and diminish milk production. In early stages of the disease, the interdigital skin of affected feet is moist, hyperemic, and superficially necrotic. Later, and beginning at the skin-horn junction near the axial bulbar notches, the heel bulbs, soles, and axial and abaxial walls show undermining and loosening of the corneum (Fig. 15-1). Removal of the loose horn reveals pultaceous tissue, from which a fetid odor emanates. Old cases, after healing, may show hoof deformities with cavities, cracks, and pits extending into the corneum of bulbs and soles. The morbidity in affected flocks commonly reaches 70%, but the mortality is negligible. The course among untreated sheep ranges from several weeks to 3 months or longer.

Fig. 15-1. Undermined soles and walls of hooves from sheep with contagious foot rot. The loose soles have been removed. × 1.0.

A mild form is caused by some strains that closely resemble the severe form, except a smaller proportion of sheep and feet are involved, regression is more frequent, and chronicity is lacking. Benign and mild forms of foot rot have little effect on body weight and wool production, whereas the severe form reduces wool growth and body weight appreciably.

DIAGNOSIS. Veterinarians diagnose CFR when undermining of the corneum of the bulbs, soles, and walls of hooves occurs in a large percentage of sheep of a flock. In case of doubt, stained smears of degenerating hoof tissue can be examined for *B. nodosus*.

The differential diagnosis requires consideration of other causes of lameness, e.g., foot abscess, strawberry foot rot, bluetongue, foot-and-mouth disease, and contagious ecthyma.

TREATMENT AND CONTROL. Effective treatment and elimination of CFR consist of separating the animals into apparently healthy and obviously affected flocks. After deeply paring all hooves of all sheep, the feet are disinfected and the flocks placed in separate clean pens or pastures. The reason for paring the hooves is to expose all foci of *B. nodosus* organisms to contact with the disinfectant.

Zinc sulfate, copper sulfate and formalin have been used for foot bathing. Zinc sulfate is currently the chemical of choice due to the undesirable side effects of copper sulfate and formalin. A 10% (W/V) zinc sulfate plus a 0.2% (V/V) anionic surfactant (preferably a detergent with a high concentration of sodium dodecyl sulphate) is prepared by dissolving technical grade $ZnSO_4$ $7H_2O$ in water to a 50% W/V concentrated solution then diluting 1:4 with water for use. Foot bathing twice weekly and holding the sheep in the footbath for at least 5 minutes improves the cure rate. Three 1-hour foot soaks at weekly intervals in the zinc sulfate is effective in association with foot paring in severe cases or without foot paring in mild and benign cases. Walk through footbaths are helpful in preventing new cases but are ineffective for treatment. *B. nodosus* is highly susceptible to penicillin. Tetracycline, erythromycin, tylosin tartrate, nitrofurazone, and dihydrostreptomycin sulfate are relatively effective. To be effective, high antibiotic levels must be maintained over an extended period of time. Use of antibiotics in large scale operations is not economically feasible. Nitrofurazone ointment followed by bandaging or fitting of a boot may be used in individual cases. Dietary zinc and organic iodides are of doubtful benefit. Commercially available pilus antigen vaccines containing the strains of *B. nodosus* common to the area are highly effective in preventing foot rot and have some therapeutic value. Two initial vaccinations 30 days apart followed by an annual booster is required. Due to the short duration of immune stimulation, the vaccination strategy must be designed to provide the highest immune response during the peak exposure period. Although the control strategy will vary with geography, environment and management practices the following factors remain constant in a control or eradication scheme:

1. Early detection, identification, and isolation of all suspected cases.

2. Early treatment consisting of paring and foot bathing or soaking in zinc sulfate.

3. Placing noninfected and recently treated sheep on pastures which have been free of sheep for 2 weeks to prevent reinfection.

4. A vaccination program with a commercial vaccine which includes the strains prevalent to the area.

5. Cull all sheep which do not respond to early treatment and those chronic cases with mishapen hoofs which act as reservoirs of infection.

6. Prevent reintroducing the disease by not mixing of sheep, not using common facilities, and not purchasing sheep from unknown sources.

Animal Health Yearbook: FAO-WHO-OIE (Italy), 1970.

Beveridge, W.I.B.: Foot rot in sheep: a transmissible disease due to infection with *Fusiformis nodosa* (n. sp.). Studies on its cause, epidemiology and control. Aust. CSIRO Bull. 140, 1941, pp. 1-53.

Cross, R.F.: Response of sheep to various topical, oral, and parenteral treatments for foot rot. JAVMA, *173*: 1569-1570, 1978.

Cross, R. and Parker, C.: Oral administration of zinc sulfate for control of ovine foot rot. JAVMA, *178*:704-705, 1981.

Cross, R. and Parker, C.: Zinc sulfate foot bath for control of ovine foot rot. JAVMA, *178*:706-707, 1981.

Deane, H.M. and Jensen, R.: The pathology of contagious foot rot in sheep. AJVR, *16*:203-208, 1955.

Egerton, J., Laing, E., and Mulley, R.: Failure of oral zinc therapy to alleviate *Bacteroides nodosus* infection in cattle and sheep. Aust. Vet. J., *62*:85-88, 1985.

Egerton, J., Ribeiro, L., Kieran, P., and Thorley, C.: Onset and remission of ovine foot rot. Aust. Vet. J., *60*:334-336, 1983.

Egerton, J.R. and Parsonson, I.M.: Benign foot rot—a specific interdigital dermatitis of sheep associated with infection by less proteolytic strains of *Fusiformis nodosa*. Aust. Vet. J., *45*:345-349, 1969.

Egerton, J.R., Parsonson, I.M., and Graham, N.P.H.: Parenteral chemotherapy of ovine foot rot. Aust. Vet. J., *44*:275-283, 1968.

Egerton, J.R., Roberts, D.S., and Parsonson, I.M.: The etiology and pathogenesis of ovine foot rot. I. A histological study of the bacterial invasion. J. Comp. Pathol., *79*:207-215, 1969.

Ellis, R., Kimberling, C., Winn, D., and Swanson, V.: The efficacy of foot vax in the control of foot rot. SID Research Digest, Winter, 1986, pp. 7-10.

Emery, D., Stewart, D., and Clark, B.: The comparative susceptibility of five breeds of sheep to foot rot. Aust. Vet. J., *61*:85-88, 1984.

Emery, D., Stewart, D., and Clark, B.: The structural integrity of pili from *Bacteroides nodosus* is required to elicit protective immunity against foot rot in sheep. Aust. Vet. J., *61*:237-238, 1984.

Every, D. and Skerman, M.: Protection of sheep against experimental foot rot by vaccination with pili purified *Bacteroides nodosus*. N.Z. Vet. J., *30*:156-158, 1982.

Every, D. and Skerman, M.: Surface structure of *Bacteroides nodosus* in relationship to virulence and immunoprotection in sheep. J. Gen. Microbiol., *129*: 225-234, 1983.

Gradin, J. and Schmitz, J.: Susceptibility of *Bacteroides nodosus* to various antimicrobial agents. JAVMA, *183*:434-437, 1983.

Graham, N.P.H. and Egerton, J.R.: Pathogenesis of ovine foot rot: the role of some environmental factors. Aust. Vet. J., *44*:235-240, 1968.

Marsh, H. and Tunnicliff, E.A.: Experimental studies of foot rot in sheep. Montana State Coll. Exp. Stat. Bull. 285, 1934.

Mohler, J.R. and Washburn, H.J.: Foot rot of sheep. USDA, Bur. Anim. Ind. Bull. 63:1-39, 1904.

Murname, D.: Foot rot in sheep. Aust. CSIRO, Bull. 6, 1933, pp. 252-259.

Roberts, D.S. and Egerton, J.R.: The etiology and pathogenesis of ovine foot rot. II. The pathogenic association of *Fusiformis nodosa* and *S. necrophorus*. J. Comp. Pathol., *79*:217-227, 1969.

Ross, A.: Formalin and foot rot in sheep. N.Z. Vet. J., *31*:170-172, 1983.

Ross, A. and Titterington, D.: Injection site lesions of foot rot vaccines in sheep. N.A. Vet. J., *32*:6-8, 1984.

Scanlan, C., Garret, P., Campbell, F.: Ovine contagious foot rot. The Compendium of Continuing Education, 7:515-518, 1985.

Simon, W., Alexander, B., and McGowan, B.: Purification, characterization and serologic characteristics of *Bacteroides nodosus* pili and use of a purified pili vaccine in sheep. Am. J. Vet. Res., *44*:1676-1681, 1983.

Skerman, T., Erasmuson, S., and Morrison, L.: Duration of resistance to experimental foot rot infection in Romney and Merino sheep vaccinated with *Bacteroides nodosus* oil adjuvant vaccine. N.Z. Vet. J., *30*:27-31, 1982.

Skerman, T., Green, R., Hughes, J., and Herceg, M.: Comparison of foot bathing treatments for ovine foot rot using formalin or zinc sulfate. N.Z. Vet. J., *31*:91-95, 1983.

Skerman, T., et al.: Failure of orally administered zinc to prevent experimentally induced foot rot in sheep. N.Z. Vet. J., *31*:54-57, 1983.

Sterk, V., Beslin, R., and Vulie, I.: Protective value of a vaccine against foot rot in sheep. Veterinski Glasnik, *30*:1009-1011, 1976.

Stewart, B., et al.: A *Bacteroides nodosus* immunogen, distinct from the pilus, which induces cross-protective immunity in sheep vaccinated against foot rot. Aust. Vet. J., *60*:83-85, 1983.

Stewart, D.: Review of foot rot. Diagnosis and the role of vaccination. Sheep Production and Preventive Medicine Proceedings, *67*:487-491, 1983.

Stewart, D.F.: The treatment of contagious foot rot in sheep by the topical application of chloromycetin. Aust. Vet. J., *30*:209-212, 1954.

Stewart, D., Clark, B., and Jarrett, R.: Differences between strains of *Bacteroides nodosus* in their effects on the severity of foot rot, body weight and wool growth in Merino sheep. Aust. Vet. J., *61*:348-352, 1984.

Stewart, D., et al.: Effect of pilus dose and type of Freund's adjuvant on antibody and protective responses of vaccinated sheep to *Bacteroides nodosus*. Res. Vet. Sci., *35*:130-137, 1983.

Stewart, D., et al.: The protection given by pilus and whole cell vaccines of *Bacteroides nodosus* strain 198 against ovine foot rot induced by strains of different serogroups. Aust. Vet. J., *62*:153-159, 1985.

Thomas, J.H.: Pathogenesis of foot rot in sheep with reference to protease of *Fusiformis nodosa*. Aust. J. Agric. Res., *15*:1001-1016, 1964.

Foot Abscess

(*FA; digital suppuration*)

Foot abscess, an acute or chronic suppurative laminitis of a single digit, is characterized by severe lameness and discharge of pus through sinuses near the coronet and is caused by bacteria. Because FA is widely distributed with modest incidence, the disease has considerable importance to the sheep industry and causes financial waste to some individual enterprises. Economic losses result from temporary incapacitation of rams and ewes, from live weight loss, and from the cost of labor and materials for prolonged treatments. The disease merits scientific research to improve understanding of most of its aspects.

OCCURRENCE. FA occurs in adult sheep of all breeds. Heavy rams and pregnant ewes 2 to 5 years of age often contract the disease while grazing wet pastures. Outbreaks are common during wet seasons where sheep are pastured on heavily contaminated ground. The incidence can be high during the dry season when animals are grazed on alfalfa stubble which damages the interdigital skin allowing an area for entry of the causative organism. Some outbreaks are associated with sheep traveling over crusted snow thus damaging the interdigital skin. Most cases develop during late spring and summer, but the disease, once established, continues into subsequent seasons. Geographically, FA commonly occurs in Australia, New Zealand, United States, Europe, and probably other sheep-producing countries.

ETIOLOGY AND PATHOGENESIS. Although *Fusobacterium necrophorum* and *Coryne-bacterium pyogenes* cause most cases of FA, other species of bacteria, such as *Streptococci* and *E. coli*, may gain entrance to infected feet. For a description of *F. necrophorum*, see the discussion of contagious foot rot. *C. pyogenes*, a nonmotile, nonsporing, noncapsulating, gram-positive, anaerobic bacillus, measures 0.2 to 0.3 × 0.5 to 2.0 μm. It grows on standard serum-containing media, and growth accelerates from reduced oxygen tension. On blood and serum agar, the small colonies cause beta hemolysis of erythrocytes and, after several days' growth, become dry and opaque. Cultures produce acid and gas from glucose, maltose, galactose, lactose, fructose, mannose, sucrose, and dextrin, but not from arabinose, xylose, inulin, salicin, dulcitol, mannitol, and glycerol. The organism is pathogenic for most domestic mammals.

The pathogenesis of FA begins with penetration of the corneum of the bulb or sole by the causative bacteria. *F. necrophorum*, a normal inhabitant of the ruminant digestive tract and subsequently a fecal contaminant, does not possess invasive properties, therefore, it is unable to colonize or invade the normal intact epidermis. Maceration of the epidermic in the interdigital space from continuous wetness as encountered during prolonged rainy seasons or abrasions to the interdigital skin from stones, stubble, mud, ice, etc. allows for a mode of entry of the causative organism. The bacteria present in the feces contaminated environment colonize in the damaged epidermis and initiate a bacterial dermatitis. *F. necrophorum* is dermonecrotic and produces a strong leukocidal exotoxin that protects it and other bacteria from phagocytosis. *Corynebacterium pyogenes*, the second bacterium of this mixed infection, is a synergistic organism which produces a factor that stimulates the growth of *F. necrophorum* allowing establishment of the interdigital infection. The invasion and necrosis of the soft tissues at the bulb of the heal produces a severe inflammation with acute lameness. The digits spread and the entire foot enlarges due to the inflammation and swelling. As the infection progresses the discharge becomes purulent in nature and eventually ruptures from a sinus tract above the coronary band.

In the progress of infection from the initial interdigital lesion to forming a sinus tract above the abaxial surface of the coronary band the axial collateral ligaments, the interdigital ligament, and the distal interphalangeal joint become infected. The infection can cause rupture of these ligaments with luxation of the distal phalanx and distal sesamoid. Infection of the distal interphalangeal joint destroys the articular cartilage exposing the subchondral bone to infection. There is a periostitis and periostial newbone growth of the distal and middle phalanx. Unless the infection is stopped at the interdigital necrotic stage the course of the infection is about 8 weeks regardless of treatment. As healing takes place the distal interphalangeal joint becomes ankylosed and exostosis of the distal and middle phalanx results in permanent enlargement. Rupture of the axial collateral ligaments and the interdigital ligament results in permanent spreading of the digits. Following recovery the enlarged and arthritic foot is functional without apparent pain or lameness.

CLINICAL SIGNS AND POSTMORTEM LESIONS. Sheep affected with FA rapidly develop severe lameness of the foot and tenderness in the digit. Nonpigmented feet may become red from hyperemia and swollen from inflammation. After a course of 7 to 10 days, one or more sinuses may spontaneously open above the coronet or on the interdigital skin and discharge pus (Fig. 15-2). Paring the bulb and sole may reveal the location, usually near the toe, of the exudate.

Infected flocks often develop a morbidity of 10%. FA rarely causes death, however, but prolonged lameness may provoke the owner to order euthanasia. Outbreaks in pregnant sheep ewes is often complicated with pregnancy toxemia. The course in untreated sheep ranges from many weeks to several months.

At necropsy, the sinuses extend into the derma of the sole and, in some feet, into the distal interphalangeal joint and bone. Ex-

Fig. 15-2. Foot abscess. × 0.8.

carpus and may involve more than one foot. Contagious ecthyma may cause skin ulcers near the coronet, but simultaneous vesicles, pustules, or crusts also develop near the mouth and eyes.

PREVENTION AND TREATMENT. Vaccine for immunizing against FA is in experimental stages. Flocks, such as rams, developing high incidence of the disease should be moved from wet pasture to drier soil or on slatted floors.

Individual cases of FA are effectively treated with surgical drainage and antibacterial compounds. The hoof should be pared to locate and drain the exudate. All hoof tissue, separated by exudate from the derma, should be removed. Sulfathiazole powder or penicillin powder or ointment should be topically applied to cleaned tissue. In addition, intramuscular injection of penicillin at the rate of 70,000 units per kg of body weight may be given. A long-acting penicillin or tetracycline may be the drug of choice in certain management schemes as they will provide therapeutic blood levels over a 48- to 72-hour period. To prevent involvement of the ligaments and distal interphalangeal joint, treatment must be initiated early, otherwise the infection will run its course regardless of the therapeutic regimen.

ostoses may have formed around the second and third phalanges, especially near infected distal interphalangeal joints.

DIAGNOSIS. Veterinarians diagnose FA from evidence in gross lesions. Lameness, swelling, and sinus openings above the coronet or onto interdigital skin of one digit justify the diagnosis.

The differential diagnosis requires consideration of contagious foot rot, strawberry foot rot, and contagious ecthyma. Contagious foot rot causes bidigital undermining of the corneum and usually occurs in two or more feet. Strawberry foot rot produces multiple raised skin crusts between the coronet and tarsus or

Gardner, D.E.: Acute laminitis in sheep caused by *C. pyogenes.* N.Z. Vet. J., *9*:59, 1961.

Gregory, T.S.: Foot rot in sheep. Aust. Vet. J., *15*:160-167, 1939.

Momberg-Jorgensen, H.C.: Malignant foot rot in sheep. Maanedsskr. Dyrlaeg, *53*:317-329, 1941.

Newson, I.E.: *Sheep Diseases.* Baltimore, Williams & Wilkins, 1952.

Scanlan, C., Garrett, P., and Campbell, I.: Ovine contagious foot rot. The Compendium on Continuing Education, 7:515-518, 1985.

West, D.: A study of naturally occurring cases of ovine foot abscess in New Zealand. N.Z. Vet. J., *31*:152-156, 1983.

West, D.: Observations on an outbreak of foot abscess in sheep. N.Z. Vet. J., *31*:71-74, 1983.

16

DISEASES OF THE MUSCULAR SYSTEM

Blackleg

(Black quarter; quarter ill; symptomatic anthrax; charbon symptomatique; rauschbrand)

An acute infectious but noncontagious disease of cattle and sheep, blackleg is characterized by focal gangrenous and emphysematous myositis and is caused by anaerobic bacteria. The disease is equally malignant in both sheep and cattle, but with sheep, because of a lower incidence, it is of less economic importance. High financial losses may accrue, however, to individual sheep enterprises from deaths, maintenance of preventive programs, and depreciation of contaminated property. In the future, the disease incidence in sheep may be lowered even further by reducing traumatic injury from shearing and by applying improved sanitary procedures when docking, tagging, castrating, and vaccinating. The name "blackleg" describes the appearance of infected limb muscles in both cattle and sheep.

OCCURRENCE. Blackleg is a disease of all breeds and ages, including fetuses, of sheep; it is encountered in both sexes, but frequently, more cases appear in young rams, possibly because of injuries received in aggressive fighting. Usually the disease follows injuries in the skin from shearing, in the genital tract from parturition, or from surgical operations, such as docking, castrating, vaccinating, and tagging. Although blackleg can develop during any season, the incidence is highest during spring, when shearing and parturitional injuries usually occur. Blackleg is far more common in cattle than in sheep. Among cattle it is a major malady. Cases also occur in deer and swine.

Geographically, the disease probably occurs in all countries where cattle and sheep industries have developed. Within individual countries, however, the disease incidence varies. In the United States, cases of blackleg of both sheep and cattle are more common among the western states than among eastern states. Because of protection of the environment against contamination, the disease incidence is lower on properties where owners promptly destroy by burning or deep burial in quicklime all cattle and sheep carcasses of animals that die from disease.

ETIOLOGY AND PATHOGENESIS. While *C. chauvoei* is the main cause of blackleg, occasionally *C. septicum* and, less commonly, *C. novyi* are also present and contribute to development of the disease. Presumably, their normal habitat is soil; there they endure as spores for prolonged periods and may, in the presence of adequate organic material, moisture, and temperature, germinate and grow. The three species are motile, anaerobic, spore-bearing and, as young cultures, gram-positive rods, with a tendency to become gram-negative in older cultures. The vegetative rods measure 0.8 to 1.5×5 to $10 \,\mu$m. The oval-shaped spores are subterminal. The fermentation of some sugars is shown in Table 16-1.

325

TABLE 16-1. *Fermentation and Morphologic Features of Clostridia**

	Glucose	Maltose	Lactose	Salicin	Bacteria From Guinea Pig Liver
C. chauvoei	AG	AG	AG	—	Mostly single
C. septicum	AG	AG	AG	AG	Mostly chains
C. novyi	AG	AG	—	—	
C. haemolyticum	AG	AG	—	—	
C. perfringens	AG	AG	AG	—	

* A = acid; G = gas.

In smears from the surface of liver from infected guinea pigs, *C. chauvoei* forms single bacilli or short chains, whereas *C. septicum* mostly forms chains; this morphologic difference is of diagnostic importance in determining species. The vegetative forms are highly susceptible to drying, high temperatures, and chemical disinfectants, whereas the spores are resistant and withstand a temperature of 120°C for 10 minutes and endure in dried infected tissues for many years. Spores are killed in 15 minutes by a 3% solution of formaldehyde.

For the three main species of *Clostridium*, the antigenic structure and toxin production have been investigated. Strains of *C. chauvoei* appear to be of a single serologic type. Although an exotoxin is produced in liquid cultures, its concentration is low and variable. The addition of blood to broth media enhances exotoxin production. Different strains of *C. septicum* can be separated into four major antigenic groups. These forms produce potent exotoxins that hemolyze erythrocytes and remain stable when exposed to oxygen. *C. novyi* contains three serologic types of organism and possibly produces six types of exotoxin.

Predisposing or contributing causes include breaks in skin and mucous membranes and necrosis in muscle tissue. Injuries commonly result from shearing, castrating, docking, and vaccinating. Necrosis may occur in contused muscle of fighting rams and in tissues damaged by parturition.

Even though the pathogenesis of ovine blackleg is incompletely understood, some factual information is available, and rational conjectures can be made. Viable spores of both ovine and bovine strains of *C. chauvoei* reside in soil. Exposure of injured sheep to soil heavily contaminated with spores of either bovine or ovine strains of *C. chauvoei* produces the disease. The bacteria enter the muscle through wounds. Exposure of normal sheep to soil heavily contaminated with spores of ovine strains also produces disease. The enhanced pathogenicity of ovine strains for sheep enables the organisms to enter the sheep through the alimentary tract and later to cause disease.

The exposure of normal sheep to soil having low concentrations of spores of bovine strains usually does not cause disease. In the injured tissues where the oxidation-reduction potential is below normal, the anaerobic spores germinate and the vegetative cells grow, ferment muscle glycogen, digest protein, and produce exotoxin. The toxin hemolyzes erythrocytes, necroses muscle cells, and at least in small amounts, enters the circulatory system. The bacteria and their products provoke a strong inflammatory reaction. Injured and dead cells, exudate and congestion, and gas from fermentation cause pain and inactivation of affected muscles.

Exotoxins from the bacteria, toxic substances from the lesions, and acute shock cause death of the animal. In the few recovered sheep, antibodies specific to *C. chauvoei* develop and protect against subsequent attacks by homologous pathogens. Following death, tissues rapidly decompose, and some bacteria sporulate and re-enter the soil.

CLINICAL SIGNS AND POSTMORTEM LESIONS. Infected sheep usually have a history of recent

injury from shearing or from surgical operations or parturition. Although the incubation
period is difficult to determine, it probably
varies from 2 to 5 days. Body temperature
rapidly rises to 41 to 42°C. Muscular stiffness
and swelling, pain, depression, disinclination
to move, and anorexia are prominent.

In animals affected in muscles of the limbs,
lameness is manifested. Infection is located in
muscles of the shoulder, thigh, neck, face,
and back. Blackleg infection following parturition results in acute and extensive swelling
throughout the perineum and extending dorsally to the pelvis and ventrally and laterally
along medial aspects of the thighs. Nonpigmented skin over affected muscles may become red or purple.

The short clinical course varies from 24 to
48 hours. The sporadic incidence commonly
becomes 2 to 5%, but a long sequence of cases
in some outbreaks may reach 10 to 20% of the
flock. Nearly all untreated animals die. In ewes
in advanced stages of pregnancy, blackleg
may develop in the fetuses; ewes so affected
with intrauterine disease develop marked distension of the abdomen, depression, and anorexia and finally die.

At necropsy, most changes are limited to affected muscles and covering skin. Lesions may
be located in any muscle, but are found more
commonly in the thigh, shoulder, back, perineum, neck, and face. Muscles in the tongue,
crura of the diaphragm, and myocardium may
be less commonly involved. The affected muscle is swollen and emphysematous. Gas bodies may accumulate under the skin, along
fascia, and between specific muscle bundles.

Where hemorrhage has occurred, affected
tissue is black, a characteristic of the disease. A
butyric odor emanates from the lesion. Frequently, the muscle is dry, but connective tissue at the periphery of the lesion and along
fasciae is edematous and hemorrhagic. The
serosanguineous transudate is more abundant
in lesions containing *C. septicum.* Skin over
the lesions is red or purple. In blackleg of the
fetus, similar changes occur, but early fetal
death and rapid decomposition of tissues obscure the characteristic pathologic changes.

Careful examination of the skin and genitalia
usually reveals the injury through which infection occurred.

Histopathologically, affected tissue shows
coagulative necrosis of muscle and other tissue, accumulation of serum and leukocytes,
and hemolyzed erythrocytes. The gram-positive rods can be found throughout the lesion,
but not uniformly. Some muscle bundles are
separated by gas bodies.

DIAGNOSIS.   The clinical diagnosis of blackleg is made from a history of exposure of affected sheep to trauma from shearing, docking,
castration, or parturition, and from the typical signs and lesions. The clinical diagnosis is
confirmed in the laboratory by isolating *C.
chauvoei* from suspect lesions.

The differential diagnosis requires consideration of malignant edema, hydrocyanic acid
poisoning, anthrax, and shipping fever.

PREVENTION AND TREATMENT.   Sheep producers and veterinarians can prevent many cases
of blackleg by exercising hygienic principles in
animal management and, under certain conditions, by vaccination. Even though *C. chauvoei* and *C. septicum* are common in the soil in
endemic areas, the degree of exposure of susceptible animals can be reduced by prompt
disposal of infected carcasses through either
burning or deep burial, and by disinfection of
contaminated surfaces with chemicals or heat.

Shearers should carefully avoid injuring the
sheep, and all veterinarians and owners should
perform surgical operations under strictly sanitary conditions. In most cases, preventive vaccination is justifiable only when veterinarians
have diagnosed the first few cases in an outbreak or when owners anticipate exposing
sheep to both injuries and heavily contaminated soil. High-quality vaccines are commercially available on the market and should be
applied several weeks in advance of exposure
to the disease.

Although prevention is more convenient
and economical, treatment becomes desirable
under certain circumstances. Each exposed or
infected sheep should receive intramuscularly
1,500,000 units of penicillin daily for several
days.

Albiston, H.E.: Blackleg in lambs following vaccination for enterotoxemia. Aust. Vet. S., 13:245-247, 1937.

Andrieu and Badano: Rev. Med. Vet., 4:283, 1919.

Armstrong, H.L. and MacNamee, J.K.: Blackleg in deer. JAVMA, 117:212-214, 1950.

Armstrong, M.C.: Blackleg or blood poisoning of sheep and cattle. N.Z. J. Agric., 87:507-511, 1953.

Bollinger, O.: Dtsch. Tiermed. Vergl. pathol. 1:297, 1875, quoted from Robertson, M.: A system of bacteriology. 3:225-297, 1929.

Buddle, M.B.: A note on penicillin treatment of experimental Clostridium chauvoei infection in sheep. N.Z. Vet. J., 1:13-14, 1952.

Butler, H.C. and Marsh, H.: Blackleg of the fetus in ewes. JAVMA, 128:401-402, 1956.

Green, W.J.B.: Immunization against anaerobes of the gas-gangrene type in South Africa by means of anatoxins. 15th Ann. Rep. Dir. Vet. Serv., South Africa, 1929, pp. 193-221.

Heller, H.H.: Etiology of acute gangrenous infections of animals: a discussion of blackleg, braxy, malignant edema and whole septicemia. J. Infect. Dis., 27:385-451, 1920.

Marsh, H.: An outbreak of blackleg in sheep. JAVMA, 56:139-321, 1919.

Marsh, H., Welsh, H., and Jungherv, E.: Blackleg in sheep. JAVMA, 74:63-88, 1928.

Miessner, H. and Albrecht: DTW, 33:179, 1925.

Miessner, H. and Meyn, A.: Zeitiger stand der gasodemfrage. DTW, 35:548-550, 1927.

Miessner, H. and Meyn, A.: Vergleichende untersuchungen uber den rinder–und schafrauschbrand. DTW, 34:571-579, 1926.

Minett, F.C.: Pathogenesis of black quarter. J. Comp. Pathol., 58:201-209; 245-258; 259-266, 1948.

Newsom, I.E. and Cross, F.: Blackleg in sheep due to shearing. Vet. Med., 28:16-20, 1933.

Ostertag, R.: DTW, 32:62, 1924.

Roberts, R.S. and McEwen, A.D.: Gas gangrene infections of sheep. J. Comp. Pathol. Ther., 44:180-191, 1931.

Scheibel, D.: DTW, 25:61, 1907.

Sedden, H.R., Belschner, H.G., and Edger, G.: Blackleg in sheep in New South Wales. Aust. Vet. J., 7:2-18, 1931.

Spiegl, A.: Untersuchungen uber den rauschbrand der schafe. DTW, 28:467, 1920.

Sterne, M. and Edwards, J.B.: Blackleg in pigs caused by Clostridium chauvoei. Vet. Rec., 67:314-315, 1955.

Stiles, G.W.: Blackleg (Clostridium chauvoei) infection in sheep. North Am. Vet., 24:354-356, 1943.

Witt, C. and Stickdorn, W.: Rauschbrand des schafes. Berl. Tieraerztl. Wochenschr., 35:199, 1919.

Wulff, F.: Uber rauschbrand und rauschbrandahnliche erkrangen. DTW, 20:625, 689, 1912.

Zeissler, J.: Der rauschbrand und verwandte erkrungen der tiere. Berl. Klin. Wochenschr., 56:107, 1919.

Sarcocystosis

(Sarco; sarcosporidiosis)

Sarcocystosis, an acute or latent intracellular parasitism, is characterized during the acute stage by fever, weakness, and anemia and is caused by an isosporoid parasite. Acute sarcocystosis is an invasion in host endothelial cells, and latent sarcocystosis is an encystment in skeletal and cardiac cells. The latent form, but not the acute form, has been known historically. The latent form has been considered innocuous and consequently has been ignored, but all latent forms acquire their positions through earlier invasions.

During recent years, veterinary scientists have observed severe and fatal illnesses—first induced and then natural—from acute sarcocystosis. These findings suggest that instances of the acute disease have been overlooked or misdiagnosed. If all animals with muscle sarcocysts are adversely affected at the time of parasite invasion, then the disease, because of high prevalence, is important. In addition to sheep, the condition develops in cattle and most other species of domestic animals.

OCCURRENCE. Sarcocystosis develops in all breeds, sexes, and ages of sheep, but more often in animals over 6 months of age and associated with canine and feline animals. The degree of infection probably ranges from slight and inconsequential to severe and fatal. Infection apparently can occur during all seasons, but free-living sporocysts probably maintain infectivity for longer periods during warm, moist seasons than during dry, hot, or cold seasons.

Geographically, the condition probably occurs in all countries of the temperate and hot climatic zones.

ETIOLOGY AND PATHOGENESIS. Sarcocystis tenella (ovicanis), a major pathogen, and S. gigantia (ovifelis), a lesser pathogen, both of the family sarcocystidae and belonging to the order Eimeriorina cause sarcocystosis. The sarcocystidae are heteroxenous, requiring one type of host (definitive host-dog-cat or other carnivore) for the sexual stage and another type (intermediate host-sheep) for the asexual stages. Oocysts develop in the lamina propria of the small intestine of the dog (S. tenella) or cat (S. gigantia). They sporulate forming 2 sporocysts each with 4 sporozoites. These are released into the lumen of the intestine and pass with the feces contaminating feed and sources. The sheep becomes infected by ingesting feed or forage contaminated with the sporocysts. The enzymes and bile in the abomasum and proximal small intestine cause excystation releasing the sporocysts. The route and mode of tissue penetration by the sporozoites is not known. Following penetration a first-generation of meronis (tachyzoites) develop within the endothelial cells of capillaries followed by some merogonous stages occurring within cells of the mononuclear phagocytic system. Finally, the last meront (sarcocyst) generation develops in the striated muscles. Here it forms metrocytes within itself. These divide repeatedly by endodyogeny to form bradyzoites, which come to live in compartments divided by septa in the mature sarcocyst. The dog and cat (definitive host) become infected by ingesting mature sarcocysts containing bradyzoites which develop into oocysts in the lamina propria of the small intestine thus complicating the life cycle. Depending on the number of ingested sarcocysts the prepatent period in the definitive host is 8 to 13 days. In the intermediate host the initiation of active infection can occur as early as 3 days following ingestion. Merozoites appear in the peripheral blood between 14 and 23 days following ingestion. Developing sarcocysts occur in striated muscle as early as 35 days post ingestion. Mature sarcocysts develop in about 60 to 90 days.

In fresh meat, the zoites survive 18 days in storage at 2°C, but not for 3 days at −20°C. They endure cooking temperatures that reach 55 to 60°C, but not 65 to 70°C.

Pathogenicity of the sporocysts varies directly with the size of the dose. As few as 5×10^3 given at one time to a sheep may cause illness, while the same number given over a period of weeks or months may have no clinical effect, but may accumulate the same number of intracellular cysts. Infected host capillaries are weakened under normal pressure and are permeable to plasma proteins. Heavy concentration of infection in cardiac muscle and Purkinje cells, in endothelial cells of blood vessels, and in neurons of the brain

may result in malfunction of those respective organs. Death is from hemorrhagic diathesis. Infection probably does not cross the placenta.

CLINICAL SIGNS AND POSTMORTEM LESIONS. Following ingestion of large doses of sporocysts over a short time, sheep become clinically ill. Both ewes and lambs develop fever, anorexia, muscular stiffness, mental depression, anemia, hypoproteinemia, reduced weight, and unthriftiness. Pregnant ewes may abort. Natural morbidity is not known, but may be high. Mortality from mild infection probably is low, but may reach 10 to 20% from heavy infection. Up to 100% of young adults may contain intracellular cysts. The course of illness extends through several weeks.

At necropsy, heart muscle, skeletal muscle, and serosal membranes contain numerous hemorrhages, and body cavities as well as intramuscular fasciae may accumulate fluids. Lymph nodes are swollen. In latent stages, esophageal muscle may contain pale cysts 10 to 10×4 to 6 mm (Fig. 16-1). During acute and intermediate stages of the disease, schizonts in endothelial cells are widespread in capillaries of viscera; in latent stages, however, sarcocysts are concentrated in muscle cells of heart, skeleton, esophagus, diaphragm, and tongue, and rarely are in neurons of the brain (Fig. 16-2).

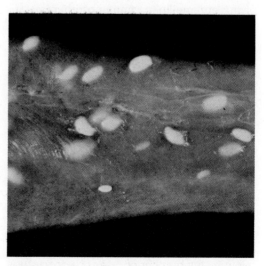

Fig. 16-1. Sarcocyst nodules in muscularis of the esophagus.

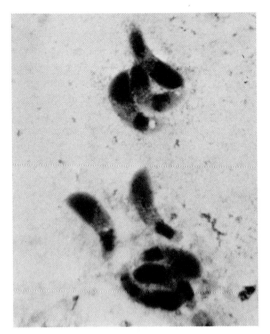

Fig. 16-2. Sarcocystis ovicanis from esophagus. Giemsa's stain. × 1412.

DIAGNOSIS. Historically, pathologists have identified latent sarcocystosis, either grossly or microscopically, at inspection or necropsy. Currently, however, practicing veterinarians, should clinically suspect acute sarcocystosis from evidence of typical signs and lesions and should confirm it in a laboratory with the aid of the enzyme-linked immunosorbent assay, the lymphocyte blastogenic assay or a significant number of endothelial schizonts. The differential diagnosis requires consideration of gastrointestinal parasitism, toxoplasmosis, eosinophilic myositis, other anemias, and chronic poisonings.

For technical assistance from a diagnostic laboratory, practitioners should submit (1) refrigerated paired sera and samples of fresh lung, kidney, and feces, (2) formalin-fixed lung, kidney, lymph node, liver, diaphragmatic crura, heart, tongue, and esophagus, and (3) fecal samples from suspect canine and feline sources of infection.

PREVENTION AND TREATMENT. Producers can minimize the number of cases of sarcocystosis by preventing dogs and cats from contaminating sheep feed and water with their feces and by strict avoidance of feeding raw viscera and muscle to dogs and cats.

Effective treatment of affected animals has not been developed, but potential benefit could result from (1) administering amprolium in feed or water to provide 25 to 50 mg/kg daily for 5 to 10 days and (2) giving intragastric fluids and nutrients as needed. Weight loss and severe clinical signs can be prevented by the chemoprophylactic use of salinomycin at the rate of 2 mg/kg/day. The medication must be administered prior to exposure as it is not effective for treatment once clinical signs appear.

Dubey, J., Speer, C., Callis, G., and Blixt, J.: Development of the sheep-canid cycle of *Sarcocystis tenella*. Can. J. Zool., *60*:2464-2476, 1982.

Erber, M.: Life cycle of *Sarcocystis tenella* in sheep and dog. Z. Parasitenkd., *68*:171-181, 1982.

Frenkel, J.K.: *Besnoitia wallacei* of cats and rodents, with a reclassification of other cyst-forming isosporoid coccidia. J. Parasitol., *63*:611-628, 1977.

Gasbarre, L., Suter, P., and Fayer, R.: Humoral and cellular immune responses in cattle and sheep inoculated with sarcocystis. Am. J. Vet. Res., *45*:1592-1596, 1984.

Gestrich, R., Schmidt, M., and Heydorn, A.O.: Pathogenicity for lambs of *Sarcocystis tenella* sporocysts from feces of dogs. Berl. Muench. Tieraeztl. Wochenschr., *87*:362-363, 1974.

Heydorn, A.O., Gestrich, R., Mehlhorn, H., and Rommel, M.: Proposal for new nomenclature of the sarcosporidia. Z. Parasitenkd., *48*:73-82, 1975.

Landsverk, T. and Bratberg, B.: Polyarteritis nodosa associated with sarcocystosis in a lamb. Acta Vet. Scand., *20*:306-308, 1979.

Leek, R.G. and Fayer, R.: Experimental *Sarcocystis ovicanis* infection in lambs: Salinomycin chemoprophylaxis and protective immunity. J. Parasitology, *69*:271-276, 1983.

Leek, R.G. and Fayer, R.: Sheep experimentally infected with sarcocystis from dogs. II. Abortion and disease in ewes. Cornell Vet., *68*:108-123, 1978.

Leek, R.G., Fayer, R., and Johnson, A.J.: Sheep experimentally infected with sarcocysts from dogs. I. Disease in young lambs. J. Parasitol., *63*:642-650, 1977.

Levine, N.: *Veterinary Protozoology*. 2nd Edition. Ames, Iowa, Iowa State Univ. Press, 1985, pp. 233-260.

O'Donoghue, P. and Ford, G.: The asexual pre-cyst development of *Sarcocystis tenella* experimentally infected specific-pathogen-free lambs. Int. J. Parasitol., *14*:345-355, 1984.

Rezakani, A., Cheema, A.H., and Edjtehadi, M.: Second degree atrioventricular block and sarcosporidiosis in sheep. Zentralbl. Veterinaermed., *24A*:258-262, 1977.

17

DISEASES OF THE CENTRAL NERVOUS SYSTEM

Rabies

*(Hydrophobia; tollwut;
le rage; lyssa)*

Rabies, an acute infection of the central nervous system and salivary glands, is characterized by a syndrome of excitation, depression, paralysis, coma, and death and is caused by a virus transmitted by the bite of a rabid animal. Although rabies occurs in all species of warm-blooded animals, especially mammals, throughout most countries, it has low sporadic incidence among sheep and, consequently, little economic importance to the sheep industry. Some losses, however, result from deaths and the cost of diagnostic and preventive programs. Because all cases of rabies, including those in people, terminate in horrifying death, the disease has public interest and public health significance.

OCCURRENCE. Although rabies occurs in all breeds, sexes, and ages of sheep, feedlot lambs, because of restricted movements within crowded pens and limited ability to retreat from intruding rabid animals, develop higher incidence than do other animal classes. Even though the disease occurs in all seasons, more cases develop during spring breeding months when carnivorous species are active and highly mobile. The number of cases of ovine rabies in the United States from 1962 through 1971 was small. In addition to sheep, the disease also occurs, with higher incidence, in cattle, dogs, cats, skunks, and foxes. Cattle, naturally inquisitive, investigate intruding animals, whereas timid sheep retreat from them; this behavorial difference may account for fewer cases of rabies among sheep.

Geographically, ovine rabies has a low sporadic incidence in southern and northern Africa, South America, North America, Europe, Middle East, and the USSR. Australia, Britain, and Scandinavia have been rabies-free for prolonged periods.

ETIOLOGY. The virus causing rabies falls into the group of Rhabdoviridae, genus lyssavirus. With the use of monoclonal antibodies the serotypes have been classified as follows: Serotype 1: Prototype strain challenge virus standard (CVS) 24; includes the majority of field viruses and laboratory strains from different parts of the world. Serotype 2: Prototype strain Lagos bat (isolated from bats in Nigeria and Central African Republic). Serotype 3: Prototype strain Mokola (isolated from schrews, man, wild and domestic animals from Africa). Serotype 4: Prototype strain Duvenhage (isolated from man and bats in Africa and Central Europe. Serotype 2, 3, and 4 are commonly referred to as rabies-related viruses. The rabies virus is enveloped with a single, non-segmented negative-strand RNA. The virus contains multiple copies of five structural proteins: the virion transcriptase (L), nucleoprotein (N), glycoprotein (G), the nucleo capsid-associated protein (NS) and matrix (M) protein. The N, NS and L proteins are non-covalently bound to the virion RNA and

331

the resulting nucleocapsid (NC) complex forms a helically coiled structure within the virion. The nucleocapsid is surrounded by a lipoprotein envelope consisting of matrix protein and surface projections of G proteins extending to the exterior of the virus. The G protein is the only protein capable of inducing and reacting with virus-neutralizing antibody which is the basis for new virus recombinant vaccines. Monoclonal antibodies have been used to distinguish between rabies and rabies-related viruses at the nucleoprotein level and have also revealed extensive antigenic variation in both the glycoprotein and nucleoproteins of laboratory and street rabies virus strains. Monoclonal antibodies are used to group an undetermined number of rabies virus strains isolated from man and animals in different parts of the world.

In media with which it is usually associated, rabies virus is sensitive to environmental adversities. In a fluid medium at 70°C, it is killed in 15 minutes, but when dried, it withstands a temperature of 100°C for 2 to 3 minutes. Contact with acids, bases, phenol, mercuric chloride, formalin, and ultraviolet light rapidly destroys the virus. Ether inactivates it, but at an inconstant rate. Storage in 50% glycerol or in the lyophilized state maintains viability for approximately 1 year.

Rabies virus can be cultivated in cell cultures of baby hamster kidneys, embryonating chicken eggs, and suckling mice.

TRANSMISSION. In sheep, rabies is transmitted exclusively by the bite of saliva-infected rabid animals. Rabid dogs, coyotes, cats, foxes, and skunks are the usual vectors in the United States, and these animals, when infected, wander widely and often fearlessly enter sheep feedlots or attack range or pastured sheep. Timid sheep retreat whenever possible, but aggressive intruders, especially dogs, may attack the confined animals and inflict saliva-infected wounds about the head and neck, and less often the limbs.

In South and Central America, hematophagous bats, often infected, transmit the disease to livestock; consequently, the incidence of livestock rabies, especially in cattle, from bat transmission has been high and costly. The common vampire bat, *Desmodus rotundus,* and the hairy-legged bat, *Diphylla ecaudata,* are transmitters, and as night feeders they attack large livestock, including sheep, and inflict tooth incisions in the skin of the head, neck, back, and limbs; the bat laps the exuding blood. In the process of biting and lapping, virus-infected saliva may contaminate the wound and inoculate the host animal.

PATHOGENESIS. Following bite inoculations, especially into muscle, rabies virus replicates locally. Unless inactivated by natural or induced defense mechanisms, the virions cross neuromuscular and neurotendinous spindles, move centripetally, and replicate along peripheral nerve axons into dorsal root ganglia and spinal cord, ascend the central nervous system, and spread centrifugally along axons of trigeminal, facial, olfactory, and glossopharyngeal peripheral nerves into salivary glands, taste buds, and olfactory cells, and hence into oral and nasal secretions. At the onset of clinical signs, virus is widespread throughout the central nervous systems (CNS) with highest concentrations in the brain stem, basal ganglion, hippocampus, and cerebellum. There is no viremia but after reaching the CNS, rabies virus is present in neurons throughout the body, an important factor making diagnosis of the condition possible from skin biopsy prior to clinical signs. Within the nervous system, only neurons, and nerve supporting cells, become infected. In the central nervous system, neurons, especially Purkinje cells, are heavily infected, and some develop inclusions. There is no viremia. All clinically affected sheep die.

CLINICAL SIGNS AND POSTMORTEM LESIONS. The course of ovine rabies is divisible into three phases: prodromal, excitative, and paralytic.

Following an incubation period of 15 days to several months, the prodromal phase begins, and in sheep it is short, inconspicuous, and undetected. Body temperature may elevate, and apprehensiveness may develop. During the excitative period, affected animals refuse feed and water, move restlessly, salivate, aggressively butt caretakers, frequently bleat, bite, and pull wool, rhythmically oscillate the tongue, faint, and show sexual excitement. With onset of paralysis, the animal becomes depressed, physically weak, and recumbent. Death usually occurs within 12 hours after initial prostration.

Morbidity ranges up to 77% of small flocks and may reach 10% of a large flock. All clinically affected sheep die. The course usually varies from 1 to 4 days.

At necropsy, organic changes are minimal and have little diagnostic importance. The dehydrated carcass may be traumatized from violent behavior during the course of the disease. The meninges and brain may be congested and edematous. Microscopically, neurons of many parts of the brain, especially the brain stem, are swollen, degenerated, and occasionally necrotic. Specific Negri bodies usually are present in the cytoplasm of some neurons of the hippocampus and Purkinje cells. Inflammation and neuronophagia may be present along the brain stem. The bizarre symptomatology and extremely high fatality rate of rabies are associated with minimal neuropathologic findings.

DIAGNOSIS.   Veterinarians diagnose ovine rabies on evidence of case history, clinical manifestations, and laboratory findings. The history of exposure to the bite of animals or residence in a rabies-endemic area is important. Typical signs during the excitative and paralytic phases direct attention to rabies; crucially significant are excitement, dysphagia, bleating, aggression, sexual excitement, and terminal paralysis.

Following natural termination of the disease, the head should be removed, refrigerated, and promptly shipped to a diagnostic laboratory for further studies. In the laboratory, smears and/or sections of the hippocampus and cerebellum are examined for specific evidence of rabies virus. The fluorescent-antibody technique possesses high accuracy and is used frequently.

Other methods, such as Seller's staining, differentiate the Negri bodies of the disease. In the absence of Negri bodies, three to five young adult Swiss mice are intracerebrally inoculated with 0.03 ml of suspected brain suspension. If rabies virus is present, the inoculated mice usually die within 7 to 10 days after inoculation. The observation period may be shortened by fluorescent antibody examination of brains of inoculated mice killed 4 days or more after inoculation. A positive diagnosis requires the identification of Negri bodies in the mouse brain or neutralization of the virus with known antibodies. Early antemortem evaluation of the rabies status of biting dogs, cats, and other animal species can be made by skin biopsies, especially skin areas containing tactile hairs which are surrounded by large concentrations of nerve fibers, with the use of immunofluorescent examination. The immunofluorescence technique or the peroxidase-antiperoxidase (PAP) method can be used for retrospective diagnosis using formalin-fixed or paraffin-embedded brain tissues.

The differential diagnosis requires consideration of polioencephalomalacia, listeriosis, and choke.

PREVENTION.   Feedlot and farm flock sheep can be protected against rabies by management practices and immunization. From feedlots of small dimensions, some rabid animals, especially dogs, can be excluded by fencing. Because rabid cats, rats, bats, and possibly some other animals cannot be mechanically excluded, a supplementary method of prevention is the regional program for control of the disease in all animals.

In rabies-endemic areas where the probability of exposure is high, immunization of sheep can be—but seldom is—practiced. In most of the world the animal reservoir of rabies is the dog. The most cost effective and logical approach to the control of the disease is via the animal reservoir host. At least 80% of dogs must be vaccinated along with control of strays to effectively control rabies in the dog population. Each ecosystem varies but wild carnivores appear to be the main transmitters of wildlife rabies with only one or two species responsible for the perpetuation of the rabies epidemic in that particular ecosystem.

Oral immunization or depopulation of the wildlife host may be necessary to eliminate rabies from infected areas. Where bats are the main host control, procedures are directed towards mass immunization of the cattle, sheep, and other domestic animals being attacked along with bat depopulation. Subunit vaccines are being developed which will greatly reduce production and handling costs, while improving the safety and efficacy. Vaccines are commercially available for domestic animals and should be used only as directed by the manufacturer to assure safety and efficacy.

Ballantyne, E.E. and O'Donoghue, J.G.: Rabies control in Alberta. JAVMA, 125:316-326, 1954.

Blender, D., Bell, J., Tsao, A., and Umott, J.: Immunofluorescent examination of the skin of rabies-infected animals as a means of early detection of rabies virus antigen. J. Clin. Microbiol., 18:631-636, 1983.

Branckaert, R. and Herin, V.: Note on rabies in a flock of sheep in Leopoldville. Ann. Med. Vet., 110:126-135, 1966.

Camargo, F.: The derriengue problem in Mexico. 59th Ann. Proc. U.S. Livestock Sanit. Assoc., 1955, pp. 313-318.

Carneiro, V., Black, J., and Koprowski, H.: Rabies in cattle. V. Immunization of cattle in Brazil against exposure to street virus of vampire bat origin. JAVMA, 127:366-369, 1955.

Gomez, C., Black, J., and Koprowski, H.: Rabies in cattle. III. Comparative studies on vaccination of cattle in Colombia with Flury virus and chloroform inactivated vaccine. JAVMA, 127:360-363, 1955.

Henderson, J.A.: An outbreak of ovine rabies. Vet. Med., 37:88-89, 1942.

Johnson, H.N.: Rabies. In *Viral and Rickettsial Infections of Man*. 3rd Edition. Edited by T.M. Rivers and F.L. Horsfall. Philadelphia, J.B. Lippincott, 1959, pp. 405-431.

Kissling, R.E.: Growth of rabies virus in non-nervous tissue culture. Proc. Soc. Exp. Biol. Med., 98:223-225, 1958.

Kleckner, M.D.: Sylvatic rabies investigations in the Southeast. Proc. CDC Conf. Teachers Vet. Public Health, 1958, pp. 204-212.

Kligler, I.J. and Bernkopf, H.: Cultivation of rabies virus in the allantois of the developing chick embryo. Proc. Soc. Exp. Biol. Med., 39:212-214, 1938.

Lafon, M. and Wiktor, T.: Antigenic sites on the ERA rabies virus nucleoprotein and non-structural protein. J. Gen. Virol., 66:2125-2133, 1985.

Lodmell, D. and Ewalt, L.: Pathogenesis of street rabies virus infection in resistant and susceptible strains of mice. J. Virol., 55:788-795, 1985.

Magendie, F. and Breschet, G.: J. Physiol. Exptl., 1:42, 1821, quoted from Stimson, A.M.: Hyg. Lab. Bull. U.S. Pub. Health Service No. 65, 1910, pp. 1-90.

Mahin, L., Chadli, M., and Marzou, A.: Clinical aspects of bovine and ovine rabies in Morocco. Maghreb Veterinaire, 1:59-63, 1983.

Murphy, F.A., et al.: Pathogenesis of rabies. Viral transit from inoculation site to CNS. Lab. Invest., 28:361-376, 1973a.

Murphy, F.A., et al.: Pathogenesis of rabies infection of CNS and centrifugal spread of virus. Lab. Invest. 29:1-16, 1973b.

Palmer, D., Ossent, P., Suter, M., and Ferrari, E.: Demonstration of rabies viral antigen in paraffin tissue sections: Comparison of the immunofluorescence technique with the unlabeled antibody enzyme method. Am. J. Vet. Res., 46:283-286, 1985.

DeQueiroz Lima, E.: A transmissao da raiva bovina pelo morcego hematophago *Desmodus rotundus*. Brazil Med., 18:38 10, 1934.

Runnels, C.F.: Rabies in sheep. Vet. Med., 34:321, 1939.

Schroeder, C.R.: Rabies in Central and South America. Proc. 89th Ann. Meeting AVMA, 89:411-412, 1952.

Starr, L.E., Clower, T.B., Bromley, C.L., and Routh, C.F.: Antirabic immunization of cattle in Georgia using living virus vaccine of chick embryo origin. Vet. Med., 49:366-370, 1954.

Thompson, R.D., Mitchell, G.C., and Burns, R.J.: Vampire bat control by systemic treatment of livestock with an anticoagulant. Science, 77:806-807, 1972.

Tierkel, E.S.: Rabies. Adv. Vet. Sci., 5:183-226, 1959.

Wachendorfer, G.: Epidemiology and symptoms of rabies in sheep. Vet. Med. Nachr., 4:275-294, 1966.

Wachendorfer, G., Forster, U., and Krekez, H.: Humoral immune response of sheep to the use of an inactivated rabies vaccine. Zentralbl. Veterinaermed., 20B: 118-126, 1973.

Webster, W., Casey, G., Charlton, K., and Wiktor, T.: Antigenic variants of rabies virus in isolates from eastern, central and northern Canada. Can. J. Comp. Med., 49:186-188, 1985.

Wiktor, T., et al.: Protection from rabies by a vaccinia virus recombinant containing the rabies virus glycoprotein gene. Proc. Natl. Acad. Sci. U.S.A., 81:7194-7198, 1984.

World Health Organization. WHO expert committee on rabies. Technical Report Series 709. WHO, Geneva, 1984.

Wunner, W., et al.: Antigenic variants of CVS rabies virus with altered glycosylation sites. Virology, 140:1-2, 1985.

Wunner, W., Dietzschold, B., Curtis, P., and Wiktor, T.: Rabies subunit vaccines. J. Gen. Virol., 64:1649-1656, 1983.

Borna Disease

(BD; infectious meningoencephalomyelitis)

Borna disease, an acute contagious encephalomyelitis, is characterized by fever and neurologic disturbances and is caused by an unclassified slow virus. Although chiefly a disease of horses, BD does occur, to a lesser extent, in sheep. Because it has limited geographic distribution and low flock incidence, the disease is of only minor importance to the entire sheep industry, but within endemic areas, it may cause considerable financial waste to some individual sheep enterprises. Economic losses result from deaths of severely affected animals and unthriftiness among convalescent sheep, and from protein deficiencies among sheep-dependent people of the Middle East. Antibodies detected by the indirect immunofluorescence focus assay in psychiatric patients in Philadelphia, U.S.A., Wurzberg and Giessen, Germany, add significant human interest to this slow virus disease. The disease derived its name from the city of Borna, East Germany, where many horses and some sheep contracted the disease.

OCCURRENCE. Borna disease occurs in all breeds and sexes of sheep, but animals 1 to 2 years of age appear to be more susceptible than other age groups. In addition to sheep, the disease naturally affects horses, rabbits, goats, and cattle, and experimentally, tree shrews, chickens, guinea pigs, rats, hamsters, cats, and rhesus monkeys. Seasonally, BD usually develops during late winter and spring, and again in autumn, but may occur sporadically during other times. Geographically, BD occurs throughout Central Europe, especially Germany, and in Syria, Lebanon, and Egypt.

ETIOLOGY AND PATHOGENESIS. The BD virus, although unclassified, may be transmitted through the tick, *Hyalomma anatolicum*. The viral particles have a diameter of 50 to 60 nm, but as determined by filtration, one component measures about 20 nm. The virus resists drying for prolonged periods, and when lyophilized and stored at $-30°$C, it retains viability for several years, and when frozen in tissue and stored at $-20°$C, it is viable for at least 1 year. It is inactivated in 30 minutes at $57°$C and in 10 minutes at $70°$C. Although the virus remains one of few conventional, unclassified agents, it is heat and acid labile and sensitive to treatment with chloroform or ether which indicates the virus has an envelope. Indications are that it contains RNA and does not possess a reversive transcriptase.

In sheep and rabbits, the virus evokes complement-fixing antibodies, but neutralizing antibodies only at low titers, if at all. Antigenicity appears to be homogeneous. Outside the natural hosts, the BD virus grows in cell cultures from a wide host spectrum including kidney, testes, brain, and spleen of the naturally infected and experimentally infected animals. In its natural environment, the virus can only be found in neural tissue and organs derived from the ectoderm. Only brain and retina, but no other organs or lymphocytes harbor the virus. The virus is located in the alimentary tract of vectoring ticks.

The mode or modes of transmission have not been established, although it is suspected that the virus is entering through the nasal region, invading cells with no signs of cell alterations and spreading slowly from cell to cell. A humoral immune response appears only irregularly, particularly in cases of natural infection. Age dependency is a factor in the persistence of the disease. Those animals infected within the first few hours of life may tolerate the infection with a lack of a host response. The virus may persist in certain species for months or years with clinical signs either missing or only developing slowly. The data collected to date suggest that BD is a process where immunologic factors are of paramount importance in tissue destruction and manifestation of disease.

CLINICAL SIGNS AND POSTMORTEM LESIONS. After an incubation period of 1 to 2 months, body temperature rises to 41 to $42°$C and may persist throughout the period of viremia. Affected sheep often carry their heads near the ground. Vision may be impaired and the conjunctivae reddened. Anorexia, salivation, and teeth-grinding often develop. Animals may show ataxia, muscular tremors of the head and neck, hyperexcitability, hyperesthesia, physical weakness, and recurring convulsions.

Eventually, recumbency, with limb-paddling, supervenes and, after several days, death or recovery occurs. The morbidity, usually low, may reach 25% of a flock, and the mortality of affected sheep approximates 50%. The length of the clinical course varies from a few days to 2 or more weeks.

At necropsy, saliva may soil the face, and ticks may parasitize the nonwooled skin. In some animals, edematous fluid infiltrates the subcutaneous or intermuscular tissues. Visceral changes include petechial hemorrhages in the subepi- and subendocardial tissues, and 100 to 200 ml of fluid fill the pericardial sac. Meningeal blood vessels are congested. Histopathologic changes—diffuse infiltration and perivascular cuffing with lymphocytes and plasma cells, focal proliferation of microglial cells, neuronal degeneration and necrosis, and neuronophagia—are located in the cortex, pons, medulla, and basal nuclei, and neurons of the hippocampus may contain Joest-Degen inclusion bodies.

DIAGNOSIS. Veterinarians diagnose BD on evidence of typical signs and laboratory findings. In endemic areas, neurologic disease in cohabitating sheep and horses and the presence of vectoring ticks strongly suggest the disease. In the laboratory, the virus can be isolated by intracerebrally inoculating suspect sheep brain tissue into rabbits or cell cultures. Borna disease virus-specific antigens can be detected by complement fixation tests, direct or indirect fluorescence antibody test. A newly developed technique using the combined principals of the enzyme-linked immunosorbent assay (ELISA) and the peroxidase-anti-peroxidase (PAP) technique and termed PELISA allows quantitation of virus as well as titration of antibodies. The presence of Joest-Degen inclusion bodies are additional diagnostic evidence. The differential diagnosis requires consideration of rabies and louping-ill. In both of these diseases, the causative viruses can be isolated in cell cultures or laboratory animals and identified by use of the indirect immunofluorescent-antibody technique.

PREVENTION. A specific vaccine is commercially available and should be annually administered to protect sheep against anticipated BD. Controlling ticks reduces exposure of susceptible sheep to the virus.

Danner, K., Luthgen, K., Herlyn, M., and Mayr, A.: Comparative studies on the demonstration and formation of serum antibodies against Borna disease. Zentralbl. Veterinaermed., 25B:345-355, 1978.

Daubney, R.: Viral encephalitis of equines and domestic ruminants in the Near East. Part II. Res. Vet. Sci., 8:419-439, 1967.

Daubney, R. and Mahlau, E.A.: Near East equine encephalomyelitis. Nature, 179:584, 1957.

Daubney, R. and Mahlau, E.A.: Viral encephalomyelitis of equines and domestic ruminants in the Near East. Part I. Res. Vet. Sci. 8:375-397, 1967.

Heinig, A.: Experimental infection of horses and sheep with the virus of Borna disease. Arch. Vet. Med., 18:753-766, 1964.

Hirano, N., Kao, M., and Ludwig, H.: Persistent tolerant or subacute infection in Borna disease virus-infected rats. J. Gen. Virol., 64:1521-1530, 1983.

Ihlenberg, H.: Beitrag zum klinischen bild der Bornaschen krankheit des schafes. Mh. Vet. Med., 14:305-306, 1959.

Ludwig, H., Becht, H., and Groth, L.: Borna disease (BD), a slow virus infection. Med. Microbiol. Immunol. (Berl.), 158:275-289, 1973.

Mayr, A. and Danner, K.: Borna—a slow virus disease. Comp. Immun. Microbiol. Infect. Dis., 1:3-14, 1978.

Metzter, A., Ehrensperger, F., and Wyler, R.: Natural Borna virus infection in rabbits. Zentralbl. Veterinaermed., 25B:101-104, 1978.

Nicolau, S. and Galloway, I.A.: Borna disease and enzootic encephalomyelitis of sheep and cattle. London. Med. Res. Counc. Bull. 121, 1928.

Pauli, G., Grunmach, J., and Ludwig, H.: Focus-immunoassay for Borna disease virus-specific antigens. Zbl. Vet. Med. B., 31:552-557, 1984.

Rott, R., et al.: Detection of serum antibodies to Borna disease virus in patients with psychiatric disorders. Science, 228:755-756, 1985.

Seffner, W.: Sheep disease statistics from nine years of postmortem examinations. Mh. Vet. Med., 21:858-866, 1966.

Ter Muelen, V. and Katz, M. (eds.): Slow Virus Infections of the Central Nervous System. New York, Springer-Verlag, 1977.

Wagner, D.: Distribution of Borna disease in Bavaria and the occurrence of serum antibodies in horses, cattle, sheep and pigs. Diss. Tieraerztl. Fak Munchen, 1970, p. 38.

Wagner, K., Ludwig, H., and Paulsen, J.: Fluorescence-serological demonstration of Borna virus antigen. Berl. Muench. Tieraerztl. Wochenschr., 81:395-396, 1968.

Zwick, W., Seifried, O., and Witte, J.: Weitere beitrage zur enforschung der gehirn und ruchenmarksentzundung der pferde (Borna krankheit). Z. Infektkrankh. Parasit. Krankh. Hyg. Haust. 30:42, 1926.

Scrapie

(Scratchie; rubbers; la tremblante; traberkrankheit)

Scrapie, a slow transmissible disease of the central nervous system in sheep and goats, is characterized by prolonged incubation, sensory and motor malfunction, depression, and death and is caused by an infectious replicating agent. The ovine and caprine forms are similar. Even though the disease incidence is low, scrapie causes major concern and financial waste to the sheep industry. Economic losses result from required extra care, eventual deaths, and necessary disposal of all affected animals, from legal constraints against domestic and international sheep commerce, and from costly eradication and research programs. During the last two decades, a great deal of research has been directed towards this ominous disease and its enigmatic cause, but despite the relevant and multiplying knowledge, scrapie still prevails and threatens the industry and the survival of some valuable ovine and caprine family lines.

The disease has exciting scientific aspects, however. Ovine scrapie, transmissible mink encephalopathy, human kuru, and human Creutzfeldt-Jakob disease are homologues, and scrapie has become the general paradigm for the slow-developing neurologic diseases. Moreover, unique features of the causative agent—resistance to physicochemical factors and failure to evoke antibodies—have attracted the attention and interest of biologic, veterinary, and medical scientists. Information obtained from the study of the agent may provide insight into the understanding of some other obscure pathogens of animals, people, and plants.

OCCURRENCE. Scrapie occurs in all sexes and probably all breeds, but in the United States, the Suffolk breed has a high incidence, whereas the Rambouillet, Targhee, and Hampshire breeds have low incidences. Most natural cases occur in animals 30 to 60 months of age, but occasionally animals 12 months younger or older are affected. The long incubation period prevents younger sheep from manifesting signs and showing lesions.

Geographically, the natural disease has been officially diagnosed in Britain, Europe, Iceland, India, Kenya, Colombia, Canada, and America, and formerly in Australia, New Zealand, and the Republic of South Africa. In the United States, over 200 outbreaks have occurred since the first discovery in 1947, and these were concentrated in Illinois, Indiana, Texas, Ohio, and California. Eradicative programs in Australia, New Zealand, Canada, and the United States have eliminated the disease from many subdivisional regions.

ETIOLOGY. The scrapie agent—a filterable, transmissible, replicating, virus-like substance—causes scrapie disease. Although classification of the scrapie agent has not been accomplished, research findings relevant to the nature of the agent have been used in formulating three hypotheses. The first, the prion hypothesis asserts that the infectious agent is composed of a maximum of three protein molecules and thought to be devoid of nucleic acid. The filamentous structures observed in scrapie preparations are interpreted as a polymeric form of this infectious protein. The second, the virino hypothesis concludes that the agent contains a small nucleic acid which does not encode protein but serves as the template for its own production and the protective protein associated with the agent is derived from the host. The third, the filamentous agent hypothesis postulates that the agent is the scrapie-associated fibril (SAF) and, as such, is the first filamentous animal virus. This hypothesis places the scrapie agent within the field of molecular virology. An understanding of the nature of the scrapie agent will assist in the study of the epidemiology and pathogenesis of scrapie and similar slow infections of animals and man.

The resistance of the scrapie agent to inactivation by heat, ultraviolet irradiation, and numerous chemical inactivants is probably due to its ability to aggregate readily and a subpopulation of the scrapie agent would appear more resistant than would the unit virus. The consensus of many researchers is that the evidence strongly suggests that the scrapie agent is a small virus with conventional sensitivities to heat and chemical inactivants.

In sheep, goats, and mice, the agent evokes neither cellular nor humoral antibodies. In affected sheep, it is located first in the tonsils, lymph nodes associated with the alimentary tract, the spleen, and lastly in the central nervous system.

TRANSMISSION. Presumably, the agent moves from infected to susceptible animals by direct and indirect contact and enters through the gastrointestinal tract. Consequently, its spread is vertical and horizontal. Lambs born to affected dams may contract the disease by contact and possibly by action of a hereditary factor, and lambs born into a contaminated environment acquire the agent through contact. Spatial spread within and among geographic units is by commercial movements of infected animals in incubative stages of the disease from infected flocks to clean flocks. Scrapie is not diagnosable during incubative stages.

PATHOGENESIS. Susceptibility to infection appears to vary inversely with age. Young animals, especially newborns, are highly susceptible and when born into a contaminated environment become inoculated with the agent during or close to birth. The scrapie agent can be isolated from the tonsils, retropharyngeal lymph and mesenteric portal lymph nodes, and intestine of clinically normal lambs (10 to 14 months) suggesting that the primary infection occurs in the alimentary tract. Following transmission through the gastrointestinal tract, the agent penetrates the small intestinal mucosa, enters the lymphatics, and moves to mesenteric lymph nodes. Here it replicates and moves, presumably through the blood, into spleen and other organs, then the spinal cord, and finally the brain. Infection of the central nervous system can occur as early as 25 months in clinically normal animals, with the highest titer of the scrapie agent in the diencephalon, midbrain, medulla oblongata, and cerebellar cortex. Following parenteral injection of the agent into mice, an orderly sequence of events occurs: after 4 weeks, the agent titer in brain tissue increases; after 12 to 14 weeks, neuronal vacuolization and astrocyte hypertrophy begin; and after 19 weeks, clinical signs start. Death probably results from neuronal dysfunction.

CLINICAL SIGNS AND POSTMORTEM LESIONS. Following an incubation period ranging from 2 to 5 years from natural exposure, and for shorter periods after experimental inoculation, neurologic signs develop insidiously and intensify slowly. During early stages, affected sheep appear apprehensive and excitable and are disturbed by routine stimuli. They may

Fig. 17-1. Suffolk ram affected with scrapie.

isolate themselves from the flock or be ostracized by their fellows. Voluntary muscles, especially of the head and neck, develop tremors, which exacerbate during excitement and abate during rest. Incoordinated movements in the caudal limbs cause a hopping gait.

In more advanced stages, affected sheep incessantly rub their backs, sides, rumps, and heads against fences, trees, and equipment. In addition, some animals scratch their sides, abdomens, and heads with their hind feet and bite the skin over their sides and rumps (Fig. 17-1). As a result of these abrasive actions, the wool may be broken and extirpated over extensive skin surfaces of the neck, sides, back, and sacrum. Dermatitis is absent, however, except that caused by mechanical excoriations. Gentle digital movements on the sensitive skin by a manipulator may reflexly stimulate the sheep to extend and oscillate its head, to make nibbling lip and licking tongue movements, to violently shake the tail and rump skin, and to bleat weakly.

Impaired vision may cause collision with fixed objects such as fences and equipment. Exacerbated incoordination of movements causes stumbling gait, high stepping, and frequent falls. During terminal stages, the physically weak but not paralyzed animal continually reclines in prostration. Throughout all stages, live weight declines despite the persistence of appetite. Ewes may abort. Some cases, especially of non-Suffolk breeds, may bypass the manifestation of pruritus.

At necropsy, no gross lesions are discernible except emaciation and areas of denuded skin. Histopathologic changes occur along the brain stem and spinal cord, but are more constantly present in the thalamus, and consist of neuronal skrinkage and vacuolization, astrocytic hypertrophy and proliferation, and spongiform degeneration. Cytoplasmic vacuoles may be large and single or small and multiple (Fig. 17-2). The spongiform degeneration consists of small holes among fibers of the ground substances and commonly is located in the cerebellar peduncles. Inflammation is absent.

The morbidity that develops in previously unexposed groups of animals placed in con-

tact with infected sheep in contaminated environments is up to about 10%; but in the progenies of those intrabred groups, it may reach 40 to 60%. After a usual course of 4 to 6 weeks, all affected animals die.

DIAGNOSIS. Veterinarians diagnose scrapie on evidence of typical signs and histopathologic changes in the brain. The long incubation period, history of exposure to scrapie, incessant rubbing, reflex nibbling and licking movements of lips and tongue, and muscular incoordination are significant and indicative signs. Laboratory confirmation is based on (1) finding characteristic histopathologic changes in the thalamus and medulla in suspect cases, and (2) if necessary, inducing characteristic disease by intracerebral inoculation of mice with suspect sheep brain.

The differential diagnosis requires consideration of bacterial, fungal, and parasitic dermatitides, and all encephalopathies such as

Fig. 17-2. Cystoplasmic vacuoles in neurons of the reticular formation of the medulla. HE stain. × 600.

listeriosis, polioencephalomalacia, and enzootic ataxia.

For assistance from a diagnostic laboratory, practitioners should submit one undecomposed frozen cerebral hemisphere and the balance of the brain fixed in ample amounts of 10% neutral formalin.

PREVENTION. Veterinarians and producers, through the authority and force of state and federal regulatory agencies, prevent scrapie by avoiding the exposure of susceptible animals to infected animals and contaminated environments. In the United States and many other countries, suspected and positively diagnosed cases of scrapie by law must be reported immediately to state or federal regulatory officers, who then assume the responsibility for confirming diagnoses, quarantining the flocks, appraising the value of the animals, eliminating the infection, and cleaning the environment.

Infected flocks (those in which scrapie has been diagnosed), source flocks (those in which no known scrapie has occurred, but has developed in some of their members within 18 months after dispersion to other flocks), and intermediate-source flocks (those through which transient animals pass before manifesting scrapie) are destroyed and burned or buried.

No preventive vaccine has been developed, and no effective treatment has been devised.

Alper, T. and Haig, D.A.: Protection by anoxia of the scrapie agent and some DNA and RNA viruses irradiated as dry preparations. J. Gen. Virol., 3:157-166, 1968.

Alper, T., Haig, D.A., and Clarke, M.C.: The exceptionally small size of the scrapie agent. Biochem. Biophys. Res. Commun., 22:278-284, 1966.

Animal Health Yearbook. FAO-WHO-OIE (Italy), 1970.

Besnoit, C. and Morel, C.: Note sur les lesions nervenses de la tremblante du mouton. Rev. Vet. Toulouse, 23:397-400, 1898, cited from Palmer, A.C.: Scrapie, a review of literature. Reviews and Annotations, 5:1-15, 1959.

Carp, R., et al.: Nature of the scrapie agent: Current status of facts and hypothesis. J. Gen. Virol., 66:1357-1368, 1985.

Chandler, R.L.: Experimental scrapie in the mouse. Res. Vet. Sci., 4:276, 1963.

Chatelain, J., Delasherie-Laupretre, N., and Cathala, F.: Scrapie in France: Some possible predisposing factors in the naturally-acquired disease of sheep. Vet. Microbiol., 8:511-515, 1983.

Cuille, J. and Chelle, P.L.: La maladie dite tremblante du mouton est-elle inoculable? C. R. Acad. Sci., 203:1552-1554, 1936.

Dees, C., Wade, W., German, T., and Marsh, R.: Inactivation of the scrapie agent by ultraviolet irradication in the presence of Chlorpromazine. J. Gen. Virol., 66:845-849, 1985.

Diener, T.O.: Is the scrapie agent a viroid? Nature; New Biology, 235:218-219, 1972.

Ehlers, B., Rudolph, R., and Diringer, H.: The reticuloendothelial system in scrapie pathogenesis. J. Gen. Virol., 65:423-428, 1984.

Field, E.J., Caspary, E.A., and Joyce, G.: Scrapie agent in blood. Vet. Rec., 83:109-110, 1968.

Gordon, W.S.: Advances in veterinary research. Vet. Rec., 58:516-518, 1946.

Gordon, W.S.: Studies on scrapie. Vet. Rec., 69:1324-1327, 1957.

Gordon, W.S.: Report on scrapie. USDA, ARS, 91-22: 1-12, 1960.

Gustafson, D.P. and Kanitz, C.L.: In vitro studies of scrapie virus. Fed. Proc., 24:248, 1965.

Hadlow, W.J.: The pathology of experimental scrapie in the dairy goat. Res. Vet. Sci., 2:289-314, 1961.

Hadlow, W.J. and Eklund, C.M.: Scrapie—a virus-induced chronic encephalopathy of sheep. In Infections of the Nervous System. Baltimore, Williams & Wilkins, 1968, pp. 281-306.

Hadlow, W., Jackson, T., and Race, R.: Experimental infection of fetal and newborn Suffolk sheep with scrapie virus. Am. J. Vet. Res., 45:2637-2639, 1984.

Hadlow, W., Kennedy, R., and Race, R.: Natural infection of Suffolk sheep with scrapie virus. J. Infect. Dis., 146:657-667, 1982.

Haig, D.A. and Clarke, M.C.: Multiplication of the scrapie agent. Nature, 234:106-107, 1971.

Hourrigan, J., Klingsporn, A., Clark, W.W., and deCamp, M.: Epidemiology of scrapie in the U.S. In Slow Transmissible Disease of the Nervous System. Edited by S.B. Prusiner and W.J. Hadlow. New York, Academic Press, 1980.

Hunter, D.G. and Millson, G.C.: Studies on heat stability and chromatographic behavior of the scrapie agent. J. Gen. Microbiol., 37:251-258, 1964.

Kimberlin, R. and Walker, C.: The antiviral compound HPA-23 can prevent scrapie when administered at the time of infection. Arch. Virol., 78:9-18, 1983.

Klingsporn, A.L., Hourrigan, J.L., and McDaniel, H.A.: Scrapie—Eradication and field trial study of the natural disease. JAVMA, 155:2172-2177, 1969.

Pattison, I.H.: Resistance of the scrapie agent to formalin. J. Comp. Pathol., 75:159-164, 1965.

Pattison, I.H., Gordon, W.S., and Millson, G.C.: Experimental production of scrapie in goats. J. Comp. Pathol., 69:300-312, 1959.

Rohwer, R.: Scrapie infectious agent is virus-like in size and susceptibility to inactivation. Nature, 308:658-661, 1984.

Stamp, J.T., et al.: Further studies on scrapie. J. Comp. Pathol., 69:268-280, 1959.

Strain, G., et al.: Serum and cerebrospinal fluid concentrations of immunoglobulin G in Suffolk sheep with scrapie. Am. J. Vet. Res., 45:1812-1813, 1984.

Wilson, D.R., Anderson, R.D., and Smith, W.: Studies in scrapie. J. Comp. Pathol., 60:267-278, 1950.

Zlotnik, I.: The histopathology of the brain stem of sheep affected with natural scrapie. J. Comp. Pathol., *68*: 148-166, 1958.

Zlotnik, I. and Rennie, J.C.: Experimental transmission of mouse passaged scrapie to goats, sheep, rats and hamsters. J. Comp. Pathol., 75:147-157, 1965.

Heartwater

(Black gall sickness; mad gall sickness; cowdriosis)

Heartwater is a noncontagious acute infection characterized by fever, hydropericardium, hydrothorax, and hydroperitoneum. It is caused by a rickettsial organism transmitted by ticks of the genus *Amblyomma*. Although heartwater was once limited to the African countries, it has been diagnosed in Guadeloupe and Antigua in the Caribbean with a potential of spread to other regions and the United States where efficient vector species of the *Amblyomma* tick exist. It causes waste of sheep, cattle, and goats in endemic areas. Economic losses from the disease result from deaths, loss of valuable exotic breeding stock, animal protein deficiencies among sheep-dependent people, and cost of tick control programs.

OCCURRENCE. Although heartwater occurs in all sexes and breeds of sheep, breeds indigenous to endemic areas and Persian sheep are more resistant than are breeds imported from other continents. Young lambs are naturally resistant, but sheep 6 months of age and older are fully susceptible. In addition to sheep, heartwater also occurs as a severe and often fatal disease in cattle and goats. For susceptible populations of cattle it is second in importance only to East Coast fever and tsetse-transmitted trypanasomiasis and has a wider distribution. Wild ruminants, including blesbok, black wildebeest, springbok, eland, and possibly others, may develop asymptomatic heartwater and form a reservoir of infecting rickettsiae.

Seasonally, heartwater occurs during months of high rainfall when the transmitting ticks actively pursue and parasitize sheep and cattle. In the process of feeding on a sheep, an infected bont tick transmits the rickettsiae.

The disease is known to occur throughout most of Africa south of the Sahara, from South Africa north to the Sudan and from Senegal in the west to Somolia in the east. Its distribution outside the African continent includes the Islands of Madagascar, LaReunion and Mauritius to the east, Sao Tome in the Atlantic Ocean, and Guadeloupe and Antigua in the Caribbean.

ETIOLOGY. *Cowdria ruminantium,* the cause of heartwater, is a diplococcal but pleomorphic rickettsia measuring 0.2 to 0.5 μm in diameter. In staining reaction, it is gram-negative, but deep blue when treated with Giemsa solution.

C. ruminantium parasitizes both mammalian and arthropod hosts. In the mammalian host it is found in the cytoplasm of vascular endothelial cells occurring in groups. The groups of rickettsia are located inside a membrane-linked vacuole in the cytoplasm of an endothelial cell. Multiplication appears to occur mainly by binary fission with some indications of multiple budding and endosporulation. In the tick *C. ruminantium* has been found only in epithelial cells of the intestine. Culture of the organism has been unsuccessful except in albino mice.

TRANSMISSION. Under experimental conditions *C. ruminantium* readily is transmitted by injecting whole blood from febrile animals into susceptible sheep, cattle, or goats. All known vectors of heartwater are three-host *Amblyomma* species in which the infection is transstadial, from larva to nymph, nymph to adult, or larva through nymph to adult, but not transovarial. At least 5 species of *Amblyomma* ticks are known natural transmitters of *C. ruminantium*: *A. gemma, A. hebraeum, A. lepidum, A. pomposum,* and *A. variegatum.* The tropical bont tick, *A. variegatum,* is the most widespread and efficient of the tick vectors. The gulf coast tick, *A. maculatum,* found in the Southeastern states bordering the Gulf of Mexico and the Atlantic Ocean is shown to be an efficient vector of *C. ruminantium* and is of extreme concern to the U.S. livestock industry. Since the rickettsia does not cross the ovary to infect tick eggs, the unfed larvae are innocuous. After feeding on infected blood, a tick retains rickettsiae throughout all successive life stages and can transmit the disease while feeding on a susceptible host. Although the role of a wildlife reservoir is unknown, one tick generation, infected in the larval stage, is able to maintain the infection for over 3 years.

The bont tick, although hardy and long-lived, survives in warm, moist, and shady habitats. It is a three-host tick; both larvae and nymphae attach to general skin of warm-blooded hosts, but adult ticks prefer denuded skin of sheep and cattle, such as perineum and axilla, where penetration may cause significant injury and dermatitis. Engorged adult females drop to the ground and, in secluded places, deposit up to 20,000 eggs.

PATHOGENESIS. The pathogenesis of heartwater is poorly understood. By feeding on an infected host, tick larvae and nymphae ingest the pathogenic rickettsia which invades the epithelial cells of the intestine where it multiplies, especially after the tick has moulted and started to feed again. This increase reaches a high level after 3 days and persists during further feeding, through to full engorgement. This concentration of rickettsia spills over into the lumen of the gut from where it is regurgitated into the mammalian host. It is hypothesized that the initial development takes place mainly in reticuloendothelial cells, beginning with the formation of dense bodies. These grow and undergo cleavage, resulting in fragments of irregular shape with poorly defined edges, around which double unit membranes develop, giving rise to mature organisms lying free in the cytoplasm and that colonies form in the cytoplasm during the febrile period. The leukocyte blood fraction is not normally infected. The only certainty in the pathogenesis is that C. ruminantium lives and multiplies in vascular endothelial cells in ruminants and occurs in the cirulating blood. The sequence of events leading to the increase in capillary permeability and passage of fluids and plasma proteins from the blood vascular system causing pulmonary edema, hydropericardium, hydrothorax, and ascites is unknown. There is a terminal decrease in arterial blood pressure associated with a terminal fall in plasma volume. In acute cases death is commonly due to asphyxiation from pulmonary edema, in other cases death may be from shock and vasocollapse. Young calves and lambs possess a resistance to infection independent of the immune status of the dam and is thought to be a function of the cell mediated immune system.

Indigenous livestock also possess a resistance factor.

CLINICAL SIGNS AND POSTMORTEM LESIONS. Following an incubation period of 7 to 14 days after experimental inoculation, 11 to 18 days after infected tick feeding, and 14 to 28 days after entering tick-infested areas, some animals suddenly develop high body temperature, convulse, and die. In most affected sheep, however, body temperature rises to 41 to 43°C for several days and then abruptly declines prior to death.

During the febrile period, appetite diminishes, body weight decreases, and diarrhea develops. Heart sounds become muffled because of hydropericardium, and breathing becomes difficult because of pulmonary edema. Neurologic signs commonly develop and include violent and repeated blinking of eyelids, walking in circles, lifting forelimbs high during walking, impaired vision, prostration, convulsions, muscular tremors, galloping limb movements, coma, and death. Most animals that develop nervous manifestations die. The disease course is approximately 6 days, and the expected mortality is 60% of affected animals.

At necropsy, affected sheep may have lost some body weight, and transmitting ticks may be attached to the skin, especially the denuded areas. Approximately 95% of all cases show hydropericardium, 66% hydrothorax, and 25% ascites. Although usually clear, the fluid may contain blood. The lungs are congested and edematous in the ventral planes. Both abomasum and small intestines are hyperemic and hemorrhagic. The spleen may be enlarged by a factor of 5. Brain hemorrhages are common (acute hemorrhagic meningoencephalitis).

Histopathologically, in tissues collected and fixed within 6 hours after death, clusters of C. ruminantium in the cytoplasm of endothelial cells are demonstrable in the brain, spleen, and glomeruli. In addition, the brain shows vasculitis, vessel necrosis, choroiditis, swollen glia, swollen axis cylinders, microcavitation, and perivascular globules.

DIAGNOSIS. Veterinarians diagnose heartwater from clinical and pathologic evidence. In endemic areas, the presence of attached bont ticks on animals showing nervous symptoms and hydropericardium, hydrothorax, and ascites is highly indicative. The histopathologic demonstration of rickettsiae in the cytoplasm of endothelial cells confirms the diagnosis. Cerebral cortex, kidney cortex, and jugular vein in smears or sections are usually examined for the organisms.

The differential diagnosis requires consideration of organophosphate poisoning, strychnine poisoning, tetanus, anthrax, and rabies.

PREVENTION AND TREATMENT. Veterinarians and producers prevent heartwater by controlling the transmitting ticks and by premunition of susceptible sheep. In some areas, the bont and related ticks cannot only be controlled, but possibly eradicated by frequent treatment of susceptible sheep and other hosts with appropriate acaricides and by regulating the availability of suitable hosts. In heavily infected areas, sheep can be immunized by injecting lambs up to 1 week of age with virulent blood from a case of heartwater—a newly developed C. ruminantium-infected tick stabilate. On the tenth to twelfth day after inoculation or preferably as soon as the febrile reaction commences, the lambs should receive oxytetracycline for 2 to 4 days at the daily rate of 10 mg/kg. The drugs of choice are oxytetracycline (Terramycin) rolitetracycline (Reverin) or doxycycline administered at the rate of 5 to 10 mg/kg with two treatments 1 to 2 days apart. To be effective, treatment must be started on the first or second day of the febrile reaction. The patient must be monitored closely for temperature relapses which require further treatment. The use of tetracyclines after nervous symptoms or a hemorrhagic diarrhea has developed is to no avail. In addition to specific antibiotic therapy, supportive symptomatic therapy and good nursing care are helpful.

Animal Health Yearbook. FAO-WHO-OIE (Italy), 1970.
Bezuidenhout, J.: Demonstration of Cowdria ruminantium in Amblyomma herbraeum by fluorescent antibody techniques, light and electron microscopy. Onderstepoort J. Vet. Res., 51:213-215, 1984.
Birnie, E., Burridge, M., Camus, E., and Barre, N.: Heartwater in the Caribbean: Isolation of Cowdria ruminantium from Antigua. Vet. Rec., 116:121-123, 1985.
Burridge, M.: Heartwater: Review of new exotic disease threat to the United States. Proc. Eighty-Sixth Annual Meeting U.S. Animal Health Association, 1982, pp. 322-325.
Clark, R.: Pathological physiology of heartwater. Onderstepoort J. Vet. Res., 29:25-33, 1962.
Cowdry, E.V.: Studies on the etiology of heartwater. I. Observations on a rickettsia, Rickettsia ruminantium (n. sp.) in tissues of animals. II. Rickettsia ruminantium (n. sp.) in the tissues of ticks transmitting the disease. J. Exp. Med., 42:231-274, 1925.
Daubney, R.: Natural transmission of heartwater of sheep by Amblyomma variegatum Fabricus, 1794. Parasitology, 22:260-267, 1930.
DePlessis, J., Bezuidenhout, J., and Ludemann, C.: The immunization of calves against heartwater: Subsequent immunity both in the absence and presence of natural tick challenge. Onderstepoort J. Vet. Res., 51:193-196, 1984.
DePlessis, J.: Colostrum-derived antibodies to Cowdria ruminantium in the serum of calves and lambs. Onderstepoort J. Vet. Res., 51:275-276, 1984.
Dixon, R.W., 1898, quoted from Henning: Animal Diseases in South Africa. 3rd Edition. South Africa, Central News Agency, 1956, p. 1155.
Karrar, G.: Further studies on the epizootiology of heartwater in the Sudan. Sudan J. Vet. Sci. Anim. Husb., 6:83-85, 1966.
Lounsbury, C.P., 1900, quoted from Henning: Animal Diseases in South Africa. 3rd Edition. South Africa, Central News Agency, 1956, p. 1155.
Mackenzie, P.: The culture of Cowdria ruminantium in mice; Significance in respect of the epidemiology and control of heartwater. Preventive Vet. Med., 2:227-237, 1984.
Mare, C.J.: The effect of prolonged oral administration of oxytetracycline on the course of heartwater (Cowdria ruminantium) infection in sheep. Trop. Anim. Health Prod., 4:69-73, 1972.
Pienaar, J.G., Basson, P.A., and Van der Merwe, J.L.de B.: Studies on the pathology of heartwater. I. Neuropathological changes. Onderstepoort J. Vet. Res., 33:115-138, 1966.
Poisson and Geoffroy, 1925, quoted from Curasson, G.: Traite de pathologie exotique veterinaire et comparee. Vol. 2. Paris, Vigot Freres, 1936, p. 317.
Steck, W.: Pathological studies on heartwater. 13th and 14th Repts. Dir. Vet. Educ. Res., 1928 pp. 283-305.
Uilenberg, G.: Heartwater (Cowdria ruminantium infection): Current status. Advances in Veterinary Science and Comparative Medicine. 27:427-480, 1983.
Webb, J., 1877, quoted from Henning: Animal Diseases in South Africa. 3rd Edition. South Africa, Central News Agency, 1956, p. 1155.
Young, E. and Basson, P.A.: Heartwater in the eland. J. S. Afr. Vet. Assoc., 44:185-186, 1973.

Botulism

(Carrion poisoning)

Usually an acute, and often fatal, intoxication, ovine botulism is characterized by ascending muscular weakness and paralysis and is caused by ingesting food or water containing a toxin of saprophytic bacteria that reside in soil and metabolize toxin in dead organic matter of animal or plant origin. Because of limited geographic distribution, the disease has little economic importance in America and most European countries, but in South African countries and Australia, botulism has more importance than elsewhere. Prior to the prevalent practice of immunization, veterinary officers of Australia estimated losses from botulism to exceed losses from all other diseases. Severe losses may still occur when circumstances preclude vaccination. Additional losses result from lamsiekte and loin disease (both bovine botulism), from duck sickness and chicken limberneck (avian botulism), and from occasional human botulism.

OCCURRENCE. All breeds and sexes of sheep are equally susceptible to botulism. Although sheep of all ages may contract the disease, animals having high mineral requirement, such as rapidly growing yearlings and pregnant ewes, more commonly develop an appetite for carrion and for that reason suffer a higher disease incidence than do other age groups.

Botulism occurs commonly during late summer and autumn, especially following a season of drought, because grasses mature and dry early and their content of phosphorus and protein declines. Although most cases of botulism in ruminants involves carrion or carrion contaminated feed or water, noncarrion associated botulism can occur from improperly fermented silages.

Geographically, ovine botulism occurs in countries of the southern part of Africa and Australia. Although isolated cases and sporadic outbreaks may develop in other regions, the incidence is low, and the economic effect is of minor importance.

ETIOLOGY AND PATHOGENESIS. *Clostridium botulinum,* an anaerobic, motile, sporing, gram-positive, saprophytic bacillus, measures 0.9 to 1.2 × 4 to 6 μm and resides in soil. The oval subterminal spore has a diameter greater than the width of the bacillus. In old cultures the organism becomes gram-negative. *C. botulinum* metabolizes eight known complex exotoxins, designated types A, B, Ca, Cb, D, E, F, G with each type differing in geographic distribution and species susceptibility. Each toxin is composed of toxic and nontoxic components with varying molecular size for the components. The nontoxic component acts as a protective device which prevents gastric and intestinal juices from destroying the toxic component. Soil type, a near neutral pH, and bacteriophages are important factors in presence of *C. botulinum* and toxin production. Toxin production is inhibited below pH 4.6 and certain toxin types depend on bacteriophages for their production. Some toxin types require trypsin for activation, while others act independently. Types A, B and E and occasionally F are associated with human botulism. Types A, B, C1, C2, D and E are associated with botulism in animals and fowl with type G being isolated from the soil. Type C usually causes botulism in sheep. Type prevalence in a geographic area is dependent on soil type and other ecologic factors.

The pathogenesis of ovine botulism involves six essential ecologic factors: bacteria, soil, carrion, toxin, forage, and sheep. The natural development of botulism in sheep requires each factor in sequence. Although the route of infection can be through wound botulism, toxicoinfectious botulism, or botulism from preformed toxin, the latter is the only route of importance in sheep. The bacterium, *C. botulinum* type C, resides as a saprophyte in alkaline soil, and although widely distributed, the organism is not ubiquitous. In South Africa and Australia, where ovine botulism is common, the soil of some districts harbors the specific organism, whereas the soil of other districts is free of it. Existing as spores, the bacteria survive for long periods, especially when sheltered against the action of direct sunlight. Under proper conditions of temperature and moisture, the organism grows in organic substrates.

The carcasses of dead rabbits, sheep, tortoises, and other animals lie and decompose on the soil surface. *C. botulinum* in the soil penetrates the carcass skin and enters muscle and other soft tissues. Under anaerobic conditions inside the carcass, the bacteria metabolize type C toxin, which diffuses throughout the carcass, including the skeleton. The toxin usually reaches maximum concentration within 5 to 10 days and then declines to innocuous levels within 30 to 40 days. Protection of the carcass causes longer persistence of the toxin. If the toxic carcass enters sheep's drinking water, the toxin may dissolve in the water and raise its toxicity to dangerous levels. Carcasses do not become toxic if *C. botulinum* is absent from the soil, if ambient temperatures are too low, or if moisture is not available. Vegetable sources of toxin include decomposing moist grass, lodged hay and grain, moldy silage, and spoiled stackhay.

Both the composition of the soil and meteorologic factors of the environment affect the composition of plants growing on the soil. The soils of some ranges and pastures may be deficient in available phosphorus. Twenty parts per million is a critical level of phosphorus in soil. Lesser amounts result in a phosphorus deficiency in grass and other plants growing on the deficient soil. During summers of drought, plants dry and mature early and commonly contain low levels of phosphorus and protein. Young growing forage plants normally contain 0.2% P. Forage plants containing only 0.05 to 0.1% P are seriously deficient.

Sheep and other ruminants subsisting for several months on forage deficient in phosphorus, proteins, and carbohydrates develop pica or a depraved appetite for abnormal foods. Growing yearlings and pregnant ewes require large amounts of mineral and protein nutrients and, because of these needs, develop pica earlier than do other groups of sheep.

Sheep with pica avidly devour partially desiccated carcasses of dead rabbits and dead sheep. If the carcass material contains botulinus toxin, the sheep eating the toxic carcass become poisoned to variable degrees. At the time of maximum concentration of toxin, 3 to 5 g of carcass tissue may be fatal to the consuming sheep.

In the sheep, the ingested toxin is absorbed from the alimentary tract and is widely distributed throughout the tissue. The toxins exert their effect on peripheral nerves with no known effect on the C.N.S. and not all muscle groups are affected equally. Muscle groups like the pharyngeal muscles with large amounts of efferent nerve fibers may paralyze more quickly. The toxin impairs the passage of stimuli across neuromuscular junctions by acting presynaptically to prevent nerve action potentials from releasing normal amounts of acetylcholine. This disruption of a threshold percentage of neuromuscular junctions causes overt paralysis, the severity of which depends upon the degree by which the threshold is exceeded. Paralyzed sheep die from respiratory failure. Approximately 50% of affected sheep recover, but do not develop immunity from the attack. Recontamination of the soil with *C. botulinum* occurs from high numbers of organisms being shed in the feces for up to 8 weeks in convalescent cases or, in fatal cases, with decomposing tissues.

CLINICAL SIGNS AND POSTMORTEM LESIONS. Sheep affected with botulism may have a history of eating or chewing debris from desiccated carcasses of rabbits and sheep. Muscle, skin, and bones may have been consumed.

The period of time between eating carrion and the beginning of symptoms varies directly with the amount of toxin consumed. Following the consumption of large doses, clinical signs may appear within 12 hours, and death may occur after a disease course of a few hours. With smaller doses of toxin, the incubation period commonly ranges from 2 to 3 days.

In early stages, the affected sheep separates from the flock and stands with its head lowered to one side and its tail rapidly oscillating from side to side. Movements are incoordinated, stiff, and forced. Saliva drips from the mouth, and swallowing is difficult. Feed may be held in the mouth, and the paralyzed tongue may protrude. Paralysis begins in the caudal limbs, and the animal may require assistance to stand.

Respiration becomes difficult and irregular. Death comes after a period of recumbency. The disease course varies from 2 to 10 days. The morbidity ranges up to 15%, and approximately 50% of affected animals die.

At necropsy, few lesions are evident. Paralysis of the pharynx and esophagus may result in the accumulation of feed in the mouth, pharynx, and esophagus. Fragments of ingested carcass may be identifiable in contents of the rumen.

DIAGNOSIS. Veterinarians diagnose botulism on the basis of history and clinical signs. Some animals of the flock may have manifested pica, and the area may have a known deficiency in phosphorus. The ascending and progressive paralysis, tail movements, and head position are highly suggestive signs. A laboratory diagnosis is accomplished by a standard mouse inoculation procedure using extracts of the suspected materials. The type of *C. botulinum* toxin can be determined by the use of specific antitoxins to protect challenged mice. The use of monoclonal antibodies with the enzyme-linked immunosorbent assay (ELISA) test or the reversed passive latex agglutination (RPLA) test facilitates a rapid determination of the presence and type of toxin.

PREVENTION AND TREATMENT. Veterinarians and producers prevent botulism by husbandry management and by immunization. Producers avoid pica by providing the sheep with a diet that is both balanced in quality and adequate in amount. All sources of toxin, such as carcasses of rabbits, sheep, tortoises, and other animals, should be removed from the grazing area and burned or buried. Finally, sheep that are expected to be exposed to botulism can be vaccinated against the disease. A few months before protection is needed, the vaccine should be given as a single dose and should be repeated annually.

In most sheep producing areas where *C. botulinum* is an endemic problem, the economic constraints preclude treatment. Treatment, when feasible, is directed at removing the source and neutralizing the circulating toxin. Antitoxins are used to neutralize the

absorbed toxins and a mild cathartic, such as mineralized oil or sodium sulfate, may be used to remove ingested toxin which has not been absorbed. Avoid the use of magnesium products. Some antibiotics, especially the aminoglycosides (gentamycin), tetracyclines, and procaine penicillin, may potentiate neuromuscular weakness. Following neutralization of the circulating toxins providing nutrition, electrolytes and water directly into the rumen is essential. Recumbent animals must be repositioned frequently and assisted to stand. Recovery may take 2 to 3 weeks.

Bekker, J.G. and Rossouw, S.D.: A note on some conditions in sheep in the Strandveld of the Bredasdorp district. 16th Ann. Rep. Dir. Vet. Serv. Anim. Ind. S. Afr., 1930, pp. 393-400.
Bennetts, H.W.: Carrion poisoning of sheep. Aust. Vet. J., 4:105-106, 1928.
Bennetts, H.W. and Hall, H.T.B.: Botulism of sheep and cattle in Western Australia: its cause and its prevention by immunization. Aust. Vet. J., 14:105-119, 1938.
Cook, C.W. and Harris, L.E.: Nutritive value of seasonal ranges. Utah Agric. Exp. Stat. Bull., 472, 1968.
Divers, T., et al.: *Clostridium botulinum* type B toxicosis in a herd of cattle and a group of mules. JAVMA, 188:382-386, 1986.
Filmer, J.F.: Botulism in domestic animals in western Australia. Aust. Vet. J., 13:170-172, 1937.
Fourie, J.M.: Persistence of botulinus toxin in carcass material with special reference to that of tortoises. J. S. Afr. Vet. Med. Assoc., 16:85-87, 1946.
Horiguchi, Y., Kozaki, S., and Sakaguchi, G.: Determination of *Clostridium botulinum* toxin by reversed passive latex agglutination. Jpn. J. Vet. Sci., 46:487-491, 1984.
Montville, T.: Interaction of pH and NaCl on culture density of *Clostridium botulinum*. 62A Appl. Environ. Microbiol., 46:961-963, 1983.
Oguma, K., et al.: Analysis of antigenicity of *Clostridium botulinum* type C and D toxins by polyclonal and monoclonal antibodies. Infect. Immun., 43:584-588, 1984.
Ohishi, I.: Oral toxicities of *Clostridium botulinum* type A and B toxins from different strains. Infect. Immun., 43:487-490, 1984.
Robinson, E.M.: The bacteria of the *Clostridium botulinum* C and D types. 16th Ann. Rep. Dir. Vet. Serv. Anim. Ind. S. Afr., 1930, pp. 107-142.
Seddon, H.R.: *Diseases of Domestic Animals in Australia*. Vol. 1. Aust. Dept. Health, 1965.
Shone, C.: Monoclonal antibody-based immunoassay for type A *Clostridium botulinum* toxin is comparable to the mouse bioassay. Appl. Environ. Microbiol., 50:63-67, 1985.
Simpson, L.: The origin, structure and pharmacological activity of botulism toxin. Pharmacol. Rev., 33:155-188, 1981.

Smith, L.: *Clostridium botulinum*: Characteristics and occurrence. Rev. Infect. Dis., *1*:637-641, 1979.

Sterne, M. and Wentzel, L.M.: A new method for the large-scale production of high-titer botulinum formoltoxoid types C and D. J. Immunol., *65*:175-183, 1950.

Theiler, A.: Cause and prevention of lamsiekte. J. Dep. Agric. S. Afr., June, 1920.

Theiler, A., et al.: Lamsiekte (parabotulism) in cattle of South Africa. 11th & 12th Reps. Dir. Vet. Educ. Res. S. Afr., 1927, pp. 821-1361.

Underwood, E.J., Beck, A.B., and Shier, F.L.: Further experiments on the incidence and control of pica in sheep in the botulism areas in western Australia. Aust. J. Exp. Biol. Med. Sci., *17*:183-192, 1939.

Wang, Y., et al.: Acute toxicity of aminoglycoside antibiotics as an aid in detecting botulism. Applied and Environmental Microbiology, *48*:951-955, 1984.

Gid

(*Coenurosis; staggers; sturdy*)

Gid, a parasitic invasion of the central nervous system of sheep, is characterized by the development of bladderworms in the brain and along the spinal cord, and is caused by the larval stage of a tapeworm of dogs, coyotes, foxes, and jackals. Because the disease has wide geographic distribution, high mortality and, in some areas, high prevalence, it is of importance to the world sheep industry, except in the United States. Economic losses result from prolonged disease course, low productive performance, costs of treatment, and deaths of most untreated sheep.

In addition to sheep, the disease affects goats, cattle, and horses.

OCCURRENCE. Gid occurs in all breeds, sexes, and ages of sheep. Although animals usually contract the disease during summer grazing seasons, the long incubation period and disease course continue the manifestations into all seasons. Geographically, the malady occurs in Europe, Republic of South Africa, USSR, New Zealand, Chile, and America. In the United States, gid occurred early during the twentieth century in New York State and northern Montana, but since those early diagnoses, the disease has declined, certainly to insignificance and possibly to extinction.

ETIOLOGY AND PATHOGENESIS. A tapeworm causes gid. The adult worm, *Taenia (Multi-ceps) multiceps,* inhabits the small intestines of dogs and other canine animals, and the larvae, *Coenurus cerebralis,* reside in the brain and spinal cord of sheep. The adult worm, measuring 40 to 100 cm in length, has a scolex about 0.8 mm in diameter, with a rostellum bearing 22 to 32 hooks. Gravid segments, 8 to 12 × 3 to 4 mm, contain eggs 30 to 36 μm in diameter. The mature bladderworm, measuring up to 5 cm in diameter, contains clear fluid and numerous scoleces attached to the germinal membrane.

The life cycle begins with expulsion of gravid segments or eggs to the exterior. When eggs are eaten by sheep in contaminated feed or water, the released embryos penetrate the small intestine, enter portal vessels, traverse capillaries of the liver and lungs, and are distributed to many organs. Those entering the central nervous system survive, but others perish. The larval parasites develop through two phases—migratory and stationary—in the brain. During the migratory phase, the larvae channel through the brain tissue and finally settle in a stationary position where, in 2 to 7 months, they grow to maturity. Following ingestion of the coenurus by a dog, the scoleces evaginate, attach to the small intestine, and grow to mature tapeworms.

Gradual enlargement of the coenurus causes pressure atrophy and necrosis of nerve tissue and even of parietal bone. Clinical signs usually persist through infection months 2 to 7.

CLINICAL SIGNS AND POSTMORTEM LESIONS. Heavy infection during the migratory phase may cause fever, hyperesthesia from meningitis, and death; the mortality, however, is low. In the stationary phase, the coenurus gradually enlarges, and the resulting pressure causes signs that correlate with location of the bladderworm. Impaired vision, walking in circles, abnormal head position, head pushing, incoordinated gait, falling, ascending paralysis, and excitability, followed by prostration, convulsions, and death, are variable signs. The mortality at this phase is high.

At necropsy, the unilateral bladderworm commonly is located in a frontal lobe of the cerebrum or in a lateral ventricle, and less commonly in other parts of the brain and spinal cord. Gyri over the coenurus are atrophied and flattened. The superimposed cranial bone may also be thinned and even perforated or bulged.

DIAGNOSIS.   Veterinarians diagnose gid in flocks by finding characteristic coenuri in the brain or along the spinal cord in some animals at necropsy. Interpretation of clinical signs is the best method of diagnosis as serologic tests are unreliable. The clinical sign also gives an indication of the location of the lesion which is an important factor when surgical removal is economically justifiable. Lesions in the frontal cortex tend to induce head pressing, circling, and depression. Cysts located in the contralateral frontal cerebral cortex cause unilateral paresis and paralysis. Circling is most likely caused by lesions in the ipsilateral cerebral cortex area or basal ganglia which causes circling to either or both sides. Head aversion is usually caused by a cyst in the cerebral cortex and most likely to the opposite side, although some cases are on the same side. Postural defects are due to cerebral cortical cysts located contralateral to the signs. Visual defects may result from tentorial herniation of either cerebral cortex or a cerebral cortical cyst. The lesion is likely to be in the contralateral cerebral cortex. Papilledema is a sign of increased intracranial pressure due to a space occupying lesion and is not necessarily associated with clinical signs. The differential diagnosis requires consideration of polioencephalomalacia, brain abscesses, brain tumors, heartwater, and louping-ill. Each disease presents characteristic signs and lesions.

PREVENTION AND TREATMENT.   Producers and veterinarians prevent gid by the same principles and procedures as they use in preventing abdominal cysticercosis. They treat cases in gid-diagnosed flocks by locating a skull perforation or bulge and aseptically inserting a needle through that point into the coenurus. Fluid is withdrawn and replaced with a mild antiseptic, such as 0.1% solution of acriflavine.

Less than half of the cases of gid can be located by softening and protrusion of the skull. It may, therefore, be necessary to conduct a thorough neurologic examination using a variety of reflex examinations to determine the location of the cyst. Once located, surgical removal is then accomplished under general anesthesia by folding back a crescent shaped flap of skin and tissue over the area, a 0.5 to 1.5 cm diameter hole is trephined through the cranium, and the meninges are incised exposing the cerebral cortex. The cyst wall with attached protoscoleces can then be removed by applying suction on the catheter sufficient to draw the cyst wall to the exterior and gentle removal with the aid of forceps. Normal postoperative care is all that is required. Economic constraints limit the surgical approach to valuable breeding animals. Slaughter of fat lambs should be considered early in the course of the disease.

Barlow, R.: Neurological disorders of cattle and sheep. Vet. Rec. Supp. In Practice, 5:77-84, 1983.
Becklund, W.W.: Current knowledge of the gid bladder worm, *Coenurus cerebralis* (—*Taenia multiceps*), in North American domestic sheep, *Ovis aries*. Proc. Helminthol. Soc. Wash., 37:200-203, 1970.
DeVilliers, S.W.: Treatment of gid in sheep. J. S. Afr. Vet. Med. Assoc., 21:155-157, 1950.
Ermolova, E.N.: Eradication of coenurus from sheep farms. Veterinariia (Moscow), 35:58-60, 1958.
Frankhauser, R., Hintermann, J., and Valette, H.: Coenurosis in sheep. Schweitz Arch. Tierheilk., 101:15-32, 1959.
Hall, M.C.: Gid, a historic review. USDA Bull. 125, 1910.
Newsom, I.E. and Cross, F.: Diseases of Colorado feeding lambs. Colorado Agric. Exp. Stat. Bull. 305, 1925.
Sherritt, G. and Stallbaumer, M.: Diagnosis on treatment of coenuriasis (gid) in sheep. Vet. Rec., 115:399-403, 1984.
Taylor, W.J. and Boynton, W.H.: Gid in sheep in New York. Ann. Rep. New York State Vet. Coll., 1908-09.

Cerebrospinal Nematodosis

(*Lumbar paralysis*)

Cerebrospinal nematodosis, an acute or chronic injury to the central nervous system, is characterized by motor deficiencies and is caused by invading larvae from unnatural parasites. In the western hemisphere, the disease is generally uncommon and for that reason causes little concern to the sheep industry, but in some enterprises it results in severe wastage. Economic losses come from prolonged partial or complete incapacitations, extra labor, and eventual deaths. Development of the disease also in goats, horses, and possibly other domestic animals enhances its economic importance.

ETIOLOGY AND PATHOGENESIS. Larvae of two species of heteroxenous nematodes—*Parelaphostrongylus tenuis* and *Setaria digitata*—cause the disease (Table 17-1). In natural hosts they are nonpathogenic, but in sheep and goats—unnatural hosts—they induce myelopathy and occasionally encephalopathy.

Adult *P. tenuis* reside in the cranial subdural space of white-tailed deer. The gravid female deposits eggs on the dura, and the first stage larvae penetrate venous vessels, transport to the lungs, enter alveoli, ascend the airways, descend the gastrointestinal tract, and discharge to the external environment. The free-living larvae then penetrate and parasitize land snails—the intermediate host—and undergo further development. When the parasitized snail is eaten as a contaminant in feed by deer, the larvae pass into the abomasum, penetrate the gastric wall, and migrate to the spinal cord. At this point, the larvae penetrate the cord and move cephalad to their definitive cranial position without inflicting significant damage to the host. In sheep and goats, the life cycle is similar to the one in deer up to the point of penetrating the spinal cord; here the larvae randomly wander, injure the cord, and provoke strong inflammatory reactions that eventually immobilize and kill the parasites.

Adult *S. digitata* normally occupy the peritoneal cavities of cattle. Microfilariae enter the circulation and are ingested in blood meals by vector mosquitoes. After about 2 weeks, the larvae reach the salivary glands and are injected into the blood of new cattle during subsequent hematophagous feeding. Eventually the larvae return to the peritoneal cavity and mature. In sheep, the microfilariae from the vectors do not induce parasitemia, but migrate into the spinal cord, where they wander and inflict injuries that are manifested after a latent period of about 1 month.

CLINICAL SIGNS AND POSTMORTEM LESIONS. Affected animals usually are mentally alert but paralyzed in one or both caudal limbs and, in some cases, one or both cranial limbs. Morbidity may reach 15%, with an average of 8%; mortality is high.

At necropsy, many cases present no gross lesions. Some, however, show small hemorrhages in the spinal cord. Histologic lesions are randomly distributed in the cord and consist of malacia, microcavitation, demyelination, degeneration and enlargement of axons, sections of viable or degenerated larvae, infiltration of leukocytes—eosinophils, macrophages, and lymphocytes—in tissue and around parasites, and gliosis.

DIAGNOSIS. Veterinarians suspect the disease in animals exhibiting characteristic signs, and they confirm the diagnosis in the laboratory by finding the specific lesions with or without the parasites. The differential diagnosis requires consideration of enzootic ataxia, bacterial spondylitis, polioencephalomalacia, focal symmetrical encephalomalacia, *Taenia multiceps* infection, and spinal cord abscesses.

TABLE 17-1. *Parasites Causing Cerbrospinal Nematodosis*

| | Larval Dimensions | Natural Hosts | | Geographic Distribution |
		Intermediate	Definitive	
P. tenuis	48–65 mm × 180–240 μm	land snails	white-tailed deer	U.S.: Northeastern states
S. digitata	40–80 mm × 240–260 μm	*Anopheles sinensis* *Armigeres obturans* *Aedes togoi*	cattle	Japan, Korea, Sri Lanka, USSR

For technical assistance from a diagnostic laboratory, practitioners should submit entire spinal cords and brains from suspect cases.

PREVENTION AND TREATMENT.　Infections with *P. tenuis* can be controlled by avoiding exposure of sheep to heavy concentrations of white-tailed deer, and infections with *S. digitata* by controlling mosquitoes. Neither of these methods may be practical.

Alden, C., Woodson, F., Mohan, R., and Miller, S.: Cerebrospinal nematodiasis in sheep. JAVMA, *166*: 784-786, 1975.

Anderson, R.C.: Pathogenesis and transmission of neurotropic and accidental nematode parasites of the central nervous system. Helminthol. Abst., *37* (Part 3):191-210, 1968.

Anderson, R.C.: Ecological relationships of meningeal worm and native cervids in North America. J. Wildl. Dis., *8*:304, 1972.

Innes, J.R.M., Shoho, C., and Pillai, C.P.: Epizootic cerebrospinal nematodiasis or setariasis. Br. Vet. J., *108*: 71-88, 1952.

Kennedy, P.C., Whitlock, J., and Roberts, S.J.: Neurofilariosis, a paralytic disease of sheep. Cornell Vet., *42*:118-123, 1952.

Nielson, S.W. and Aftosmis, J.: Spinal nematodiasis in two sheep. JAVMA, *144*:155-158, 1964.

Milkweed Poisoning

Milkweed poisoning, an acute plant intoxication of sheep, is characterized by nervous disturbances, locomotor incoordination, physical weaknesses, and difficult respirations. It is caused by several species of the genus *Asclepias,* common weeds of western ranges and pastures. Because the disease has wide distribution and moderate incidence from weed infestations of fresh and preserved diets, it adversely affects the American sheep industry and may cause serious financial waste to some enterprises. Economic losses result from deaths and incomplete use of infested ranges, pastures, and hays. Occurrence of the condition also among cattle and horses adds economic importance to the malady.

OCCURRENCE.　Milkweed poisoning occurs in all breeds, sexes, and ages of grazing sheep; range animals, however, in comparison to pastured animals, encounter the causative weeds more commonly and therefore more often develop poisoning. Even though the disease usually occurs during summers and autumns, it may also develop during winters among animals fed milkweed-infested hays. Geographically, milkweed poisoning occurs in the arid and semiarid western United States and Mexico.

ETIOLOGY.　The milkweed genus, *Asclepias,* contains numerous species; of these, at least five cause poisoning. Table 17-2 presents minimal lethal doses and distributions. The milkweeds, perennial herbs with milky saps, form erect stems with opposite or whorled leaves. The umbellate flowers contain corollas with two whorls of petals arranged about the stigma, and each of the podded seeds bears a tuft of silky hairs (Fig. 17-3). Some species, perhaps all, contain toxic cardiac glycosides (cardenolides) in their aerial parts. Generally the narrowed leafed species of milkweed contain the highest concentrations of glycosides.

TABLE 17-2.　*Species of Asclepias*

Species	MLD (% body weight)	Distribution
A. labriformis (labriform)	0.05	Four Corners: Arizona, New Mexico, Utah, Colorado
A. subverticillata (*A. galioides*) (western)	0.2	Kansas and Oklahoma west to Utah; Arizona and south into Mexico
A. eriocarpa (wooly pod)	0.2	California into Mexico
A. fascicularis (*A. mexicana*) (mexican whorled)	2.0	Washington and Idaho south into Mexico
A. pumila (dwarfed)	2.0	U.S.: high plains

Fig. 17-3. Mexican whorled milkweed, *Asclepias fascicularis*. × 0.1.

These compounds have a digitalis-like action on the heart. They are synthesized in the plants and persist at dangerous levels in dried forage and preserved hay.

Milkweeds grow in disturbed soil and depleted ranges and pastures. Overgrazed areas, such as corrals, marching routes, roadsides, fence lines, ditch banks, and abandoned orchards, are their common habitats. Sheep usually find asclepias unpalatable, especially in the growing state, and reject them in forage mixtures. Under circumstances of urgent hunger and abundant mildweed, animals readily consume toxic and lethal doses.

CLINICAL SIGNS.   Following the ingestion of toxic or lethal doses of milkweed, sheep sicken within 12 to 24 hours. In early stages, affected animals become depressed and decline feed, and after a few hours they are weak and incoordinated and tremble, stumble, and fall. Paralysis follows ataxia, especially in the hind limbs; some animals, propelling with their front limbs, drag their back parts; but immobility and prostration finally supervene. Muscular spasms and repetitive convulsions develop. The pupils dilate, the weak pulse accelerates, and the body temperature elevates. Respiration decelerates and becomes labored, oral, and gasping. Some animals show cyanosis and diarrhea. Fatal cases pass into coma and die.

The morbidity ranges up to 60% or more, and the mortality reaches 80% of affected sheep when *A. labriformis* or *A. subverticillata* are the poisoning species. The clinical course varies from 10 to 90 hours.

At necropsy, no specific lesions exist, but fragments of ingested milkweed may be identified in the ruminal contents. The kidneys may show tubular nephrosis and glomerulonephrosis.

DIAGNOSIS.   Veterinarians diagnose milkweed poisoning on evidence of herd history and clinical signs. Identifying causative asclepias in ruminal contents confirms the diagnosis. The differential diagnosis requires consideration of other acute poisonings, such as those from cyanogenic plants, oxalate-containing weeds, pesticides, and mineral compounds.

PREVENTION.   Producers prevent milkweed poisoning by denying hungry sheep access to large amounts of the plant. Supplementary feed should be provided before marching over asclepias-infested routes and after unloading animals from transport vehicles onto infested ranges or pastures. Even after accidental access to and consumption of milkweed, a full meal of nutritious feed dilutes the ingested plant, ameliorates its effect, and minimizes losses. No specific treatment is known.

Benson, J.M., Seiber, J.N., Keller, R.F., and Johnson, A.E.: Studies on the principle of *Asclepias eriocarpa* and *Asclepias labriformis*. In *Effects of Poisonous Plants on Livestock*. Edited by R.F. Keeler, K.R. VanKampen, and L.F. James. New York, Academic Press, 1978, pp. 273-284.

Benson, J.M., et al.: Effects on sheep of milkweeds *Asclepias eriocarpa* and *Asclepias labriformis* and of cardiac glycoside-containing material. Toxicon, *17*: 155-165, 1979.

Clark, J.C.: Whorled milkweed poisoning. Vet. Hum. Toxicol., *21*:431, 1979.

Fleming, C.E., et al.: Narrow-leafed milkweed poisoning in Nevada. Univ. Nevada Agric. Exp. Stat. Bull. 99, 1920, pp. 1-32.

Glover, G.H., Newsom, I.E., and Robbins, W.W.: New poisonous plant: whorled milkweed. Colorado Agric. Exp. Stat. Bull. 246, 1918, pp. 1-16.

Marsh, C.D. and Clawson, A.B.: Mexican whorled milkweed (*Asclepias mexicana*). USDA Bull. 969, 1921.

Marsh, C.D. and Clawson, A.B.: Wolly-pod milkweed (*Asclepias eriocarpa*). USDA Bull. 1212, 1924, pp. 1-13.

Marsh, C.D., Clawson, A.B., Couch, J.F., and Eggleston, W.W.: Whorled milkweed (*Asclepias galioides*). USDA Bull. 800, 1920.

May, W.L.: Whorled milkweed. Colorado Agric. Exp. Stat. Bull. 255, 1920, pp. 1-39.

Steyn, D.C.: Plant poisoning and tolerance in stock. Onderstepoort J. Vet. Sci. Anim. Ind., *1*:149-156, 1933.

Progressive Retinal Degeneration

(*PRD; bright blindness*)

Progressive retinal degeneration is a slow neuropathy of both eyes, is characterized by unresponsive pupils, tapetal photoreflection, and blindness, caused by prolonged consumption of bracken fern. It results in biologic waste and economic losses to producers from partial incapacitations and early culling of affected sheep, and from reduced values of associated pastures and ranges.

OCCURRENCE.   The disease develops in British breeds, such as Herdwick, Swaledale, and Suffolk, usually females ranging in age from 1 to 7 years and averaging about 4 years. Most cases develop during autumn. Geographi-

cally, it is recognized in Great Britain, especially in highland grazing flocks, but possibly it may occur in other countries.

ETIOLOGY.   Bracken, *Pteridium aquilinum*, as a significant part of the diet over several continuous months causes PRD. The specific toxin in the plant responsible for retinal degeneration is not known. Bracken fern does not contain thiaminase, a carcinogen capable of inducing urinary bladder tumors in cattle, and factors which cause thrombocytopenia in cattle. This perennial erect fern with many fronds reproduces by spores formed at the undersurface margins of leaves as well as by rhizomes and may reach 1 to 2 m in height (Fig. 17-4). It grows in highlands, forests, and forest openings on dry, drained, sandy soil and is distributed throughout the world's temperate zones. In the U.S., it is prevalent except in the arid southwest.

CLINICAL SIGNS AND POSTMORTEM LESIONS. Early signs are impaired vision progressing to bilateral blindness. The pupils are round, dilated, and unresponsive to light. The tapetum lucidum is smooth and reflective. Ophthalmoscopic examinations reveal narrowed and darkened retinal major vessels. Most affected animals have thrombocytopenia and leukopenia. They remain mentally alert. Morbidity ranges from 4 to 35%. Blindness is permanent.

Histologically, the rods and cones as well as the outer nuclear layer gradually atrophy and finally disappear from the retina except at its peripheries. Changes in specific activity of lactate dehydrogenase isoenzyme as well as

Fig. 17-4. Bracken fern (*Pteridium aquilinum*) showing typical leaf structure.

increases in specific activity of glucose-6-phosphate dehydrogenase have been reported.

DIAGNOSIS. Veterinarians suspect PRD in sheep with impaired vision and long access to bracken, and they confirm the diagnosis by ophthalmoscopic and histologic examinations of affected eyes for typical lesions. The differential diagnosis requires consideration of polioencephalomalacia, early cerebral coenuriasis (gid), cataract, pregnancy disease, and keratitis.

PREVENTION AND TREATMENT. Producers prevent the disease by avoiding continuous feeding on bracken either on pasture or in hay. Treatment for blindness is not effective.

Barnett, K.E. and Watson, W.A.: Bright blindness in sheep. A primary retinopathy due to feeding bracken fern (*Pteris aquilina*). Res. Vet. Sci., *11*:289-290, 1970.

Mason, J., Barnett, K.C., Blackmore, W.F., and Evans, E.T.R.: Biochemical observations on primary PRD in sheep. Exp. Eye Res., *15*:51-60, 1973.

Watson, W.A., Barlow, R.M., and Barnett, K.C.: Bright blindness—a condition prevalent in Yorkshire hill sheep. Vet. Rec., *77*:1060, 1965.

Watson, W.A., Barnett, K.C., and Terlecki, S.: PRD (bright blindness) in sheep. Vet. Rec., *91*:665-670, 1972.

Watson, W.A., et al.: Experimentally produced progressive retinal degeneration in sheep. Brit. Vet. J., *128*:457, 1972.

Lightning Stroke

Lightning stroke, the conductance of enormous electric current from thunderclouds through animals to earth, is characterized by cutaneous and nervous injuries. This violent phenomenon often causes flock damages because of ovine propensities to cluster for rest and protection under superstructures such as trees and buildings that project cloudward from the earth's surface.

OCCURRENCE. Lightning stroke occurs in all breeds, sexes, and ages. Most strike events develop in summer, when thunderclouds are prevalent, and they probably occur in all sheep-producing countries of hot and temperate climatic zones. Occasionally, groups of animals are killed in close proximity to trees, fences, or other structures which may show evidence of damage.

ETIOLOGY AND PATHOGENESIS. The powerful electric current, moving along a voltage gradient from cloud to earth, causes lightning stroke. The bolt first strikes the superstructure and then the animal group. Occasionally, individual uncovered sheep are struck on open pasture. The great force may break, ignite, or explode the tree or building and kill or disable the animals. Shock and heat cause malfunction and necrosis of animal cells.

CLINICAL SIGNS AND LESIONS. The sudden injuries and deaths have histories of developing near the time of violent thunderstorms and are often accompanied by breakage of associated physical structures. Nonfatal cases may suffer temporary coma and, after prehension, hold feed in their mouths. They may show visual

Fig. 17-5. Singe streaks (*a*) in hair of skin on limb of bovine from lightning stroke.

and ambulatory impairments as well as skeletal fractures. If lightning injures an animal its effects are instantaneous. Both killed and surviving animals may have wide and diffuse or linear and branched singe marks on hair of faces, ears, and medial surfaces of limbs. Singed hairs are twisted, curled, and browned or blackened (Fig. 17-5). Scorchings are variable and affect 20 to 90% of struck animals. Dry—but not wet—hair singes. The only consistent finding in the respiratory system is hemorrhage into the trachea. Hemorrhage and hyperemia are common in the superficial lymph nodes, whereas the internal lymph nodes are normal. Small pinpoint hemorrhages may occur in the fascia between the muscles. Hemorrhages are occasionally found in the central nervous system.

DIAGNOSIS. Veterinarians diagnose lightning stroke on evidence of typical history, signs, and lesions. Each involved animal should be thoroughly examined for singe marks and skin burns. The differential diagnosis requires consideration of wire electrocutions, bloat, acute poisonings, shootings, collisions with moving vehicles, predation, and other sudden death syndromes. Diagnoses are often legally examined for payments of casualty insurance claims. Therefore, a diagnosis must be made from a thorough postmortem examination.

Prevention and treatment are not effective.

Barr, M.: Stroke of lightning. Vet. Rec., 79:170-172, 1966.

Mory, W.: Lightning stroke in the field. Wien. Tierztliche Monatsschrift, 62:170-174, 1975.

Ramsey, F.K. and Howard, J.R.: Diagnosis of lightning strike. JAVMA, 156:1472-1474, 1970.

Ramsey, F.K., et al.: Responsibility in lightning losses in livestock. Vet. Med., 57:809-814, 1962.

Ramsey, F. and Howard, J.: Lightning strike and electrocution. In Current Veterinary Therapy. 2. Food Animal Practice. Edited by J. Howard. Philadelphia, W.B. Saunders Co., 1986, pp. 458-459.

18

DISEASES OF THE BLOOD AND BLOOD-FORMING SYSTEM

Anaplasmosis

Anaplasmosis, a subacute infectious but noncontagious disease, is characterized by fever, anemia, weakness, and icterus and is caused by a rickettsia. Even though anaplasmosis sporadically occurs in many major sheep-producing countries, this mild and often undiagnosed disease has minor importance to the sheep industry. Some economic losses, however, result from unthriftiness, reduced live weight, and occasional deaths. Experimentally, the disease develops in sheep following their inoculation with heavily infected blood and after splenectomy; consequently, it has scientific interest and investigative use. Unlike ovine anaplasmosis, bovine anaplasmosis is a major disease that annually attacks 50,000 cattle and costs $100 million in the United States alone.

OCCURRENCE. Anaplasmosis occurs in all breeds and sexes, but sheep 1 year of age and older probably have higher susceptibility than do animals of younger age groups. Outbreaks usually develop during spring and early summer when vectoring ticks are active. A second surge in incidence may develop during autumn months of high rainfall. Ovine anaplasmosis also occurs in goats and bovine anaplasmosis in cattle and deer.

Geographically, the incidence of anaplasmosis is widespread among sheep of South Africa, Morocco, and Algeria, and sporadic in the USSR, the United States, Bulgaria, Tur-

key, Rhodesia, Argentina, Lebanon, Israel, Jordan, Iran, and India.

ETIOLOGY AND PATHOGENESIS. *Anaplasma ovis,* the specific cause of ovine anaplasmosis, is a rickettsia. Within the erythrocyte, 65% of the organisms occupy a peripheral position, and the balance occupy a central location. Consisting of a dense globular mass, the organism colors basic with Giemsa's stain and Wright's stain, and measures 0.3 to 1.0 μm in diameter (Fig. 18-1).

As seen under the electron microscope, each anaplasma body consists of a colony of up to eight subunits or initial bodies, each subunit ranging in size from 0.16 to 0.27 × 0.24 to 0.52 μm. Division is by fission, and the initial body is the infective unit. A three-layered membrane, 130 to 239 Å thick, surrounds each colony.

Infective blood, when mixed with citrate solution or with glucose, saccharose, and citrate solution and stored at 3°C, retains viability for 82 and 350 days, respectively. In general, species of anaplasma are host-specific, but A. ovis affects both sheep and goats, and in the complement-fixation test, A. ovis and A. marginale show some cross-antigenicity.

The Dutch have identified another anaplasma in sheep that parasitizes the margin of 30% of the red blood cells. The isolate has cross-immunity with A. ovis and is transmitted by ticks. They have proposed the name *Anaplasma mesaeterum.*

355

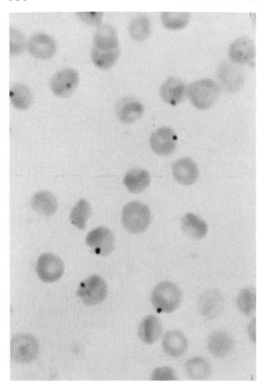

Fig. 18-1. *Anaplasma ovis* in erythrocytes of sheep. Giemsa's stain. × 1500.

The means of natural transmission of ovine anaplasmosis has been investigated very little. In southern Russia, the tick *Haemaphysalis sulcata* is a vector, but in the United States, seven species of tick—*Argas persicus, Dermacentor andersoni, D. variabilis, D. occidentalis, D. albipictus, Rhipicephalus sanguineus,* and *Ixodes scapularis*—transmit bovine anaplasmosis, and possibly some of these species transmit the sheep disease. Vectors acquire infection by feeding on infected or carrier sheep and transmit the disease by subsequently feeding on susceptible sheep.

In the process of transmission, infective initial bodies, along with vector saliva, enter the susceptible host, move to capillaries of visceral organs, multiply, and eventually enter the peripheral circulation. Anemia results from destruction of infected erythrocytes and from suppression of erythropoiesis. After parasitizing erythrocytes, the initial body increases in size and divides by fission into two to eight new

initial bodies, and a colony of these forms the marginal body.

Eventually, the initial bodies are liberated from the parasitized erythrocyte, and the process is repeated. Growth of the anaplasma is accompanied by reduction in the amount of phospholipid within the erythrocyte stroma and by development of erythrocyte fragility. Although cell fragility and anemia reach peaks at about the same time, hemolysis does not occur in the plasma. Gradually, the parasitized and injured erythrocytes are recognized by immunologic means and removed from the circulation through erythrophagia by the reticuloendothelial cells of bone marrow, spleen, liver, and lymph nodes. The erythrocyte count may decline from 9 to 12, the normal range, to 5 to 7 million/cmm. Many clinical signs result from hypoxia. Death seldom occurs unless other pathogens intervene. Recovered sheep are permanent carriers.

CLINICAL SIGNS AND POSTMORTEM LESIONS. After an incubation period ranging from 20 to 30 days, the body temperature rises and fluctuates. Affected sheep are physically weak, anemic, and icteric. Unthriftiness, anorexia, and loss of live weight are prominent. Hematologic studies reveal the reduction in erythrocytes, hemoglobin, and packed cell volume. Furthermore, anaplasma can be identified in many erythrocytes; the organisms are discernible for 20 to 60 days from beginning infection.

Although the morbidity may reach 10 to 20%, the mortality is usually low and seldom exceeds 5% of affected animals. Deaths are caused by combined action of anaplasma and other pathogens, such as piroplasmas, babesiosis, eperythrozoonosis, and conditions such as malnutrition, trace-element deficiencies, and intoxications.

At necropsy, anemia and infection are evident in the form of pale membranes, thin blood, icterus, and swollen spleen. In blood films and tissue sections, anaplasmata are discernible in erythrocytes.

DIAGNOSIS. Veterinarians diagnose anaplasmosis on evidence of typical signs and laboratory findings. Anemia, weakness, and icterus strongly suggest the disease, and finding anaplasmata in 0.5% or more of the erythrocytes confirms the clinical diagnosis. Serologic testing can be done by the complement fixation test where antigen for *A. ovis* is available. The differential diagnosis requires consideration of chronic copper poisoning, leptospirosis, eperythrozoonosis, yellow lamb disease, and some plant poisonings. Each of these diseases contains characteristic features, and none shows anaplasmata in erythrocytes.

PREVENTION AND TREATMENT. Since anaplasmosis is a mild disease and causes deaths when exacerbated by other conditions, prevention of complications usually protects sheep against anaplasmosis. Presumably an inactivated vaccine, similar to the bovine product, could be prepared and administered in two doses. The drug of choice for treatment is long-acting oxytetracycline administered at the rate of 20 mg/kg. Elimination of the carrier state, in cattle, by the use of long-acting tetracyclines even with a 4-dose regimen has not been totally successful. This regimen has not been fully investigated in sheep.

Animal Health Yearbook. FAO-WHO-OIE (Italy), 1970.

Dyakonov, L.P. and Avakyan, A.A.: Ultrastructure of *Anaplasma ovis*. Veterinariia (Moskow), No. 11:43-45, 1970.

Goksu, K.: A review of anaplasmosis and observations on infections in sheep and goats in Turkey. Turk. Vet. Hekim. Dern. Derg., *35*:399-417, 1965.

Hadani, A., et al.: A case of apparent suppression of *Anaplasma marginale* infection by eperythrozoonosis (*Eperythrozoon teganodes*). Vet. Parasitol., *9*:267-272, 1982.

Konyukhov, M.P.: Pathogenesis of anaplasmosis in sheep. Tr. Vses. Inst. Eksp. Vet., *21*:155-173, 1957.

Kyurtov, N.: Piroplasmal infections in sheep and goats. II. Anaplasmosis. Vet. Med. Nauki (Sofia), *5*:81-86, 1967.

Magonigle, R. and Newby, T.: Elimination of naturally acquired chronic *Anaplasma* marginale infection with a long-acting oxytetracycline injectable. Am. J. Vet. Res., *43*:2170-2173, 1982.

Myalo, I.I.: Mixed *Anaplasma* and *Babesia* infections in sheep. Tr. Vses. Inst. Eksp. Vet., *21*:177-194, 1957.

Obi, T. and Akinboade, O.: West African Dwarf sheep: Clinical syndrome, packed cell volume, erythrocyte and haemoglobin levels in naturally-occurring babesiosis and anaplasmosis. Int. Goat Sheep Res., *3*: 197-201, 1984.

Rakhimov, T.K.: Epidemiology of ovine anaplasmosis in Uzbekistan. Tr. Vses. Inst. Eksp. Vet., *31*:302-304, 1965.

Ryff, J.F., Gilbert, C.S., Weibel, J.L., and Breen, H.: Anaplasmosis and concurrent copper poisoning in sheep. JAVMA, *133*:312-315, 1958.

Sharma, S. and Bansal, G.: Chemoprophylaxis of *Anaplasma ovis* infection in sheep with a long-acting oxytetracycline. Vet. Parasitol., *17*:255-258, 1984/85.

Splitter, E.J., Anthony, H.D., and Twiehaus, M.J.: *Anaplasma ovis* in the United States. Experimental studies with sheep and goats. AJVR, *17*:487-491, 1956.

Stepanova, N.I. and Kazakov, N.A.: Invasive and immunogenic properties of *Anaplasma ovis*. Veterinariia (Moscow), No. 6, 57-58, 1970.

Uilenberg, G., van Vorstenbosch, C.J.A.H.V., and Pierie, N.M.: Blood parasites of sheep in the Netherlands. I. *Anaplasma mesaeterum* sp n. (*Ricketsiales, Anaplasmataceae*). Vet. Q., *1*:14-22, 1979.

Eperythrozoonosis

Eperythrozoonosis, a subacute infectious but noncontagious disease, is characterized by anemia and physical weakness in lambs and is caused in part by a rickettsia. Even though eperythrozoonosis occurs sporadically in most major sheep-producing countries, this mild and often undiagnosed disease is of minor importance to the sheep industry. Some economic losses, however, result from unthriftiness and occasional deaths among lambs. The disease has scientific interest because experimentally, it develops in lambs following their inoculation with adult blood and, in mature sheep, after splenectomy.

OCCURRENCE. Eperythrozoonosis occurs in all breeds and sexes of sheep, but animals up to 1 year of age develop a higher incidence than do other age groups. The premunitive state among adult sheep appears to be common. In Australia, the disease develops during late winter and early spring. Geographically, eperythrozoonosis occurs in South Africa, Algeria, Nigeria, the United States, Scandinavia, Australia, Japan, India, Iran, Ireland, and Germany. In addition to sheep, similar diseases attack cattle and swine.

ETIOLOGY AND PATHOGENESIS. *Eperythrozoon ovis*, the cause of the disease, is a rickettsia. This pleomorphic organism takes the form of cocci, rods, rings, triangles, and dumbbells. Under scanning electron microscope the rod form measures 0.2 to 0.6 μm in length, while the ring form measures 0.2 to 0.4 μm in diameter with both forms being located at the concave regions of erythrocytes. The organism is composed of a single limiting membrane and ribosome-like granular material with high electron density in the inner layer. When stained with Giemsa's solution, it is blue to pink, and negative with gram stain. The parasite inhabits the surface of erythrocytes and the plasma. The mode of attachment of *E. ovis* to erythrocytes is not fully understood. Although related forms attack other domestic animals—*E. wenyoni* in cattle and *E. suis* in swine—each species is host-specific, except that *E. ovis* will transfer to goats.

E. ovis, like other species of the genus, possesses low pathogenicity and usually causes clinical manifestations and parasitemia in sheep debilitated from malnutrition, trace-element deficiencies, helminthosis, and subacute intoxications, in sheep inoculated with heavily infected blood, and in sheep with incapacitated reticuloendothelial systems, such as from splenectomy. Transmission of *E. ovis* is by the ticks, *Haemaphysalis plumbeum* and *Rhipicephalus bursa.* The sheep ked, *Malophagus ovinus,* has been incriminated as a vector. The mosquitoes, *Aedes camptorhynchus* and *Culex annulirostris,* are efficient vectors and possibly other biting insects. The exact pathogenesis is unknown, but the bone marrow may be a main organ for multiplication as the parasitic rate of *E. ovis* approximates 4% in the peripheral blood and 35% in the bone marrow. In the bone marrow, the *E. ovis* attaches to reticulocytes, erythroblasts, and "ghost cells" at an early stage of infection. In the peripheral blood, erythrocytes are destroyed causing a hemolytic anemia. Following clinical recovery, the host animal develops permanent premunition and occasionally experiences short remissions. Deaths result from the combined effects of eperythrozoa, other pathogens, and additional inimical conditions such as pneumonia.

CLINICAL SIGNS AND POSTMORTEM LESIONS. After an incubation period ranging from 4 to 21 days, affected lambs become unthrifty, weak, anemic, and in some cases mildly icteric. Episodes of remission occur, and body temperatures fluctuate. Hematologic studies reveal hypochromic anemia with numeric reduction of erythrocytes by as much as 28% from normal levels, and large numbers of the causative organisms on the surface of erythrocytes and in plasma (Fig. 18-2). Both morbidity and mortality are low. At necropsy, the spleen is swollen, the blood thin, and the tissues icteric.

In experimentally infected lambs, the incubation period is inversely proportional to the inoculating dose, but the resulting disease is not influenced by the infecting dose. The time required to reach a maximum degree of anemia is similar for all infecting doses and as such is not directly associated with parasitization of the red blood cells.

DIAGNOSIS. Veterinarians diagnose eperythrozoonosis on evidence of unthriftiness, anemia, and the presence of many eperythrozoa in stained blood films. The inoculation of infected blood into susceptible splenectomized sheep provokes systemic infection.

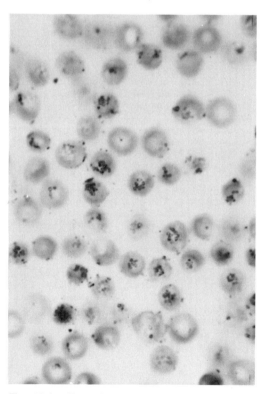

Fig. 18-2. *Eperythrozoon ovis* on sheep erythrocytes. Giemsa's stain. × 1220.

The complement fixation test is an effective screening tool detecting flock infection but may not identify carrier animals due to undetectable antibody levels. The differential diagnosis requires consideration of helminthosis, malnutrition, trace-element deficiencies, and anaplasmosis.

PREVENTION AND TREATMENT. The maintenance of lambs on balanced and adequate rations and relative freedom from internal and external parasites help prevent naturally acquired eperythrozoonosis, and disinfection of instruments between surgical operations, such as castration and docking, prevents artificial transmission. Immunizing agents have not been developed. Affected sheep should be treated by correcting the primary or predisposing causes.

Animal Health Yearbook. FAO-WHO-OIE (Italy), 1970.

Campbell, R.W., Sloan, C.A., and Harbutt, P.R.: Observations on the mortality of lambs in Victoria associated with Eperythrozoon ovis. Aust. Vet. J., 47:538-541, 1971.

Daddow, K.: A serological survey of Eperythrozoon ovis antibody in Queensland sheep. Queensland J. Agric. Anim. Sci., 38:55-59, 1981.

Daddow, K.: Culex annulirostris as a vector of Eperythrozoon ovis infection of sheep. Vet. Parasitol., 7:313-317, 1980.

Daddow, K.: The protection of lambs from eperythrozoon infection while suckling Eperythrozoon ovis carrier ewes. Vet. Parasitol., 10:41-45, 1982.

Daddow, K.N. and Dunlop, L.B.: The serological and microscopic monitoring of a natural outbreak of eperythrozoon infection in sheep. Queensland J. Agric. Anim. Sci., 33:233-236, 1976.

Donatiens, A. and Lestoquard, F.: The existence of Eperythrozoon ovis in Algeria. Bull. Soc. Pathol. Exot., 28:423-426, 1935.

Friedhoff, K., Drommer, W., and Wolfhagen, M.: Eperythrozoon ovis infections in sheep in North Germany. Berl. Muench. Tieraerztl. Wochenschr., 19:361-368, 1971.

Gordon, D., Cole, M., and Larkin, H.: Occurrence of eperythrozoonosis in sheep in Ireland. Irish Vet. J., 39:25-26, 1985.

Ichijo, S., Hosokawa, S., Kim, D., and Konishi, T.: Scanning and transmission electron microscopic observations of Eperythrozoon ovis (E. ovis). Jpn. J. Vet. Sci., 44:127-132, 1982.

Jensen, R.: Eperythrozoonosis in cattle and sheep of Louisiana; preliminary report. Louisiana Bull. 366, 1943.

Littlejohns, I.R.: Eperythrozoonosis in sheep. Aust. Vet. J., 36:260-265, 1960.

Neitz, W.O., Alexander, R.A., and DuToit, P.I.: Eperythrozoon ovis (n. sp) infection in sheep. Onderstepoort J. Vet. Sci., 3:263-271, 1934.

Nikolskii, S.N. and Slipchenko, S.N.: Experimental transmission of Eperythrozoon ovis by the ticks Hyalomma plumbeum and Rhipicephalus bursa. Veterinariia (Moscow), No. 5, 46, 1969.

Overas, A.J.: Eperythrozoon ovis—a new blood parasite in sheep in Norway. Nord. Vet. Med., 11:791-800, 1959.

Overas, A.J.: Studies on Eperythrozoon ovis infection in sheep. Acta Vet. Scand., 28:Suppl. 148, 1969.

Sinada, M., Tekahashi, K., Tamura, T., and Koriva, M.: Clinical and hematological observation on spontaneous and experimental cases of eperythrozoon infection in sheep. J. Jpn. Vet. Med. Assoc., 30:374-379, 1977.

Sutton, R.H. and Jolly, R.D.: Experimental Eperythrozoon ovis infection in sheep. N.Z. Vet. J., 21:160-166, 1973.

Anthrax

(Splenic fever; charbon; milzbrand)

An acute contagious septicemia, anthrax is characterized by splenic swelling and blood exudations from body openings and is caused by a sporing bacterium that commonly resides in alkaline soil. The disease attacks all homeothermic animals, including man, but in the United States, anthrax is a disease primarily of cattle and sheep. The combined annual losses to the national cattle and sheep industries have been conservatively estimated at several hundred thousand dollars. In some other countries where animal disease control is underdeveloped, annual losses from anthrax may be high. Economic losses result from animal deaths, property depreciation, quarantine enforcement, and the cost of immunization programs, treatment practices, and dead animal disposal. Additional losses come from incapacitation of people affected with the disease.

OCCURRENCE. Although anthrax is a disease of all breeds, sexes, and ages of sheep, it occurs more commonly in adult animals than in lambs. This difference may be due, in part, to eating habits that provide a greater opportunity for grazing adults to ingest spores from the soil. Although anthrax is uncommon in feedlot lambs, the disease occurs occasionally as a result of contaminated feed or water. In addition to sheep, cattle and horses are highly susceptible. People and swine possess considerable resistance, whereas dogs, cats, birds, and wild animals develop anthrax only under certain conditions. In the laboratory, mice, guinea pigs, and rabbits can be infected. Geographically, anthrax occurs in all countries where sheep and/or cattle production are major industries. The disease is common in Asia, southern Europe, Africa, South America, and North America. In the United States, the incidence is high and recurring in South Dakota, Arkansas, Missouri, Louisiana, Texas, and California. From 1916 to 1944, the number of states reporting anthrax increased from 21 to 37. From 1945 through 1954, 3447 outbreaks occurred in 17,604 animals from 39 states. Approximately 65% of these cases were cattle and sheep.

In 1957, 1627 head of livestock on 741 premises died of anthrax in northeastern Oklahoma and southeastern Kansas. Since that time, only 3 major outbreaks with losses over 100 animals have been reported. During the period 1980–1983 only 7 states (California, Colorado, Idaho, New Mexico, North Dakota, South Dakota, and Texas) had laboratory-confirmed cases of anthrax. The reporting statistics indicate a decline in the prevalence of animal and human anthrax.

Probably because grazing provides opportunity for ingesting anthrax spores from contaminated soil, food, and water, and partly because of summer multiplication of the organism in soil, anthrax occurs more commonly during July, August, and September of dry hot summers preceded by periods of high rainfall.

ETIOLOGY. *Bacillus anthracis,* the causative bacterium of anthrax, is a nonmotile, capsulated, spore-bearing, cylindric, truncated, aerobic rod whose dimensions are 1 to 1.2 × 3 to 8 μm. The elliptic spore is located centrally within the cell. While young cultures are gram-positive, older ones tend to decolorize easily. In the tissues of infected animals, especially the blood, the organism forms heavily capsulated chains.

In the laboratory, the organism grows on many common artificial media. Virulent organisms commonly form rough colonies. Freshly isolated virulent strains, grown on serum agar in an atmosphere of carbon dioxide, form smooth mucoid colonies. On serum agar, in the presence of increased CO_2 tension, virulent strains form smooth mucoid colonies consisting of fully virulent encapsulated organisms. Continued cultivation in an atmosphere of carbon dioxide produces rough outgrowth, subcultures from which give rough, and non-mucoid colonies that consist of non-encapsulated bacilli. Non-encapsulated bacilli are uniformly avirulent. Encapsulation is considered to be one of the factors that determines virulence of *B. anthracis. B. anthracis* possesses two primary virulence factors: a poly-D-glutamic acid capsule, which protects the organism from phagocytosis and lytic antibodies, and a triportite toxin composed of edema factor (EF), protective antigen (PA), and lethal factor (LF). These factors independently are innocuous but the combination of PA and LF produces lethality in some species. These toxin components are produced by the encapsulated strains, from early logarithmic through stationary phases of growth and are not a product of secondary metabolism. Synthesis of the capsule is regulated by plasmids. A 114-megadalton plasmid designated pX01 carries the structural genes for protective antigen. A 60-megadalton plasmid, designated pX02, is responsible for the capsule formation. Rough variants that are non-encapsulated and thus avirulent can revert to the capsulated form only if they have retained the pX02 plasmid.

On exposure to oxygen, anthrax bacilli form spores that are highly resistant to the adversity of chemical and physical agents. Some controversy exists over the length of time *B. anthracis* spores survive in the soil. One postulation is that under usual soil conditions, *B. anthracis* spores compete poorly with other soil microorganisms and may be eliminated in a few months to 3 to 4 years. In "incubator areas" of alkaline soil (pH > 6.0) where there is periodic flooding and decomposition of plant material the spores vegetate, multiply, and resporulate. *B. anthracis* spores have been recovered after 37 years from soil with a pH 4.2 to 4.7 which contains profuse natural aerobic spore forming microflora with a cool climate which supports the theories of the long persistence of *B. anthracis* spores in soil. Freshly prepared 5% sodium hydroxide is an effective disinfectant and kills spores after prolonged action. Spores die after 15 minutes in 10% formaldehyde. Resistance to heat varies with the method of heating and with the medium carrying the spores. In a water bath, spores from different strains endure 5 to 30 minutes at 80°C but are destroyed in 2 minutes at 100°C. In flowing steam from an Arnold sterilizer at 101°C, spores are killed in 5 to 15 minutes, and in the autoclave at 6.8 kg steam pressure per 25 mm² at 120°C, they are also killed in 5 to 15 minutes. Dry spores are destroyed by dry heat at 150°C in 60 minutes.

TRANSMISSION.   Anthrax is transmitted from soil of endemic regions to sheep and cattle by ingested spores penetrating the wall of the alimentary tracts through points of injury or by spores contaminating skin injuries. Transmission may also occur by animal ingestion of spore-contaminated bone meal or other feed or water, and by biting insects that feed in rapid succession on the blood of infected animals and then on the blood of susceptible animals.

Transmission by insects is a mechanical process in which the piercing mouth parts, while feeding on the blood of an infected animal, take up *B. anthracis* and then inject the bacteria into susceptible animals during subsequent feedings on blood. Following death of sheep or cattle, carnivorous animals, such as dogs, cats, coyotes, and birds, may become contaminated while feeding on infected tissue and carry spores to distant areas, including feedlots.

PATHOGENESIS.   In the United States, most outbreaks of anthrax develop in endemic areas, and the causative organisms presumably come as spores from infective soil. A tenable hypothesis for the pathogenesis has been formulated. Anthrax spores, resistant to heat and dryness, remain viable for prolonged periods. Soil pH values higher than 6, ambient temperature higher than 15.5°C, and stagnant mixtures of water and dead grass favor anthrax

endemia. Calcareous soil provides the optimum pH, dry hot months of July, August, and September maintain the correct temperature, and high precipitation during spring supplies the water and devitalized grass that accumulate in topographic depressions. Under these conditions, the spores germinate and form vegetative bacteria which, acting on the grass substrate, grow and multiply. As the water evaporates, the soil dries and the bacteria sporulate in large numbers and thus replenish the soil. Wind, flash floods, and moving vehicles may disperse the spores onto edible forage and into potable water.

Sheep and cattle occupying the endemic area may contract the disease. Virulent spores from soil, feed, or water gain entrance into tissues through abrasions of the skin, or more probably, through injuries along the alimentary tract. In the invaded tissues of susceptible animals, the spores germinate, and the bacteria multiply and form capsules that protect them against phagocytosis. The elaboration of the toxic edema factor causes local edema, which protects the bacteria against anthracidal substances in normal plasma, leukocytes, and tissues.

The organisms continue to multiply rapidly in the edematous fluid and are carried through afferent lymphatics into regional lymph nodes, where lymphoid tissue is injured. Passing along efferent lymphatics, the organisms ultimately reach the circulating blood. Rapid multiplication results in a severe septicemia, with the production of fantastically large numbers of organisms. The toxins contain the lethal factor (LF) and the protective factor (PF). The combined effects of the LF and PF act through the central nervous system causing fatal respiratory failure. Death in some cases may be attributed to respiratory distress as a result of increased capillary permeability with a resulting fluid loss into the lungs.

During the clinical course, blood and bacteria may exude from the body openings, and if necropsy is performed, blood escapes from the vessels. On exposure to atmospheric oxygen, the bacteria form spores and may return to the soil.

CLINICAL SIGNS AND POSTMORTEM LESIONS. The signs of anthrax vary with the acuteness of the disease. After a variable incubation period of from 1 to 14 days, animals without the observation of previous illness may be found dead. Body temperature rises to a range of 41 to 42°C. Aggressive movements, such as shaking of the head, bleating, stamping the feet, and butting, are manifested. Some animals show generalized depression and muscular tremors. Following the loss of appetite, rumination ceases and bloating develops. Small amounts of blood may be mixed with nasal excretions, urine, and feces. The oral mucous membranes and conjunctivae are congested and cyanotic.

The course of anthrax also varies according to acuteness. In the acute and peracute forms, the course is usually from 10 to 36 hours, but in exceptional cases, especially in early stages of an outbreak, death may occur after 1 to 2 hours. The morbidity varies from low to high, and the mortality is approximately 90%.

At necropsy of acute cases, the feces, urine, and nasal excretions are stained with blood, and blood may actually exude from the skin. The systemic blood is dark and has a prolonged clotting time. The mucous membrane of the alimentary tract may be irregularly hemorrhagic and eroded, especially at Peyer's patches. Serosa of the endocardium and epicardium and the subcutaneous tissues contain multiple petechial and ecchymotic hemorrhages. Usually the spleen is enlarged by a factor of 2 to 4, and the parenchyma is soft and exudes from the cut surface. Lymph nodes, especially in the area of entering infection, are swollen and hemorrhagic.

Histopathologically, the blood shows large numbers of bacteria, many in chains, of *B. anthracis*. The leukocyte count may be reduced. Blood capillaries and veins tend to be distended, and hemorrhage is common. Germinal centers of lymph nodes and splenic corpuscles are depleted of lymphocytes. In the spleen, the red pulp is filled to capacity with blood. Many erythrocytes are fragmented and hemolyzed. Frequently, vast numbers of bacteria are distributed throughout the spleen.

Animals with anthrax submitted for salvage slaughter should be condemned and all contaminated instruments, equipment, and surfaces thoroughly disinfected.

DIAGNOSIS. The clinical diagnosis of anthrax is made on the basis of typical signs and is usually supplemented with laboratory procedures. Important clinical signs in animals of anthrax-endemic areas are the high fever, bloody discharges, and short courses. Although necropsy should be avoided in sheep and cattle suspected of anthrax, the acute splenitis, lymphadenitis, and edema are of diagnostic importance if necropsy is performed.

In the laboratory, confirmation of the diagnosis can be obtained by the study of blood smears, by bacterial cultures, and by laboratory animal inoculations. Blood smears should be obtained near the time of death and stained with Giemsa or Wright's stain. In typical cases of anthrax, encapsulated single bacterial cells and chains of cells are demonstrable. With these stains, the capsule is purplish pink. Blood smears prepared after considerable autolysis are unsatisfactory for diagnosis.

A sample of jugular blood submitted in the collecting syringe, heart blood, or spleen, if the animal has been necropsied, is recommended. Using blood or spleen the laboratory can conduct the string-of-pearls test which can give a tentative diagnosis in 2 to 4 hours. To confirm the diagnosis the sample is plated onto tryptose blood agar and phenylethanol blood agar plates and incubated 12 to 18 hours at 37°C. Any suspicious colonies can be rechecked with the string-of-pearls test and at the same time the bacteriophage lysis and penicillin sensitivity tests are conducted. Using these techniques a confirmation can be made in 24 hours. In case of heavy contamination of tissues, mouse or guinea pig inoculations may be necessary. Inoculated guinea pigs usually die from anthrax in 36 to 48 hours, and *B. anthracis* can be isolated and identified from the tissues. The enzyme-linked immunosorbent assay can be used for determining anthrax antibodies in serum samples.

The differential diagnosis requires consideration of acute bloat, malignant edema, blackleg, black disease, acute poisoning, and lightning strike.

PREVENTION AND TREATMENT. Following an outbreak of anthrax in an endemic area, the sheep and cattle should be immunized with a viable, avirulent, noncapsulated spore vaccine, such as the Stern-strain spore vaccine. Considerable immunity is established within 1 week from the time of administration. A single vaccination should provide protection throughout the entire grazing season. Following an outbreak and to avoid disease spread, the premises should be quarantined according to state health regulations. All sick or febrile sheep and cattle should be isolated for treatment. Under no circumstances should necropsies be performed within the pens.

Dead animals, bones, skin, manure, and bedding should be removed and disposed of by incineration or deep burial in quicklime. All pen surfaces, including soil, fences, walls, feeding equipment, watering equipment, and machinery, should be disinfected by liberal application of a pressurized spray of freshly prepared 5% aqueous lye solution. Following a few weeks of vacancy and exposure to sunshine, the cleaned pen can be reoccupied. Potentially transmitting arthropods, such as ticks and biting flies, should be controlled.

Often the treatment of peracute anthrax is not feasible because of death after a short course. In many animals, however, treatment is practical and may be administered on either an individual or herd basis. The early stages of anthrax are more amenable to individual treatment. Penicillin should be administered daily at the rate of 5000 units per kg. The antibiotic treatment can be supplemented with the use of 50 to 100 ml of antianthrax serum given subcutaneously and repeated at 6- to 12-hour intervals.

Adami, G.F.: *Inflammation.* London, The Macmillan Company, 1909.

Beall, F.A. and Dalldorf, F.G.: The pathogenesis of the lethal effect of anthrax toxin in the rat. J. Infect. Dis., *116*:377-389, 1966.

Bloom, L., Watson, D.W., Cromartie, W.J., and Freed, M.: Studies on infection with *Bacillus anthracis.* IV. Preparation and characterization of an anthracidal substance from various animal tissues. J. Infect. Dis., *80*:41-52, 1947.

Ezzell, J., Ivins, B., and Leppla, S.: Immuno-electrophoretic analysis, toxicity and kinetics of *in vitro* production of the protective antigen and lethal factor components of *Bacillus anthracis* toxin. Infect. Immun., *45*:761-767, 1984.

Green, B., et al.: Demonstration of a capsule plasmid in *Bacillus anthracis.* Infect. Immun., *49*:291-297, 1985.

Ivanovics, G. and Bruckner, V.Z.: Chemical and immunological studies on the mechanism of anthrax. Immun. Forsch., *90*:304, 1937.

Johnson-Winegar, A.: Comparison of enzyme-linked immunosorbent and indirect hemagglutination assays for determining anthrax antibodies. J. Clin. Microbiol., *20*:357-361, 1984.

Koch, R.: Beitr. Biol., *2*:277, 1876.

Losses in Agriculture. USDA/ARS Handbook 291, 1965.

Merchant, I.A. and Packer, R.A.: *Veterinary Bacteriology and Virology.* 7th Edition. Ames, Iowa, Iowa University Press, 1967.

Pasteur, L. and Joubert, C.R.: Acad. Sci., Paris, *84*:900, 1877.

Personeus, G., Cooper, M.S., and Percival, R.C.: Studies on an anthrax vaccine prepared for noncapsulated variants of *Bacillus anthracis.* AJVR, *17*:153-156, 1956.

Preisz, H.: Experimentelle studien uber virulenz empfanglichkeit und immunitat beim milzbrand. Abl. Bakt., *49*:341, 1909.

Rayer, P.F.O. and Davaine, C.: Inoculation of splenic blood. Bull. Soc. Biol. Paris. Ser. 1, *2*:141, 1850.

Remmele, N.S., et al.: Anthrax toxin: preliminary site of action. J. Infect. Dis., *118*:104-113, 1968.

Schlingman, A.S., et al.: Immunizing activity of alum-precipitated protective antigen of *Bacillus anthracis* in cattle, sheep, and swine. AJVR, *17*:256-261, 1956.

Smith, D.T., Conant, N.F., and Overman, J.R.: *Zinsser Microbiology.* 13th Edition. New York, Appleton-Century-Crofts, 1964, p. 676.

Smith, H. and Keppie, J.: Studies on the chemical basis of the pathogenicity of *Bacillus anthracis* using organisms grown *in vivo.* Mechanisms of pathogenicity. 5th Symp. Soc. Gen. Microbiol. London, Cambridge Univ. Press, 1955, pp. 126-155.

Smith, H., Keppie, J., and Stanley, U.L.: The chemical basis of the virulence of *Bacillus anthracis.* I. Properties of bacteria grown *in vivo* and preparation of extracts. Br. J. Exp. Pathol., *34*:477-485, 1953.

Stableforth, A.W. and Galloway, I.A.: *Infectious Diseases of Animals. Diseases Due to Bacteria.* Vol. 1. New York, Academic Press, 1959, pp. 2-52.

Stein, C.D.: Anthrax in livestock during the first three quarters of 1955 and a review of its incidence and control during the past decade, 1945 to 1954. Proc. U.S. Livestock Sanit. Assoc., 1955, pp. 105-114.

Sterne, M.: The effects of carbon dioxide concentrations on the growth of virulent anthrax strains. Pathogenicity and immunity tests on guinea pigs and sheep with anthrax variants derived from virulent strains. Onderstepoort J. Vet. Sci. Anim. Ind., *9*:49-67, 1937a.

Sterne, M.: The use of anthrax vaccines prepared from avirulent (uncapsulated) variants of *Bacillus anthracis.* Onderstepoort J. Vet. Sci. Anim. Ind., *13*:307-312, 1939.

Sterne, M.: Variation in *Bacillus anthracis*. I. Some effects of carbon dioxide on the formation of capsules and spores by *B. anthracis*. Onderstepoort J. Vet. Sci. Anim. Ind., *8*:272-278, 1937b.

Sterne, M.: Variations in *Bacillus anthracis*. II. Some correlations between colony variation and pathogenicity in strains of *Bacillus anthracis*. Onderstepoort J. Vet. Sci. Anim. Ind., *8*:279-349, 1937c.

Uchida, I., Sekizaki, T., Hashimoto, K., and Terakado, N.: Association of the encapsulation of *Bacillus anthracis* with a 60 megadalton plasmid. J. Gen. Microbiol., *31*:363-367, 1985.

Van Ness, G.B.: Ecology of anthrax. Science, *172*:1303-1307, 1971.

Van Ness, G.B., Plotkin, S.A., Huffaker, R.H., and Evans, W.G.: The Oklahoma-Kansas epizootic of 1957. JAVMA, *134*:125-129, 1959.

Welker, J.S., Lincoln, R.E., and Klein, F.: Proc. Conf. Progress in the Understanding of Anthrax. Beaumont House, FASEB, Bethesda, Md., 1967.

Whitford, H.: Anthrax: Update and overview. Am. Assn. Vet. Lab. Diagnosticians. 26th Annual Proc., 1-12, 1983.

Trypanosomiasis

(Nagana; tsetse fly disease)

Trypanosomiasis, an acute or chronic disease, is characterized by remittent fever, anemia, reduced weight, and physical weakness, and is caused by three hemoflagellate protozoans. The disease has no direct economic importance to the livestock industry in North America. It does, however, affect the industry to some degree in Central and South America, but in tropical Africa it excludes livestock production, and this impoverishes regional economics and causes malnutrition among people. The infection of humans in tropical Africa causes "sleeping sickness" making trypanosomiasis an extremely important zoonotic disease.

OCCURRENCE. Trypanosomiasis is prevalent throughout tropical Africa from the Ivory Coast on the Atlantic side to the Indian Ocean on the east and from the sub-Sahara to South Africa. Trypanosomiasis was introduced into the western hemisphere in 1830 when Zebu cattle were imported from French Guiana and the Antilles from Senegal. The subsequent distribution includes all Latin American countries with an Atlantic coastline from Panama to the west Indian islands of Guadalupe and Martinique. The three species of trypanosomes, *Trypanosoma congolense, T. brucei,* and *T.*

vivax vary in their geographic distribution with *T. brucei* and *T. congolense* dependent upon the tsetse fly (*Glossinia*) for development and transmission. *T. vivax* has a distribution outside the *Glossinia* zone due to its ability to persist by mechanical transmission.

ETIOLOGY AGENT. There are three main species of Trypanosome, *T. brucei, T. congolense,* and *T. vivax. T. brucei* is divided into three subspecies: *T.B. brucie,* which attacks cattle, sheep and goats and *T.B. rhodesiense* and *T.B. gambiense* which attacks humans. Natural infection of *T. vivax* occurs in sheep and goats. Although relatively uncommon, they may be found in areas where it is impossible to keep cattle. All three species infect domestic ruminants with *T. brucie* being the prevalent Trypanosome in sheep (Table 18-1).

TRANSMISSION AND PATHOGENESIS. Trypanosomiasis is transmitted by the bite of infected tsetse flies. *T. brucie* and *T. congolense* are dependent upon the tsetse fly for development and transmission, whereas *T. vivax* can be by the tsetse fly vector or other mechanical means. The life cycle is complex, although all species share the same basic life-style, each behaves differently and are capable of surviving vastly different environments of the insect vectors gut, mammalian skin, and the host blood stream. In the tsetse fly the trypanosome develops in the proboscis and/or the proventriculum, through the noninfective forms (amastigote, promastigote, and epimastigote). As the trypanosome develops for invasion into the mammalian host (trypomastigote or metacyclic form), it develops a thick surface coat of glycoprotein antigens to protect it from the mammalian host antibodies. The infective trypanosome is regurgitated and injected into the mammalian host, or in the case of *T. vivax* it can also be transmitted mechanically by the bite of the tsetse fly. Upon entering the blood stream trypanosomes have the ability to vary the molecular structure of the glycoprotein coat and alter its antigens to stay a step ahead of the host's antigens. These variable antigens can now be identified using monoclonal antibody techniques. Multiplication occurs within the blood stream. Depending on the number

TABLE 18-1. *Pathogenic Hemoflagellates of Genus Trypanosoma and Section Salivaria*

Species	Cell Morphology	Vectors	Hosts	Geographic Distribution
T. congolense	small, monomorphic; nucleus central; flagellum free	tsetse flies	domestic and game mammals	Central and South Africa
T. vivax	large, monomorphic; nucleus antero-central; flagellum free	tsetse flies	domestic and game mammals	Central, S. Africa; Central, S. America
T. brucei	polymorphic	tsetse flies	domestic and game mammals, man	Central, S. Africa

of trypanosomes in the infective dose the incubation period may vary from 4 to 12 days experimentally or 2 to 4 weeks under natural infection. In the case of *T. vivax* multiplication and existence is mainly within the blood stream, whereas *T. brucei* or *T. congolense* commonly invade tissues outside the blood stream, causing extensive tissue damage. The life cycle is completed when the trypanosome is once again ingested by a feeding tsetse fly and the parasite sloughs the glycoprotein protective coat becoming noninfective once more. Within the mammalian host the parasite multiplies within the blood and tissues developing several waves of parasitemia which are separated by a parasitemic or low parasitemic periods. The early high parasitemic phase may last up to 12 weeks. Sheep with acute or subacute disease usually die during the initial period of high parasitemia. The characteristic high fever of the disease is usually associated with the parasitemic wave. In case of *T. vivax* during the parasitemic wave an anemia, the most common feature of the disease, arises from extravascular destruction of red blood cells in the spleen, liver, and lungs. There is also a depression of reticulocytes, a depression of the bone marrow, leukopenia associated with lymphopenia and neutropenia, hypoglycemia, and uremia. There is a disseminated intravascular condition with formation of fibrin thrombi, par-

ticularly in the brain, kidney and testicles. *T. brucei* in its ability to invade tissues produces extensive tissue damage. All forms of trypanosomiasis cause a severe immunodepression.

CLINICAL SIGNS AND LESIONS. Three clinical forms—peracute, acute, and chronic—develop in the same and different animals. After an incubation period of 2 to 4 weeks, body temperatures rise up to 42°C and repeatedly remit and exacerbate. Anemia develops, often with the production of regenerative erythrocytes, and affected animals lose weight, become weak, and have accelerated pulse and respiration. Edema of limbs, scrotum, and eyelids forms and fluids may accumulate in body cavities.

Photophobia with keratoconjunctivitis and, in some cases, panophthalmitis and blindness develop. Neurologic disturbances from nonpurulent encephalitis and meningitis also become noticeable, except possibly from infections with *T. congolense*. Salivation, lacrimation, and nasal discharge are prominent. Peripheral lymph nodes are enlarged from edema and lymphoid hyperplasia.

In addition to the clinical signs of acute infections, the non-fatal chronic and subclinical infections cause weight loss, decreased milk production, abortions, stillbirths, infertility due to testicular and cystic ovarian degeneration, and an increased susceptibility to other infections. Morbidity and mortality vary depending on the strain involved, the nutritional status of the animal, concurrent infections with such diseases as anaplasmosis, babesiosis, theileriosis, and bacterial diseases. Certain breeds or locally selected sheep have a greater resistance to infection.

DIAGNOSIS.   Veterinarians suspect trypanosomosis in endemic areas from typical signs and lesions, and they confirm the diagnosis in the laboratory by finding the causative parasites in smears of blood and lymph nodes (Fig. 18-3) or serology. Identifying the parasite in the laboratory is by examination of wet, thin and thick blood films, and of lymph node smears, as well as the buffy coat or hematocrit method and the hypotonic shock test. Inoculation of susceptible laboratory animals, including healthy sheep, with the suspect blood and tissue, may be necessary. The serologic tests of choice are the indirect fluorescent antibody test (IFAT) and the indirect hemagglutination test.

PREVENTION AND TREATMENT.   Trypanosomiasis can be prevented and possibly eliminated in some areas by applying integrated programs with combinations of the following procedures:

1. Control tsetse flies by

    (a) removing from a geographic region trees and brush under which the flies obtain protection against drought and other environmental adversities,

    (b) systematically spraying wide areas with insecticide compounds such as DDT to eliminate or numerically reduce fly populations and thus lower the exposure rate of livestock to the disease, and

    (c) grazing livestock only during night hours when flies are inactive and protecting them during day hours when flies actively feed.

2. Clean and disinfect all instruments—needles, knives, saws—between individual animal applications of surgical procedures—vaccinations, castrations, dockings, dehornings—to prevent mechanical transfer of infective blood and tissue from diseased to clean animals.

3. Eliminate or reduce reservoir hosts in the wild fauna and thereby lower the opportunity for area flies to obtain infected blood meals.

The International Laboratory for Research on Animal Diseases (ILRAD) in Kenya has successfully cultured trypanosomes and has made great strides in developing a vaccine. The drugs of choice for treatment are Berenil (diaminazene aceturate), Samorin (isometamidium chloride), and Novidium (homidium

A

B

Fig. 18-3. Blood smears with *T. congolense* (*A*) and *T. brucei* (*B*). × 1200.

chloride). Berenil used at 3.5 to 7.0 mg/kg body weight, and Novidium at 1.0 mg/kg are preferred for treatment, while Samorin at 0.5 mg/kg is recommended for chemoprophylaxis. Good nutritional and nursing care are essential for prompt and uncomplicated recovery. Treatment of any concurrent disease is also necessary.

Anosa, V.: Diseases produced by *Trypanosoma vivax* in ruminants, horses and rodents. Zbl. Vet. Med., *30*: 717-741, 1983.

Anosa, V.O. and Isoun, T.T.: Pathology of experimental *trypanosoma vivax* infection in sheep and goats. Zbl. Vet. Med., *30*:685-700, 1983.

Anosa, V.O. and Isoun, T.T.: Serum proteins, blood and plasma volumes in experimental *T. vivax* infections in sheep and goats. Trop. Anim. Health Prod., *8*:14-19, 1976.

Askonas, B.: Interference of general immune function by parasite infections: African trypanosomiasis as a model system. Parasitology, *88*:633-638, 1984.

Crowe, J., et al.: All metacyclic variable antigen types of *Trypanosoma congolense* identified using monoclonal antibodies. Nature, *306*:389-391, 1983.

Dwinger, R.: Studies on the influence of non-steroidal anti-inflammatory drugs upon trypanosomiasis in goats and sheep. J. Vet. Pharmacol. Therap., *7*:293-301, 1984.

Glick, D. and Jones, F.: *In vivo* analysis of impaired macrophage bactericidal capacity during experimental African trypanosomiasis. Infect. Immun., *46*:663-667, 1984.

Habtemariam, T.: Application of a linear programming model to the control of African trypanosomiasis. Prevent. Vet. Med., *3*:1-14, 1984/85.

Henning, M.W.: *Animal Diseases in South Africa.* 3rd Edition. Onderstepoort, Central News Agency LTD, 1956, p. 718.

Ikede, B.O.: Genital lesions in experimental chronic *T. brucei* infections in rams. Res. Vet. Sci., *26*:145-151, 1979.

Ikede, B.O.: Ocular lesions in sheep infected with *T. brucei.* J. Comp. Pathol., *84*:203-213, 1974.

Ikede, B.O. and Losos, G.J.: Pathogenesis of *T. brucei* infection in sheep. J. Comp. Pathol., *85*:23-31; 33-36; 37-44, 1975.

Ikede, B.O. and Losos, G.J.: Pathology of the disease in sheep produced experimentally with *T. brucei.* Vet. Pathol., *9*:278-289, 1972.

Johnstone, B.: A vaccine for trypanosomiasis. New Scientist, 30 October 1984.

Levine, N.D.: *Protozoan Parasites of Domestic Animals and Man.* 2nd Edition. Minneapolis, Burgess Publishing, 1973, p. 36.

MacKenzie, P.K.I. and Cruickshank, J.G.: Phagocytosis of erythrocytes in sheep infected with *T. congolense.* Res. Vet. Sci., *15*:256-262, 1973.

Parish, N., Morrison, W., and Pearson, T.: Identification of an antigen specific to *Trypanosoma congolense* by using monoclonal antibodies. J. Immunol., *134*:593-597, 1985.

Theileriosis

Ovine theileriosis includes a generic pair of diseases that result in invasion and destruction of blood cells. Even though the clinical signs are similar and the causative protozoans are morphologically indistinguishable, the diseases are classified as two entities—malignant and benign—because the two are immunologically distinct.

Benign ovine theileriosis, a mild and nonfatal form of theileriosis, is caused by *Theileria ovis.* The disease occurs in Africa, northern Europe, southeastern Europe, southern USSR, Iran, and India. Anemia, hemoglobinuria, icterus and swelling of the spleen and liver are absent. Clinically recovered sheep are susceptible to malignant theileriosis.

Malignant theileriosis, the main focus of this discussion, is an acute infectious but noncontagious disease of sheep and goats and is characterized by fever, icterus, and enlargement of lymph nodes and is caused by a sporozoan parasite transmitted by ticks. In endemic areas, the disease causes economic losses from deaths of affected sheep, from the cost of tick control, and from protein deficiencies among sheep-dependent people.

OCCURRENCE. Malignant theileriosis occurs in all breeds and sexes of sheep, but is milder in lambs than in other age groups. Most cases develop during spring months, and less commonly during autumn months, when vectoring ticks are active. Geographically, malignant theileriosis occurs in Africa, southeastern Europe, southern USSR, Asia Minor, and India.

ETIOLOGY. *Theileria hirci,* the sporozoan parasites causing malignant ovine theileriosis, inhabit the erythrocytes as piroplasms and lymphocytes as schizonts. The erythrocyte forms are round or oval, rod-shaped and anaplasma-like. The predominating round forms measure 0.6 to 2 μm in diameter. Binary or quadruple fission takes place in the erythrocytes. Schizonts in nodal or splenic lymphocytes measure 4 to 10 μm and contain numerous chromatin granules.

The vector is unknown, but the ticks *Rhipicephalus bursa* and *Hyalomma anatolicum* are suspect. Clinically recovered sheep are susceptible to benign theileriosis.

CLINICAL SIGNS AND POSTMORTEM LESIONS. After an incubation period of unknown length, affected sheep develop fever ranging from 42 to 43°C, lose appetite, and show swelling of the prescapular lymph nodes. Clinically recovered sheep are premune. There is no cross immunity with *T. ovis*.

T. hirci is highly pathogenic for sheep and goats. Mortality ranges from 46 to 100%, and the course varies from 5 to 40 days. The disease is relatively mild in young lambs. Affected animals are anemic and frequently icteric. There is a transitory hemoglobinuria. Erythrocytes of sick sheep contain *T. hirci* at the rate of 10 to 20 or more per 1000 cells.

At necropsy, the lymph nodes, spleen, and liver are swollen. The kidneys may contain infarcts and the lungs, edematous fluid. There are petechiae on the mucosa of the abomasum and irregularly disseminated red patches on the intestinal mucosa, particularly in the cecum and large intestine.

DIAGNOSIS. Veterinarians diagnose malignant theileriosis on evidence of typical signs and lesions and upon identification of the parasites in stained blood, lymph node, or spleen smears. In contrast to *T. ovis* the erythrocyte stages are usually present in relatively large numbers. The indirect fluorescent antibody test has been applied for the detection of circulating antibodies in *T. hirci*.

PREVENTION. The incidence of malignant theileriosis can be reduced by controlling ticks, especially *R. bursa,* through systematic use of pesticides.

Hawa, N., Latif, B.M.A., and Bakir, F.A.: Application of the indirect fluorescent antibody test for the diagnosis of *Theileria hirci* infection in sheep, using cell culture schizont antigen. Trop. Anim. Health Prod., *8*:97-101, 1976.

Hooshmand-Rod, P. and Hawa, N.S.: Transmission of *Theileria hirci* in sheep by *Hyalomma anatolicum anatolicum.* Trop. Anim. Health Prod., *5*:103-109, 1973.

Kyurtov, N.: Incidence of theileria carriers among sheep and goats. Vet. Sbir. (Sofia), *67*:23-25, 1969.

Levine, N.D.: *Protozoan Parasites of Domestic Animals and Man.* Minneapolis, Burgess Publishing, 1973.

Neitz, W.O.: Theileriosis. Adv. Vet. Sci., *3*:241-297, 1959.

Rafyi, A. and Maghami, G.: In *Rep. FAO/OIE Int. Conf. Sheep Diseases.* FAO (Rome), 1966, pp. 60-66.

Babesiosis

(*Ovine piroplasmosis; red water disease*)

Ovine and caprine babesiosis, an acute or chronic infectious but noncontagious disease, is characterized by fever, anemia, hemoglobinuria, and icterus and is caused by two hemosporidian parasites transmitted by ticks. Because of wide geographic distribution, high incidence, and elevated mortality, the disease in some areas causes serious financial waste. Economic losses result from deaths among affected sheep and goats, from unthriftiness of chronic cases, from the cost of preventive and treatment programs, from restricted movements of animals during tick season, and from inadequate protein in the diets of sheep-dependent people. Babesias of cattle and horses, although similar in some respects, do not transfer to sheep and goats.

OCCURRENCE. Babesiosis occurs in all breeds and sexes of sheep and goats, but animals 6 to 12 months old have higher incidence than animals of other age groups. Most cases develop during spring months when vectoring ticks are abundant and vigorously active. Geographically, babesiosis from *B. motasi* occurs in Zambia, Portugal, Rumania, Cyprus, Israel, Jordan, Iraq, Iran, Afghanistan, and India, and from *B. ovis* in Algeria, Morocco, Libya, Somalia, Zambia, Madagascar, Italy, USSR, Rumania, Bulgaria, Turkey, Syria, Lebanon, Israel, Jordan, Iraq, Iran, and India.

ETIOLOGY. *Babesia motasi* and *B. ovis,* the antigenically different causes of babesiosis, are hemosporozoan parasites. *B. motasi,* usually more virulent of the two pathogens, occurs singly or paired in erythrocytes; pairs form an acute angle. The piriform bodies occupy the centers of erythrocytes and measure 2.5 to 4 × 2 μm. *B. ovis,* single or paired, occupies the cell periphery and measures 1 to 2.5 μm in length; paired organisms form an obtuse angle (Fig. 18-4). Following recovery from either disease, immunity is incomplete, and most animals carry a latent infection.

Natural transmission of both parasites occurs through the tick, *Rhipicephalus bursa,*

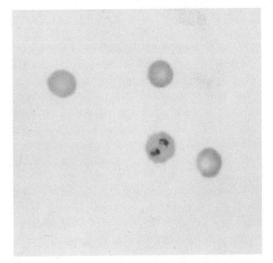

Fig. 18-4. Blood smear with *Babesia ovis*. × 1200.

and within the vector, both transovarian and trans-stadial transmission takes place. In addition, intrauterine transmission of *B. ovis* occurs.

CLINICAL SIGNS AND POSTMORTEM LESIONS. In acute babesiosis, affected sheep experience fever, anemia, hemoglobinuria, icterus, and weakness. Thirty to 40% of affected animals die. Chronically infected sheep usually are symptomless, except for parasitemia and unthriftiness. At necropsy, the spleen and lymph nodes are swollen, and babesias infect many erythrocytes of the peripheral circulation. Morbidity may reach 30% and the mortality, 25%.

DIAGNOSIS.   In endemic areas, veterinarians diagnose babesiosis from evidence of typical signs and lesions and from finding the piriform bodies in erythrocytes of stained blood films. Blood collected at different times and from different sheep may be necessary for demonstrating the protozoa.

The differential diagnosis requires consideration of anthrax, anaplasmosis, and theileriosis.

PREVENTION AND TREATMENT.   Ovine and caprine babesiosis can be reduced and controlled in some areas by systematic use of pesticides during spring months. Imidocarb dihydrochloride administered subcutaneously in divided doses of 2 mg/kg for 3 days is effective in eliminating experimental babesiosis.

An experimental live vaccine attenuated in splenectomized sheep produces solid immunity for over 6 months.

Animal Health Yearbook. FAO-WHO-OIE (Italy), 1970.

Hashemi-Fesharki, R.: Studies on imidiocarb dihydrochloride in experimental *Babesia ovis* infection in splenectomized lambs. Br. Vet. J., *133*:609-614, 1977.

Kyurtov, N.: Testing a live vaccine against babesiasis in sheep. Vet. Med. Nauki, *14*:25-30, 1977.

Neitz, W.O.: Classification, transmission and biology of piroplasms of domestic animals. Ann. N.Y. Acad. Sci., *64*:56-111, 1956.

Rafyi, A. and Maghami, G.: In *Rep. FAO/OIE Int. Conf. Sheep Diseases*. FAO (Rome), 1966, pp. 61-62.

Suleimanov, S.A.: Intrauterine infection of a sheep fetus with *Babesia ovis*. Dagestan and Turkmenia. Tr. Vses. Eksp. Vet., *31*:307-308, 1965.

Weisenhutter, E.: Coccidia and piroplasms in sheep and goats in Syria. Berl. Muench. Tieraerztl. Wochenschr., *78*:247-249, 1965.

Schistosomiasis

(Bilharziasis)

Schistosomiasis, a chronic phleboparasitism, is characterized by reduced weight, anemia, and emaciation and is caused by blood flukes. The disease occurs primarily in Africa and the Far East. In endemic areas, it causes serious economic losses to producers of both sheep and goats from inefficient feed conversion, expensive treatments, and deaths; to meat packers from condemnations of infected organs and carcasses; and to sheep- and goat-dependent people from loss of animal protein for food, and animal fiber for clothing. Occurrence of the disease also in other species of domestic animals and people adds both economic importance and public health significance to the malady.

ETIOLOGY AND PATHOGENESIS.   Six species of the genus *Schistosoma*, listed in Table 18-2, cause schistosomiasis. These unisexual elongate trematodes range in lengths from 5 to 25 mm for males and 5 to 28 mm for females. The male holds the female in his gynaecophoral groove (Fig. 18-5).

The life cycles are similar and begin with expulsion of eggs mixed with feces to the external environment. They hatch immediately on contact with fresh water at about 22°C. The

Fig. 18-5. Two pairs of *Schistosoma japonicum* in a branch of the mesenteric vein. The large males embrace the small females. (Cross section)

resulting miracidia, measuring about 120 × 50 μm, swim about and are chemically attracted to their respective host snails, which they penetrate. In the snail livers, they develop two generations of sporocysts. After about 30 days of parasitism, the second generation produces and releases bifid-tailed cercariae. These motile forms seek their definitive hosts and, on contact, penetrate the skin, lose their tails, and thus become schistosomules. Such organisms move to the host lungs, mostly by transport in venous blood, but possibly some by migration through tissue. There many die, but survivors enter the systemic circulation and eventually localize in hepatic portal veins. After maturation they migrate mostly to mesenteric veins, but some to pelvic veins, their definitive locations. Gravid females deposit eggs in the lamina propria of the intestines. The prepatent

period ranges from 35 to 50 days, and the egg output per female in feces is approximately 50.

In the pathogenesis, host albumin and erythrocytes leak into the intestinal lumen and thereby cause hypoalbuminemia and anemia. Fluke eggs accumulate in intestinal wall, liver, lymph nodes and, less commonly, in other organs such as lungs. Host tissue reactions against the eggs vary with egg densities and with hosts. Generally, however, they lead to granulomas and later to calcification.

CLINICAL SIGNS AND POSTMORTEM LESIONS. Cercarial penetration of host skin produces transient papules at the sites—usually the digits. After several weeks, a normochromic, normocytic anemia and hypoalbuminemia develop. Anorexia and diarrhea with mucus and blood in the feces result in reduced growth rate or even weight loss and broken wool and hair. Progression of the disease leads to emaciation, ascites, exhaustion, and finally death. During patency, fluke eggs can be recovered from host feces. Morbidity varies with numbers of cercariae in the environment and may reach high levels, and mortality from heavy infections is also high. The course ranges from 12 to 25 weeks. Infections with *S. nasalis*, "snorter disease," is manifested by dyspnea, stertor, and oral breathing.

At necropsy, fat depots are depleted, and ascites may be present. Infected small and large intestines are focally or generally thickened and contain numerous discrete and some confluent granulomatous nodules that may be partially calcified. Veins, especially subserosal, are thickened and tortuous. Livers may be focally fibrosed and pigmented, particularly in portal areas, and in advanced stages, cirrhotic and nodular. Infections with *S. mattheei* commonly result also in pulmonary lesions. In animals with nasal infection, the thickened mucosa contains both discrete and confluent granulomas, and veins have pairs of *S. nasalis*.

Histologic sections of gross lesions reveal aggregates of fluke eggs surrounded by eosinophils, macrophages, multinucleated giant cells, fibrous tissue and, in advanced stages, calcification. Pigment, some phagocytized, accompanies the egg deposits. Infected veins

TABLE 18-2. *Schistosomes of Sheep and Goats*

Species	Intermediate (Snails)	Definitive	Geographic Distribution
S. japonicum	*Oncomelania* (sp)	sheep, goats, cattle, buffalo, horse, swine, man	China, Japan, Philippines, Thailand
S. indicum	*Indoplanorbis exustus*	sheep, goat, cattle, camel, horse	India
S. spindale	*Planorbis* (sp) *Indoplanorbis* (sp)	sheep, goats, cattle, buffalo, antelope, horse	India, Sumatra
S. nasalis	*Limnaea luteola, L. acuminata, Indoplanorbis exustus*	sheep, goats, cattle	India
S. bovis	*Physopsis nasuta, P. africans, P. globosa, Bulinus contortus, B. truncata*	sheep, goats, cattle, antelope, horse	Africa, Mediterranean basin, Iraq, Iran
S. mattheei	*Physopsis africana*	sheep, cattle	Africa
S. mansoni	*Biomphalaria*	sheep, ruminants, wild animals, man	Africa, Caribbean, Mediterranean, Brazil, Venezuela

may contain flukes (Fig. 18-5) and show phlebitis, thrombosis, medial hypertrophy, and intimal proliferation.

DIAGNOSIS. Veterinarians suspect schistosomiasis in endemic areas from the presence of typical signs and lesions, and they confirm the diagnosis by identifying eggs in feces and/or in histosections of affected tissue. In some cases, moving schistosomes can be detected with transmitted light in mesenteric veins at necropsy of dead animals or inspection of slaughtered animals. A kinetic-dependent enzyme-linked immunosorbent assay has been developed as a diagnostic aid for schistosomiasis. The differential diagnosis requires consideration of other forms of gastrointestinal parasitism, liver fluke disease, paratuberculosis, chronic pneumonias, malnutrition, and chronic intoxications.

PREVENTION AND TREATMENT. An effective treatment for ruminants is the oral administration of praziquantel at the rate of 20 mg/kg. Praziquantel is also an effective human treatment. A vaccine produced with irradiated cercariae or schistosomula is effective against homologous species and in some cases gives resistance to heterologous species.

Bushara, H., Hussein, M., Majid, M., and Taylor, M.: Effects of praziquantel and metrifonate on *schistosoma bovis* infections in Judanese cattle. Res. Vet. Sci., *33*:125-126, 1982.
Dargie, J.D. and MacLean, J.M.: Pathophysiology of ovine schistosomiasis. III. Plasma protein metabolism in experimental *S. mattheei* infection. J. Comp. Pathol., *83*:543-557, 1973.
Gameel, A.D.: Clinico-pathological study on naturally occurring *A. bovis* infection in sheep. Acta Vet. (Yugoslavia), *24*:277-285, 1974.
Hussein, M.F., Buchara, H.O., and Ali, K.E.: Pathology of experimental *S. bovis* infection in sheep. J. Helminol., *50*:235-241, 1976.
Lawrence, J.A.: *S. mattheei* in sheep: host-parasite relationship. Res. Vet. Sci., *17*:263-264, 1974.
McCauley, Majud, A. and Tayeb, A.: Economic evaluation of the production impact of bovine schistosomiasis and vaccination in the Sudan. Prevent. Vet. Med. *2*:735-754, 1984.
Massoud, J.: Pathology of *O. turkistanicum* and *S. bovis* in cattle, sheep, and goats in Iran. Trans. R. Soc. Trop. Med. Hyg., *65*:431, 1971.
Massoud, J.: Parasitological and pathological observations on *S. bovis* in calves, sheep, and goats. J. Helminol., *47*:155-164, 1973.

Monrad, J.: Clinical pathology of *Schistosoma bovis* infection in sheep. Res. Vet. Sci., *33*:382-383, 1982.

Preston, J.M. and Dargie, J.D.: Pathophysiology of ovine schistosomiasis. V. Onset of development of anemia in sheep infected with *S. mattheei.* J. Comp. Pathol., *84*:73-81, 1974.

Preston, J.M., Dargie, J.D., and MacLean, J.M.: Pathophysiology of ovine schistosomiasis. I. Clinicopathological study of *S. mattheei* infections. II. Observations on the sequential changes in blood volume. J. Comp. Pathol., *83*:401-428, 1973.

Soulsby, E.J.L.: *Textbook of Veterinary Clinical Parasitology.* Philadelphia, F.A. Davis, 1965, pp. 595-601.

Chronic Copper Poisoning

(*CCP*)

Chronic copper poisoning, a slow-developing but rapidly acting intoxication, is characterized by hemolysis, anemia, icterus, and hemoglobinuria. It is caused by gradual accumulation in the liver of large stores of copper and its sudden release into the blood. Because CCP, caused by agricultural chemicals or grazing forages normal in copper but low in molybdenum, occurs in all sheep producing countries and causes extensive financial waste, the disease is of major concern to the entire sheep industry. Economic losses result from deaths of most affected sheep and from the cost of preventive programs.

OCCURRENCE. CCP occurs in all breeds and sexes of sheep beyond weaning age, but mature ewes of British breeds develop the disease more commonly than do other classes and ages of animals. In the United States, CCP occurs in the western states of the intermountain region during autumn and winter. Sheep transferred from certain mountain ranges to agricultural pastures of crop residues often contract this disease.

Geographically, the malady occurs in Australia, New Zealand, America, Britain, Norway, South Africa, USSR, and possibly other sheep-producing countries.

ETIOLOGY AND PATHOGENESIS. The accumulation of copper in the tissues, mainly the liver, over a period of a few weeks to more than a year with no clinical signs followed by a sudden release of hepatic copper causes clinical CCP. Accumulation of toxic levels of copper in the liver is a complex interaction between copper, molybdenum and sulfate with magnesium, zinc, and iron also playing a role in this interrelationship. Chronic copper poisoning can be primary from excessive intake of copper or secondary from normal dietary copper intake associated with low intake of molybdenum, calcium, zinc, and sulfate, or following liver damage. Sources of excess copper intake can be related to forages with high copper levels from soils high in copper or that have been fertilized or sprayed with copper containing products. Some feed stuffs, such as corn distiller grains and soybean meal, are naturally high in copper. In Australia, and possibly other areas, forages such as subteranean clover may accumulate abnormally high levels of copper and no molybdenum. Chronic copper poisoning can be seen on pastured forages which are normal to low in copper but are extremely low in molybdenum and sulfate, thus a dietary imbalance of the copper-molybdenum-sulfate ratio allows copper to accumulate. Liver damage from plants containing pyrrolizidine alkaloids, *Heliotropium euporaeum* and *Echium plantagineum,* damage livers and case these organs to assiduously collect and continuously accumulate copper from consumed feed. If sheep are fed a diet containing normal amounts of copper (8 to 11 ppm) with no molybdenum, copper toxicity may result. Conversely, the same dietary copper intake may lead to a copper deficiency in areas where there is an excess of molybdenum and sulfate. Levels of 4 to 6 mg cu/kg in feed on a dry matter basis are necessary to prevent copper deficiency, whereas toxicity can occur when sheep are grazing pastures with 10 to 20 mg cu/kg on a dry matter basis. Vitamin-mineral preparations containing copper but no molybdenum may elevate the copper concentration in the ration to as much as 25 to 35 ppm. Normal concentrations of molybdenum in the feed is low (1 to 2 ppm), thus the vitamin-mineral supplementation without molybdenum may cause toxicity. The site of copper absorption is from the large intestine. Upon reaching the liver copper is distributed among soluble hepatic metal-binding proteins.

The sheep accumulates copper in the liver more readily than other animals and over a period of time critical levels of 1000 to 3000 ppm DW may be reached. During this accumulation the blood-copper level maintains normal values at 0.10 to 0.20 mg/dl. Toxicity is usually associated with stress situations and death of liver cells which release copper into the blood. The plasma copper levels increase 10 to 20 times followed by an increase in copper concentration of red cells causing damage and hemolysis, production of methemoglobin and formation of Heinz bodies. Elevated blood copper levels of 500 to 2000 mg/dl precede clinical signs by 24 to 48 hours. Serum lactic dehydrogenase and glutamic oxaloacetic transaminase (GOT) increase 6 to 8 weeks prior to the hemolytic crisis indicating that liver damage is taking place during the accumulation phase. At the time of hemolytic crisis a further increase in GOT occurs by enzymes released from the red cells and further liver and kidney damage. The serum creatine phosphakinase (CPK) remains normal until the time of hemolytic crisis when it increases markedly (100 fold) and then falls rapidly indicating that the effect on muscle is short lived. Liver damage prior to the crisis also indicated by increase in arginase, sorbitol dehydrogenase, and glutamate dehydrogenase. Morphologic and histochemical changes start to occur in liver parenchymal and Kuppfer cells several weeks prior to the hemolytic crisis. These changes include nuclear vacuolation and increased acid phosphate activity and marked copper disposition in the Kuppfer cells.

CLINICAL SIGNS AND POSTMORTEM LESIONS. At the same time of crisis, the anemic animals accelerate breathing and circulation, thirst for water, and, because of weakness, fall behind the moving flock. The skin and membranes become bright yellow and the urine dark brown. At the time of intravascular hemolysis, plasma creatine kinase becomes elevated, and these levels return to normal following the crisis. After a short period of recumbency, most animals die.

The morbidity often reaches 20%, and the mortality of affected sheep is high. The clinical course ranges from 1 to 4 days.

At necropsy, the blood is thin, and the hemoglobin may have descended to 4 g/dl. Most tissues are yellow, but the kidneys are black and the spleen dark and soft (Fig. 18-6). The liver is yellow-brown and friable. Some cases show gastroenteritis. Histopathologically, there is a centrilobular fatty degeneration and necrosis in the liver with a hyperplasia of bile ducts. In the kidney, the lesions consist of a nephrosis of the proximal convoluted tubules and swollen Bowman's capsule.

DIAGNOSIS.   Veterinarians diagnose CCP on evidence of history, signs, lesions, and laboratory findings. Anemia, icterus, brown urine, and normal temperatures are indicative signs, and prolonged grazing on potentially contaminated forage or hepatotoxic plants is suggestive history. At necropsy, the characteristic liver and spleen changes give additional evidence and histologic findings of hemoglobinuric nephrosis. Copper levels of 1 to 2 mg/dl in the blood and/or 1000 to 3000 ppm DW in the liver confirm the diagnosis.

Fig. 18-6. Blackened kidney from sheep with chronic copper poisoning. × 0.8.

The differential diagnosis requires consideration of leptospirosis, yellow lamb disease, piroplasmosis, and lupinosis.

PREVENTION AND TREATMENT. Producers and veterinarians avoid CCP by preventing sheep from grazing copper-contaminated forage or hepatotoxic plants. In areas low in molybdenum or when using feedstuff and forages with high levels of copper-molybdenum ratio, a balance of 1 part molybdenum to 6 to 10 parts of copper prevents toxicity. Increasing dietary zinc concentration of 200 to 420 mg/kg may also be used to avoid copper poisoning. If CCP develops, a flock should be daily treated with 50 to 100 mg of ammonium molybdate and 0.5 to 1.0 g of sodium sulfate per animal for 3 weeks. An aqueous solution of the two salts should be sprayed onto the feed.

Urinary excretion of copper is increased 10- to 20-fold in intoxicated sheep by the administration of 52 mg/kg of D-penicillamine daily for 6 days.

Albiston, H.E., Bull, L.B., Dick, A.T., and Keast, J.C.: A note on the etiology of enzootic jaundice of sheep in Australia. Aust. Vet. J., 16:233, 1940.

Bischoff, O. and Haun, F.: Poisoning from copper and arsenic in domestic animals. DTW, 47:442-447, 1939.

Boughton, I.B. and Hardy, W.T.: Chronic copper poisoning in sheep. Texas Agric. Exp. Stat. Bull., 1934, p. 499.

Bull, L.B.: Toxemic jaundice in sheep of Australia: chronic copper poisoning and pyrrolizidine alkaloids. Vict. Vet. Proc., 22:17-20, 1963/64.

Cunningham, I.J.: Copper deficiency in sheep in New Zealand. N.Z. J. Agric., 69:559, 1944.

Dick, A.T.: Control of copper storage in liver of sheep by inorganic sulfate and molybdenum. Aust. Vet. J., 29:233-238, 1953.

Doherty, P.C., Barlow, R.M., and Angus, K.W.: Spongy changes in the brains of sheep poisoned by dietary copper. Res. Vet. Sci., 10:303-304, 1969.

Eden, A.: Observations on copper poisoning. J. Comp. Pathol., 53:90-111, 1940.

Ellenberger and Hofmeister: The physiologic effects of copper on ruminants. Arch. Wiss. Prokt. Tierheilk, 9:325, 1883.

Froslie, A., Norheim, G., and Soli, N.: Levels of copper, molybdenum, zinc and sulfur in concentrates and mineral feeding stuffs in relation to chronic copper poisoning in Norway. Acta Agriculturae Scandinavia 33:261-267, 1983.

Froslie, A. and Norheim, G.: Copper, molybdenum, zinc and sulfur in Norwegian forages and their possible role in chronic copper poisoning in sheep. Acta Agriculturae Scandinavia 33:97-104, 1983.

Gooneratne, S.R. and Howell, J. McC.: Creatine kinase release and muscle changes in chronic copper poisoning in sheep. Res. Vet. Sci., 28:351-361, 1980.

Hidrioglou, M., Heaney, D., and Hartin, K.: Copper poisoning in a flock of sheep. Copper excretion patterns after treatment with molybdenum and sulfur or penicillamine. Can. Vet. J., 25:377-382, 1984.

Hubbs, R. and Oehme, F.: Understanding chronic copper poisoning in sheep. Bovine Practice, 3:15-22, 1982.

MacPherson, A. and Hemingway, R.G.: Merits of various blood analyses and liver tests in early diagnosis of chronic copper poisoning. Br. Vet. J., 125:213-221, 1969.

Maclachlan, G. and Johnston, W.: Copper poisoning in sheep from north Ronaldsay maintained on a diet of terrestrial herbage. Vet. Rec., 111:299-301, 1982.

Muth, O.H.: Chronic copper poisoning in sheep. JAVMA, 120:148-149, 1952.

Pearson, J.K.L.: Copper poisoning in sheep fed a copper supplement. Vet. Rec., 68:766-768, 1956.

Pierson, R.E. and Aanes, W.A.: Treatment of chronic copper poisoning in sheep. JAVMA, 133:307-311, 1958.

Pryor, W.J.: Copper poisoning in sheep following top-dressing of pasture. Aust. Vet. J., 35:366-369, 1959.

Report of Investigating Committee: Etiology and control of enzootic jaundice of sheep. Aust. Vet. J., 26:229-232, 1949/1950.

Sali, N.E., Froshe, A., and Aaseth, J.: The mobilization of copper in sheep by chelating agents. Acta Vet. Scand., 19:422-429, 1978.

Schaper and Luetje: Copper poisoning in sheep from fruit tree spray of copper sulfate. Berl. Tieraerztl. Wochenschr., 47:36-39; 49-54, 1931.

St. George-Grambauer, T.D. and Rac, R.: Hepatogenous copper poisoning in sheep from Echium plantagineum in Australia. Aust. Vet. J., 38:288-293, 1962.

Suttle, N.: Effects of molybdenum concentration in fresh herbage, hay and semi-purified diets on copper metabolism of sheep. J. Agric. Sci. Lamb, 100:651-656, 1983.

Suttle, N. and Field, A.: Effects of dietary supplements of thiomolybdates on copper and molybdenum metabolism in sheep. J. Comp. Path., 93:379-389, 1983.

VanRyssen, J., Botha, W., and Stielau, W.: Effect of a high copper intake and different levels of molybdenum on the health of sheep. J. S. Afr. Vet. Assn., 53:167-170, 1982.

VanRyssen, J. and Stielau, W.: The influence of dietary sulfur on copper and molybdenum in sheep. S. Afr. J. Anim. Sci., 10:49-57, 1980.

Caseous Lymphadenitis

(CL; pseudotuberculosis)

Caseous lymphadenitis, a chronic contagious disease of adult sheep, is characterized by unilateral enlargement and suppuration of lymph nodes and occasionally lungs and spleen. Because the disease insidiously occurs with high incidence, CL causes extensive waste and major concern to the sheep industry. Economic losses result from unthriftiness and death of some sheep and from condemnation of infected carcasses and parts of carcasses at slaughter. During the year 1981, 5,671,620 sheep and lambs were slaughtered in abattoirs under federal inspection of the United States. Condemnations of whole carcasses due to CL amounted to 5528 (0.097%) under federally inspected slaughter. There were 401,000 mature cull sheep slaughtered under federal inspection in 1981, although a summary of condemnations for this subgroup is not available. Studies on prevalence of CL suggest that this condition is the most prevalent and economically significant disease condition of mature culled sheep in the U.S. The occurrence of the disease also in goats, deer, cattle, and rarely in people adds both economic importance and public health significance to the malady.

OCCURRENCE.   Although CL occurs in all breeds and sexes, Merinos, because of wrinkled skin, suffer numerous shearing wounds and, for this reason, develop many lesions. The disease incidence steadily increases with age because infections from successive shearings are cumulated up to 4 years. In the United States, range herds usually develop higher infection rates than do farm flocks. The chronic lesions of CL occur at all seasons. From a population of 37,383 mature culled sheep, federally inspected for human consumption, 4089 randomly selected individuals had a prevalence rate for CL of 42.41%. Lesions occurred in the thoracic viscera, skeletal tissues, and abdominal viscera in 1,021 (24.97%), 944 (23.09%), and 482 (11.79%) respectively. The region of origin in the U.S. influences these prevalence rates.

Geographically, CL is widespread or sporadic in Australia, New Zealand, the United States, Argentina, Peru, Mexico, South Africa, Sudan, Egypt, Norway, Spain, Italy, Iran, and the Philippines.

ETIOLOGY AND PATHOGENESIS.   *Corynebacterium pseudotuberculosis,* the specific cause of CL, is a nonmotile, nonspore-forming, noncapsulating, aerobic, gram-positive coccoid bacillus measuring 0.5 to 0.6 × 1.0 to 3.0 μm.

It commonly resides in manure, soil, and intestines, on the skin, and in infected organs, especially lymph nodes.

The organism may survive for up to 20 weeks in discharging purulent material in shaded areas of a shearing shed. In the laboratory the organism abundantly grows on serum agar, where it produces opaque, dry, crumbling, concentrically ringed, red to pink colonies. All strains produce acid without gas from glucose, fructose, maltose, mannose, and sucrose, but do not ferment arabinose, xylose, raffinose, lactose, inulin, salicin, dulcitol, or starch. The strains do not liquefy solid serum, but do form hemolysin and exotoxin. The latter is lethal to guinea pigs, rabbits, and sheep.

Studies on the pathogenesis of CL indicate that infection may occur after penetration of the organism through unbroken skin or mucous membranes; in most cases it probably begins with superficial skin wounds from shearing clippers, grass awns, wood splinters, dog bites, docking, and castrating. The causative bacteria living on skin surface, manure, shearing blades, and shearing pens contaminate and infect the wounds. The proliferating bacteria enter afferent lymphatic vessels and gradually move into the regional lymph nodes, where they continue to grow and multiply. In the lymphoid tissue, leukocytes, especially neutrophils, accumulate around and among the bacteria, and fibrocytes and capillaries form at the periphery of the infection. Toxic bacterial metabolites, including the exotoxin, slowly but continuously kill the leukocytes and tissue.

The typical lesion of CL, therefore, consists of a central mass of necrotic tissue surrounded by a wall of connective tissue and capillaries. The bacteria, uncontrolled by the wall, enter the capillaries and form colonies that occlude and thrombose the vessels. The resulting ischemia and toxins kill the cells of the inner part of the connective tissue wall and, thus, add a new layer to the necrotic mass. New connective tissue proliferates to reinforce the wall. By this slow repetitive process, successive layers add to the necrotic mass. As live bacteria escape from the lesion, they spread through efferent lymphatics, penetrate other nodes

Fig. 18-7. Laminated caseous necrosis in a lymph node from a sheep with caseous lymphadenitis. × 1.0.

CLINICAL SIGNS AND POSTMORTEM LESIONS. Following a prolonged incubation period, infected superficial lymph nodes, especially prescapular, precrural, and popliteal, unilaterally enlarge and, in approximately 10% of affected sheep, discharge pus into the wool. As the disease advances, emaciation develops, and breathing may become accelerated and difficult. Among infected flocks the morbidity ranges up to 15% with most cases in animals 4 to 5 years of age. The eventual mortality of affected sheep is high. The course varies from months to years.

The abdominal organ most frequently affected with CL lesions is the liver then the kidney (Fig. 18-8). Thoracic lesions involve lung parenchyma or lymph nodes with bronchial and mediastinal lymph nodes most frequently involved (Fig. 18-7). Lesions of the lung parenchyma are mostly multiple and vary from a few millimeters to those that occupy an entire lung. Each lesion consists of a central mass of laminated caseative necrosis surrounded by a wall of connective tissue. The necrotic tissue, often converted to green tenacious pus, contains discernible layers of recently added necrotic tissue. Sinus tracts may

along the chain, eventually enter the venous blood, and go to the lungs. Organisms passing through the lungs may cause lesions in any invaded organ. In an infected node, liquefaction of necrotic tissue and abscess formation result from entrance of neutrophils and release of proteolytic enzymes and from invasion by other species of pyogenic bacteria. The connective tissue wall may rupture and discharge pus and bacteria to the environment, or into the blood stream or airways.

Abortion has been caused by the intravenous inoculation of *C. pseudotuberculosis* in the second half of gestation. The visceral form of CL is one of the major factors involved in the debilitating condition called "thin ewe syndrome." The route of entry and exposure dose of the *C. pseudotuberculosis* organism will influence the incubation period, the tissues involved, and the number of abscesses produced.

Fig. 18-8. Laminated lesion of caseous lymphadenitis in a kidney. × 0.08.

discharge pus onto the surface. Histopathologically, a wall of connective tissue surrounds the caseative necrosis. Colonies of *C. pseudotuberculosis* are discernible in the necrotic tissue and in the lumina of capillaries in the wall.

DIAGNOSIS. Veterinarians diagnose CL from typical signs, lesions, and laboratory findings. Unilateral enlargement of prescapular and/or precrural lymph nodes with, in some cases, a discharge of green pus, suggests the disease. Laminations of the necrotic nodes give substantiating evidence. Isolating *C. ovis* from lesions confirms the diagnosis.

The enzyme-linked immunosorbent assay (ELISA) test for detection of the antitoxin will detect infections as early as 30 to 60 days. The test is both sensitive and specific and easy to conduct. The ELISA can be used as a diagnostic and eradication tool.

The differential diagnosis requires consideration of actinobacillosis and tuberculosis. Purulent exudate from lesions of actinobacillosis contains rosettes and gram-negative bacteria, and tubercles contain acid-fast bacilli that can be isolated and identified.

PREVENTION AND TREATMENT. Producers prevent or reduce CL by avoiding injuries and by practicing sanitation. Shearers should avoid cutting the skin, and the pen fences should be freed of traumatizing nails and wire. Shearing should be sanitized by: disinfecting the hands, machines, and floors at daily or more frequent intervals; sequential shearing of sheep aged 1, 2, 3, 4, and 5 years; cleaning and disinfecting holding pens; disinfecting the more serious wounds; and moving newly shorn sheep to pasture or range as soon as possible. The mechanism of immunity against *C. pseudotuberculosis* is not yet fully understood. However, continued research is being conducted to improve the efficacy of present vaccines. In some countries vaccines are available, although an absolute immunity has not yet been established. Treating sheep for CL is not practical.

Addo, P.B.: Pathology and bacteriology of abortion in sheep experimentally infected with Corynebacterium pseudotuberculosis. Bull. Anim. Health Prod. Afr., 27:257-262, 1979.

Aktas, H.: Isolation of Corynebacterium pseudotuberculosis ovis from abscesses in the lymph nodes of sheep slaughtered at Ankora Meat and Fish Company. Turk. Ask. Vet. Hekim. Derg., 48:4-19, 1971.

Brogden, K., Cutlip, R., and Lehmkuhl, H.: Comparison of protection induced in lambs by Corynebacterium pseudotuberculosis whole cell and cell wall vaccines. Am. J. Vet. Res., 45:2393-2395, 1984.

Brogden, K., Cutlip, R., and Lehmkuhl, H.: Experimental Corynebacterium pseudotuberculosis infection in lambs. Am. J. Vet. Res., 45:1532-1534, 1984.

Cameron, C. and Bester, F.: An improved Corynebacterium pseudotuberculosis vaccine for sheep. Onderstepoort J. Vet. Res., 51:263-267, 1984.

Federal Meat Inspection: Statistical Summaries. USDA, 1967-1971.

Hunter, A.H.: Caseous lymphadenitis: results of six years' observations. Vet. Rec., 13:952-953, 1933.

McGrath, T.T.: On the presence of the bacillus of Preisz-Nocard in infected shear-cut wounds in sheep. Aust. Vet. J., 5:148-149, 1929.

Maki, L., et al.: Diagnosis of Corynebacterium pseudotuberculosis infections in sheep, using an enzyme-linked immunosorbent assay. Am. J. Vet. Res., 46: 212-214, 1985.

Norgaard, V.A. and Mohler, J.R.: The nature, cause and economic importance of ovine caseous lymphadenitis. USDA 16th Ann. Rep. Bur. Anim. Ind., 1899, pp. 638-662.

Preisz and Guinard: J. Med. Vet. Zootech., Lyons, 1891.

Seddon, H.R.: Caseous lymphadenitis (Preisz-Nocard disease: "cheesy-gland" disease). In Bacterial Diseases. Vol. I. Aust. Dept. Health, 1965, pp. 109-114.

Seddon, H.R., Belschner, H.G., Rose, A.L., and Blumer, C.: Further observations on the method of infection in caseous lymphadenitis of sheep. Aust. Vet. J., 5:139-148, 1929.

Stoops, S., Renshaw, H., and Thilsted, J.: Ovine caseous lymphadenitis: Disease prevalence, lesion distribution, and thoracic manifestations in a population of mature culled sheep from western United States. Am. J. Vet. Res., 45:557-561, 1984.

Woodruff, H.A. and Gregory, T.S.: Observations on the age and sex incidence in an infected flock in relation to possible routes of infection. Aust. Vet. J., 5:134-139, 1929.

Woodruff, H.A. and Oxer, D.T.: An experimental inquiry as to the common modes of natural infection in sheep. Aust. Vet. J., 5:130-134, 1929.

INDEX

Page numbers in *italics* indicate figures; page numbers followed by "*t*" indicate tables.

visceral. *See* Visceral cysticercosis
Cysticercus ovis, 190
Cysticercus tenuicollis, 167

Damalinia ovis, 305*t,* 314
Death camas poisoning, 244-245, 244*t, 244*
  clinical signs of, 245
  diagnosis, prevention, and treatment of, 245
  etiology of, 244-245, 244*t, 244*
  occurrence of, 244
Deer
  Parelaphostrongylus tenuis infestation of, 349
Demodex ovis, 304*t,* 306
Dental attrition, 211-212, *212*
  clinical signs and lesions of, 211-212, *212*
  diagnosis and prevention of, 212
  occurrence, etiology, and pathogenesis of, 211
Dermacentor andersoni, 123, 301*t*
Dermatitis
  contagious pustular, 135. *See also* Contagious
    ecthyma
Dermatophilosis, 291-293
  clinical signs and lesions of, 292-293
  diagnosis, prevention, and treatment of, 293
  etiology and pathogenesis of, 292
Dermatophilus congolensis, 292
Dermatosis
  ulcerative. *See* Ulcerative dermatosis
Desmodus rotundus
  rabies transmission from, 332
Diamphenethide
  for liver fluke disease, 98
Diaphragm
  eosinophilic myositis of, 188, *188*
Diarrhea
  calf, 80
  colibacillosis and, 76, 77-78
  hemorrhagic, 159. *See also* Coccidiosis
Dicrocoelium dendriticum, 94*t,* 96
Dictyocaulus filaria
  verminous pneumonia and, 99-100
Diet(s)
  calcium-deficient
    dental attrition and, 211
  high-copper, 372
  high-oxalate, 247
  imbalance of
    calculosis and, 205
Digestive system disease(s)
  in adult sheep, 211-263, *212-214, 217-220, 239,*
    240, 241t, 244, 244t, 246, 247, 249, 254t, 258,
    259, 261
  fatal
    in lamb feedlots, 132*t*
  in feedlot lambs, 135-171, *136, 143, 145, 147, 148,*
    149t, 150, 151, 156, 157, 160t, 162, 165, 168,
    169, 170, 171
  in nursing lambs, 73-99, *75, 77, 85t, 86, 87, 90, 94t,*
    96, 97
  See also names of specific diseases
Digital suppuration, 321. *See also* Foot abscess
Diphylla ecaudata
  rabies transmission from, 332
Dirt-eating disease, 81. *See also* Enterotoxemia

Distomatosis, 93. *See also* Liver fluke disease
Dugaldia hoopesii, 239, *239*
Dysentery
  coccidial, 159. *See also* Coccidiosis
  lamb. *See* Lamb dysentery
  salmonellal. *See* Salmonellal dysentery

Echinococcosis, 257-259, *258, 259*
  clinical signs and postmortem lesions of, 258, *259*
  diagnosis of, 258
  etiology and pathogenesis of, 258, *258*
  occurrence of, 257-258
  prevention of, 259
Echinococcus granulosus, 258, *258*
Ecthyma
  contagious. *See* Contagious ecthyma
Ectrin
  use of, 313
Edema
  malignant, 102-104, *103*
    clinical signs and postmortem lesions of, 103, *103*
    diagnosis of, 103-104
    occurrence, etiology, and pathogenesis of, 102
    prevention and treatment of, 104
    swelled head vs., 291
Ehrlichia phagocytophilia
  tick-borne fever and, 43
Eimeria ahsata, 159, 160*t*
Eimeria ovina, 159, 160*t,* 160
Eimeria ovinoidalis
  coccidiosis from, 159, 160*t,* 160, 161, *162*
Elaeophora schneideri larvae
  facial dermatitis and keratitis from, *298,* 299
  stomatitis from, 299, *299*
Elaeophorosis, 298-300, *298, 299*
  clinical signs and postmortem lesions of, *298,* 299,
    299
  diagnosis of, 299-300
  etiology and pathogenesis of, 298-299
  occurrence of, 298
  prevention of, 300
Encephalitis
  listeric, 195, 198
Encephalomalacia
  focal symmetrical. *See* Focal symmetrical
    encephalomalacia
Encephalomyelitis
  ovine, 112. *See also* Louping-ill
Enteropathogenic *E. coli* (EPEC), 76
Enterotoxemia (ET), 149-151, 149*t, 150, 151*
  clinical signs and postmortem lesions of, 150-151,
    150, 151
  diagnosis and prevention of, 151
  etiology and pathogenesis of, 149-150
  focal symmetrical encephalomalacia and, 200
  hemorrhagic, 73-75, *75*
    clinical signs and postmortem lesions of, 74, *75*
    diagnosis of, 75
    etiology and pathogenesis of, 73-74
    occurrence of, 73
    prevention of, 75
  infectious, 149
  occurrence of, 149
  of suckling lambs, 81-83